OBSTETRICS AND GYNAECOLOGY

Dr. Kedir Yahya Yasin

ALLIED
HEALTH
PRESS

Obstetrics and Gynaecology

Author: **Dr. Kedir Yahya Yasin**

Allied Health Press
4164 Lakeshore Road
Burlington ON L7L 1A4
Canada
www.alliedhealthpress.com
Email: orders@arclereducation.com

ISBN: 978-1-77956-257-9

ABOUT THE AUTHOR

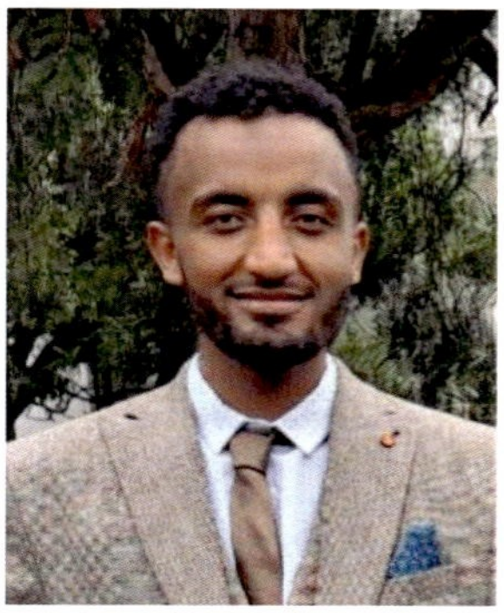

Dr. Kedir Yahya is a young medical doctor who is currently working in Asella teaching and referral hospital. He embarked on a journey to explore various fields within the medical landscape. With a versatile skill set and a commitment to lifelong learning, he has made significant contributions to healthcare across diverse specialities. Whether it's clinical practice, research, or teaching, he continues to strive for excellence in improving patient care and advancing medical knowledge.

Word Roots, Prefixes, and Suffixes by Chapter

Chapter 1 Maternal Anatomy

"-ectomy" (surgical removal)
"-graphy" (process of recording)
"-gram" (record or picture)
"-itis" (inflammation)

Chapter 2 Maternal Changes During Pregnancy

Para Multipara
Uter Uterine
Placenta Placental
Lact Lactation
Mamm Mammary

Chapter 3 Prenatal Care

angio- vessel
anti- attacks, treats condition
cardio- related to the heart
cephal- head
-cyst related to the bladder

Chapter 4 Physiology of Labor and Puerperium

cervic/o cervix
glact/o milk
gravid/o pregnancy
gynec/o woman

Chapter 5 Complications of Pregnancy

abdomin(o)-, of or relating to the abdomen
-emia, blood condition
ect(o)-, outer, outside
encephal(o)-, of or pertaining to the brain
endo-, denotes something as 'inside' or 'within'

Chapter 6 Medical Diseases Complicating Pregnancy

peri- surrounding
endo-within
dys- painful, difficult, abnormal, labored
cervic/o cervix
endometri/o endometrium

Chapter 7 The Newborn Infant

neo- Neonatal
peri- Perinatal
partum Antepartum
pre- Prenatal
post- Postnatal

Chapter 8 Abnormal Labor

algia pain
dys- abnormal
hem(ato)- blood
plasty surgical repair
hypo- low, depressed

Chapter 9 Gynecological Diagnosis

Gyn-/Gyne-/Gynec- woman" or "female."
-logy "the study of."
Hyster- "uterus."
Metr-/Metro-/Metri- "uterus."
-ectomy "surgical removal."

Chapter 10 Gynecological Diagnosis

Ped/o Pediatric
Men/o Menarche
Hyster/o Hysteroscopy
Vagin/o Vaginitis
Ovari/o Ovarian

PREFACE

For many years, it was believed that the differences between males and females were minimal, and knowledge about men could be applied to women as well. However, an evolving understanding has led to the recognition that women's health encompasses more than just reproductive health and the absence of gynecological issues. These changes are discussed further in the following paragraphs.

Changing lifestyles have led to smaller family sizes. The female-to-male sex ratio has declined, and instances of selective female foeticide present unique challenges to gynecologists, involving ethical, moral, and medical considerations. Additionally, there has been a rise in the number of divorced women and single mothers, leading to specific problems such as sexually transmitted diseases (STDs) and sexual dysfunction. The increased life expectancy means that women now spend a significant portion of their lives post-menopause, requiring gynecologists to effectively address their postmenopausal issues and expectations. The level of education attained by women in any society is correlated with their health, and today more women are literate than ever before. However, education also makes women more aware of their health issues, demanding a more responsive approach from physicians caring for women's health.

Careers have become increasingly important for women today, leading to later marriages and family planning at non-peak reproductive ages. This trend poses challenges such as subfertility, prompting patients to turn to assisted reproduction techniques. Advanced age itself is a risk factor for many pregnancy-related medical disorders, including gestational diabetes mellitus, gestational hypertension, and the need for operative interventions.

The rate of smoking among women is rising, with smoking having multifaceted effects including a higher incidence of heart disease and cancer. Smoking during pregnancy poses serious risks to the fetus, including low birth weight. Similarly, alcohol consumption not only causes psychological dependence but is also particularly harmful during pregnancy, leading to birth defects, developmental disorders, and fetal alcohol syndrome.

Drug abuse has increased among the young population, and while the percentage of pregnant women using illicit drugs is relatively low, the effects can be severe for both mother and fetus, including growth restriction, placental abruption, and fetal demise.

A woman's ability to control fertility is fundamental to her health. Although contraceptive acceptance has increased across all socioeconomic strata, it has not reached the desired levels. Emergency contraception has provided women with occasional exposure to greater freedom. Safe abortion services are now more accessible and well-utilized in cases of contraceptive failure, although some argue that it has led to increased promiscuity among women.

Women experience higher rates of psychological distress, depression, and physical morbidity compared to men. Increased workforce participation, rising divorce rates, single parenthood, and an aging population have significantly increased stress levels in women. Stress can impact neurohormonal and endocrinological pathways, leading to menstrual irregularities or altered reproductive behavior.

Changes in dietary habits and reduced physical activity have contributed to an obesity epidemic. When associated with obesity, polycystic ovarian syndrome poses specific challenges such as subfertility and hirsutism. Obesity is more prevalent among women of childbearing age than among older women. Obese patients have a higher incidence of heart disease, cardiac problems, endometrial cancer, and postmenopausal breast cancer. Overweight and obesity are serious concerns during pregnancy, increasing the risk of all pregnancy-related complications. Body image, or how a woman perceives her own body, is particularly important in the relational aspects of sexuality. Being overweight and obesity have significantly affected women's self-body image, leading many to adopt rigorous exercise routines, dietary regimens, and unnecessary cosmetic procedures.

This book on Obstetrics and Gynecology aims to provide a comprehensive text for scientists and clinical professionals working in the field. It covers topics related to obstetrics, maternal-fetal medicine, general gynecology, gynecologic oncology, urogynecology, reproductive medicine and infertility, reproductive endocrinology, and sexual medicine. This book serves as a valuable reference for obstetricians and gynecologists, providing them with the latest information and guidelines to enhance their clinical practice and patient care. Medical residents and trainees in obstetrics and gynecology will find this book to be a valuable learning tool, helping them build a solid foundation of knowledge in the field.

Nurses and midwives working in obstetrics and gynecology will benefit from the practical insights and guidelines provided in this book, enhancing their ability to provide quality care to women.

Chapter 1

MATERNAL ANATOMY

Contents

Introduction

Maternal anatomy encompasses the intricate physiological and anatomical adaptations in a woman's body to support pregnancy and childbirth. This specialized branch of anatomy focuses on the changes in the reproductive, cardiovascular, respiratory, musculoskeletal, gastrointestinal, urinary, endocrine systems during pregnancy. These adaptations are critical for nurturing and protecting the developing fetus and preparing the mother for labor and delivery.

Orientation and Directional Terms

Term	Definition	Illustration
Pelvic floor	The pelvic floor muscles are located between the tailbone (coccyx) and the pubic bone within the pelvis. They support the bowel and bladder (as well as the uterus and vagina in females).	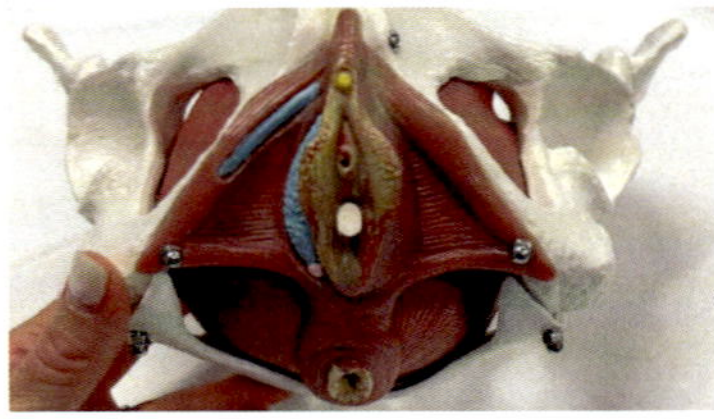
Anal Triangle	The anal triangle is formed by the coccyx, sacrotuberous ligaments, and an imaginary line between the ischial tuberosities. The anal triangle contains the anal canal and two ischiorectal (ischioanal) fossae that lie on either side of the anal canal.	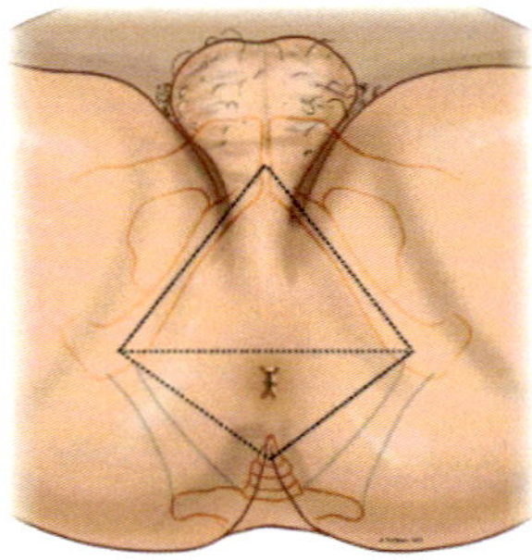
Bulbospongiosus muscles	The bulbospongiosus muscles (in older texts bulbocavernosus and, for female muscle, constrictor cunni) are a subgroup of the superficial muscles of the perineum. They have a slightly different origin, insertion and function in males and females. In males, these muscles cover the bulb of the penis, while in females, they cover the vestibular bulbs.	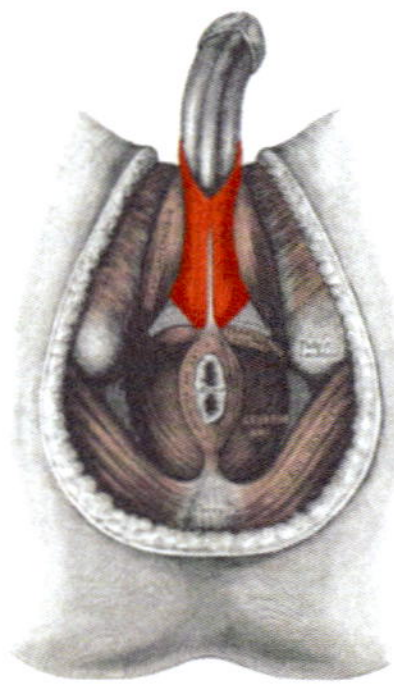
Suprapiriform foramen	Suprapiriform foramen should be considered as a fascio-osseous canal, as it is 4–4.5 cm long and 0.6–1.0 cm wide. It is formed by the upper margin of the greater sciatic notch covered with a thin fascia, fasciae of the gluteal and piriform muscles and the parietal layer of the pelvic fascia.	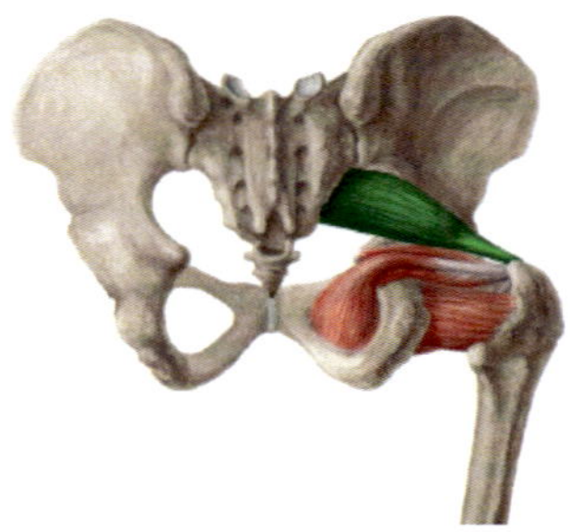
Levator ani muscle	The levator ani muscle, also known as the pelvic diaphragm, is a broad muscle group that forms the greater part of the floor of the pelvic cavity. It is composed of three striated muscles on each side: the iliococcygeus, pubococcygeus, and the puborectalis muscles.	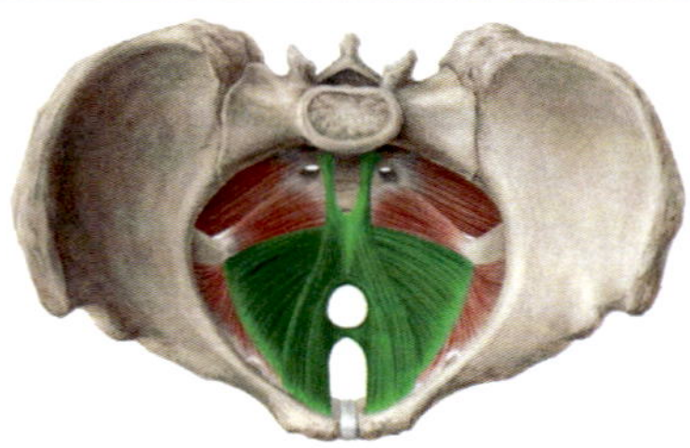

1.1. Anatomy of the Pelvis

The anatomy of the pelvis is complex and includes bones, joints, muscles, ligaments, and other structures that provide support and facilitate movement. The pelvis plays a crucial role in weight bearing, movement, and childbirth.

1.1.1. Area of the Pelvis

1.1.1.1. The Perineum

One part of the pelvis' anatomy is the perineum. This part of the pelvic outlet is the most inferior and is situated between the thighs. The pelvic floor divides the perineum superiorly from the pelvic cavity. This area is crucial for processes like micturition, defecation, sexual activity, and childbirth because it houses structures that support the gastrointestinal and urogenital systems (White, Black, and Folkens, 2011) (Figure 1.1).

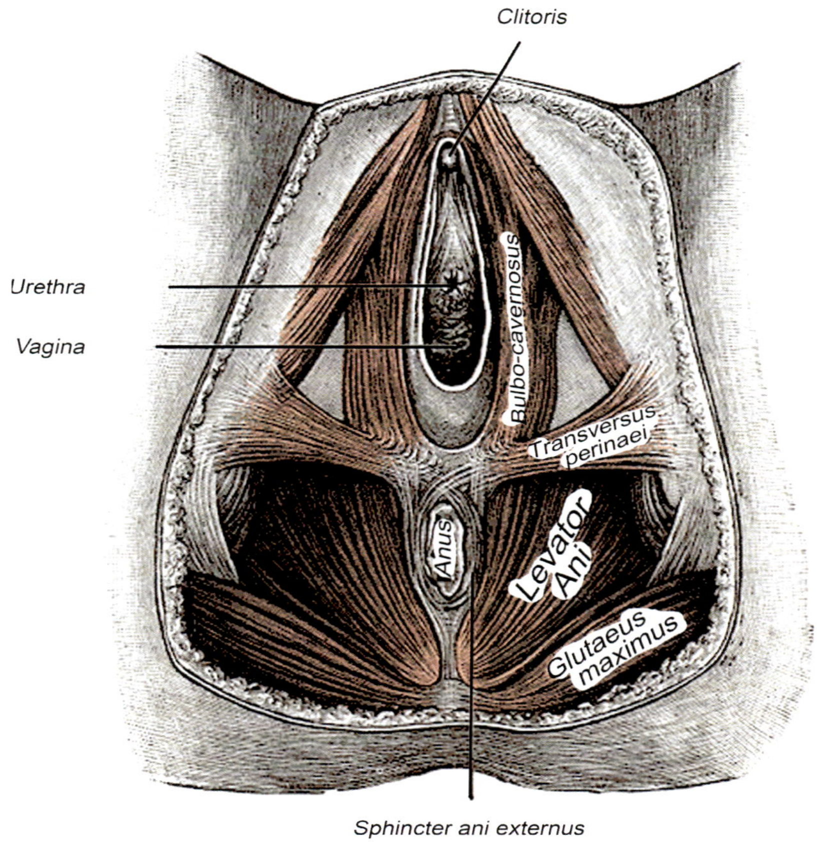

Figure 1.1. *The perineum is located between the thighs.*

Source: By Henry Vandyke Carter – Henry Gray (1918) Anatomy of the Human Body (See "Book" section below) Bartleby.com: Gray's Anatomy, Plate 408, Public Domain, https://commons.wikimedia.org/w/index.php?curid=531382.

1.1.1.1.1. Boundaries

In clinical practice, the region between the external genitalia and the anus is commonly referred to as the "perineum." Nonetheless, the anatomical structure of the perineum is shaped like a diamond. There are two primary methods for characterizing the perineum's boundaries. While the surface borders outline the perineum's surface anatomy, the anatomical borders relate to the precise bony margins of the structure (Figure 1.2).

1. **Anatomical Borders:** The anatomical borders of the perineum are:

    - Anterior – pubic symphysis.
    - Posterior – tip of the coccyx.
    - Laterally – inferior pubic rami and inferior ischial rami, and the sacrotuberous ligament.
    - Roof – pelvic floor.
    - Base – skin and fascia.

    A theoretical line drawn transversely between the ischial tuberosities subdivides the perineum, creating the anterior urogenital triangle and the posterior anal triangle. These triangles correspond to distinct components of the perineum.

2. **Surface Borders:** The surface boundaries are best shown when the lower limbs are abducted, and a diamond shape is depicted:

    - Anterior – mons pubis in females, base of the penis in males.
    - Laterally – medial surfaces of the thighs.
    - Posterior – superior end of the intergluteal cleft.

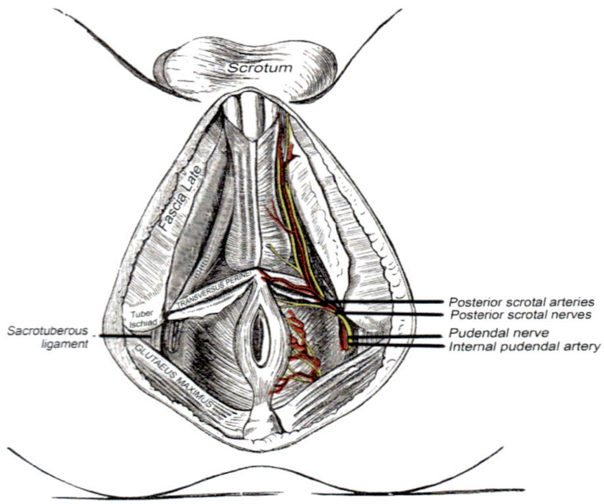

Figure 1.2. *Anatomical and surface borders of the perineum.*

Source: By Henry Vandyke Carter – Henry Gray (1918) Anatomy of the Human Body (See "Book" section below) Bartleby.com: Gray's Anatomy, Plate 542, Public Domain, https://commons.wikimedia.org/w/index.php?curid=541089.

1.1.1.1.2. Contents

A theoretical line drawn transversely between the ischial tuberosities can be used to divide the perineum into smaller sections. The anterior urogenital and posterior anal triangles are formed by this split.

1. **Anal Triangle:** The back half of the perineum is known as the anal triangle. The coccyx, the sacrotuberous ligaments, and a hypothetical line that separates the ischial tuberosities are its boundaries.

    The main contents of the anal triangle are:

- Anal aperture – the opening of the anus.
- External anal sphincter muscle – voluntary muscle responsible for opening and closing the anus.

- Ischioanal fossae (x2) – spaces located laterally to the anus.

The ischioanal fossae are on either side of the anal aperture, which is situated in the triangle's center. The anal canal can expand during defecation because of the fat and connective tissue found in these fossae. They stretch from the inferior skin of the anal region to the superior skin of the pelvic diaphragm.

Inside the anal triangle, the pudendal nerve is another significant anatomical structure that supplies somatic fibers to the entire perineum (Figure 1.3).

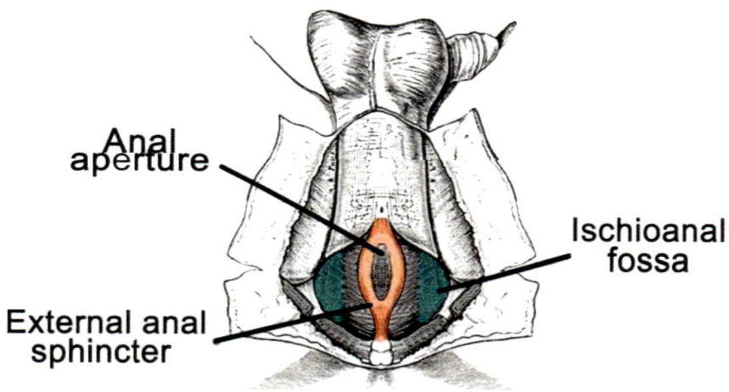

Figure 1.3. *Contents of the anal triangle.*

Source: https://teachmeanatomy.info/pelvis/areas/perineum/.

2. **Urogenital Triangle:** The urogenital triangle is the front portion of the perineum and is defined by the pubic symphysis, ischiopubic rami, and an imaginary line connecting the two ischial tuberosities. This area contains the external genitalia and urethra, which are part of the urogenital system (Figure 1.4).

The urogenital triangle has a complex structure with several fascial layers and pouches. The perineal membrane is an extra layer of robust deep fascia that separates the urogenital triangle from the anal triangle. There are pouches on the superior and inferior surfaces of this membrane.

The layers of the urogenital triangle (deep to superficial):

- **Deep Perineal Pouch**: a possible gap between the inferior perineal membrane and the deep fascia of the pelvic floor. It includes a portion of the female vagina, the external urethral sphincter, and the urethra. It also houses the deep transverse perineal muscles and bulbourethral glands in males.
- **Perineal Membrane:** a layer of strong fascia that is broken through by the vagina in females and the urethra in males. The membrane's function is to serve as an attachment point for the external genitalia's muscles.
- **Superficial Perineal Pouch**: a possible gap between the superficial perineal fascia (inferiorly) and the perineal membrane (superiorly). Together with three muscles—the ischiocavernosus, bulbospongiosus, and superficial transverse perineal muscles—it houses the erectile tissues that make up the penis and clitoris. There is also a larger vestibular gland (also known as Barneolin's glands) in the superficial perineal pouch. The perineal body forms the posterior boundary of the pouch.
- **Perineal Fascia:** a continuity of the abdominal fascia that has two components:

o **Deep Fascia:** covers the superficial perineal muscles and protruding structures (e.g., penis & clitoris).

o Superficial fascia is composed of a further two layers of fascia:

  - Superficial layer – continuous with Camper's fascia of the anterior abdominal wall

- Deep layer (Colles' fascia) – continuous with Scarpa's fascia of the anterior abdominal wall

- **Skin:** The urethral and vaginal orifices open out onto the skin.

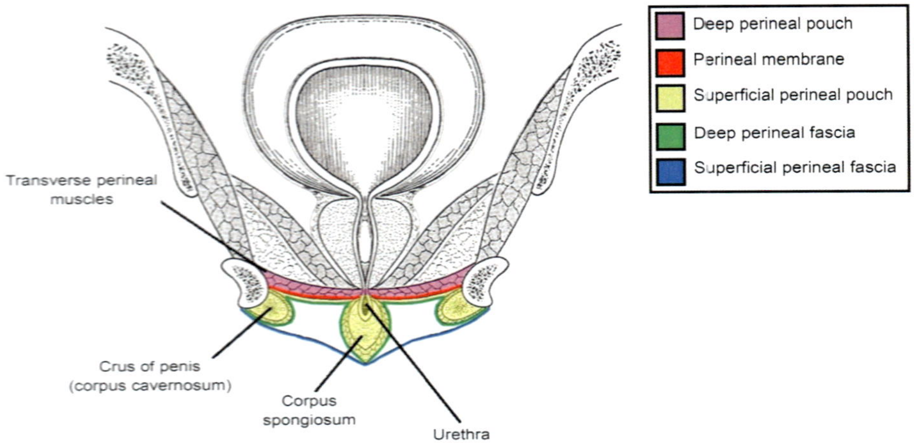

Figure 1.4. *Coronal section of the male pelvis, showing the layers of the urogenital triangle.*

Source: https://teachmeanatomy.info/pelvis/areas/perineum/.

3. **The Perineal Body:** An asymmetrical mass of fibromuscular tissue is the perineal body. It is situated at the perineum's central point, the intersection of the urogenital and anal triangles. Skeletal muscle, smooth muscle, and collagenous and elastic fibers are all present in this structure.

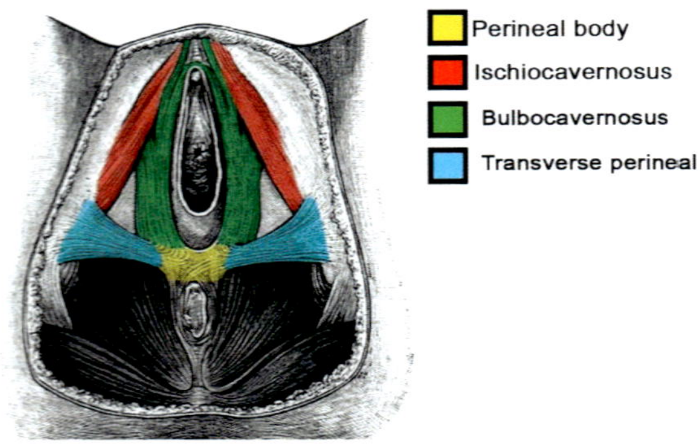

Figure 1.5. *Muscles attaching to the perineal body.*

Source: https://teachmeanatomy.info/pelvis/areas/perineum/.

Anatomically, the perineal body lies just deep into the skin. It acts as a point of attachment for muscle fibers from the pelvic floor and the perineum itself:

- Levator ani (part of the pelvic floor).
- Bulbospongiosus muscle.

- Superficial and deep transverse perineal muscles.
- External anal sphincter muscle.
- External urethral sphincter muscle fibers.

It supports the posterior portion of the vaginal wall against prolapse in women by functioning as a tear-resistant body between the vagina and the external anal sphincter. It is located in the male between the anus and the penis bulb (Figure 1.5).

1.1.1.2. The Sciatic Foramina

There are two apertures in the posterior aspect of the pelvis called the greater and lesser sciatic foramina. The sacrospinous ligament divides the larger, greater sciatic foramen from the smaller, lesser sciatic foramen (Meindl and Lovejoy, 1985).

1.1.1.2.1. Greater Sciatic Foramen

The greater sciatic foramen provides a passageway for structures to pass from the pelvis into the gluteal region (Figure 1.6).

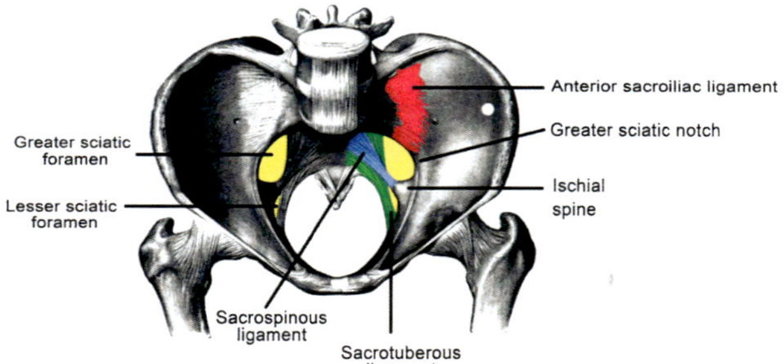

Figure 1.6. *The borders of the greater sciatic foramen.*

Source: https://teachmeanatomy.info/pelvis/areas/sciatic-foramen/.

1. **Borders:** The greater sciatic foramen is bordered by:

- Superior – anterior sacroiliac ligament
- Posteromedial – sacrotuberous ligament
- Anterolateral – greater sciatic notch of the ilium
- Inferior – sacrospinous ligament and ischial spine

2. **Contents:** The suprapiriform and infrapiriform foramina of the greater sciatic foramen are separated by the presence of the piriformis muscle (Figure 1.7).

- Suprapiriform foramen:
    - o Superior gluteal artery and vein
    - o Superior gluteal nerve
- Infrapiriform foramen:
    - o Sciatic nerve
    - o Pudendal nerve
    - o Inferior gluteal artery and vein
    - o Inferior gluteal nerve
    - o Posterior femoral cutaneous nerve
    - o Nerve to obturator internus
    - o Nerve to quadratus femoris

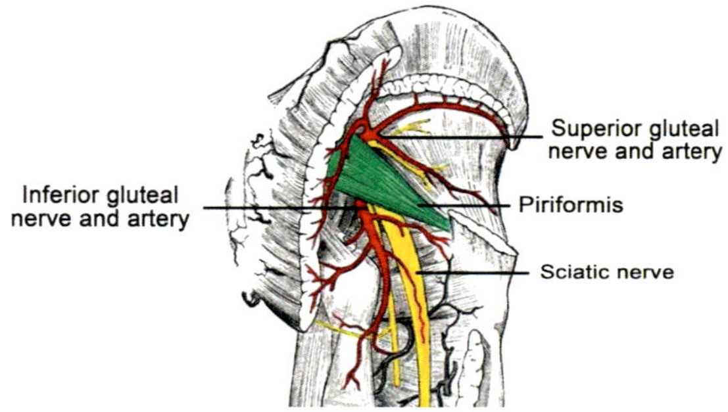

Figure 1.7. *The piriformis divides the greater sciatic foramen into two – the supra- and infrapiriform foramina.*

Source: https://teachmeanatomy.info/pelvis/areas/sciatic-foramen/.

1.1.1.3. Lesser Sciatic Foramen

There is communication between the gluteal region and the pelvic perineum through the lesser sciatic foramen. In relation to the pelvic floor, it is inferior (Figure 1.8).

1. **Borders:** The lesser sciatic foramen is bordered by:
   - Superior – sacrospinous ligament and ischial spine
   - Anterior – ischial spine, lesser sciatic notch and ischial tuberosity
   - Posterior – sacrotuberous ligament
2. **Contents:** The following structures pass through the lesser sciatic foramen:
   - Internal pudendal artery and vein
   - Pudendal nerve (note the pudendal nerve first leaves the pelvis via the greater sciatic foramen, and then re-enters via the lesser sciatic foramen)
   - Obturator internus tendon
   - Nerve to obturator internus

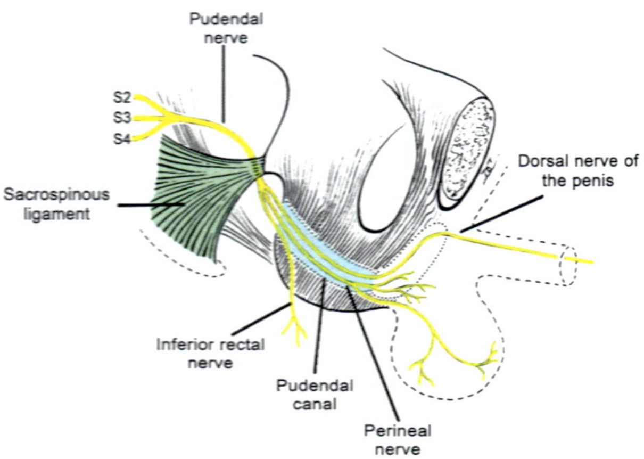

Figure 1.8. *The pudendal nerve first leaves the pelvis via the greater sciatic foramen, and then re-enters via the lesser sciatic foramen.*

Source: https://teachmeanatomy.info/pelvis/areas/sciatic-foramen/.

1.1.2. The Pelvic Floor

The pelvic cavity, also known as the true pelvis, is home to the pelvic viscera, which include the bladder, rectum, pelvic genital organs, and terminal portion of the urethra. This cavity is situated below the pelvic brim in the lesser part of the pelvis. The obturator internus and the piriformis muscle, which also forms the posterior wall, are two of the muscles that contribute to the cavity's walls.

We shall look at the individual roles of these muscles, their innervation and blood supply, and any clinical correlations (Figure 1.9).

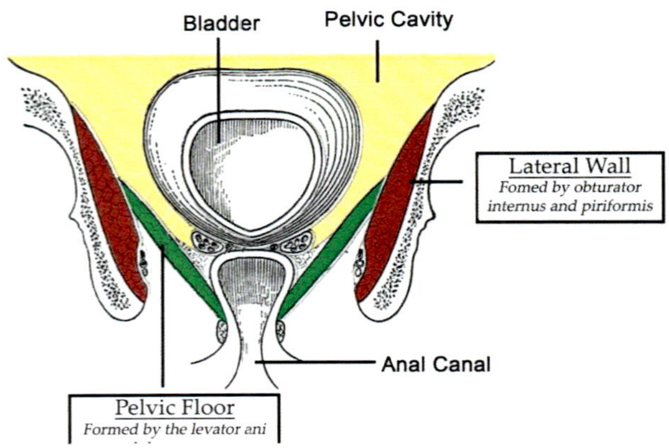

Figure 1.9. *An overview of the pelvic cavity and its walls. Note the funnel shape of the pelvic floor.*

Source: https://teachmeanatomy.info/pelvis/muscles/pelvic-floor/.

1.1.2.1. Pelvic Floor Structure

The pelvic floor is a structure that resembles a funnel. It connects to the walls of the smaller pelvis, dividing the inferior perineum—the area containing the genitalia and anus—from the pelvic cavity.

In order to allow for urination and defecation, there are a few gaps in the pelvic floor. There are two 'holes' that have significance:

i **Urogenital Hiatus**: an anteriorly situated gap, which allows passage of the urethra (and the vagina in females).

ii. **Rectal Hiatus:** a centrally positioned gap, which allows passage of the anal canal.

1.1.2.2. Functions

These muscles, which form the floor of the pelvic cavity, are crucial to the proper operation of the viscera in the abdomen and pelvis.

The roles of the pelvic floor muscles are:

- Support to the tonic contraction of the abdominopelvic viscera.
- Resistance to intra-pelvic/abdominal pressure rises brought on by actions like coughing or lifting large objects.
- The rectum and urethra are sphinctered by the muscle fibers, which maintains urinary and fecal continence. They loosen up to permit urinating and feces.

1.1.2.3. Muscles

It is essential to remember the funnel shape when studying the muscles of the pelvic floor. The pelvic floor consists of three primary components (Figure 1.10):

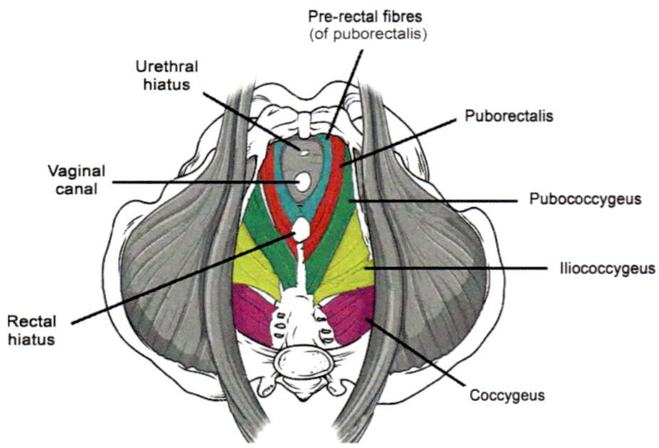

Figure 1.10. *Superior (bird's eye) view of the pelvic floor. Note the pre-rectal fibers of the puborectalis.*

Source: https://teachmeanatomy.info/pelvis/muscles/pelvic-floor/.

i. Levator ani muscles (largest component).

ii. Coccygeus muscle.

iii. Fascia coverings of the muscles.

1.1.2.3.1. Levator Ani Muscles

The levator ani is a large muscle sheet. It is made up of the pubococcygeus, puborectalis, and iliococcygeus, three distinct paired muscles (Figure 1.11).

- **Puborectalis:** The puborectalis muscle is crucial in the levator ani group for ensuring fecal continence.
  - **Attachments:** Originates on the pubic posterior surface. It wraps around the anal canal in the shape of a U and attaches to the pubis on the opposite side.
  - **Actions:** The anal canal is bent anteriorly by tonic contraction, forming the anorectal angle that helps with fecal continence. This contraction is voluntarily stopped during defecation.
  - **Innervation:** Nerve to levator ani and pudendal nerve.
- **Pubococcygeus:** The majority of the levator ani complex is made up of the pubococcygeus. It is situated on the pelvic floor, in between the iliococcygeus and the puborectalis.
  - **Attachments:** Originates on the pubic posterior surface. It merges with the pelvic floor's contralateral muscle in the midline.
  - **Actions:** Stability and support

of abdominal and pelvic organs.

- **Innervation:** Nerve to levator ani and branches of the pudendal nerve.

- **Iliococcygeus:** The posterolateral portion of the levator ani muscle group is made up of the slender iliococcygeus muscle.
  - **Attachments:** Originates from the internal obturator fascia's posterior tendinous arch and ischial spines. It attaches to the anococcygeal ligament, perineal body, and coccyx. Additionally, it combines with the contralateral muscle fibers in the pelvic floor's midline.
  - **Actions:** Elevates the pelvic floor and anorectal canal.
  - **Innervation:** Nerve to levator ani and branches of the pudendal nerve.
- **Coccygeus:** A small triangular muscle, the coccygeus is situated behind the levator ani muscle group.
  - **Attachments:** It originates from the ischial spines and attaches to the lower part of the sacrum and coccyx.
  - **Actions:** Supports the pelvic viscera and flexes the coccyx.
  - **Innervation:** Sacral nerves and branches of the pudendal nerve(S3,S4,55).
  - **Blood Supply:** Inferior vesical, inferior gluteal and pudendal arteries.

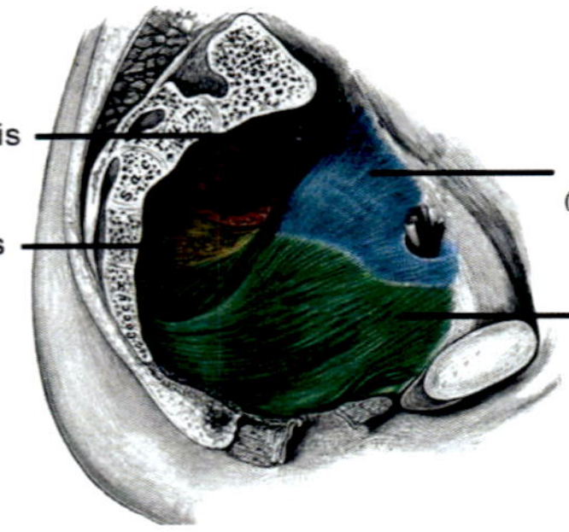

Figure 1.11. *Sagittal cut through the pelvis, showing a lateral view of the pelvic floor and walls.*

Source: https://teachmeanatomy.info/pelvis/muscles/pelvic-floor/.

1.1.3. Difference Between Male and Female Pelvis

The differences between male and female pelvises are primarily due to the requirements of childbirth in females. These differences can be observed in their shape, size, and structural features. Here's a detailed comparison:

1.1.3.1. General Shape and Structure

- **Male Pelvis**:
  - o **Shape**: Generally, the male pelvis is narrower, more robust, and more heart-shaped.
  - o **Bones**: The bones are heavier and thicker to support a heavier body build.
  - o **Pelvic Inlet**: The pelvic inlet (the upper opening of the pelvic cavity) is more heart-shaped or narrower.
  - o **Pelvic Outlet**: The pelvic outlet (the lower opening of the pelvic cavity) is relatively smaller.
  - o **Overall Structure**: More vertical and compact.
- **Female Pelvis**:
  - o **Shape**: The female pelvis is wider,

shallower, and more oval or circular.

- o **Bones**: The bones are lighter and thinner to allow for greater flexibility during childbirth.
- o **Pelvic Inlet**: The pelvic inlet is wider and more circular or oval.
- o **Pelvic Outlet**: The pelvic outlet is larger to facilitate childbirth.
- o **Overall Structure**: Broader and more spacious.

1.1.3.2. Specific Features

- **Ilium**:
- o **Male**: The iliac crests are higher, causing the male pelvis to look taller and more upright.
- o **Female**: The iliac crests are lower and more flared outward, contributing to a broader pelvis.
- **Sacrum**:
- o **Male**: The sacrum is longer, narrower, and more curved.
- o **Female**: The sacrum is shorter, wider, and less curved, providing a larger pelvic cavity.
- **Ischial Spines**:
- o **Male**: The ischial spines are longer, sharper, and point more medially, making the pelvic cavity narrower.
- o **Female**: The ischial spines are shorter, farther apart, and point more outward, allowing a larger space for the birth canal.
- **Pubic Arch/Subpubic Angle**:
- o **Male**: The subpubic angle is narrower, typically less than 70 degrees, forming a more acute angle.
- o **Female**: The subpubic angle is wider, typically greater than 80 degrees, forming a more obtuse angle.
- **Acetabulum**:
- o **Male**: The acetabula are larger and closer together.
- o **Female**: The acetabula are smaller and set farther apart.
- **Obturator Foramen**:
- o **Male**: The obturator foramen (the large opening created by the ischium and pubis bones) is rounder.
- o **Female**: The obturator foramen is more oval.

1.1.3.3. Functional Differences

- **Childbirth**: The most significant functional difference is related to childbirth. The wider pelvis in females provides more space for the passage of the newborn during delivery.
- **Locomotion**: The shape of the male pelvis supports a more stable and efficient walking and running gait, with the narrower structure aiding in the alignment of the legs.

1.2. Anatomy of Human Placental Development

The trophectoderm (TE), the outer layer of the pre-implantation embryo, forms approximately ~5 days after fertilization (dpf) and is where the human placenta develops. The pre-implantation embryo, also known as a blastocyst, is now divided into the inner cell mass (ICM) and the telosperm (TE). The endometrium, which is the surface epithelium of the uterine mucosa, is where the polar TE—the portion of the TE that is contiguous with the underlying ICM—attaches. The morphological observations of early pregnant hysterectomy specimens and higher primates suggest that the TE fuses to form a primary syncytium after attachment to the uterine surface epithelium at approximately ~6–7 dpf, even though the earliest stages of implantation have not been seen in humans. This is the placental prelacunar phase (Figure 1.12).

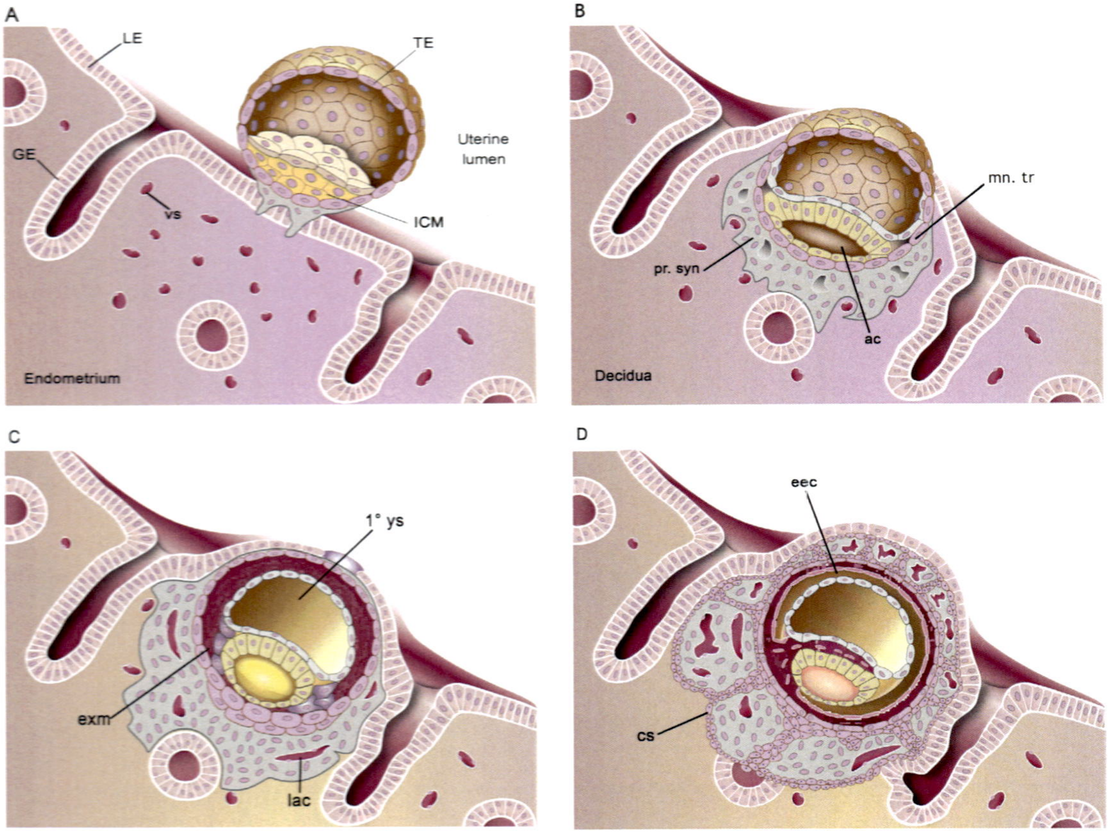

Figure 1.12. *The early stages of human placental development.*

Source: https://journals.biologists.com/dev/article/146/22/dev163428/223131/Development-of-the-human-placenta.

After implantation, the primary syncytium infiltrates the underlying endometrium rapidly through the surface epithelium, developing into the specialized tissue known as decidua during pregnancy. The blastocyst is fully embedded in the decidua and covered in surface epithelium by the time of the first missed menstrual period (approximately ~14 dpf). The syncytial mass then becomes divided into a system of trabeculae by fluid-filled spaces (lacunae) that grow and merge. The lacunar stage is this. Additionally, as the syncytium erodes into decidual glands, secretions can cover the syncytial mass (Hertig et al., 1956).

In the villous stage of development, the trophoblast cells beneath the syncytium—referred to as cytotrophoblast cells—are initially not in direct contact with maternal tissue but quickly multiply to form projections that push through the primary syncytium to form primary villi, which are composed of a cytotrophoblast core and an outer layer of syncytiotrophoblast, or SCT. Further proliferation and branching create villous trees, and the lacunae turn into the intervillous space. Eventually, cytotrophoblast cells break through the primary syncytium and combine laterally to form a continuous cytotrophoblast shell between the decidua and the villi that encircles the conceptus. Three layers now cover the blastocyst: the cytotrophoblast shell in contact with the decidua, the villi divided by the intervillous space, and the inner chorionic plate in contact with the original cavity.

Extraembryonic mesenchymal cells break through the villous core shortly after, on days 17–18, to form secondary villi. Fetal capillaries begin to emerge within the core by day 18 dpf, signifying the emergence of tertiary villi. By gradually branching out from the chorionic plate, the villous tree keeps growing quickly until it forms a network of villous trees. Individual cytotrophoblast cells leave the shell to invade the decidua as extravillous trophoblasts (EVT), a process that resembles the epithelial-mesenchymal transition (EMT), where the cytotrophoblast shell meets the decidua (the maternal-fetal interface). In this manner, the placenta's blueprint is set by the end of the first trimester.

1.2.1. Cell Types of the Human Placenta

1.2.1.1. Trophoblast Cells

Trophoblast cells carry out the placenta's primary tasks. The trophoblast's emergence is a crucial evolutionary development that distinguishes placental mammals. The Dutch embryologist Ambrosius Arnold Willem Hubrecht coined the term "trophoblast" in 1889 to refer to the cells that carry nutrients and serve as a barrier of protection between the mother and the fetus. He also noted that decidua is necessary for the trophoblast to develop because it is a highly invasive, or "corrosive," cell type by nature. A multitude of human trophoblast subtypes have been discovered since these initial investigations. These consist of the EVT subtypes, the SCT, and the villous cytotrophoblast (VCT).

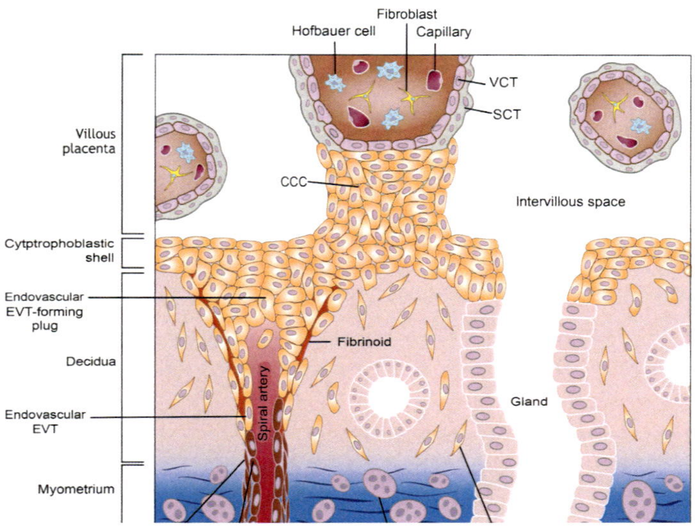

Figure 1.13. *The maternal-fetal interface and trophoblast subtypes.*

Source: https://journals.biologists.com/dev/article/146/22/dev163428/223131/Development-of-the-human-placenta.

The placental villi's outer lining, or SCT, comes into direct contact with the glandular secretions of the mother and, later, with her blood as it enters the intervillous space (Figure 1.13). It is the primary location of the gas and nutrient exchange between the mother and fetus that is required for the feto-placental unit to grow. The surface area of the SCT is increased by five to seven times due to its highly polarized epithelial layer that is densely covered in microvilli. The SCT is multinucleated and lacks cell borders, as confirmed by microinjection of fluorescein-labeled dextrans, most likely to aid in diffusion throughout the entire structure and shield the fetus from infections. Proteomic analyzes of SCT membranes reveal a high density of growth factor and hormone receptors in the microvilli. Transporter proteins that efflux xenobiotics and transport amino acids and glucose are abundant in the apical and basal membranes of the SCT. A significant endocrine organ, the SCT drives the physiological and metabolic changes associated with pregnancy by secreting hormones and proteins into the mother's bloodstream. Moreover, SCT serves as a defensive immunological barrier since it never expresses human leukocyte antigen (HLA) molecules. This means that circulating immune cells won't recognize the SCT as "non-self" even in the presence of the allogeneic fetus. The neonatal Fc receptor (FcRn), which enables the transfer of maternal IgG antibodies to the fetal circulation, is also expressed by the SCT. Digalactosylated IgG1 molecules are the antibodies that bind to FcRn on the SCT preferentially. These molecules are useful in stimulating fetal natural killer (NK) cells to safeguard the neonate prior to birth (Jennewein et al., 2019).

On a basement membrane, the mononuclear VCT is positioned below the SCT (Figure 1.13). Because the VCT are mitotic and express proliferative markers, they have historically been referred to as the trophoblast's "germinative" layer. When the VCT forms a continuous layer in the early stages of pregnancy, they are cuboidal cells with a high ratio of nucleus to cytoplasm. When only a thin syncytial layer divides the majority of the villous core from maternal blood, the VCT layer becomes discontinuous and covers only 25% of the villous surface by term as the villous trees grow (Benirschke et al., 2012).

The cytotrophoblast shell becomes discontinuous as the placenta grows, and cytotrophoblast cell columns (CCCs) appear at the distal tips of the anchoring villi when they come into contact with the decidua (Figure 1.13). The columnar cells are round, tightly packed, and abundant in glycogen. The endovascular trophoblast EVT (eEVT) travels down the inside of the spiral arteries, while the interstitial EVT (iEVT) migrates through the decidual stroma towards the maternal spiral arteries. The EVT migrates from the shell, and later the anchoring villi, into the decidua along two differentiation pathways. The iEVT are non-cycling, exhibit alterations in senescence, and have a pleomorphic and fusiform morphology with tetraploid nuclei in the decidua. They move in the direction of the spiral arteries, forming a cuff of neighboring cells. This is linked to the "fibrinoid" change in histology, which is caused by the loss of actin in the smooth muscle cells of the artery media and its replacement by amorphous eosinophilic material. Loss of vasoactivity and transformation into a vessel with high conductance at low pressure are the results of this trophoblast-mediated artery transformation, which is a necessary adaptation for a healthy pregnancy. The inner third of the myometrium, or the muscular layer of the uterine wall, is where the iEVT invade and are believed to fuse to form placental bed giant cells. Following the arterial transformation, the eEVT descends the artery retrogradely to create a plug that stops blood from entering the intervillous space until the end of the first trimester, at which point the entire hemopoietic circulation is established (Boyd and Hamilton, 1970; Burton et al., 1999; Hustin and Schaaps, 1987).

1.2.1.2. Other Placental Cells

In addition to trophoblast cells, the placenta is made up of fibroblasts, immune, and vascular cells that are located in the stromal core of the villi (Figure 1.13). It is believed that all of these cells originated from the extra-embryonic mesenchyme, the origin of which is unknown in humans. There are two theories as to where it comes from: either the VCT that goes through EMT, or the hypoblast, which is the endodermal derivative of the ICM, with the embryonic mesoderm contributing after gastrulation (Boss et al., 2018).

The first-trimester villi's single cell RNA-sequencing (scRNA-seq) revealed the existence of at least two distinct fibroblast populations based on the imprinted gene DLK1's presence or absence. $DLK1^+$ cells may be involved in the development of new blood vessels and resemble pericytes. A network of canals that feed into the extra-embryonic coelom is formed by the fibroblasts joining together. Hofbauer cells are placental macrophages found in these canals. Hofbauer cells are generated from haemangioblastic cells in extra-embryonic tissue, which is likely why they are the only immune cells in the placenta. They appear in the villous core from about day 18 postcoitum, before there is any vascular connection to the embryo itself. Their roles in influencing trophoblast and placental vascular development, safeguarding the fetus against vertical infections, and delivering nutrients to the extra-embryonic coelom have not been thoroughly studied. Additionally, by the end of the first trimester, the vascular system connects to the fetus via the umbilical cord, having developed from haemangioblastic populations in the mesenchyme. The pattern of gene expression in these immature endothelial cells is distinct, e.g., Their expression of EGFL7 is associated with the regulation of vascular morphogenesis.

1.2.2. Molecular Mechanisms Underpinning Human Placental Development

Trophoblast cells are distinct from all other cell types due to a multitude of unique features, such as global hypomethylation, differential microRNA expression, atypical patterns of HLA molecule expression, and endogenous retroviral product expression. Of the 92 human imprinted genes, 75 are expressed in the placenta. Imprinted genes, which are preferentially expressed from one parental allele, are also significant in placental development. In the trophoblast, the C19MC cluster, which codes for microRNAs, is expressed paternally. Chromosome 19q13.4 contains several other genes involved in reproduction besides the C19MC cluster, even though these miRNAs are expressed in hESCs, with trophoblast expression being significantly higher. Genes encoding nucleotide-binding oligomerization domain, killer-cell immunoglobulin-like receptors (KIRs), leukocyte immunoglobulin-like receptors (LILRs), pregnancy-specific glycoproteins (PSGs), choriogonadotropin subunit β (CGB), and leucine-rich repeat and pyrin domain-containing family (NLRP) members are among them. In addition, a large number of X chromosome genes manage to evade X inactivation within the human placenta. This results in transcriptional variations between male and female pregnancies, which could potentially account for the sex-based variations in pregnancy disorders. Trophoblast and tumor cells are remarkably similar as well. For instance, trophoblast cells display focal hypermethylation and widespread hypomethylation at CpG islands, including the promoters of tumor suppressor genes, as well as invasive proclivities and the capacity to evade harmful inflammatory or immune responses (Nordor et al., 2017).

Because long-term, genetically normal human trophoblast cell lines were unavailable until recently, studies of the molecular changes that occur during human placental development have primarily been descriptive. However, these investigations have shed light on the molecular mechanisms underlying trophoblast growth and placentation. We go over these studies below, emphasizing relevant mouse data and human data when available, with a particular focus on studies that have used primary trophoblast cells to validate the work. It is stated if additional in vitro instruments were utilized.

1.2.2.1. Establishment of the Trophoblast Lineage

In mice, TE lineage commitment is determined by a hierarchy of transcription factors (TFs). This process starts when Hippo signaling upregulates Tead4 in a subset of cells during the morula stage of preimplantation development. Tead4 in turn drives the expression of Cdx2 in the TE that develops later. At the eight-cell stage, Tcfap2c is already expressed, and it also binds to the enhancer of Cdx2 to control its expression. To sustain its own expression, Cdx2 represses Oct4, and Gata2/Gata3 function simultaneously to promote trophoblast development. The epigenetic regulation of Elf5, whose expression is reinforced by a positive-feedback loop involving Cdx2 and Eomes, locks the trophoblast lineage's identity in place (Ng et al., 2008).

The timing and expression pattern of these TFs differ in human embryos, indicating the presence of additional regulatory mechanisms from the outset of TE specification. In humans, lineage segregation between the ICM and TE occurs later in development; OCT4 is expressed in the TE until day 6, whereas CDX2 is only expressed at the blastocyst stage. In mice, there is a clear differential expression of Oct4 and Cdx2 in the ICM and TE, respectively. Even on day 7, some ICM cells maintain their TE identity. As a result, the human TE lineage appears to be more flexible before implantation. The deletion of OCT4 at the diploid zygote stage hampered the development of both the ICM and the TE in a ground-breaking study of CRISPR/Cas9 gene editing of human embryos, highlighting the molecular distinctions between humans and mice during these early fate decisions (Fogarty et al., 2017).

1.2.2.2. VCT and CCC Formation

It is clear that much remains unknown about the molecular processes in humans that take place between implantation and villous formation. Trophoblast populations most likely originate from the polar TE since these are the cells that undergo initial implantation. The placenta's proliferative compartment, or VCT, expresses the trophoblast TFs—GATA2, GATA3, TFAP2C/A, and TEAD4—found in mouse TSCs but not EOMES. In fact, in human pluripotent stem cells, four of these factors—GATA2, GATA3, TFAP2A, and TFAP2C—can induce cells that are thought to be of the trophoblast lineage. Similar to mice, humans express ELF5, whose hypomethylated promoter is found in the VCT. Since there is no ELF5 protein, its expression must be regulated by other mechanisms even though the ELF5 promoter is still hypomethylated in the EVT. Early in the first trimester and continuing through term, there is also widespread expression of TP63, a transcription factor that is typical of epithelial stem cells. In proximity to the chorionic plate, some TP63+ cells express CDX2 (. During the first trimester, CDX2 expression is then downregulated in the VCT throughout the majority of the placenta, except for cells that are near the chorionic plate, where residual expression is observed. The absence of CDX2 expression in hTSCs raises questions about whether this protein serves as a marker for trophoblast stem cells in the human placenta.

In addition, the VCT expresses a variety of surface markers that set it apart from other trophoblast populations, including EGFR, MET, and particular members of the Wnt family. The isolation of proliferative trophoblasts has confirmed the significance of these signaling pathways for VCT proliferation. Early in the first trimester, proliferative cells are also found in CCCs; by about ~12 weeks, their number has gradually decreased and they are primarily confined to the base of the CCCs. This so-called "generative niche" was first identified more than fifty years ago, and more recently, it was discovered that the trophoblast cells in this area expressed Notch1, ITGA2, and CD31, and had a different transcriptome from the VCT and EVT. By the end of the first trimester, Notch1 expression is limited to the CCC's base (Haider et al., 2016). It is unknown if cells in this niche produce VCT and/or EVT alone.

1.2.2.3. SCT Differentiation

Terminal differentiation occurs in the SCT covering the villi, and SCT fragments are constantly lost into the mother's bloodstream. The BeWo choriocarcinoma line, primary trophoblast cells capable of fusing in vitro, and placental explants have all been used to study the process of SCT regeneration from the underlying VCT. Human endogenous retroviral proteins (HERVs), like SYNCYTIN-1 (HERV-W env), have been identified in these studies as important regulators of this process. Retroviral elements are remnants of viral genes that have been incorporated into the human genome and used as enhancers or promoters. In the case of the placenta, these elements also encode retroviral proteins. HERVs are present in about 8% of the human genome. Particularly favorable conditions exist for HERV expression in the placenta, where various species have appropriated various retroviral families for the same purpose (Harris, 1991; Frendo et al., 2003a).

Acquiring fusion competence—a prerequisite for syncytialization—requires the VCT to break free from the cell cycle. It is unknown if the same process happens after syncytial damage and whether the signal that starts this event comes from the VCT or the SCT. After VCT cells upregulate fusion genes, cell membranes break down and the cytoplasm is incorporated into the SCT. An important step in this process was found using choriocarcinoma lines to increase cyclic AMP via protein kinase A (PKA) signaling. This upregulates GCM1 expression, which then triggers the expression of the fusion proteins syncytin 1 and syncytin 2. Fusion of the cell membranes and mixing of the contents of the cell are necessary for the last stage of syncytialization (Gerbaud and Pidoux, 2015).

Syncytins facilitate the fusion of the VCT with the SCT employing particular receptors called ASCT2 (for syncytin 1) and MFSD2 (for syncytin 2). While MFSD2 is expressed on the SCT, ASCT2 is limited to the VCT. Moreover, SCT generates hCG, which stimulates cyclic AMP signaling and, upon binding to the LH-CG receptor, upregulates both hCG and syncytial gene expression. Thus, in a positive feedback loop, the SCT itself reinforces the procedure. PKA signaling via hCG is also connected to connexin 43 (Cx43) phosphorylation via ezrin, which causes gap junctions to open and fusogenic signals to move from the VCT to the SCT. Syncytialization may also be influenced by several other factors, including the GM-CSF signaling pathway, the MAPK signaling pathway, which acts through EGFR and EGF, and the activin A signaling pathway, which acts through SMAD4. Conversely, TGFβ generated by the SCT appears to offer a signal that counteracts the syncytialization process by preventing fusion. Notably, interferons generated through infection function to stop other nearby cells from becoming infected. When infections like CMV or rubella are present, one interferon-stimulated gene, IFITM3, prevents syncytin-mediated trophoblast fusion into SCT, which may lead to pregnancy failure (Buchrieser et al., 2019).

1.2.2.4. EVT Differentiation

Studies on global transcriptomes clearly distinguish the VCT from the EVT. Features typical of EMT are seen when the EVT migrates from the CCCs into the decidua. Several changes occur in the epithelium, such as decreased expression of E-cadherin and tight junction proteins like ZO-1, altered apical-basal polarity, altered integrin expression from laminin-binding α6β4 to fibronectin-binding α1β1 and α1β5, increased cell size, and glycogen accumulation. Additionally, endothelial markers like VE-cadherin, MCAM, the laminin α4 receptor, and the metalloproteinases MMP2, MMP3, and MMP9 are all upregulated by the EVT. Upregulation of both HLA-C and the non-classical MHC class I molecule HLA-G is a characteristic of EVT differentiation. Many growth factor receptors exhibit altered expression as well: ERBB2 is upregulated and EGFR, MET (the HGF receptor), prolactin receptor (PRLR), and the BMP receptor BMPR1A are all downregulated. Alongside these modifications are changes in the expression of cell cycle regulators and a decrease in proliferation as measured by Ki67 expression. Tetraploid cells are produced by endoreduplication, which is another characteristic of EVT differentiation.

TGFβ1, follistatin, and hyper-glycolsylated hCG are among the proteins and hormones that EVT cells themselves produce. In contrast to the mouse, where it promotes the proliferation of trophoblast stem cells, activin A stimulates the differentiation of EVT in placental explants. (Caniggia et al., 1997; Erlebacher et al., 2004).

Fusion to giant cells in the placental bed is the final stage of iEVT differentiation. These massive multinucleated cells, which are found deep within the decidua basalis and the inner third of the myometrium, the typical limit of iEVT infiltration, generate human placental lactogen. It is unknown which signals and transcription factors (TFs) drive EVT differentiation into eEVT or iEVT. The morphology of the cells in the spiral artery EVT plugs differs greatly from that of the iEVT cells. So far, only two distinct phenotypic differences have been identified: eEVT express CD56 (NCAM); additionally, it is believed that signals from maternal blood may stimulate eEVT differentiation because occasionally CD56+ cells appear within the shell covering the artery openings. Conversely, PLAC8, a protein known to be involved in EMT, is specifically expressed by iEVT (Chang et al., 2018).

Owing to the presence of eEVT plugs in the spiral arteries, the conceptus is in a physiologically low-oxygen environment before ~10 weeks gestation; this is not be confused with hypoxia, which refers to a non-physiological state of insufficient oxygen. The metabolic consequences of this are a reliance on glycolysis, preservation of carbon skeletons used for synthesis of cellular components and protection from damage by free radicals. The subsequent dissolution of the eEVT plugs (at ~10 weeks) and the onset of the maternal circulation correlate with changes in oxygen levels, from 2.5% to around 8%. The onset of circulation occurs more in the center than at the periphery of the placentation site because of the more pronounced trophoblast invasion and arterial transformation centrally. The villi regress at the periphery, resulting in the formation of the chorion laeve (fetal membranes composed of amnion and chorion superimposed on decidua parietalis) and the definitive placenta. Disturbance of this orderly process can result in miscarriage and abnormal placental membranes, predisposing to preterm labor and placental abruption. The hypoxic environment of the first few weeks of gestation might induce EVT differentiation through HIF1A; indeed, more HLA-G+ EVT is generated *in vitro* when cultured in 2% O_2 with upregulation of the imprinted bHLH factor ASCL2, a WNT target involved in EMT.

1.3. Fetal Development

As you may remember, from the ninth week of pregnancy until delivery, a developing human is referred to as a fetus. The structures and functions of the immature organ systems formed during the embryonic period are fully developed during this 30-week period of development, which is characterized by continued cell growth and differentiation. When fetal development is complete, a newborn is produced who, despite being immature in many aspects, can survive outside the womb.

1.3.1. Sexual Differentiation

The onset of sexual differentiation occurs in weeks 9–12 of the fetal period. Despite their genetic differences, embryonic males and females have the same morphology (Figure 1.14). Müllerian and Wolffian ducts connect bipotential gonads, or gonads that have the potential to develop into either male or female sexual organs, to the cloaca, a central cavity. The primitive gut extends into the cloaca. During this time, several things lead to sexual differentiation.

In a developing male fetus, the bipotential gonads develop into the testes and the accompanying epididymis. Müllerian ducts become less functional. The urethra and rectum are formed from the cloaca, and the Wolffian ducts become the vas deferens. The bipotential gonads give rise to the ovaries in a female fetus. It degenerates into Wolffian ducts. The Müllerian ducts develop into the uterine tubes, uterus, and part of the vagina, while the cloaca contributes to the formation of the urethra and rectum.

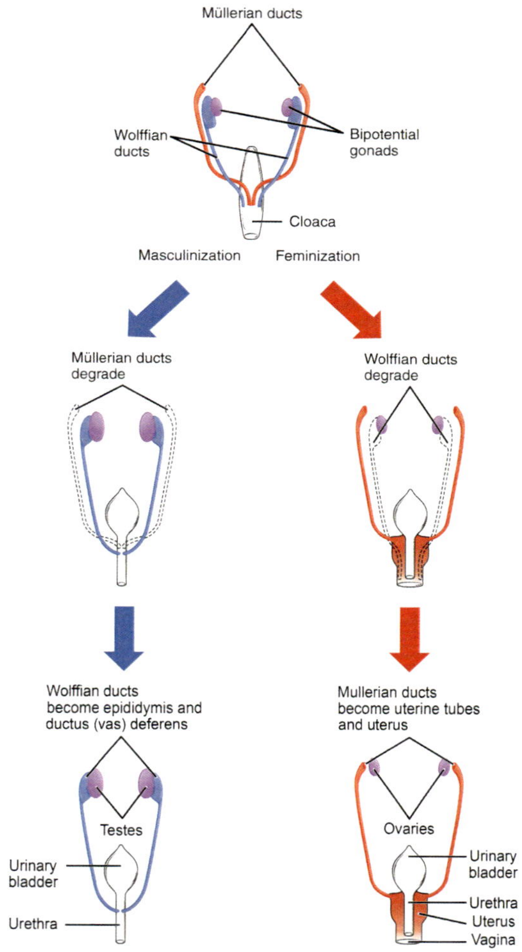

Figure 1.14. *Sexual differentiation: Differentiation of the male and female reproductive systems does not occur until the fetal period of development.*

Source: https://open.oregonstate.education/aandp/chapter/28-3-fetal-development/.

1.3.2. The Fetal Circulatory System

In order for the fetus to receive oxygen and nutrients from the placenta during prenatal development, the fetal circulatory system and placenta are integrated via the umbilical cord. But after delivery, the baby's circulatory system needs to be adjusted because the umbilical cord is severed. The heart begins life as two parallel tubes made of mesoderm that are lined with endothelium before fusing together in the embryo. The tube-shaped heart folds and further differentiates into the four chambers of a mature heart as the embryo grows into a fetus. The fetal cardiovascular system, however, also has circulatory shunts, or short cuts, in contrast to an adult cardiovascular system. An anatomical (or occasionally surgical) diversion known as a shunt permits blood flow to circumvent developing organs like the liver and lungs until childbirth.

Through the umbilical vein, the placenta gives the fetus the nutrition and oxygen it needs to survive. (Recall that blood travels through veins toward the heart. Because it is coming from the placenta in this instance, the blood going to the fetal heart is oxygenated). Since the respiratory system is still developing, it is unable to oxygenate blood on its own. Through the ductus venosus shunt, oxygenated blood from the umbilical vein travels toward the inferior vena cava, essentially avoiding the developing liver (Figure 1.15). The liver is only given a small amount of blood, which is sufficient for its immature, partially functional state. Along the way, blood from the inferior vena cava and fetal venous blood mix as it travels to the right atrium.

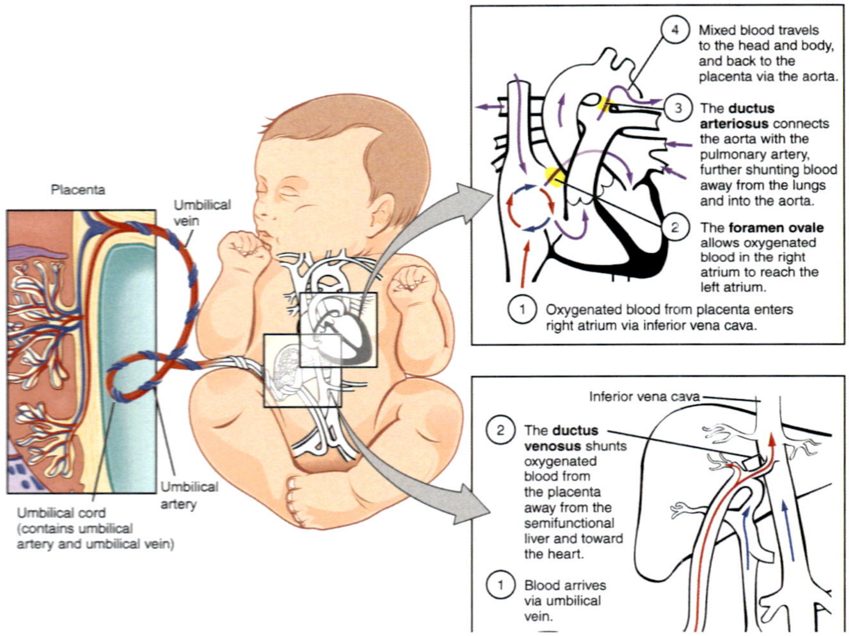

Figure 1.15. *Fetal circulatory system: The fetal circulatory system includes three shunts to divert blood from undeveloped and partially functioning organs, as well as blood supply to and from the placenta.*

Source: https://open.oregonstate.education/aandp/chapter/28-3-fetal-development/.

The fetal lungs are nonfunctional, while the liver is partially functional. Because of this, part of the blood in the fetal circulation avoids the lungs entirely by passing through the foramen ovale, a shunt that connects the right and left atria directly. The majority of the remaining blood is pumped into the right ventricle, where it enters the pulmonary trunk and divides into the pulmonary arteries. But part of this blood is diverted into the aorta by the ductus arteriosus, a shunt located within the pulmonary artery. This guarantees that the immature pulmonary circuit, which has minimal metabolic needs, only receives a tiny amount of oxygenated blood. Uninflated lung blood vessels have a high flow resistance, which promotes blood flow to the aorta, which has a far lower flow resistance. After passing through the foramen ovale and entering the left atrium, the oxygenated blood combines with the now-deoxygenated blood that is returning from the pulmonary circuit. After that, the blood enters the left ventricle and is pumped into the aorta. A portion of this blood travels to the heart via the coronary arteries, while the remaining portion travels to the brain via the carotid arteries.

Blood that has been partially oxygenated and partially deoxygenated is transported to the lower body parts by the descending aorta. Eventually, it enters the umbilical arteries via internal iliac artery branches. As the deoxygenated blood flows through the fetal body and back to the umbilical cord, it gathers waste. Thus, blood with low oxygen content, high carbon dioxide content, and fetal wastes are carried by the two umbilical arteries. Wastes from this blood are filtered by the placenta and then released into the mother's bloodstream. The process is repeated when nutrients and oxygen from the mother permeate into the placenta and then into the blood of the fetus.

1.3.3. Other Organ Systems

The brain continues to grow, the body elongates, and ossification proceeds during weeks 9–12 of fetal development. During this time, fetal movements are frequent but uncontrollably jerky. Erythrocyte production, which the liver handled during the embryonic stage, starts to be handled by the bone marrow. Bile is now secreted by the liver. By swallowing the amniotic fluid and excreting urine, the fetus circulates it. At this point, the eyes are fully formed, but the eyelids are fused shut. The growth of nails starts on the fingers and toes. The fetus measures about 9 cm (3.5 in) from crown to rump by the end of week 12. Development of the sensory organs is prominent in weeks 13–16. The eyes get closer to one another and start to blink, but they stay closed. There are sucking motions on the lips. The ears elevate themselves and rest more comfortably on the head. Hair starts to grow on the scalp. The excretory system is also growing; the kidneys are fully developed, and the intestines start to fill with meconium or fetal excrement. Meconium is made up of bile, mucus, cellular debris, and ingested amniotic fluid.

The mother may experience quickening, or fetal movements, during weeks 16–20 as the fetus grows and its limb movements become more powerful. These movements are, however, restricted by space, which usually forces the developing fetus into the "fetal position," which involves crossing the arms and bending the legs at the knees. The waxy, protective substance known as vernix caseosa, which is coated by sebaceous glands, protects, moisturizes, and may even lubricate the skin during childbirth. During weeks 17–20, a silky hair known as langugo also covers the skin; however, as the fetus grows, it sheds. Infants born very early may occasionally still have residual lanugo.

Rapid weight gain occurs during weeks 21–30 of development, which is crucial for preserving a stable body temperature after birth. The erythrocyte synthesis process is entirely taken over by the bone marrow, and the spinal cord's axons start to become myelinated, or covered in the electrically insulating glial cell sheaths required for effective nervous system operation. (Myelination is not fully developed until adolescence. The fetus grows eyelashes at this time. The eyelids can now be opened and closed and are no longer fused together. Before birth, the lungs start to produce surfactant, a chemical that lowers surface tension in the lungs and promotes healthy lung expansion. Premature babies who produce insufficient surfactant may develop respiratory distress syndrome, which may necessitate surfactant replacement therapy, extra oxygen, or continuous positive airway pressure (CPAP) chamber maintenance in the early days or weeks of life. Near the end of this stage in male fetuses, the testes descend into the scrotum. The fetus is still significantly thinner at 30 weeks, with a measured length of 28 cm (11 in) from crown to rump, roughly resembling the body proportions of a full-term newborn.

Subcutaneous fat is still being laid down by the fetus from week 31 until delivery. The skin becomes softer and more pink as the extra fat fills in the hypodermis, replacing the red and wrinkled texture. The nails grow to the tips of the fingers and toes, and lanugo is shed. The fetus weighs roughly 2.5–4 kg (5.5–8.8 lbs) at birth, with an average length of 35.5–40.5 cm (14–16 in). After birth, the baby is measured from head to toe rather than from crown to rump because they are no longer restricted to the fetal position. The average length at birth is roughly 51 cm (20 in).

1.4. Fetal Circulation

The circulatory system of a fetus differs greatly from that of an adult. The fetus can receive nutrients and oxygenated blood from the placenta thanks to this complex system. It is made up of the umbilical cord, which has two umbilical arteries and one umbilical vein, and the blood vessels in the placenta. Through a shunt called the ductus arteriosus, fetal circulation avoids the lungs. The ductus venosus bypasses the liver, and the foramen ovale allows blood to pass from the right atrium to the left atrium. Fetal heart rates typically range from 110 to 160 beats per minute. Fetuses have less contractility and less ventricular filling than adults do.

After birth, the fetal circulation quickly changes to accommodate life outside the uterus. Fetal sheep provided the first insights into the workings of human understanding of fetal circulation, but detailed information is now available thanks to prenatal ultrasound and magnetic resonance imaging (MRI). There are clear variations in fetal circulation that can result in diseases in childhood or adulthood if they are not properly formed.

1.4.1. Issues of Concern

Babies are more viable than ever at earlier gestational weeks thanks to advancements in medical technology; the effects of an immature heart's transition to newborn circulation last a lifetime. Research on adults who were born prematurely revealed that they had shorter heart chambers, more cardiac muscle mass, and worse cardiac function. Compared to those born at term, those born profoundly prematurely were found to have 50% more ventricular cardiac muscle mass, indicating that these impairments are more severe. Heart failure and ischemic heart disease are more likely to affect these patients. Failure of some shunts to close after birth raises additional concerns because the newborn may have congenital heart defects that manifest in a variety of ways (Finnemore & Groves, 2015).

1.4.2. Cellular Level

Erythropoiesis is started by the yolk sac, which continues until the liver takes over at five weeks of gestation. At six months of gestation, the bone marrow finally contributes. Fetal blood's ability to absorb oxygen is enhanced by the relative hypoxia, which occurs when compared to the mother. This activation of hypoxia-inducible factor-1 causes the kidneys to produce more erythropoietin. In addition, fetal hemoglobin has a greater affinity for oxygen than maternal hemoglobin. Fetal tissue, however, has evolved strategies to release the oxygen from the higher affinity hemoglobin by generating an acidic environment. The baby will have no fetal hemoglobin and an adult hemoglobin level by the time they are 4 to 6 months old. Erythropoiesis will also slow down after birth.

1.4.3. Development

The fetal heart starts beating at 22 days, marking the beginning of fetal circulation. Initially, gas exchange happens in the yolk sac before eventually being taken over by the placenta around ten weeks into pregnancy. The maternal oxygenated blood mixes with the low-oxygen placental blood before being delivered to the fetus. This mixing results in the fetus having lower oxygen levels compared to the mother's blood.

The baby's cardiovascular system changes dramatically and quickly after birth. As a result of the oxygen that is now in the lungs and the physical act of breathing, the baby's pulmonary vascular resistance significantly decreases with its first breath. Blood flow toward the lungs is aided by an increase in systemic vascular resistance following delivery, which occurs when the umbilical cord clamps. The ductus arteriosus flows in ten minutes from left to right. In response to oxygen, the smooth muscle in the ductus arteriosus increases the activity of its calcium channels, which results in constriction and, eventually, shunt closure. The left atrium experiences greater pressure than the right atrium due to the elevated systemic resistance, which results in the closure of the foramen ovale.

1.4.4. Organ Systems Involved

The mother's uterus provides the perfect conditions for the growth of the fetus and the health of the placenta. During fetal circulation, every organ system plays a role in supplying the growing fetus with oxygen and nutrients through the blood. Unlike the liver and lungs, which are bypassed, waste products from these organs are still received by the fetal arterial system.

1.4.5. Function

The fetal circulatory system provides the fetus with nutrients and oxygen while removing waste products and carbon dioxide from fetal circulation.

1.4.6. Mechanism

The circulatory systems of the mother and fetus are connected by the placenta. The growing fetus receives oxygen and nutrients from the mother through the placenta. Additionally, it uses the umbilical cord's blood vessels to drain the fetus of carbon dioxide and metabolic wastes. The placenta gives rise to the umbilical cord, which is then joined to the fetus. The placenta receives its oxygenated blood supply from the mother. The mother and fetus exchange gases, nutrients, and other things through the placental membrane. The syncytiotrophoblast, cytotrophoblast, endothelium of fetal blood vessels, and embryonic connective tissue (Wharton's jelly) combine to form the membrane. With an estimated oxygen saturation of 70–80%, fetal blood passes through the umbilical vein and is primarily distributed into the inferior vena cava (IVC), avoiding the liver via the ductus venosus. A portion of the blood also travels to the fetal hepatic circulation.

Blood from the IVC travels through the right atrium of the heart before being directed through a shunt into the left atrium. In fetal circulation, there is higher pressure in the right atrium than in the left atrium. This causes most of the oxygenated blood to pass from the right atrium to the left atrium through an opening known as the foramen ovale. Meanwhile, a combination of oxygenated blood from the IVC and deoxygenated blood from the SVC results in partially oxygenated blood in the right atrium. Consequently, the left atrium has an estimated oxygen saturation of 65%, higher than the 55% saturation in the right atrium.

After reaching the left atrium, the oxygenated blood passes through the left ventricle and into the coronary arteries and aorta. The aorta then branches to supply the brain with the highest concentration of oxygenated blood before the ductus arteriosus, a shunt from the pulmonary artery, allows the partially oxygenated blood to be combined with the blood supply, which will then flow to the systemic circulation with an estimated oxygen saturation of 60%. The blood in the right atrium that is partially oxygenated, as previously mentioned, can also pass into the right ventricle and subsequently the pulmonary artery. The ductus arteriosus allows blood to flow from the pulmonary artery into the aorta, largely avoiding the lungs due to the high resistance to blood flow in the lungs.

After blood enters the systemic circulation, the deoxygenated blood—which has an estimated oxygen saturation of 40%—recycles via the umbilical arteries back to the placenta, where the mother oxygenates it once more (Morton & Brodsky, 2016).

1.4.7. Related Testing

It is possible to conduct tests to find congenital cardiac defects while pregnant. As early as 16 weeks of pregnancy, the fetal heart can be seen on a fetal echocardiogram. Certain flaws don't show up until after birth. An echocardiography, a possible cardiac catheterization, and a comprehensive history and physical examination make up the evaluation process in these situations. By using a noninvasive technique called near-infrared spectroscopy (NIRS), doctors can determine the oxygenation of fetal tissues and subsequently compute oxygen delivery and blood flow. Further testing may be necessary based on the symptoms and signs that are currently present.

On a chest X-ray, a boot-shaped heart caused by right ventricular hypertrophy may be seen in patients with tetralogy of Fallot. Patients with coarctation of the aorta may show rib notching on chest X-rays due to the enlargement of the intercostal arteries with age. Any structural or valve abnormalities in the fetal or newborn heart will be visible on an echocardiogram.

1.4.8. Pathophysiology

The right side of the heart experiences greater pressure than the left during fetal circulation. The shunts can stay open because of this pressure differential. After the baby inhales for the first time, the placenta's blood flow stops and pulmonary resistance lowers in postnatal circulation. The left side of the lungs experiences greater pressure than the right as blood starts to flow through them. The aforementioned shunts close as a result.

Shunts that don't close after birth result in congenital heart defects. Anatomical abnormalities in the heart can also affect how blood should flow normally. Both cyanotic and acyanotic defects are possible. The most common cause of cyanotic heart defects is postnatal right-to-left shunts in the blood. When deoxygenated blood bypasses the lungs and enters the systemic circulation, the baby may appear blue at birth. Tetralogy of Fallot (TOF), transposition of the great arteries (TGA), tricuspid atresia, persistent truncus arteriosus, and total anomalous pulmonary venous return (TAPVR) are a few examples of cyanotic heart defects. After birth, acyanotic heart defects are usually associated with left-to-right shunts in the blood. No deoxygenated blood enters the systemic circulation because the blood on the left side is oxygenated. Instead, some blood that has been oxygenated passes through the lungs once more and then enters the right side of the heart. The infant does not initially appear blue at birth as a result. Acyanotic heart defects include patent ductus arteriosus (PDA), ventricular septal defect (VSD), atrial septal defect (ASD), and patent foramen ovale (PFO).

On the other hand, if the left-to-right shunt is not corrected, the shunt may revert in later life. Because of the increased blood flow caused by the left-to-right shunt, the right heart may be severely overworked, increasing pulmonary vascular resistance and ultimately leading to pulmonary hypertension. After a while, the right ventricle hypertrophies and the right side of the heart experiences greater pressure than the left. The shunt thus turns around and moves from right to left. When deoxygenated blood begins to enter the bloodstream, the infant may exhibit cyanosis. Eisenmenger syndrome is the term used to describe this left-to-right shunt reversing to a right-to-left shunt.

It is crucial to develop endocardial cushions to comprehend the development of specific cardiac defects. The conotruncal septum, the atrioventricular septa, the mitral and tricuspid valves, and the atrial and ventricular septa are all influenced by the endocardial cushions. ASD and VSD are two cardiac malformations that can result from an endocardial cushion defect. Patients with fetal alcohol syndrome and trisomy 21 also frequently have these abnormalities. When there is an opening in the atrial septum after birth, ASDs develop. Communication between the left and right atria is facilitated by an ASD. The primum form of ASD is less common than the secundum type and is caused by insufficient endocardial cushion development. When there is a breach in the ventricular septum after birth, VSD develops. Communication between the left and right ventricles is facilitated by a VSD.

The causes of persistent truncus arteriosus, TGA, and TOF are conotruncal septal defects. A single artery trunk arises from the left and right ventricles in patients with persistent truncus arteriosus. It is unable to dissect laterally into the pulmonary artery and aorta. This defect is caused by a failure of neural crest cell migration, which prevents the formation of conotruncal ridges. As a result, blood from the left ventricle mixes with the deoxygenated blood from the right ventricle, resulting in cyanosis. The aorta and pulmonary artery exchange positions during TGA. In this instance, the left ventricle gives rise to the pulmonary artery, while the right ventricle gives rise to the aorta. This prevents the conotruncal septum from spiraling during development, which leads to the mixing of two separate blood circuits. Blood that has lost oxygen leaves the body through the aorta and returns to the right side of the heart.

Conversely, blood that has been oxygenated leaves the lungs and passes through the pulmonary artery before returning to the left side of the heart. In this scenario, the body is not receiving enough oxygenated blood, so a shunt is necessary for survival. The conotruncal septum has an anterior displacement in TOF. Pulmonary stenosis, a VSD, an overriding aorta, and right ventricular hypertrophy are its defining features. Right ventricular hypertrophy results from the deoxygenated blood being forced by pulmonary stenosis to pass through the ventricle into the left side. The infant exhibits early cyanosis as a result of the deoxygenated blood entering the systemic circulation.

Congenital defects may also be caused by vascular malformations. When the aortic arch narrows distal to the point where the subclavian artery splits off, coarctation of the aorta occurs. The terms “pre-ductal” and “post-ductal” denote the position of the constriction relative to the ductus arteriosus and the ductus arteriosus, respectively. Deoxygenated blood passes through the pulmonary artery after leaving the right atrium and entering the right ventricle in the pre-ductal coarctation of the aorta. The deoxygenated blood passes beyond the point of constriction into the aorta due to the presence of a PDA. Deoxygenated blood passes through the pulmonary artery after leaving the right atrium and entering the right ventricle in post-ductal coarctation of the aorta. The deoxygenated blood does not move to the left side because there is no PDA.

1.4.9. Clinical Significance

There is a correlation between the hole's size and the clinical presentation of infants with ASD. Patients frequently show no symptoms at all, and a murmur is the only way to identify them. A patient with a significant ASD, however, might show up with persistent lung infections, heart failure, or failure to thrive. Since A2 occurs before P2, the right atrial and right ventricular volumes increase, which in turn increases flow through the pulmonic valve and delays closure, the murmur linked to ASD is a fixed splitting of S2.

The size of the defect also affects how a baby with VSD presents clinically. Small VSDs frequently show no symptoms. Congestive heart failure and failure to thrive can result from larger VSDs with significant left-to-right shunting because the heart cannot pump enough blood to meet the body's needs. The lower left sternal border was auscultated for a holosystolic murmur. When newborns with PDA are examined physically, the patients exhibit a continuous, machine-like murmur that is loudest at S2. It is associated with congenital rubella or prematurity and is best auscultated in the left infraclavicular area.

In TOF, a child commonly presents with "Tet spells." These spells mean that cyanosis may develop when a child is agitated. Upon physical exam, the patient will have a blue tint to their lips and around their mouth, their skin will be damp or warm, and breathing will be rapid.

A child may exhibit differential cyanosis in addition to pre-ductal coarctation of the aorta. Because the aortic branches that supply the upper extremities with blood are not receiving deoxygenated blood, cyanosis will only occur in the lower extremities. Since there is no PDA in post-ductal coarctation of the aorta, cyanosis will not manifest in a child. A child who has an aortic coarctation may also exhibit high blood pressure in their upper limbs before constriction and low blood pressure in their lower limbs following the point of constriction.

1.4.10. Treatment

Prostaglandins from the placenta keep the ductus arteriosus open. During birth, the shunts usually close due to the loss of prostaglandins from placental separation and increased oxygen due to respiration. However, in the management of PDA, NSAIDs like indomethacin may be given to close the shunt because it blocks the production of prostaglandins.

Except in cases where there is another cardiac defect that permits blood to mix, TGA is incompatible with life. Prostaglandins can be administered to keep the ductus arteriosus open, allowing oxygenated and deoxygenated blood to mix.

Squatting can help with TOF symptoms. The femoral arteries become kinked by squatting, which raises systemic vascular resistance. The shunt is reversed as a result of the left heart's pressure being higher than the right heart's. On the other hand, early surgical correction is advised.

A Closer Look

Disorders of the Developing Fetus

Throughout the second half of gestation, the fetal intestines accumulate a tarry, greenish-black meconium. The newborn's first stools consist almost entirely of meconium; they later transition to seedy yellow stools or slightly formed tan stools as meconium is cleared and replaced with digested breast milk or formula, respectively. Unlike these later stools, meconium is sterile; it is devoid of bacteria because the fetus is in a sterile environment and has not consumed any breast milk or formula. Typically, an infant does not pass meconium until after birth. However, in 5–20% of births, the fetus has a bowel movement in utero, which can cause major complications in the newborn.

The passage of meconium in the uterus signals fetal distress, particularly fetal hypoxia (i.e., oxygen deprivation). This may be caused by maternal drug abuse (especially tobacco or cocaine), maternal hypertension, depletion of amniotic fluid, long labor or difficult birth, or a defect in the placenta that prevents it from delivering adequate oxygen to the fetus. Meconium passage is typically a complication of full-term or post-term newborns because it is rarely passed before 34 weeks of gestation when the gastrointestinal system has matured and is appropriately controlled by nervous system stimuli. Fetal distress can stimulate the vagus nerve to trigger gastrointestinal peristalsis and relaxation of the anal sphincter. Notably, fetal hypoxic stress also induces a gasping reflex, increasing the likelihood that meconium will be inhaled into the fetal lungs.

Although meconium is a sterile substance, it interferes with the antibiotic properties of the amniotic fluid and makes the newborn and mother more vulnerable to bacterial infections at birth and during the perinatal period. Specifically, inflammation of the fetal membranes, inflammation of the uterine lining, or neonatal sepsis (infection in the newborn) may occur. Meconium also irritates delicate fetal skin and can cause a rash.

The first sign that a fetus has passed meconium usually does not come until childbirth, when the amniotic sac ruptures. Normal amniotic fluid is clear and watery, but amniotic fluid in which meconium has been passed is stained greenish or yellowish. Antibiotics given to the mother may reduce the incidence of maternal bacterial infections, but it is critical that meconium is aspirated from the newborn before the first breath. Under these conditions, an obstetrician will extensively aspirate the infant's airways as soon as the head is delivered, while the rest of the infant's body is still inside the birth canal.

Aspiration of meconium with the first breath can result in labored breathing, a barrel-shaped chest, or a low Apgar score. An obstetrician can identify meconium aspiration by listening to the lungs with a stethoscope for a coarse rattling sound. Blood gas tests and chest X-rays of the infant can confirm meconium aspiration. Inhaled meconium after birth could obstruct a newborn's airways leading to alveolar collapse, interfere with surfactant function by stripping it from the lungs, or cause pulmonary inflammation or hypertension. Any of these complications will make the newborn much more vulnerable to pulmonary infection, including pneumonia.

Summary

- Maternal anatomy refers to the study of the anatomical and physiological changes and structures in a woman's body that occur during pregnancy, childbirth, and the postpartum period. These changes are critical to support the developing fetus, prepare the mother for labor and delivery, and facilitate postnatal recovery and breastfeeding.
- The perineum is an anatomical region in the pelvis. It is located between the thighs and represents the most inferior part of the pelvic outlet. The perineum is separated from the pelvic cavity superiorly by the pelvic floor.
- The urogenital triangle is the anterior half of the perineum. It is bounded by the pubic symphysis, ischiopubic rami, and a theoretical line between the two ischial tuberosities. The triangle is associated with the structures of the urogenital system – the external genitalia and urethra.
- The human placenta develops from the trophectoderm (TE), the outer layer of the pre-implantation embryo, which forms at ~5 days post fertilization (dpf). At this stage, the pre-implantation embryo (termed a blastocyst) is segregated into two lineages: the inner cell mass (ICM) and the TE.
- The cytotrophoblast shell becomes discontinuous and cytotrophoblast cell columns (CCCs) emerge from the distal tips of the anchoring villi in contact with the decidua. The cells in the columns are rounded, cohesive and rich in glycogen.
- Sexual differentiation does not begin until the fetal period, during weeks 9–12. Embryonic males and females, though genetically distinguishable, are morphologically identical. Bipotential gonads, or gonads that can develop into male or female sexual organs, are connected to a central cavity called the cloaca via Müllerian ducts and Wolffian ducts.
- The descending aorta carries partially oxygenated and partially deoxygenated blood into the lower regions of the body. It eventually passes into the umbilical arteries through branches of the internal iliac arteries. The deoxygenated blood collects waste as it circulates through the fetal body and returns to the umbilical cord.

References

1. Abbas, Y., Oefner, C. M., Polacheck, W. J., Gardner, L., Farrell, L., Sharkey, A., Kamm, R., Moffett, A., & Oyen, M. L. (2017). A microfluidics assay to study invasion of human placental trophoblast cells. *Journal of the Royal Society Interface, 14*(20170131). https://doi.org/10.1098/rsif.2017.0131.
2. Abou-Kheir, W., Barrak, J., Hadadeh, O., & Daoud, G. (2017). HTR-8/SVneo cell line contains a mixed population of cells. *Placenta, 50*, 1–7. https://doi.org/10.1016/j.placenta.2016.12.007.
3. Al-Lamki, R. S., Skepper, J. N., & Burton, G. J. (1999). Are human placental bed giant cells merely aggregates of small mononuclear trophoblast cells? An ultrastructural and immunocytochemical study. *Human Reproduction, 14*(2), 496–504. https://doi.org/10.1093/humrep/14.2.496.
4. Amita, M., Adachi, K., Alexenko, A. P., Sinha, S., Schust, D. J., Schulz, L. C., Roberts, R. M., & Ezashi, T. (2013). Complete and unidirectional conversion of human embryonic stem cells to

trophoblast by BMP4. *Proceedings of the National Academy of Sciences, 110*(E1212–E1221). https://doi.org/10.1073/pnas.1303094110.

5. Aplin, J. D., Charlton, A. K., & Ayad, S. (1988). An immunohistochemical study of human endometrial extracellular matrix during the menstrual cycle and first trimester of pregnancy. *Cell and Tissue Research, 253*(2), 231–240. https://doi.org/10.1007/BF00221758.
6. Apps, R., Gardner, L., Sharkey, A. M., Holmes, N., & Moffett, A. (2007). A homodimeric complex of HLA-G on normal trophoblast cells modulates antigen-presenting cells via LILRB1. *European Journal of Immunology, 37*(7), 1924–1937. https://doi.org/10.1002/eji.200737089.
7. Apps, R., Murphy, S. P., Fernando, R., Gardner, L., Ahad, T., & Moffett, A. (2009). Human leucocyte antigen (HLA) expression of primary trophoblast cells and placental cell lines, determined using single antigen beads to characterize allotype specificities of anti-HLA antibodies. *Immunology, 127*(1), 26–39. https://doi.org/10.1111/j.1365-2567.2008.03019.x.
8. Apps, R., Sharkey, A., Gardner, L., Male, V., Trotter, M., Miller, N., North, R., Founds, S., & Moffett, A. (2011). Genome-wide expression profile of first trimester villous and extra villous human trophoblast cells. *Placenta, 32*(1), 33–43. https://doi.org/10.1016/j.placenta.2010.10.010.
9. Arias-Stella, J. (1954). Atypical endometrial changes associated with the presence of chorionic tissue. *AMA Archives of Pathology, 52*(2), 112–128.
10. Baczyk, D., Dunk, C., Huppertz, B., Maxwell, C., Reister, F., Giannoulias, D., & Kingdom, J. C. P. (2006). Bi-potential behaviour of cytotrophoblasts in first trimester chorionic villi. *Placenta, 27*(4–5), 367–374. https://doi.org/10.1016/j.placenta.2005.03.006.
11. Barchitta, M., Maugeri, A., Quattrocchi, A., Agrifoglio, O., & Agodi, A. (2017). The role of miRNAs as biomarkers for pregnancy outcomes: A comprehensive review. *International Journal of Genomics, 2017*, 1–11. https://doi.org/10.1155/2017/8067972.
12. Barker, D. J. P. (1995). The fetal and infant origins of disease. *European Journal of Clinical Investigation, 25*(7), 457–463. https://doi.org/10.1111/j.1365-2362.1995.tb01730.x.
13. Benirschke, K., Burton, G. J., & Baergen, R. N. (2012). *Pathology of the Human Placenta* (6th ed.). Springer.
14. Bernardo, A. S., Faial, T., Gardner, L., Niakan, K. K., Ortmann, D., Senner, C. E., Callery, E. M., Trotter, M. W., Hemberger, M., Smith, J. C., & Pedersen, R. A. (2011). BRACHYURY and CDX2 mediate BMP-induced differentiation of human and mouse pluripotent stem cells into embryonic and extraembryonic lineages. *Cell Stem Cell, 9*(2), 144–155. https://doi.org/10.1016/j.stem.2011.06.015.
15. Blakeley, P., Fogarty, N. M. E., del Valle, I., Wamaitha, S. E., Hu, T. X., Elder, K., Snell, P., Christie, L., Robson, P., & Niakan, K. K. (2015). Defining the three cell lineages of the human blastocyst by single-cell RNA-seq. *Development, 142*(21), 3613–3626. https://doi.org/10.1242/dev.131235.
16. Boroviak, T., Stirparo, G. G., Dietmann, S., Hernando-Herraez, I., Mohammed, H., Reik, W., Smith, A., Sasaki, E., Nichols, J., & Bertone, P. (2018). Single cell transcriptome analysis of human, marmoset and mouse embryos reveals common and divergent features of preimplantation development. *Development, 145*(19), dev167833. https://doi.org/10.1242/dev.167833.
17. Boss, A. L., Chamley, L. W., & James, J. L. (2018). Placental formation in early pregnancy: How is the centre of the placenta made? *Human Reproduction Update, 24*(6), 750–760. https://doi.org/10.1093/humupd/dmy030.

18. Boyd, J. D., & Hamilton, W. J. (1970). *The Human Placenta*. W. Heffer & Sons Ltd.

19. Brosens, I., Pijnenborg, R., Vercruysse, L., & Romero, R. (2011). The "Great Obstetrical Syndromes" are associated with disorders of deep placentation. *American Journal of Obstetrics and Gynecology, 204*(3), 193–201. https://doi.org/10.1016/j.ajog.2010.08.009.

20. Brosens, I., Robertson, W. B., & Dixon, H. G. (1967). The physiological response of the vessels of the placental bed to normal pregnancy. *Journal of Pathology and Bacteriology, 93*(2), 569–579. https://doi.org/10.1002/path.1700930218.

21. Buchrieser, J., Degrelle, S. A., Couderc, T., Nevers, Q., Disson, O., Manet, C., Donahue, D. A., Porrot, F., Hillion, K. H., Perthame, E., et al. (2019). IFITM proteins inhibit placental syncytiotrophoblast formation and promote fetal demise. *Science*, *365*(6455), 176–180. https://doi.org/10.1126/science.aav5316.

22. Bulmer, J. N., & Lash, G. E. (2015). The role of uterine NK cells in normal reproduction and reproductive disorders. In R. Moffett & C. King (Eds.), *Reproductive Immunology* (pp. 95–126). Springer. https://doi.org/10.1007/978-3-319-16185-9_6.

23. Burrows, T. D., King, A., & Loke, Y. W. (1994). Expression of adhesion molecules by endovascular trophoblast and decidual endothelial cells: Implications for vascular invasion during implantation. *Placenta*, *15*(1), 21–33. https://doi.org/10.1016/S0143-4004(05)80233-4.

24. Burton, G. J. (1987). The fine structure of the human placental villus as revealed by scanning electron microscopy. *Scanning Microscopy*, *1*(4), 1811–1828.

25. Burton, G. J. (2009). Oxygen, the Janus gas; its effects on human placental development and function. *Journal of Anatomy*, *215*(1), 27–35. https://doi.org/10.1111/j.1469-7580.2008.00978.x.

26. Burton, G. J., & Jauniaux, E. (2017). The cytotrophoblastic shell and complications of pregnancy. *Placenta*, *60*, 134–139. https://doi.org/10.1016/j.placenta.2017.06.007.

27. Burton, G. J., Jauniaux, E., & Charnock-Jones, D. S. (2007). Human early placental development: Potential roles of the endometrial glands. *Placenta*, *28*(Suppl. A), S64–S69. https://doi.org/10.1016/j.placenta.2007.01.007.

28. Burton, G. J., Jauniaux, E., & Murray, A. J. (2017). Oxygen and placental development; parallels and differences with tumor biology. *Placenta*, *56*, 14–18. https://doi.org/10.1016/j.placenta.2017.01.130.

29. Burton, G. J., Jauniaux, E., & Watson, A. L. (1999). Maternal arterial connections to the placental intervillous space during the first trimester of human pregnancy: The Boyd collection revisited. *American Journal of Obstetrics and Gynecology*, *181*(3), 718–724. https://doi.org/10.1016/S0002-9378(99)70518-1.

30. Burton, G. J., Redman, C. W., Roberts, J. M., & Moffett, A. (2019). Pre-eclampsia: Pathophysiology and clinical implications. *BMJ*, *366*, l2381. https://doi.org/10.1136/bmj.l2381.

31. Burton, G. J., Watson, A. L., Hempstock, J., Skepper, J. N., & Jauniaux, E. (2002). Uterine glands provide histotrophic nutrition for the human fetus during the first trimester of pregnancy. *The Journal of Clinical Endocrinology & Metabolism*, *87*(6), 2954–2959. https://doi.org/10.1210/jcem.87.6.8563.

32. Burton, G. J., Woods, A. W., Jauniaux, E., & Kingdom, J. C. P. (2009). Rheological and physiological consequences of conversion of the maternal spiral arteries for uteroplacental blood flow during human pregnancy. *Placenta, 30*(6), 473–482. https://doi.org/10.1016/j.placenta.2009.02.009.

33. Caniggia, I., Lye, S. J., & Cross, J. C. (1997). Activin is a local regulator of human cytotrophoblast cell differentiation. *Endocrinology, 138*(9), 3976–3986. https://doi.org/10.1210/endo.138.9.5403.

34. Cao, Z., Carey, T. S., Ganguly, A., Wilson, C. A., Paul, S., & Knott, J. G. (2015). Transcription factor AP-2 induces early Cdx2 expression and represses HIPPO signaling to specify the trophectoderm lineage. *Development, 142*(9), 1606–1615. https://doi.org/10.1242/dev.120238.

35. Carter, A. M. (2011). Comparative studies of placentation and immunology in non-human primates suggest a scenario for the evolution of deep trophoblast invasion and an explanation for human pregnancy disorders. *Reproduction, 141*(3), 391–396. https://doi.org/10.1530/REP-10-0530.

36. Carter, A. M., & Enders, A. C. (2004). Comparative aspects of trophoblast development and placentation. *Reproductive Biology and Endocrinology, 2*(1), 46. https://doi.org/10.1186/1477-7827-2-46.

37. Carter, A. M., & Enders, A. C. (2013). The evolution of epitheliochorial placentation. *Annual Review of Animal Biosciences, 1*(1), 443–467. https://doi.org/10.1146/annurev-animal-031412-103653.

38. Carter, A. M., & Pijnenborg, R. (2011). Evolution of invasive placentation with special reference to non-human primates. *Best Practice & Research Clinical Obstetrics & Gynecology, 25*(3), 249–257. https://doi.org/10.1016/j.bpobgyn.2010.10.010.

39. Castellucci, M., Celona, A., Bartels, H., Steininger, B., Benedetto, V., & Kaufmann, P. (1987). Mitosis of the Hofbauer cell: Possible implications for a fetal macrophage. *Placenta, 8*(1), 65–76. https://doi.org/10.1016/0143-4004(87)90040-3.

40. Castellucci, M., Kosanke, G., Verdenelli, F., Huppertz, B., & Kaufmann, P. (2000). Villous sprouting: Fundamental mechanisms of human placental development. *Human Reproduction Update, 6*(5), 485–494. https://doi.org/10.1093/humupd/6.5.485.

41. Chan, C. C. W., Lao, T. T., & Cheung, A. N. Y. (1999). Apoptotic and proliferative activities in first trimester placentae. *Placenta, 20*(3), 223–227. https://doi.org/10.1053/plac.1998.0375.

42. Chang, W. L., Liu, Y. W., Dang, Y. L., Jiang, X. X., Xu, H., Huang, X., Wang, Y. L., Wang, H., Zhu, C., Xue, L. Q., et al. (2018). PLAC8, a new marker for human interstitial extra villous trophoblast cells, promotes their invasion and migration. *Development, 145*(14), dev148932. https://doi.org/10.1242/dev.148932.

43. Chavan, A. R., Griffith, O. W., & Wagner, G. P. (2017). The inflammation paradox in the evolution of mammalian pregnancy: Turning a foe into a friend. *Current Opinion in Genetics & Development, 47*, 24–32. https://doi.org/10.1016/j.gde.2017.08.004.

44. Clevers, H. (2016). Modeling development and disease with organoids. *Cell, 165*(7), 1586–1597. https://doi.org/10.1016/j.cell.2016.05.082.

45. Collins, S. L., Birks, J. S., Stevenson, G. N., Papageorghiou, A. T., Noble, J. A., & Impey, L. (2012). Measurement of spiral artery jets: General principles and differences observed in small-for-

gestational-age pregnancies. *Ultrasound in Obstetrics & Gynecology*, *40*(2), 171–178. https://doi.org/10.1002/uog.10149.

46. Conrad, K. P., Rabaglino, M. B., & Post Uiterweer, E. D. (2017). Emerging role for dysregulated decidualization in the genesis of preeclampsia. *Placenta*, *60*, 119–129. https://doi.org/10.1016/j.placenta.2017.06.005.
47. Damsky, C. H., Fitzgerald, M. L., & Fisher, S. J. (1992). Distribution patterns of extracellular matrix components and adhesion receptors are intricately modulated during first trimester cytotrophoblast differentiation along the invasive pathway, *in vivo*. *The Journal of Clinical Investigation*, *89*(1), 210–222. https://doi.org/10.1172/JCI115565.
48. Damsky, C. H., Librach, C., Lim, K. H., Fitzgerald, M. L., McMaster, M. T., Janatpour, M., Zhou, Y., Logan, S. K., & Fisher, S. J. (1994). Integrin switching regulates normal trophoblast invasion. *Development*, *120*(12), 3667–3666.
49. Deglincerti, A., Croft, G. F., Pietila, L. N., Zernicka-Goetz, M., Siggia, E. D., & Brivanlou, A. H. (2016). Self-organization of the *in vitro* attached human embryo. *Nature*, *533*(7602), 251–254. https://doi.org/10.1038/nature17948.
50. Dempsey, E. W. (1972). The development of capillaries in the villi of early human placentas. *American Journal of Anatomy*, *134*(2), 221–237. https://doi.org/10.1002/aja.1001340207.
51. Finnemore, A., & Groves, A. (2015). Physiology of the fetal and transitional circulation. *Seminars in Fetal and Neonatal Medicine*, *20*(4), 210–216. https://doi.org/10.1016/j.siny.2015.05.003.
52. Gerbaud, P., Pidoux, G., Guibourdenche, J., Pathirage, N., Costa, J. M., Badet, J., Frendo, J. L., Murthi, P., & Evain-Brion, D. (2011). Mesenchymal activin-A overcomes defective human trisomy 21 trophoblast fusion. *Endocrinology*, *152*(12), 5017–5028. https://doi.org/10.1210/en.2011-1193.
53. Hertig, A. T., Rock, J., & Adams, E. C. (1956). A description of 34 human ova within the first 17 days of development. *American Journal of Anatomy*, *98*(3), 435–493. https://doi.org/10.1002/aja.1000980306.
54. Lewis, C. L., Laudicina, N. M., Khuu, A., & Loverro, K. L. (2017). The human pelvis: Variation in structure and function during gait. *The Anatomical Record*, *300*(4), 633–642. https://doi.org/10.1002/ar.23556.
55. Meindl, R. S., Lovejoy, C. O., Mensforth, R. P., & Don Carlos, L. (1985). Accuracy and direction of error in the sexing of the skeleton: Implications for paleo demography. *American Journal of Physical Anthropology*, *68*(1), 79–85. https://doi.org/10.1002/ajpa.1330680110.
56. Morton, S. U., & Brodsky, D. (2016). Fetal physiology and the transition to extrauterine life. *Clinics in Perinatology*, *43*(3), 395–407. https://doi.org/10.1016/j.clp.2016.04.001.
57. Ng, R. K., Dean, W., Dawson, C., Lucifero, D., Madeja, Z., Reik, W., & Hemberger, M. (2008). Epigenetic restriction of embryonic cell lineage fate by methylation of Elf5. *Nature Cell Biology*, *10*(11), 1280–1290. https://doi.org/10.1038/ncb1786.
58. Nordor, A. V., Nehar-Belaid, D., Richon, S., Klatzmann, D., Bellet, D., Dangles-Marie, V., Fournier, T., & Aryee, M. J. (2017). The early pregnancy placenta foreshadows DNA methylation alterations of solid tumors. *Epigenetics*, *12*(10), 793–803. https://doi.org/10.1080/15592294.2017.1342912.
59. White, T. D., Black, M. T., & Folkens, P. A. (2011). *Human Osteology* (3rd ed.). Academic Press.

Chapter

MATERNAL CHANGES DURING PREGNANCY

2

Contents

Introduction

Pregnancy induces a series of profound and multifaceted changes in a woman's body, encompassing physiological, hormonal, and anatomical adaptations. These changes are essential for supporting the developing fetus and preparing the mother's body for childbirth and breastfeeding.

One of the most notable changes is the increase in blood volume, which can rise by up to 50% to meet the needs of the growing fetus and placenta. This increase supports enhanced nutrient and oxygen delivery while also preparing the body for the blood loss that occurs during delivery. The cardiovascular system adapts with an increased heart rate and cardiac output, while blood pressure typically decreases in the first two trimesters before returning to pre-pregnancy levels or slightly higher in the third trimester.

Hormones play a pivotal role throughout pregnancy. Human chorionic gonadotropin (hCG), produced by the placenta, supports the corpus luteum in the ovary to maintain the production of progesterone and estrogen in early pregnancy. Progesterone relaxes the uterine muscles to prevent contractions, while estrogen promotes the growth of the uterus and enhances blood flow. Both hormones also contribute to changes in the breasts, preparing them for lactation. Additionally, relaxin, another hormone, loosens the ligaments in the pelvis and softens the cervix in preparation for childbirth.

The expanding uterus exerts pressure on surrounding organs, which can cause symptoms such as frequent urination, heartburn, and shortness of breath. The abdomen stretches to accommodate the growing fetus, which may result in skin changes such as stretch marks. The musculoskeletal system also adapts, with a shift in the center of gravity leading to changes in posture and potential lower back pain.

The maternal body undergoes extensive changes during pregnancy to support fetal development and prepare for delivery. Understanding these changes can help expectant mothers anticipate and manage the physical and emotional experiences associated with pregnancy, ultimately contributing to better maternal and fetal health outcomes.

Orientation and Directional Terms

<table>
<tr><th>Term</th><th>Definition</th><th>Illustration</th></tr>
<tr><td>Hydronephrosis</td><td>Hydronephrosis is a condition where one or both kidneys swell due to a buildup of urine.</td><td>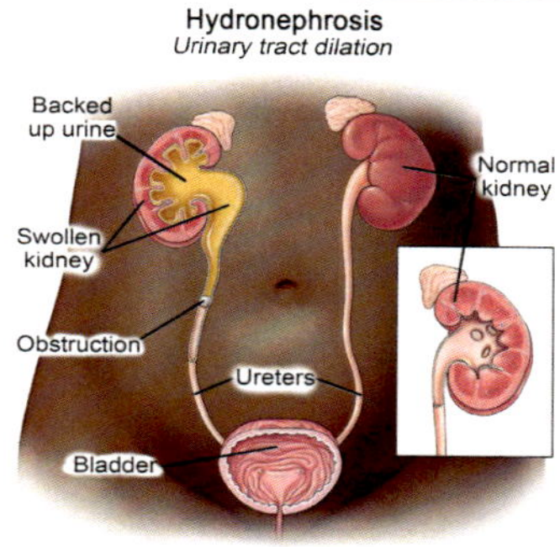
</td></tr>
<tr><td>Pulmorary edema</td><td>Pulmonary edema is a condition caused by too much fluid in the lungs.</td><td>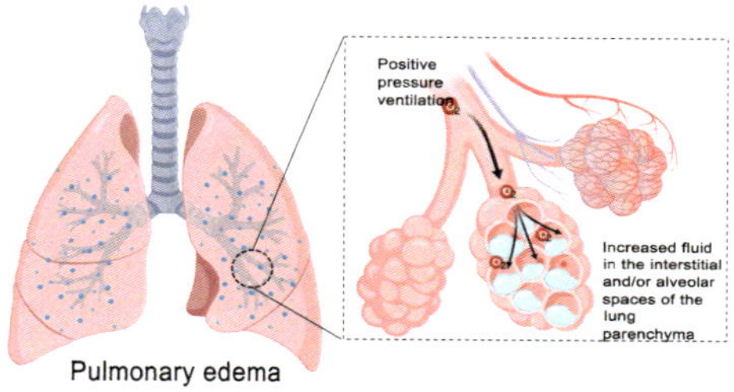
</td></tr>
<tr><td>Vasodilatory state</td><td>A vasodilatory state is a medical condition where blood vessels are extremely dilated, or relaxed, and the body can't get enough blood to the heart, brain, and kidneys.</td><td>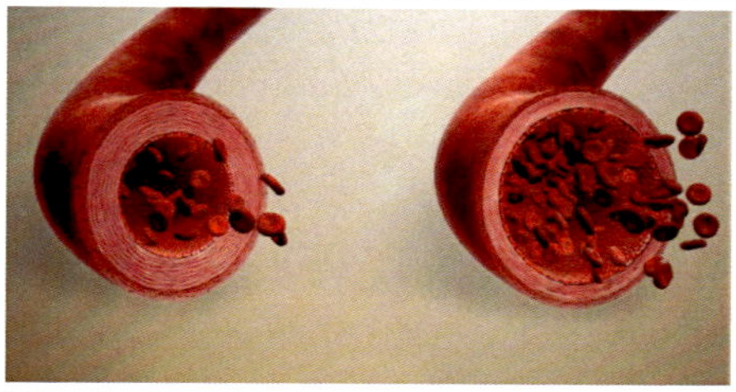</td></tr>
<tr><td>Uteroplacental perfusion</td><td>Uteroplacental perfusion is the process by which the body increases blood flow to the placenta and fetus during pregnancy to deliver oxygen and nutrients.</td><td>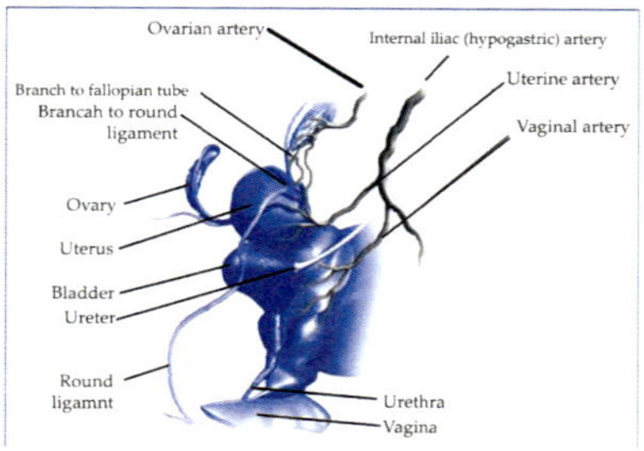
</td></tr>
<tr><td>Placental steroidogenesis</td><td>Placental steroidogenesis is the process by which the placenta synthesizes and secretes steroid hormones to establish pregnancy.</td><td>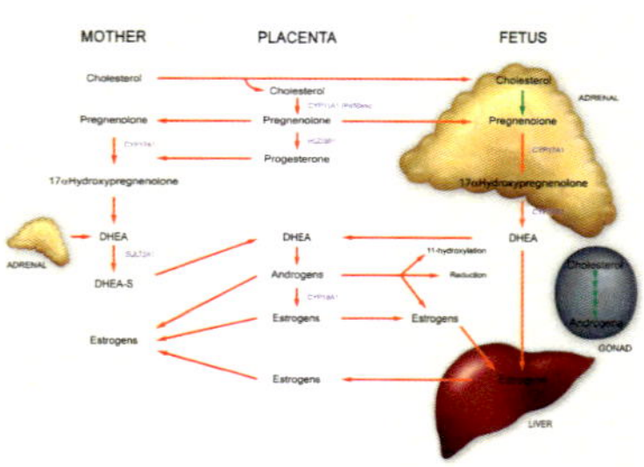
</td></tr>
</table>

2.1. Physiological Changes in Pregnancy

The expectant mother experiences notable physiological and anatomical changes in order to support and care for the growing fetus. These alterations impact all of the body's organ systems and start after conception. Most women who have an easy pregnancy experience these changes ending with little to no aftereffects. Knowing the physiological changes that are typical during pregnancy will help you distinguish between normal adaptations and abnormal ones.

The volume of plasma gradually rises during a typical pregnancy. The majority of this 50% increase happens by 34 weeks of gestation and is correlated with the baby's birthweight. The concentration of hemoglobin, hematocrit, and red blood cell count decrease because the expansion of plasma volume surpasses the growth in red blood cell mass. There is typically no change in mean corpuscular volume (MCV) or mean corpuscular hemoglobin concentration (MCHC) in spite of this hemodilution.

During a typical pregnancy, the platelet count typically falls gradually but stays within normal ranges. A small percentage of women (5–10%) will see counts of 100–150 × 10^9 cells/l by term, even in the absence of any pathological processes. In actuality, therefore, a pregnant woman's platelet count must be less than 100 × 10^9 cells/l before she is diagnosed as thrombocytopenic.

The amount of iron needed during pregnancy increases two to three times, as it is needed for the fetus as well as for the synthesis of certain enzymes and hemoglobin. The requirements for folate have increased by ten to twenty times, while those for vitamin B12 have increased by two times. Pregnancy-related changes to the coagulation system result in a physiologically hypercoagulable state (in preparation for postpartum hemostasis). Certain clotting factors, mainly VIII, IX, and X, have higher concentrations. There is a notable 50% increase in fibrinogen levels accompanied by a decrease in fibrinolytic activity. Endogenous anticoagulants like protein S and antithrombin have declining concentrations. Pregnancy therefore modifies the coagulation system's equilibrium to favor clotting, making pregnant and postpartum women more vulnerable to venous thrombosis. This elevated risk exists starting in the first trimester and lasts for a minimum of 12 weeks after delivery. In the absence of anticoagulants or a coagulopathy, the results of in vitro coagulation tests (activated partial thromboplastin time; APTT), prothrombin time; and thrombin time; TT) remain normal.

Lower limb venous stasis is linked to venodilation and reduced flow, with a greater degree of the latter, observed in the left limb. This results from the ovarian artery and left iliac artery compressing the left iliac vein. The iliac artery does not pass through the vein on the right.

2.1.1. Cardiac Changes

Pregnancy causes significant changes to the cardiovascular system, which start early in the process. By eight weeks of gestation, the cardiac output has already increased by 20%. It is most likely peripheral vasodilatation that is the main event. The synthesis of nitric oxide, which is stimulated by estradiol and potentially vasodilatory prostaglandins (PGI2), is one of the endothelium-dependent factors that mediate this. Systemic vascular resistance decreases by 25–30% as a result of peripheral vasodilation; during pregnancy, cardiac output rises by about 40% to make up for this. This is mostly accomplished by raising the stroke volume, though an increase in heart rate also plays a role. The maximum cardiac output occurs between weeks 20 and 28 of pregnancy. At term, there is very little fall. The early increase in ventricular wall muscle mass and end-diastolic volume (but not end-diastolic pressure) observed during pregnancy may contribute to an increase in stroke volume. Physiological dilation of the heart occurs, and myocardial contractility is raised. The mother's heart rate rises (10–20 bpm) even though the stroke volume decreases as she approaches term, maintaining her higher cardiac output. In the first and second trimesters, blood pressure falls; however, in the third trimester, it rises to non-pregnant levels.

Maternal position toward term has a significant impact on both the mother's and the fetus's hemodynamic profile. When a woman is supine, her weight puts pressure on her inferior vena cava (IVC), which lowers the amount of blood returning to her heart and, as a result, her cardiac output and stroke volume. A quarter of the cardiac output may be lost when turning from the lateral to the supine position. Therefore, whenever possible, nursing should be done with the pregnant woman in the left or right lateral position. To maximize cardiac output and uteroplacental blood flow, the pelvis should be rotated if the woman must be kept on her back. This will cause the uterus to drop to the side and off the IVC. Decreased cardiac output is linked to decreased placental perfusion, which could endanger the fetus. It also results in decreased uterine blood flow.

Pregnancy causes an increase in blood volume and stroke volume, but not in central venous pressure or pulmonary capillary wedge pressure. Similar to systemic vascular resistance (SVR), pulmonary vascular resistance (PVR) also dramatically drops during a typical pregnancy. Serum colloid osmotic pressure decreases by 10–15% while pulmonary capillary wedge pressure (PCWP) remains unchanged. Pregnant women are more vulnerable to pulmonary edema due to a roughly 30% reduction in the colloid osmotic pressure/pulmonary capillary wedge pressure gradient. Increased pulmonary capillary permeability, as in pre-eclampsia, or an increase in cardiac pre-load, such as fluid infusion, will cause pulmonary edema, or both.

Further increases in cardiac output (15% in the first stage and 50% in the second stage) are linked to labor. Additionally, uterine contractions cause an auto-transfusion of 300–500 ml of blood back into the circulation, and the sympathetic nervous system's reaction to pain and anxiety raises blood pressure and heart rate even more. Heart rate rises both during and in between cardiac contractions.

After delivery, the uterus contracts, releasing blood into the systemic circulation, and the inferior vena cava obstruction is relieved, resulting in an instant increase in cardiac output. After delivery, cardiac output rises by 60–80%, but it quickly drops to pre-labor levels within an hour or so. The extravascular space's fluid is transferred, which further raises the stroke volume and venous return.

Therefore, the second stage of labor and the first few days after giving birth are the times when women who have cardiovascular compromise are most vulnerable to pulmonary edema. Two weeks after delivery, cardiac output has almost entirely recovered to pre-pregnancy levels, despite some pathological alterations (e.g., hypertension in pre-eclampsia) that could require a lot more time.

For those who are not familiar with pregnancy, the aforementioned physiological changes can cause changes on a cardiovascular examination that are misinterpreted as pathological. A bounding or collapsing pulse and an ejection systolic murmur, which affect more than 90% of pregnant women, are examples of possible changes. The first heart sound and maybe a third heart sound can be clearly heard in a loud murmur that can be heard throughout the precordium. Peripheral edema and ectopic beats could be present. Normal findings on ECG in pregnancy that may partly relate to changes in the position of the heart include:

- atrial and ventricular ectopics
- Q wave (small) and inverted T wave in lead III
- ST-segment depression and T-wave inversion in the inferior and lateral leads
- left-axis shift of QRS.

2.1.2. Adaptive Changes in Renal Vasculature

By week six of pregnancy, there is a noticeable decrease in systemic vascular resistance (SVR), which serves as the main adaptive mechanism. The renal vasculature is also impacted by the 40% decrease in SVR. Because 85% of the plasma volume is in the venous circulation during pregnancy, even with a significant increase in plasma volume, the massive decrease in SVR results in a state of arterial under-filling. This under-filling of the arteries is specific to pregnancy. In contrast to other conditions of arterial under-filling, such as cirrhosis, sepsis, or arterio-venous fistulas, the decrease in SVR is accompanied by an increase in renal blood flow.

During pregnancy, the corpus luteum, decidua, and placenta produce the peptide hormone relaxin, which is crucial for controlling water and hemodynamic metabolism. After conception, serum relaxin concentrations rise to a peak at the end of the first trimester and then decline to an intermediate value during the second and third trimesters. Serum relaxin concentrations are already elevated during the luteal phase of the menstrual cycle. Relaxin promotes endothelin synthesis, which facilitates nitric oxide (NO) synthesis and renal artery vasodilation.

Even though the renin-angiotensin-aldosterone (RAA) system is activated in the early stages of pregnancy, there is a concurrent development of relative resistance to angiotensin II, which counteracts the vasoconstrictive effect and permits significant vasodilatation. The effects of progesterone and vascular endothelial growth factor-mediated prostacyclin production, along with changes in the angiotensin I receptors during pregnancy, could account for this insensitivity to angiotensin II. Other vasoconstrictors, like adrenergic agonists and arginine vasopressin (AVP), may also share the vascular refractoriness to angiotensin II. The placental vasodilators may play a more significant role in maintaining the vasodilatory state during the second half of pregnancy.

2.1.3. Changes in Renal Anatomy and Function

Renal plasma flow and glomerular filtration rate (GFR) rise 40–65 and 50–85%, respectively, in response to renal vasodilatation when compared to non-pregnant levels. Furthermore, a rise in GFR results from a decrease in glomeruli's oncotic pressure brought on by the increase in plasma volume. Due to the reduction of vascular resistance in the renal afferent and efferent arterioles, glomerular hydrostatic pressure stays constant, preventing the development of glomerular hypertension, even in the face of a massive increase in renal plasma flow. Serum creatinine and urea concentrations drop to mean values of roughly 44.2 μmol/l and 3.2 mmol/l, respectively, as GFR increases.

Renal size increases by 1–0.5 cm as a result of the increased renal blood flow, reaching its maximum size by the middle of pregnancy. The ureters are mechanically compressed, which causes the kidney, pelvic, and calyceal systems to dilate. These anatomical changes are mediated by progesterone, which also lowers contraction pressure, peristalsis, and ureteral tone. Urinary dead space, renal vasculature, and interstitial volume all increase in tandem with increasing renal size. In more than 80% of women, there is also dilation of the ureters, renal pelvis, and calyces, which results in physiological hydronephrosis. Because of the anatomical way in which the right ureter crosses the iliac and ovarian vessels at an angle before entering the pelvis, there is frequently a right-sided predominance of hydronephrosis. Pregnant women who have bacteriuria without any symptoms are at risk of developing pyelonephritis due to urinary stasis in the dilated collecting system.

The tubular handling of nutrients and wastes is also altered. In the glomerulus, glucose is freely filtered, just like it is not pregnant. The proximal and collecting tubules' ability to reabsorb glucose is less efficient and excretes glucose in different ways during pregnancy. 90% of expectant mothers with normal blood sugar excrete one to ten grams of glucose daily. Protein excretion also increases, and the fractional excretion of protein may rise to 300 mg/day as a result of increases in both GFR and glomerular capillary permeability to albumin. The total protein content of urine does not rise above the upper normal limit during healthy pregnancies. Increased GFR and/or decreased tubular reabsorption also lead to an increase in uric acid excretion.

2.1.4. Body Water Metabolism

Pregnancy-related arterial under-filling stimulates arterial baroreceptors, which in turn triggers the sympathetic nervous system and the RAA. As a result, the hypothalamus releases AVP in a non-osmotic manner. These modifications cause the kidneys to retain water and salt, which results in the hypervolemic, hypoosmolar condition that is typical of pregnancy. Both plasma and extracellular volume rise by 30–50% and 30%–40%, respectively. Maternal blood volume rises to 1,200–1,600 ml above non-pregnant values, a 45% increase. By the end of the third trimester, the volume of plasma has increased by over 50–60% while the mass of red blood cells has not increased as much. As a result, the osmolality of plasma has decreased by 10 mosmol/kg. During pregnancy, uteroplacental perfusion, blood pressure, and circulating blood volume are all crucially maintained by the increase in plasma volume.

When the RAA system is activated, the distal tubule and collecting duct retain more salt and water due to elevated aldosterone plasma levels. Early in pregnancy, the ovaries and uteroplacental unit produce an inactive precursor protein of renin in addition to the kidneys' increased renin production. In addition, the placenta secretes estrogens that cause the liver to produce angiotensinogen, which raises aldosterone levels relative to renin. Aldosterone levels in the plasma gradually increase during pregnancy and have a strong correlation with estrogen levels. The rise in plasma volume during pregnancy is caused by an increase in aldosterone. Aldosterone can retain sodium, but progesterone, a strong antagonist of aldosterone, permits natriuresis. Increased distal sodium delivery from a higher GFR enables the excretion of extra sodium. Because of the anti-kaliuretic effects of progesterone, changes in tubular reabsorption cause potassium excretion to remain constant throughout pregnancy, resulting in an increase in total body potassium.

Early in pregnancy, elevated relaxin levels cause an increase in hypothalamic AVP release. AVP uses the aquaporin 2 channels in the collecting duct to mediate an increase in water reabsorption. Pregnancy induces the hypo-osmolar state by resetting the thresholds for thirst and hypothalamic secretion of AVP to lower plasma osmolality levels. Human chorionic gonadotropin (hCG) and relaxin mediate these changes.

The placenta produces an aminopeptidase called vasopressinase, which increases fourfold in middle and late pregnancy. These modifications control the amounts of active AVP and improve vasopressin's metabolic clearance. A temporary form of diabetes insipidus can arise in situations where there is an increased production of vasopressinase by the placenta, such as in twin pregnancies or pre-eclampsia. Atrial natriuretic peptide secretion rises by 40% in the third trimester and continues to rise during the first week postpartum as a result of this volume expansion. Pregnant women with pre-eclampsia and chronic hypertension have greater levels of natriuretic peptides (Castro et al.,1994).

2.1.5. Respiratory Changes

The oxygen requirement rises noticeably during a typical pregnancy. This is brought on by a 15% rise in metabolic rate and a 20% increase in oxygen consumption. The minute ventilation has increased by 40–50%, primarily as a result of an increase in tidal volume as opposed to a rise in respiratory rate. As a result of the mother's hyperventilation, serum bicarbonate falls to 18–22 mmol/l and arterial pO_2 rises and arterial pCO_2 falls. Therefore, during pregnancy, a mild fully compensated respiratory alkalosis (arterial pH 7.44) is normal (Table 2.1).

Table 2.1. Reference Ranges for Respiratory Function in Pregnancy

	Normal Values	
Investigations	**Pregnant**	**Non-Pregnant**
pH	7.40–7.47	7.35–7.45
pCO_2, mmHg (kPa)	≤ 30 (3.6–4.3)	35–40 (4.7–6.0)
pO_2, mmHg (kPa)	100–104 (12.6–14.0)	90–100 (10.6–14.0)
Base excess	No change	+2 to −2
Bicarbonate (mmol/l)	18–22	20–28

Source: https://www.ncbi.nlm.nih.gov/pmc/articles/PMC4928162/table/T1/?report=objectonly.

Diaphragmatic excursion and thus vital capacity are unaffected by diaphragmatic elevation in late pregnancy, but functional residual capacity is reduced. Due to an increase in tidal volume early in pregnancy, the inspiratory reserve volume decreases; however, in the third trimester, this volume increases due to a decrease in functional residual capacity. Pregnancy has no effect on forced expiratory volume in one second (FEV1) or peak expiratory flow rate (PEFR) (Figure 2.1).

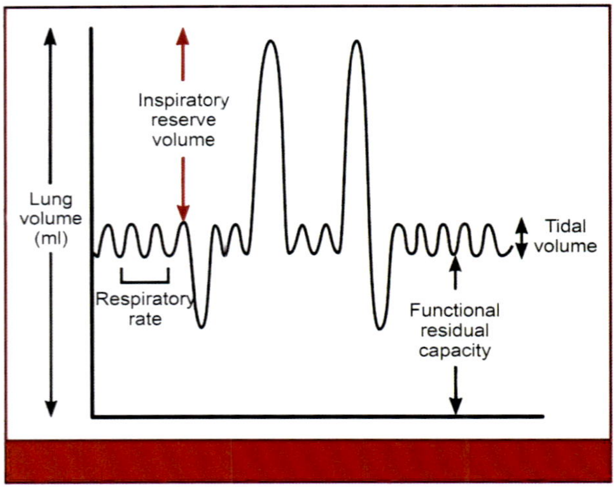

Figure 2.1. *Physiological changes in respiratory function in pregnancy.*

Source: https://www.ncbi.nlm.nih.gov/pmc/articles/PMC4928162/bin/cvja-27-92-g001.jpg.

In addition to hypoxia, a subjective sensation of dyspnea may also accompany pregnancy. Although it can begin at any point during pregnancy, this is a physiological condition that is most prevalent in the third trimester.

Traditionally, dyspnea occurs while the person is at rest or when they are speaking, and it may ironically go better with light exercise.

2.1.6. Adaptive Changes in the Alimentary Tract

In between 50 and 90% of pregnancies, nausea and vomiting are among the most common complaints during pregnancy. This may be an adaptive pregnancy mechanism designed to keep expectant mothers from ingesting foods that could cause teratogenic effects, like strongly-tasting fruits and vegetables. Pregnancy-related hormones like progesterone, estrogen, and human chorionic gonadotropin (hCG) may play a role in the etiology, though the precise underlying mechanism is unknown. When the trophoblast is most actively producing hCG at the end of the first trimester, the levels of hCG peak, which corresponds with the nausea symptoms. Additionally, nausea is more common in pregnancies with elevated hCG levels, like twin pregnancies.

There is a strong correlation between abnormal thyroid function tests and nausea, suggesting that thyroid hormones may also play a role in the development of nausea symptoms. Due to their similar biomolecular structures, hCG and thyroid-stimulating hormone (TSH) interact to stimulate the thyroid gland. It has been suggested that nutritional deficiencies, immunological factors, psychological issues, genetic incompatibility, and Helicobacter pylori infection are the etiological factors of nausea and vomiting during pregnancy.

Usually, the nausea symptoms go away by week 20, but in 10–15% of cases, the symptoms persist past week 20 and in some cases, until the end of the pregnancy. Most of the time, monitoring electrolyte balance and making small dietary adjustments are sufficient. Hyperemesis gravidum, a severe form of nausea and vomiting that affects 0.3–3% of pregnant women, can lead to dehydration, electrolyte imbalance, ketonuria, weight loss, and vitamin and mineral deficiencies. In these situations, intravenous hydration and vitamin replacement are frequently necessary. It's critical to take thiamine supplements to prevent Wernicke's encephalopathy from developing.

The growing uterus causes mechanical changes in the alimentary tract as pregnancy advances. The stomach shifts upward more and more, changing the axis and raising intragastric pressure. Additionally, there is a decrease in the tone of the esophageal sphincter, which may increase the risk of reflux symptoms, nausea, and vomiting.

The structural changes in the gastrointestinal tract are also influenced by variations in estrogen and progesterone levels. These include irregularities in the smooth muscle and gastric neural activity that result in gastroparesis or gastic dysrhythmia. Women who have had gastric bypass surgery, inflammatory bowel disease, diabetic gastroparesis, or gastroesophageal reflux disease already exhibit more marked changes.

2.1.7. Thyroid

Thyroxine (T_4) and tri-iodothyronine (T_3) levels rise as a result of the liver producing more thyroxine-binding globulin (TBG) than usual. Although slightly changed, serum-free T_4 (fT_4) and T_3 (fT_3) levels are typically not clinically significant. However, during the second and third trimesters of pregnancy, there is a slight decrease in free T_3 and T_4 levels, with a reduction in the normal ranges. The physiologically significant hormones, free T_3 and T_4, are the primary indicators of euthyroid status in patients (Glinoer, 1997).

Under the first trimester, thyrotropic effects of elevated human chorionic gonadotropin levels cause a slight decrease in serum TSH concentrations. At the end of the first trimester, TSH levels rise once more, and the upper limit is raised to 5.5 μmol/l during pregnancy as opposed to 4.0 μmol/l during non-pregnancy (Table 2.2).

Table 2.2. Reference Ranges for Thyroid Function in Pregnancy (Nelson-Piercy C. 2015)

Thyroid function	*Non-pregnant*	*1st trimester*	*2nd trimester*	*3rd trimester*
fT_4 (pmol/l)	9-26	10–16	9–15.5	8–14.5
fT_3 (pmol/l)	2.6–5.7	3–7	3–5.5	2.5–5.5
TSH (mU/l)	0.3–4.2	0–5.5	0.5–3.5	0.5–3.5

Source: https://www.ncbi.nlm.nih.gov/pmc/articles/PMC4928162/table/T2/?report=objectonly.

There is a relative iodine deficiency linked to pregnancy. Increased iodine excretion in the urine and active transport of iodine from the mother to the fetal-placental unit are the causes of this. Increased iodine intake during pregnancy is advised by the World Health Organization from 100 to 150–200 mg/day. The size of the thyroid gland does not change if iodine intake is maintained during pregnancy, so goiter should always be looked into. Patients with low iodine levels have a 25% larger thyroid gland.

2.1.8. Adrenal Gland

The adrenal glands produce mineralocorticoids, glucocorticoids, and sex steroids, which are three different kinds of steroids. Reductions in blood pressure and vascular resistance activate the RAA system, which leads to an increase in aldosterone levels of three times in the first trimester and ten times in the third. Angiotensin II levels are two to four times higher and renin activity is three to four times higher than non-pregnant levels. Serum levels of deoxycorticosterone, corticosteroid-binding globulin (CBG), adrenocorticotropic hormone (ACTH), cortisol, and free cortisol also rise during pregnancy. A state of physiological hypercortisolism is brought on by these alterations, which can be clinically shown as striae, facial plethora, elevated blood pressure, or decreased glucose tolerance. By the end of the first trimester, total cortisol levels rise, reaching a three-fold increase over non-pregnant values by the end of the pregnancy. One of the factors that lead to the start of labor, the placenta's production of corticotropin-releasing hormone, also contributes to hypercortisolism in late pregnancy. Cortisol and ACTH levels follow regular daily cycles. Pregnancy blunts the hypothalamic-pituitary axis's response to exogenous glucocorticoids.

2.1.9. Pituitary Gland

The primary cause of the pituitary gland's enlargement during pregnancy is the anterior lobe's proliferating prolactin-producing cells. In the first trimester, serum prolactin levels rise, and by term, they are ten times higher. Most likely, rising serum estradiol concentrations during pregnancy are the cause of the prolactin increase. Because of the negative feedback from high levels of estrogen, progesterone, and inhibin, follicle-stimulating hormone (FSH) and luteinizing hormone (LH) are not detectable during pregnancy. Growth hormone produced by the placenta causes a decrease in pituitary growth hormone production and an increase in serum growth hormone levels.

Both arginine vasopressin (AVP) and oxytocin are produced by the posterior pituitary. During pregnancy, oxytocin levels rise and reach their peak at term. Antidiuretic hormone (ADH) levels don't change during pregnancy, but osmolality does due to a drop in sodium concentration. Osmoreceptors for ADH release and thirst are consequently reset.

2.1.10. Glucose Metabolism

Since pregnancy is a diabetogenic condition, the changes in glucose metabolism during pregnancy enable the transfer of glucose to the fetus to support growth while preserving the mother's nutritional needs. During early pregnancy, increased insulin sensitivity and secretion are caused by hyperplasia of insulin-secreting pancreatic beta-cells, which is followed by progressive insulin resistance.

During the second and third trimesters, maternal insulin resistance peaks. This is the outcome of the increased release of hormones known to cause diabetes, including prolactin, growth hormone, progesterone, cortisol, and human placental lactogen. These hormones interfere with insulin receptor signaling, which lowers insulin sensitivity in peripheral tissues like skeletal muscle and adipocytes. Postpartum, a sharp decline in insulin resistance indicates the impact of placental hormones on insulin sensitivity.

Insulin levels are increased in both the fasting and postprandial states in pregnancy. Fasting glucose levels are however decreased due to:

- increased storage of tissue glycogen
- increased peripheral glucose use
- decrease in glucose production by the liver
- uptake of glucose by the fetus.

Lipolysis, which is brought on by insulin resistance and relative hypoglycemia, enables the expectant mother to use fat more preferentially as fuel, preserving the access to glucose and amino acids and reducing protein catabolism in the fetus. The placenta is impermeable to large lipids but permits the transfer of glucose, amino acids, and ketones to the developing fetus. Gestational diabetes arises when a woman's endocrine pancreatic function is compromised and she is unable to overcome the insulin resistance that comes with pregnancy.

2.1.11. Lipid Metabolism

Pregnancy raises the levels of triglycerides and total serum cholesterol. Reduced lipoprotein lipase activity and increased hepatic synthesis are the primary causes of the elevated triglyceride levels, which in turn slows the breakdown of adipose tissue. Moreover, levels of low-density lipoprotein (LDL) cholesterol rise and eventually reach 50% at term. Although concentrations of high-density lipoprotein are 15% higher than those of non-pregnant individuals, they rise during the first half of pregnancy and decline during the third trimester.

Lipid metabolism alterations to meet the growing fetus's needs. Elevated levels of triglycerides meet the energy requirements of the mother, saving glucose for the developing fetus. Placental steroidogenesis is impacted by the rise in LDL cholesterol.

2.1.12. Protein Metabolism

Pregnant women need to consume more protein during their pregnancy. The placenta actively transports amino acids to meet the demands of the growing fetus. Protein catabolism is reduced during pregnancy because fat reserves are used to fuel energy metabolism.

2.1.13. Calcium Metabolism

About 30 g of calcium is needed by the average fetus to maintain its physiological functions. The majority of this calcium comes from the mother's increased dietary absorption and is given to the fetus during the third trimester. During pregnancy, the total serum calcium concentration decreases. This is mostly because hemodilution causes a drop in serum albumin levels, which in turn causes a drop in the albumin-bound fraction of calcium. Serum ionized calcium, a physiologically significant fraction, does not alter, though. As a result, during pregnancy, the mother's serum calcium levels remain constant, and the fetus's requirements are satisfied by increased intestinal absorption, which doubles at 12 weeks of gestation. However, the third trimester is the only time when the demand for calcium peaks. The mother's skeleton may be able to store calcium ahead of time thanks to this early increase in calcium absorption.

The increase in 1.25-dihydroxyvitamin D is directly responsible for the increase in intestinal calcium absorption. Serum levels of 25-hydroxyvitamin D rise, and this is further metabolized into 1.25-dihydroxyvitamin Ddot.

Increased calcium excretion in the urine is correlated with increased calcium absorption, and these changes start to occur at 12 weeks. Urinary calcium levels are low or normal during fasting periods, indicating that hypercalciuria is the result of increased absorption. Thus, kidney stones are a risk factor associated with pregnancy.

2.1.14. Skeletal and Bone Density Changes

The impact of pregnancy on the loss of bone in mothers is a topic of debate. Studies refute the link between parity and osteoporosis in later life, even though pregnancy and lactation are linked to reversible bone loss. When the fetal calcium needs increase in the third trimester, bone turnover rises from low levels in the first trimester. Skeletal calcium that has been previously stored is the source of the calcium in the third trimester.

Pregnancy has been found to alter the micro-architectural pattern of bone, but not the total mass of bone, according to a study on bone biopsies. The alterations are a result of the growing fetus's requirement for the mother's skeleton to be resistant to biochemical stresses and bending forces.

Other musculoskeletal changes seen in pregnancy include:

- exaggerated lordosis of the lower back, forward flexion of the neck and downward movement of the shoulders
- joint laxity in the anterior and longitudinal ligaments of the lumbar spine
- widening and increased mobility of the sacroiliac joints and pubic symphysis.

2.2. Physiological Adaptation of the Hematological System to Pregnancy

The physiological adaptation of the hematological system during pregnancy seeks to support fetal hematopoiesis, compensate for blood loss at delivery, protect the mother and fetus against blood pressure changes and impaired venous return, and ensure adequate blood supply to the new vascular bed and gravid uterus and its contents. As early as four weeks into the pregnancy, the body adapts hematopoieticly. This includes progressive alterations in red blood cell and plasma volume (physiological anemia), leukocyte and immunological function, thrombocyte levels, coagulation, and fibrinolysis. The hormonal milieu changes associated with pregnancy and puerperium act as a mediating factor for the physiological changes in the hematological system.

2.2.1. Plasma Volume

During pregnancy, the mother's blood volume increases by 1.5 liters, reaching a level that is roughly 50% higher than that of non-pregnant women at term. Of this, 1 l is found in the placenta's maternal blood spaces and the uterus. At 6–12 weeks of gestation, plasma volume rises by 10–15%. It then grows quickly until 30–34 weeks, at which point it rises only slightly to an average of 100 ml/kg. Renal sodium retention and an increase in total body water are the results of the renin-angiotensin-aldosterone mechanism, which is activated by the direct action of progesterone and estrogen on the kidney, resulting in the release of renin. The vasculature becomes less sensitive to angiotensin when the renin-angiotensin system is activated during pregnancy. Pregnancy preserves the competitive relationship between the renin-aldosterone system and atrial natriuretic peptide (ANP) in controlling fluid volume and sodium balance. Angiotensin-precontracted vascular smooth muscle relaxes when exposed to ANP. The regulation of ANP secretion occurs around a new volume set-point, whereby blood volume is increased and maintained during pregnancy, even though the levels of ANP in the blood decrease. All of this suggests that rather than actual blood volume expansion, the elevation in plasma volume during pregnancy may be the result of an underfilled vascular system caused by systemic vasodilatation and an increase in vascular capacitance. Given that women with hydatidiform moles have shown an increase in blood volume, the presence of a fetus is not necessary for hematological abnormalities.

By the third week after giving birth, the plasma volume regresses to a level that is roughly 10–15% higher than that of the non-pregnant state, and by the sixth week, it has returned to its typical non-pregnant level.

2.2.2. Red Blood Cells

At 8–10 weeks of gestation, red blood cell (RBC) mass starts to rise, and by the end of the pregnancy, it has consistently increased to 15–20% above non-pregnant levels (average of 250–450 ml). When compared to the non-pregnant state, women who take iron supplements have a 20–30% greater increase in red blood cell mass at term. Red cell and hemoglobin mass increase peak between weeks 12 and 28 of pregnancy. Physiological or dilutional anemia of pregnancy is the term used to describe the modest decrease in hemoglobin concentration, hematocrit, and RBC count that occurs in healthy pregnant women due to a greater expansion of plasma volume relative to the increase in hemoglobin mass and erythrocyte volume. Hemoglobin levels usually drop by 1–2 g/dl by the end of the second trimester and then stabilize in the third trimester due to a decrease in the mother's plasma volume. In a typical pregnancy, mean corpuscular volume (MCV), mean corpuscular hemoglobin concentration (MCHC), and RBC indices do not significantly alter despite this hemodilution.

Additionally, the RBCs' average lifespan is marginally shortened. Compared to women who do not take hematinic supplements, those who take iron supplements experience less noticeable changes in hemoglobin. The MCV falls to an average of 80–84 feet in women who are not taking iron supplements, but it is typically 4 feet higher in iron-replete women, without indicating a folate or vitamin B12 deficiency. The increased MCV is logically explained by increased RBC production to meet the demands of pregnancy, with a higher proportion of young, larger-sized RBCs. Hemoglobin levels of less than 11 g/dl in the first and third trimesters and less than $10^{2}5$ g/dl in the second trimester are considered anemia in pregnancy. When a mean corpuscular volume is less than 84 fl and the hemoglobin concentration is less than 9.05 g/dl, it is likely a sign of iron deficiency or another illness (José Peña-Rosas et al., 2012) (Table 2.3).

Table 2.3. Normal Reference Range of Hematological Variables in Pregnancy

Variable	Non-pregnant Adult	First Trimester	Second Trimester	Third Trimester
Hemoglobin (g/dl)	12.0–15.8	11.6–13.9	9.7–14.8	9.5–15.0
Hematocrit (%)	35.4–44.4	31.0–41.0	30.0–39.0	28.0–40.0
Mean corpuscular hemoglobin (MCH) (pg/cell)	27–32	30–32	30–33	29–32
Mean corpuscular volume (MCV) (μm^3)	79–93	81–96	82–97	81–99
Red blood cell count (RBC) ($\times 10^6/mm^3$)	4.00–5.20	3.42–4.55	2.81–4.49	2.71–4.43
Red cell distribution (RDW) (%)	<14.5	12.5–14.1	13.4–13.6	12.7–15.3
Platelets ($\times 10^9/L$)	165–415	174–391	155–409	146–429
Mean platelet volume (MPV) (μm^3)	6.4–11.0	7.7–10.3	7.8–10.2	8.2–10.4
White blood cells (WBC) ($\times 10^3/mm^3$)	3.5–9.1	5.7–13.6	5.6–14.8	5.9–16.9
Neutrophils ($\times 10^3/mm^3$)	1.4–4.6	3.6–10.1	3.8–12.3	3.9–13.1
Monocytes ($\times 10^3/mm^3$)	0.1–0.7	0.1–1.1	0.1–1.1	0.1–1.4
Lymphocytes ($\times 10^3/mm^3$)	0.7–4.6	1.1–3.6	0.9–3.9	1.0–3.6
Eosinophils ($\times 10^3/mm^3$)	0–0.6	0–0.6	0–0.6	0–0.6
Basophils ($\times 10^3/mm^3$)	0–0.2	0–0.1	0–0.1	0–0.1
Ferritin (ng/ml)	10–150	6–130	2–230	0–116
Iron, serum ($\mu g/dl$)	41–141	72–143	44–178	30–193
Iron, total binding capacity (TIBC) ($\mu g/dl$)	251–406	278–403	Not reported	359–609
Transferrin (mg/dl)	200–400	254–344	220–441	288–530
Erythropoietin (U/L)	4–27	12–25	8–67	14–222
Folate, serum (ng/ml)	5.4–18.0	2.6–15.0	0.8–24.0	1.4–20.7

Source: Vinturache A, Khalil A, Glob. libr. women's med.,ISSN: 1756-2228; DOI 10.3843/GLOWM.411323.

Due to the increased metabolic oxygen requirement during pregnancy, erythropoietin levels rise by 50%, which helps to explain moderate bone marrow erythroid hyperplasia and elevated reticulocyte count. The combination of a low maternal pCO_2 and a reduced maternal RBC oxygen affinity from an elevated 2,3 diphosphoglycerate results in increased transportation of oxygen across the placenta. By four to six months after giving birth, hemoglobin levels return to those of non-pregnant women. A non-pregnant woman's normal total body iron content is about 2 g, with an additional 300 mg in her iron stores. The amount of iron needed during pregnancy is increased two to three times for the fetus, hemoglobin synthesis, and the synthesis of some enzymes. During pregnancy, about 1000 mg of iron supplements are required: 500 mg for the growth of the mother's red blood cell mass, 300 mg for the fetus and placenta, and 200 mg for iron excretion through the skin, urine, and feces. For the prevention of anemia, it is recommended to take 30–60 mg of elemental iron per day; the amount needed for treatment depends on the severity of maternal anemia. The requirements for folate and vitamin B12 increase by 10–20 times and 2 times, respectively, during pregnancy.

2.2.3. White Blood Cells

Increases in the number of white blood cells (WBCs) are linked to pregnancy. Leucocytosis with neutrophilia can start as early as the second month of pregnancy and then tends to get worse from there. The range of neutrophil counts is 5 to 12,000/μL; during the third trimester, these levels may rise to 15,000/μL, and in response to the stress of labor and delivery, they may reach 25,000/μL or higher. The WBC count returns to levels comparable to those of healthy, non-pregnant women four weeks after delivery. In the first and second trimesters of pregnancy, lymphocyte count decreases; in the third trimester, it increases. During pregnancy, the monocyte count rises, particularly in the first trimester, but falls as the pregnancy progresses. As a result, during pregnancy, the monocyte-to-lymphocyte ratio rises noticeably. There is proof that monocytes, via PGE2-mediated immunosuppression, penetrate decidual tissue between the seventh and twentieth week of gestation and help prevent fetal allograft rejection. Pregnancy does not cause a significant change in basophil or eosinophil counts.

2.2.3.1. Immunological Function

The immune system adapts to various changes during pregnancy, preparing the mother's body to receive the graft from the fetus. As a result, humoral or antibody-mediated immunity rises while cell-mediated immunity declines. The second and third trimesters are marked by an increase in complement factors C3 and C4. Pregnancy raises the level of C-reactive protein (CRP), which rises even more during labor and delivery.

Tumor necrosis factor, interleukin-2, interferon-gamma, and interferon-alpha levels are all reduced when T-helper 1 and T-cytotoxic 1 cells are suppressed. Interleukin 4, 6, and 13 levels rise in response to up-regulation of T-helper 2 and T-cytotoxic 2 cell function. There have also been reports of an increase in immunoglobulin A and G levels as well as the ratio of CD8 to CD4 T lymphocytes.

2.2.4. Platelets

With increased platelet activity and consumption, pregnancy is a relatively hypercoagulable state. While it may be slightly lower than in healthy non-pregnant women, the platelet count typically falls gradually during a typical pregnancy and stays within normal bounds. In 5–10% of women, if there is no pathological process, the count could reach levels of 100–150 × 10^9 cells/l by term. Pregnancy causes a drop in platelet count, especially in the third trimester. In late pregnancy, 100 × 10^9 cells is the generally accepted lower limit for platelet count. Hemodilution and enhanced platelet activation and accelerated clearance are two contributing factors to gestational thrombocytopenia. Babies do not usually experience severe thrombocytopenia (platelet count <20,000/mm^3) or complications associated with it.

Similar to other blood cell lineages, as gestation progresses, the platelet volume distribution width rises noticeably and steadily.

As pregnancy goes on, the mean platelet volume loses some of its sensitivity as a gauge of platelet size. The increased platelet consumption during the delivery process causes the platelet count to rise after delivery.

2.2.4.1. Coagulation and Fibrinolysis

Considered a procoagulant state, pregnancy is linked to notable alterations in the hemostatic profile. The coagulation cascade is activated, resulting in a 20–200% increase in fibrinogen and factors II, VII, VIII, X, XII, and vWF levels. Before pregnancy, fibrinogen levels are roughly 300 mg/dl; at term, they are roughly 600 mg/dl (average 450 mg/dl). Coagulation factors XI and XIII are present at lower levels. Rising estrogen levels cause increased protein synthesis, which in turn causes higher levels of coagulation factors.

One is prothrombotic when pregnant. Throughout pregnancy, the plasma of expectant mothers gradually raises the levels of fibrinolytic inhibitors like plasminogen activator inhibitor types 1 and 2 (PAI-1 and 2) and thrombin cleavage products, as well as thrombin generation. Factors V, IX, antithrombin, and protein C remain largely unaltered, despite a decrease in fibrinolysis and the anticoagulant protein S. The duration of blood clotting and bleeding remains unaltered. Pregnancy-related reductions in activated partial thromboplastin time (aPTT) can occur by as much as 4 s in the third trimester, primarily because of the hormone-induced rise in factor VIII. Prothrombin time (PT) and thrombin time (TT) do not significantly alter.

The overall goal of the coagulation profile modifications is to prevent both the myometrial contraction and thrombus formation-related postpartum hemorrhage. The risk of venous thromboembolism (VTE) is elevated when the coagulation process is activated. After giving birth, hypercoagulation lasts for three weeks before going away six to eight weeks later. Pregnancy is associated with notable elevations in D-dimer and erythrocyte sedimentation rate, with late pregnancy typically having a reference range that is ten times higher than early pregnancy or the non-pregnant state. As such, their diagnostic utility in pregnancy is restricted. Because of increased thrombin generation, increased fibrinolysis, or a combination of the two, pregnancy-related increases in total fibrin are reflected in the rise in D-dimers.

2.3. Physiological Adaptation of the Cardiovascular System to Pregnancy

The cardiovascular system undergoes substantial anatomical and physiological remodeling during pregnancy. The cardiovascular load is increased by the increased volume of maternal blood in circulation, the fetal nutritional requirement, and the addition of the new placental circulatory system. The renin-angiotensin-aldosterone system, prostaglandins (PGE1 and PGE2), progesterone, nitric oxide, and other vasoactive chemicals all play a role in mediating the adaptation. Pre-existing medical conditions may affect homeostasis and cause a noticeable clinical decline during pregnancy, even though in the majority of women the increased demands are met without compromising. Throughout the intrapartum and postpartum phases, the mother's cardiovascular system is further modified. Furthermore, poor uteroplacental circulation and fetal compromise can result from inadequate maternal hemodynamic adaptation. As a result, the cardiovascular system of the mother must strike a balance between her needs and those of the fetus.

The cardiovascular parameters that change during pregnancy include blood pressure and heart rate, systemic vascular resistance, plasma and total blood volume, cardiac output and stroke volume, and regional blood flow. When comparing pregnant women to non-pregnant women, the results of cardiac examinations and investigations differ due to hemodynamic changes as well as physical and anatomical changes.

2.3.1. Anatomical and Physical Changes

The shape of the abdomen and thorax, the strength of the anterior abdominal wall muscles, and the size and location of the uterus all affect how much the cardiovascular system changes anatomically during pregnancy. Pregnancy-induced remodeling of the heart and blood vessels mediates the changes in cardiac and vascular compliance. The diaphragm is moved upward in response to the gravid uterus's growing size, which causes the heart to move laterally and upward, closer to the chest wall. There is an increase in cardiac compliance, myocardial contractility, ventricular wall mass, and chamber size. There is an increase in the compliance of the entire vasculature, with increases in venous blood volume and compliance as well as the aortic size and compliance, through mechanisms that are still not fully understood but may include vascular smooth muscle hypertrophy and collagen softening. Additionally, there is an increase in capillary permeability, which, combined with the rise in femoral venous pressure and the drop in colloid osmotic pressure, causes edema formation, which is typical during pregnancy.

Up to 90% of pregnant women may have abnormalities in their auscultation of heart sounds. From 12 weeks of pregnancy until 2–4 weeks after delivery, there is a noticeable increase in the volume and breadth of the first sound. This alteration is brought about by an earlier closure of the mitral valve and an increased flow across it. About one-third of women have mild mitral regurgitation and the majority have regurgitation of the tricuspid and pulmonary valves. There is a continuous splitting of the aortic and pulmonary components of the second heart sound during the final 10 weeks of pregnancy. Up to 90% of expectant mothers have a third heart sound. More than 90% of pregnant women exhibit a mid-systolic murmur near the left sternal border during the final two trimesters of their pregnancy, which is a sign of an increased blood ejection load from the left ventricle into the brachiocephalic arteries or from the right ventricle into the pulmonary trunk.

Changes in cardiovascular parameters point to pregnancy-related changes in the ECG. The physiological responses to pregnancy, which include shifting the position of the heart, altering the organs' spatial arrangement in the chest, and changing the electrical characteristics of the myocardium under the influence of the sympathetic nervous system and hormone modulation of progesterone and epinephrine, are responsible for the majority of the ECG changes that occur during pregnancy. Pregnancy increases the risk of arrhythmias, including supraventricular tachycardia and atrial and ventricular ectopics.

Due to increased blood volume and diastolic filling, echocardiography performed during the second and third trimesters reveals increased left ventricle systolic and diastolic dimensions as well as wall thickness. The right atrium, right ventricle, and left atrium may all moderately increase in size along with the left ventricle's changes, and the velocities of the left and right ventricles' outflow obstructions may also rise (Gei et al., 2001) (Table 2.4).

Table 2.4. Effects of Pregnancy on Cardiovascular Investigations

Investigation	Changes
Electrocardiography	Heart rate ↑ 10–15% Right axis deviation of QRS Inverted T-wave in lead III Small Q-wave in lead III and AVF Non-specific ST changes: ST-segment depression and T-wave inversion in the inferior and lateral leads
Echocardiogram	Trivial tricuspid regurgitation Pulmonary regurgitation Mitral valve regurgitation at term (28%) Increase in left ventricular mass (52%) Increase in left ventricular end-diastolic diameter (12%) Increase in left ventricular end-systolic diameter (20%) Increase in left ventricular posterior wall diameter during diastole (22%) Increase in left ventricular posterior wall diameter during systole (13%) Increase in left intraventricular septum diameter during diastole (15%) Increase in left intraventricular septum diameter during systole (19%)

Source: Vinturache A, Khalil A, Glob. libr. women's med., ISSN: 1756–2228; DOI 10.3843/GLOWM.411323.

2.3.2. Hemodynamic Changes

Table 2.5 provides a summary of the hemodynamic alterations brought on by the cardiovascular adaptation that occurs during pregnancy. During pregnancy, systemic vascular resistance, pulmonary vascular resistance, and colloid osmotic pressure decrease, while stroke volume, heart rate, and cardiac output increase. The most notable hemodynamic alteration during pregnancy is the rise in cardiac output, which by the third trimester rises to 30–50% above the baseline in the non-pregnant state. The majority of these changes happen early in pregnancy; by eight weeks of gestation, there has been a 50% increase, and by the end of the first trimester, there has been a 75% increase.

The reduction in preload, increase in stroke volume, and decrease in systemic vascular resistance are the main mechanisms mediating these significant changes in cardiac output. Between weeks 28 and 32 of pregnancy, cardiac output reaches a plateau; it does not significantly change until delivery. The rise in cardiac output that occurs during the third trimester is mainly sustained by an increase in heart rate. By five to eight weeks of gestation, the heart rate and stroke volume start to change. Stroke volume rises by 25–30%, reaches a low point at 16–24 weeks, and then starts to fall toward the levels seen in non-pregnant women by term.

Table 2.5. Physiological Changes of the Cardiovascular System in Pregnancy

Parameter	Direction of Change	Magnitude of Change	Peak of Change
Myocardial contractility:			
Heart rate (HR)	↑	↑ 10–20% from 80 bpm to 90–100 bpm	28–32 weeks
Stroke volume (SV)	↑	↑ 30% to a maximum 85 mL	20–24 weeks
Cardiac output (HR × SV)	↑	↑ 30–50% from 4.5 l/min to ~6 l/min Plateaus at 24–30 weeks ↓ to pre-pregnancy level after delivery (variable time)	28–32 weeks
Systolic blood pressure	↓	↓ 5 mmHg	from 8 to 36 week
Diastolic blood pressure	↓	↓ 10 mmHg	24–32 weeks
Systemic vascular resistance	↓	↓ 20–30%	16–24 weeks
Pulmonary vascular resistance	↓	↓ ~30%	34 weeks
Pulmonary capillary wedge pressure	~	No significant change	
Colloid osmotic pressure	↓	↓ 14%	
Uteroplacental circulation	↑	Greater than 1000%	Term

Source: Vinturache A, Khalil A, *Glob. libr. women's med., ISSN: 1756–2228; DOI 10.3843/GLOWM.411323.*

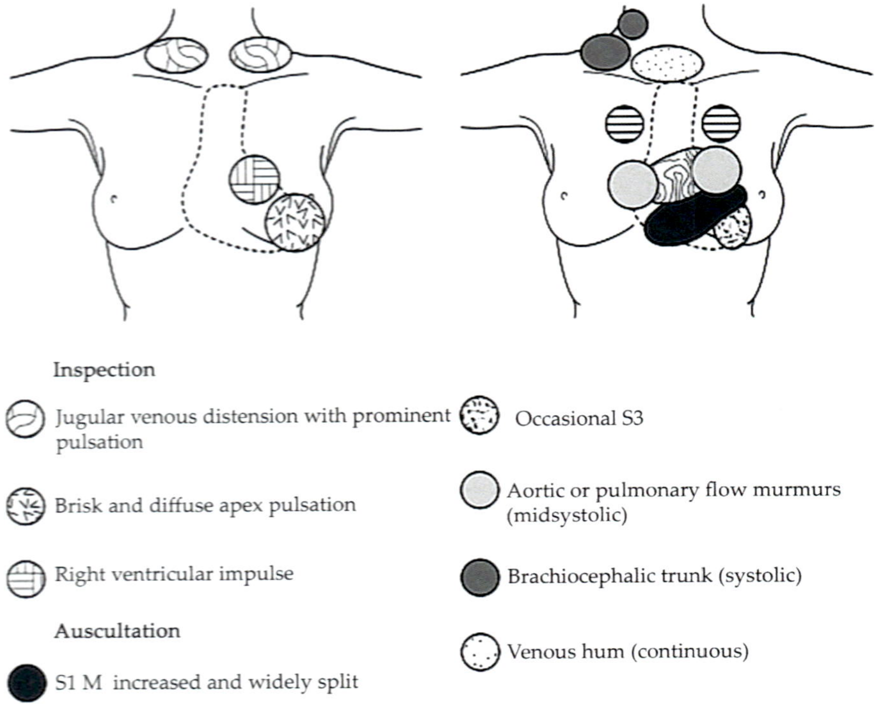

Figure 2.2. *Findings of cardiovascular examination in the pregnant women. M, mitral; P, pulmonary; S1, first sound; S2, second sound; S3, third sound.*

Source: Vinturache A, Khalil A, Glob. libr. women's med., ISSN: 1756-2228; DOI 10.3843/GLOWM.411323.

The rise in end-diastolic volume and ventricular mass mediates the increase in stroke volume. A few weeks following delivery, cardiac output returns to levels not associated with pregnancy. When there are multiple pregnancies, the cardiac output increases, with a slightly larger peak increase than when there is only one pregnancy. (Kametas et al., 2003) (Figure 2.2).

By 32 weeks of pregnancy, the heart rate rises by 10–20% (averaging 10–20 beats per minute), most likely as a result of an increase in myocardial alpha receptors brought on by estrogen. When a woman has multiple pregnancies, her heart rate rises earlier and peaks at a rate 40% higher than when she is not pregnant. (Cunningham F. William, 2009) (Figure 2.3).

Early in pregnancy, blood pressure drops due to the vasodilatory effects of progesterone, nitric oxide, and prostaglandins, resulting in physiological hypotension. It is reported that during the first trimester, both the diastolic and systolic blood pressures decrease by 10 to 15 mmHg, and that they then return to baseline during the second half of pregnancy. By 24 to 32 weeks of gestation, the decline in systolic and diastolic blood pressure reaches a nadir, and by term, it returns to a non-pregnant state. The pulse pressure widens because the diastolic blood pressure drops more than the systolic (Caulin-Glaser, 2004) (Figure 2.4).

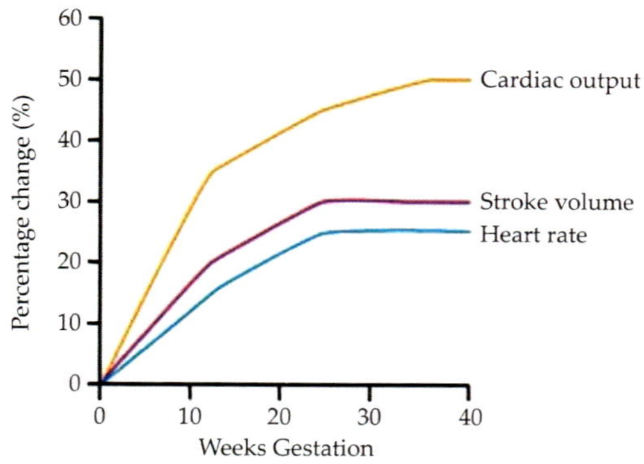

Figure 2.3. *Maternal cardiovascular changes in cardiac output, stroke volume, and heart rate during pregnancy. (Adapted from Anesthesia UK, http://www.frca.co.uk/).*

Source: Vinturache A, Khalil A, Glob. libr. women's med., ISSN: 1756-2228; DOI 10.3843/GLOWM.411323.

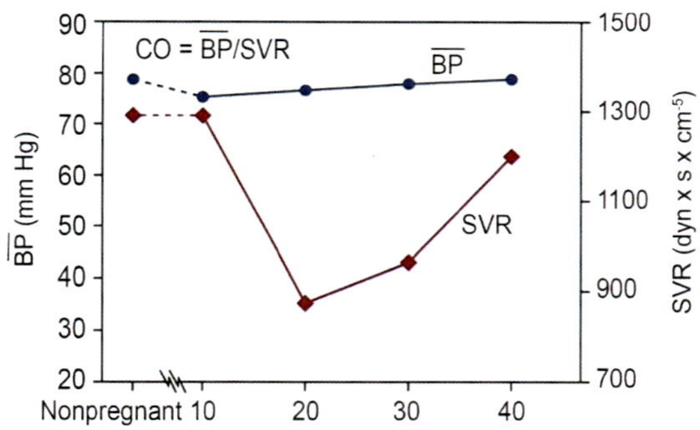

Figure 2.4. *Maternal physiological changes in blood pressure and systemic vascular resistance during pregnancy. CO, cardiac output; BP, mean blood pressure; SVR, systemic vascular resistance.*

Source: Vinturache A, Khalil A, Glob. libr. women's med., ISSN: 1756-2228; DOI 10.3843/GLOWM.411323.

The venous pressure does not change significantly during pregnancy due to the increased blood volume that is balanced by the increased compliance and capacitance, as well as the effects of progesterone and nitric oxide on collagen and vascular smooth muscle. During pregnancy, there is a 20–30% decrease in total peripheral resistance, which coincides with a drop in blood pressure. Systemic vascular resistance falls by five weeks, peaks between weeks 26 and 34, and then gradually rises to term. The hypertrophy of vascular smooth muscle, the softening of collagen fibers, the retention of fluid, and the addition of the low-resistance uteroplacental circulation all contribute to the vascular remodeling that occurs during pregnancy. The vasodilatory effects of nitric oxide, prostacyclin, prostaglandins, and progesterone intensify these alterations.

From the beginning of pregnancy, uterine blood flow increases tenfold. The Uterine blood flow increases to about 500–700 ml/min at term from around 50 ml/min by 10 weeks. By the end of the first trimester, the renal blood flow has increased and then begins to decline until term. The blood flow to the liver and brain remains relatively unchanged, while the blood flow to the kidneys rises by 50%. Prostacyclin, nitric oxide, and atrial natriuretic factor act as mediators to lower renal vascular resistance. Overall, the percentage of cardiac output that supplies blood to the kidneys stays about the same—roughly 18%—as it does for women who are not pregnant. The glomerular filtration rate rises by 40–50% as a result of the increased renal blood flow. The pulmonary vascular resistance decreases to offset the increase in pulmonary blood flow. Breast tissue, skeletal muscle, and the splanchnic bed experience a decrease in blood flow. On the other hand, during pregnancy, the cerebral blood flow does not change from its baseline levels.

The maternal blood volume in circulation rises 30- 40% above non-pregnant volumes beginning at 7–8 weeks of gestation and reaches its maximum at 28–34 weeks. Hemodilutional anemia and a drop in serum colloid osmotic pressure are the results of this as well as the decrease in serum albumin concentration. Uncertainty surrounds the mechanism underlying the increase in blood volume. Hypervolemia and the retention of water and salt may result from arginine vasopressin production being elevated, nitric oxide-mediated vasodilatation, and mineralocorticoid activity. Pregnant women are thought to benefit from pregnancy-induced hypervolemia, which shields them from hemodynamic instability brought on by blood loss during delivery.

The plasma volume accounts for up to 75% of the increase in total blood volume. In comparison to values that are not pregnant, there is a 45–50% increase in plasma volume. Up until the second trimester, the increase is rapid (6–8 weeks), and after that, it becomes progressively slower. By 32 weeks of pregnancy, plasma volume has increased to 4700–5200 ml. This increase is caused by the renin-angiotensin–aldosterone system, which is mediated by prostaglandins, progesterone, nitric oxide, and estrogen.

2.4. Physiological Adaptation of Respiratory System to Pregnancy

The goal of the physiological modifications to the respiratory system during pregnancy is to increase gas exchange and air volume in order to eliminate carbon dioxide and increase the availability of oxygen. The mother, fetus, and neonate are all affected by changes in acid-base homeostasis that result from changes in the respiratory system caused by mechanical, hormonal, and biochemical factors.

2.4.1. Anatomical and Mechanical Factors

The diaphragm's resting position rises by about 4–5 centimeters as the uterus gradually enlarges. Pregnancy causes the diaphragm to expand by roughly 2 cm, switching from thoracic to abdominal breathing. The relaxin-induced relaxation of the thoracic muscles and cartilage permits a 2 cm increase in transverse diameter and a 5–7 cm increase in thoracic circumference in addition to the rise in intra-abdominal pressure. The subcostal angle rises from 69° to 103° by 37 weeks as the pregnancy goes on. The shifting of the contents of the abdomen to make room for the expanding uterus is made possible by the anatomical changes. (Torgersen, 2006) (Figure 2.5).

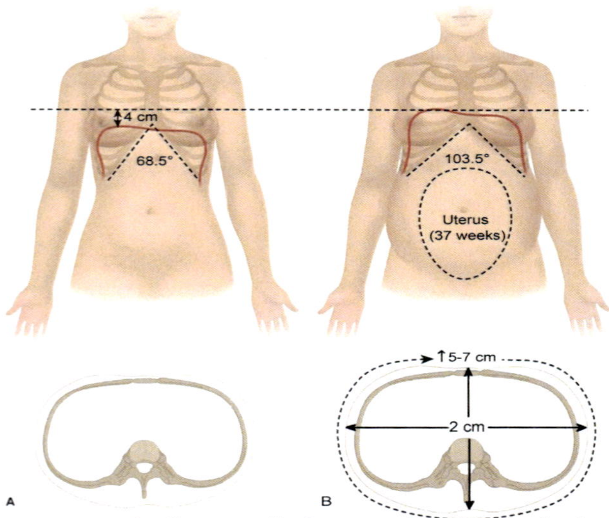

Figure 2.5. *Chest wall changes that occur during pregnancy.*

Source: Vinturache A, Khalil A, Glob. libr. women's med., ISSN: 1756–2228; DOI 10.3843/GLOWM.411323.

Lung volumes are significantly impacted by changes in the thoracic configuration and an increase in intra-abdominal pressure. The diaphragm shifts upward, causing basilar atelectasis, collapse of the basilar alveoli, and a 5–10% reduction in the total lung capacity and a 10–25% reduction in functional residual capacity. Residual volume decreases as a result of decreased chest wall compliance.

The nasopharynx, larynx, trachea, and bronchi are all impacted by changes in airway caliber and capillary engorgement, which cause changes in the upper respiratory tract. Hormonal changes, including an increase in estrogen, blood volume, edema, hyperglandular secretion, and phagocyte activity, mediate these effects. Vascular pooling is facilitated by increased blood volume and progesterone. Progesterone-induced smooth muscle relaxation adds even more to the vascular pooling. The upper respiratory tract's mucosa is swollen and erythematous. This makes it harder to breathe through your nose, increases snoring, aggravates obstructive sleep apnea, and can cause spontaneous epistaxis, hoarseness, nasal congestion and rhinitis symptoms. The discomfort that women may feel from minor upper respiratory tract infections can be significantly increased by the aforementioned symptoms.

2.4.2. Lung Volume and Function

Lung volume changes begin early in the first trimester and continue through the second trimester as the baby approaches term. Tidal volume increases by 30–50% (from 500 to 700 ml) and progressive decreases in expiratory reserve volume (15–20%), residual volume (20–25%), and functional residual capacity (20–30%) are linked to pregnancy. A functional residual capacity shortfall of about 500 milliliters results from a 200–300 milliliter drop in residual volume and a 200-milliliter decrease in expiratory reserve volume.

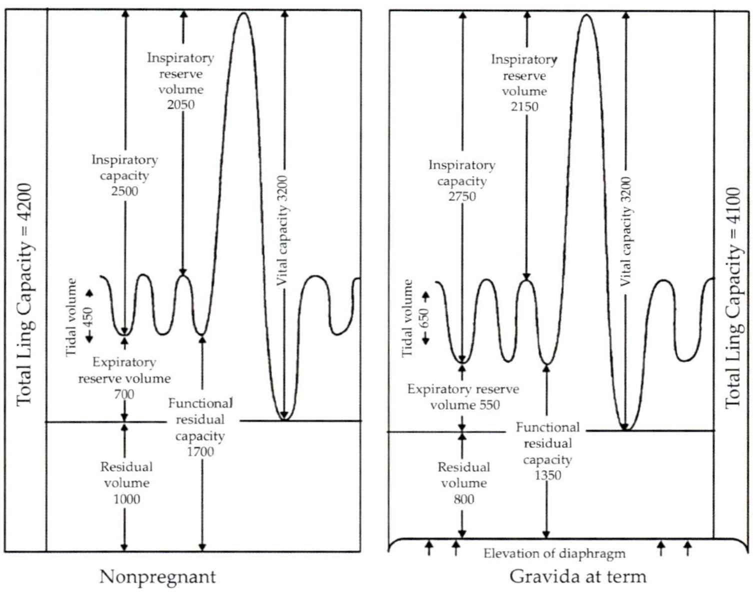

Figure 2.6. *Lung volume changes in pregnancy (ml).*

Source: Vinturache A, Khalil A, Glob. libr. women's med., ISSN: 1756–2228; DOI 10.3843/GLOWM.411323.

Minute ventilation is noticeably elevated (30–50%), despite the respiratory rate remaining unchanged from the non-pregnant state. The inspiratory capacity increases by 5–10% in tandem with the rise in tidal volume, maintaining a stable total lung capacity. The inspiratory reserve volume and vital capacity (VC) remain unchanged, but the physiological dead space rises by 60 milliliters. The ratio of FEV1/VC and the forced expiratory volume in one second (FEV1) remain unchanged. During pregnancy, peak inspiratory and expiratory flow rates typically decrease (Whitty, 2009) (Figure 2.6).Changes in ventilation, airflow, and diffusing capacity are all part of the lung function changes. Beginning around 8 weeks gestation, early in pregnancy, there are alterations in minute ventilation. A 30- to 50% increase translates into an increase from 6–7.5 l/min in the early stages of pregnancy to 10–10.5 l/min at term. Rather than variations in the relatively constant respiratory rate, the rise in minute ventilation is caused by changes in the tidal volume. During pregnancy, lung compliance and airway resistance do not change.

Increases in basal metabolism, oxygen consumption, and carbon dioxide production are linked to pregnancy. In a singleton pregnancy, oxygen consumption increases by approximately 15–20 percent. In multiple pregnancies, the increase may be even greater to accommodate the growing fetus's increased demand on the mother. An increase in basal metabolic rate and energy expenditure results in a 15–20% increase in carbon dioxide production.

Due to a rise in paO_2 and a decrease in $paCO_2$, pregnant women experience compensated respiratory alkalosis. The arterial partial pressure of carbon dioxide ($paCO_2$) falls from 35–45 mmHg to 27–32 mmHg, while the arterial partial pressure of oxygen (paO_2) rises from 90–100 mmHg to 104–108 mmHg. A gradient between the mother's and the fetus'spCO_2 is produced by the decrease in $paCO_2$, allowing CO_2 to freely diffuse from the fetus into the mother through the placenta and into the mother's lungs, where it can be expelled. A slight increase in maternal arterial blood pH from 7.35–7.45 to 7.40–7.45 is consistent with a mild respiratory alkalosis, which makes it easier for the fetus to transfer carbon dioxide to the mother.

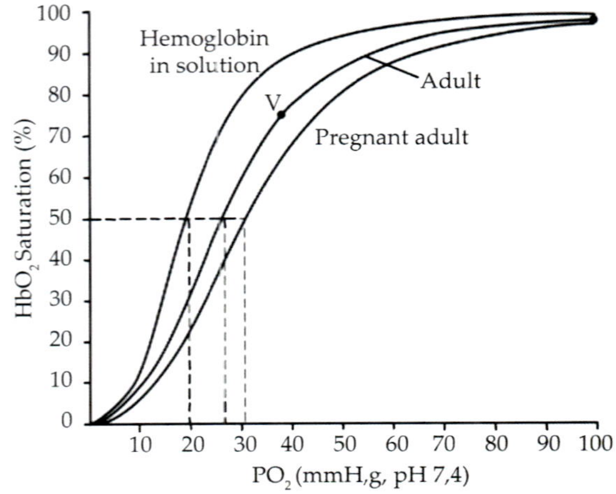

Figure 2.7. *Oxygen–hemoglobin dissociation curve. The graph shows the curve for pregnant and non-pregnant adult in normal conditions and the dissociation curve of hemoglobin in solution.*

Source: Vinturache A, Khalil A, Glob. libr. women's med., ISSN: 1756–2228; DOI 10.3843/GLOWM.411323.

Table 2.6. Arterial Blood Gases in Pregnancy

Arterial Blood Gas Measurement	Non-Pregnant State	Pregnancy
pH	7.35–7.45	7.40–7.45
paO_2 (mmHg)	90–100	104–108
$paCO_2$ (mmHg)	35–45	27–32
Serum HCO_3 (mEq/l)	22–26	18–21

Source: Vinturache A, Khalil A, Glob. libr. women's med.,ISSN: 1756–2228; DOI 10.3843/GLOWM.411323.

Increased renal excretion of bicarbonate causes a partial correction of this alkalosis, resulting in a decrease in serum bicarbonate levels from 22–26 mEq/L to 18–21 mEq/L and a decreased buffering capacity. The oxygen-hemoglobin dissociation curve is slightly shifted to the right by this partially compensated respiratory alkalosis, favoring oxygen dissociation to improve oxygen transfer across the placenta and oxygen release to the fetus (Tsaiet al., 1982) (Figure 2.7).

Table 2.6 provides a summary of the normal arterial blood values during pregnancy at sea level.The various respiratory adaptations that take place help the mother breathe more comfortably, enhance the excretion of HCO_3 through the kidneys, and improve oxygen availability for the growing fetus.

2.4.3. Hormonal and Biochemical Changes

As a respiratory stimulant, progesterone appears to mediate the changes in ventilation during pregnancy by raising minute ventilation and improving the respiratory centers' ability to respond to hypercapnia by lowering their carbon dioxide threshold. These processes could account for the sensation of dyspnea and hyperventilation that many women encounter. Water retention in the lung brought on by progesterone reduces the lung's capacity for diffusion, which in turn forces hyperventilation to keep paO_2 levels stable. Progesterone promotes easier breathing by reducing airway resistance through the relaxation of the bronchiolar smooth muscle. Prostaglandins control the smooth muscles in the bronchi, with PGF2α acting as a constrictor and PGE1 and PGE2 acting as bronchodilators. Prostaglandins raise tidal volume and decrease $paCO_2$, which aid in respiratory adaptations.

2.5. Physiological Adaptation of the Renal System to Pregnancy

All parts of the urinary tract are affected by pregnancy as early as six weeks after conception. Long recognized are the anatomical changes that result in the enlargement of the kidneys and the dilatation of the renal pelvis, ureters, and caduceus. Vasodilation and volume expansion follow modifications in the renal vascular and tubular responsiveness to the circulating hormones to define renal and systemic hemodynamics. Pregnancy has a broad functional impact on kidney physiology, affecting all aspects of kidney function, including changes to the renin-angiotensin system (RAS), tubular handling of water, electrolytes, and other substances, and glomerular filtration. (Cheung et al., 2013) (Table 2.7).

Table 2.7. Renal Hemodynamic and Functional Adaption of the Renal System in Normal Human Pregnancy

Parameters	Change	Significance
Collecting system (calyces, pelvis, and ureters)	Dilatation (predominant on the right) Hypertonicity, decreased motility, elongation	Hydronephrosis Increased risk of urinary tract infections Altered accuracy of 24 hours urine collection
Kidney	Size increase by 1 cm	

Bladder	Decreased tone Increased capacity Hyperemic and edematous mucosa Displaced in late pregnancy Incompetence of vesicoureteral valve	Urinary frequency and incontinence Altered accuracy of 24 hours urine collection Increased risk of urinary tract infection Risk of trauma and reflux Risk of urinary retention and inadequate emptying
Renal blood flow (RBF)	Vasodilation Increase by 50–80% by second trimester then decrease to term	Increase in renal plasma flow (RPF) Increase in glomerular filtration rate (GFR) Increase solute delivery to the kidney
Glomerular filtration rate (GFR)	Increases by 40–60%	Inadequate assessment of creatinine clearance due to altered accuracy of urine collection Increased filtration and excretion of water and solutes Predominant natriuretic effect Increased urine volume and flow Decreased serum creatinine, blood urea nitrogen, uric acid Altered renal excretion of drugs
Renal tubular function	Increased reabsorption of solutes Increased renal excretion of proteins, amino acids, glucose, urea, uric acid, calcium, phosphate, bicarbonate, hydrogen ions, water-soluble vitamins Retention of sodium and water	Maintain homeostasis with expanded extracellular volume Prevent solute and water loss Tendency to proteinuria, glucosuria Decreased serum bicarbonate levels Compensate for respiratory alkalosis Accumulation of sodium and water Increased nutritional needs, including calcium and water-soluble vitamins

Renin–angiotensin–aldosterone system	Upregulation of all components of the system Reduced sensitivity to the pressor effects of angiotensin II (ANG II)	Decrease in systemic and renal vascular resistance Retention of water and sodium Reduced excretion of sodium Maintain the blood pressure
Arginine-vasopressin and osmolarity regulation	Osmostat reset at lower baseline of osmolarity	Decrease in plasma osmolarity Expansion of plasma and extracellular volume Maintain volume homeostasis

Source: Vinturache A, Khalil A, Glob. libr. women's med.,ISSN: 1756–2228; DOI 10.3843/GLOWM.411323.

2.5.1. Anatomical Changes

The growing uterus causes a cephalad displacement of the kidneys. Additionally, during pregnancy, the kidneys' length increases by 1–2.5 cm, and after giving birth, it returns to pre-pregnancy measurements after six months. 30% more renal volume is produced. Dead space, increased interstitial volume, and an increase in the vasculature are likely the causes of the kidney's growth. Studies have shown growth in kidney volume in women without evidence of renal pelvic dilatation, although this growth was first linked to hydronephrosis.

Due to the effects of progesterone and compression of the ureters at the pelvic brim, the renal collecting system begins to dilate as early as six weeks into pregnancy in the first trimester. The renal pelvis and the upper segment of the ureters up to the pelvic brim are affected by these alterations. Due to a combination of mechanical compression from the enlarging, dextrorotated uterus and progesterone-mediated smooth muscle relaxation, hydroureteronephrosis is more common on the right side. The sigmoid colon increases the ureteral compression on the left side during the last trimester and aids in the uterus's dextroversion. By approximately 30 weeks of gestation, the ureter's compression at the pelvic brim reaches its maximum. PGE2-mediated hypertonicity, hypomotility, and a decrease in peristaltic movements are linked to ureteral lumen dilatation. The elongated and tortuous ureters are laterally displaced by the growing uterus as pregnancy goes on.

Progesterone causes the bladder's tone to drop and its capacity to rise, nearly doubling at term. The hyperplasia and hypertrophy of bladder smooth muscle are mediated by elevated estrogen. The mucosa of the bladder becomes edematous and hyperemic, making it more susceptible to injury and infection. The second trimester causes the bladder to shift anteriorly and superiorly. It also modifies the position of the ureters' intravesical portion, which raises the possibility of vesicoureteral reflux. Women who are pregnant experience more frequent, urgent, and incontinence urination. The fetal head's engagement in the pelvis during the third trimester exacerbates these symptoms. The amount of pee produced rises. The mean urine output increases from 1475 to 1919 ml/24 hours after changes in sodium excretion. There are also more voids every day.

2.5.2. Renal Hemodynamics

Renal hemodynamic changes are regulated by multiple hormones and are associated with a decrease in systemic vascular resistance and systemic vasodilatation. By the middle of the second trimester, renal blood flow (RBF) has increased by 50–80%, and it then slightly declines until term. Effective renal plasma flow (RPF) and glomerular filtration rate (GFR) rise as a result of renal vascular dilatation and increased blood flow to the kidney. By mid-pregnancy, effective renal plasma flow rises by 60–80%. While the growth in RPF and GFR are similar, in the early stages of pregnancy, the RPF increases more than the GFR (60–80% versus 40–60%) until it falls off quickly in the third trimester. Because of this, during pregnancy, the filtration fraction and the ratio of GFR to RPF vary. In the first half of pregnancy, the filtration fraction decreases, and in the latter stages of gestation, it increases. (Odutayo et al., 2012) (Figure 2.8).

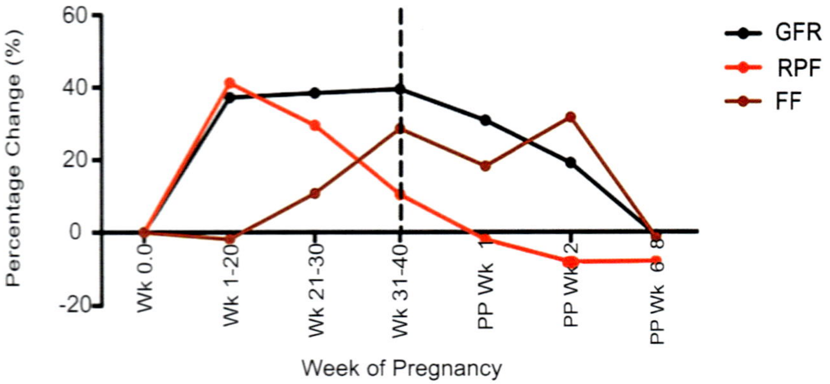

Figure 2.8. *Percentage change from baseline of glomerular filtration rate (GFR), renal plasma flow (RPF), and filtration fraction (FF) throughout pregnancy and postpartum. Mean values are measured by inulin or isothalamate and p-aminohippurate clearance, respectively, at different points during gestation and postpartum (PP).*

Source: Vinturache A, Khalil A, Glob. libr. women's med., ISSN: 1756–2228; DOI 10.3843/GLOWM.411323.

Local and systemic hormonal influences are responsible for the changes in renal hemodynamics. Progesterone can detect increases in RPF and GFR during pregnancy, but it is unable to explain the extent of these changes in the two renal variables. The placenta and deciduas secrete maternal blood relaxin, which steadily increases during pregnancy and decreases during the postpartum phase. It is unknown how relaxin affects renal vasodilation in people.

The hypothesis was that relaxin may mediate vasodilatation through an increase in nitric oxide production via upregulation of vascular gelatinase activity, which acts through the endothelial endothelin B receptor-nitric oxide pathway. However, no significant correlations between relaxin levels and renal hemodynamic variables in gestation or postpartum have been found. Pregnancy is characterized by vasodilation and a drop in systolic blood pressure, despite the renin-angiotensin system being upregulated. Hormones and other vasoactive factors, such as progesterone, vascular endothelial growth factor, prostacyclins, nitric oxide, and decreased responsiveness of the angiotensin 1 (AT1) receptors, may account for the insensitivity to elevated levels of ANG II. Prostacyclin, atrial natriuretic factor (ANF), human placental lactogen, and human chorionic gonadotropin are additional variables that might be involved.

2.5.3. Changes in Glomerular Function

By the end of the first trimester, the GFR rises by 40–60%, reaching a peak of 180 ml/min. Around six weeks into pregnancy, the increase in GFR starts, coming before the expansion of the plasma volume and the rise in cardiac output. The GFR level reaches its maximum at 16 weeks of gestation and stays there until 36 weeks. GFR levels during pregnancy, as determined by creatinine clearance, typically range from 110 to 150 ml/min. By 4 weeks of gestation, creatinine clearance rises by 25%, and by 9 weeks, it increases by 45%. The increase in glomerular blood flow, glomerular capillary hydrostatic pressure, and the drop in colloid osmotic pressure that follows the decrease in plasma proteins are likely the mechanisms mediating the secondary vasodilatation of afferent and efferent arterioles, which leads to the increase in GFR. Certain studies have indicated that elevated GFR at 36 weeks may be caused by a combination of increased RPF, decreased oncotic pressure, and increased ultrafiltration coefficient, even though the contribution of other GFR determinants is unclear in the first and second trimesters.

Urinary excretion of protein and albumin is increased due to changes in the electrical charge selectivity of the glomerular membrane and an increase in GFR.

The volume of fluid delivered into the tubular lumen and the solute concentration are both increased by 50–100% when the GFR rises. As a result, tubular reabsorption rises to prevent the retention of these materials and the depletion of sodium, potassium, chloride, glucose, and water.

2.5.4. Changes in Tubular Function

The way nutrients and waste are handled by the tubules changes during pregnancy. Pregnancy causes an increase in the excretion of proteins, amino acids, and urea. By 8–10 weeks of gestation, increased urea clearance during pregnancy causes plasma urea nitrogen levels to drop, reaching 63% of non-pregnant levels by the third trimester. By 16 weeks of pregnancy, there is a 30% increase in uric acid filtrate, which is accompanied by increased GFR-induced secretion and decreased reabsorption. As a result, by 22–24 weeks, serum uric acid levels drop by 25–35% (2–3 mg/dl), and by term, they gradually rise to normal. To manage the increased production from the placenta and fetus, there needs to be an increase in uric acid clearance.

Normal pregnancy is characterized by an increase in albumin and total urine protein excretion, particularly after 20 weeks. During a normal pregnancy, an average of 100–300 mg of protein are excreted daily. During pregnancy, the majority of the proteins expelled in urine are Tamm-Horsfall glycoprotein, with trace amounts of albumin and other circulating proteins. There is a significant daily variance, and there is some evidence that albuminuria rises in the latter stages of pregnancy, though not to a level that is higher than the upper limit of normal. Although there is no correlation between the severity of renal disease and protein excretion, values of proteinuria greater than 300 mg/24 hours are deemed abnormal. Although selective changes in glomerular charge and an increase in GFR during the third trimester are partially responsible for proteinuria in pregnancy, the exact mechanism underlying this condition remains unclear. soluble antiangiogenic factors in circulation i.e., due to disruptions in the podocyte slit diaphragm, soluble fms-like tyrosine kinase

1 (sFlt-1) and vascular endothelial growth factor (VEGF) levels rise late in a typical pregnancy, which could account for late-term elevations in proteinuria.

Pregnancy-related glucoseuria is frequently observed and is believed to result from an increased filtered glucose load that surpasses the maximum tubular reabsorptive capacity. The proximal tubule, loop of Henle, or collecting ducts cannot handle the combined effects of increased GFR and less efficient glucose reabsorption, which results in glucosuria with normoglycemia or physiological glucosuria. Urinary glucose excretion varies; values can be anywhere from 10 to 100 times higher than those of non-pregnant individuals (Table 2.8).

Table 2.8. Laboratory Values of Renal Function in Pregnancy

Variable/ Test	Non-pregnant Values	Pregnant Values	Values in Pregnancy That Require Further Investigation	Average Values in Pregnancy
Plasma creatinine	0.65 ± 0.14 mg/dl	0.46 ± 0.13 mg/dl	>0.80 mg/dl	0.5 mg/dl
Creatinine clearance	85–120 ml/min	10–150 ml/min	–	–
Blood urea nitrogen	13 ± 3 mg/dl	8.7 ± 1.5 mg/dl	>14 mg/dl	9.0 mg/dl
Plasma urate	4–6 mg/dl	2.5–4 mg/dl	>5.8 mg/dl	2–3 mg/dl
Serum sodium	136–146 mEq/l	133–148 mEq/l	<128 mEq/l	135 mEq/l
Serum potassium	3.5–5.0 mEq/l	3.6–5.0 mEq/l	>5.1 mEq/l	3.8 mEq/l
Serum chloride	102–109	97–109	>110 mEq/l	103 mEq/l
Serum bicarbonate	27–28 mEq/l	20–22 mEq/l	<20 mEq/l	18–20 mEq/l
Plasma osmolality	275–295 mOsm/kg H_2O	276–289 mOsm/kg H_2O	>290 mOsm/kg H_2O	270 mOsm/kg H_2O
Urinary glucose	20–100 mg/24 h	>100 mg/24 h	–	–
Urinary protein	<100–150 mg/24 h	<250–300 mg/24 h	>300 mg/24 h	–
Urinary amino acids	–	Up to 2 g/24 h	>2 g/24 h	–

Source: Vinturache A, Khalil A, Glob. libr. women's med.,ISSN: 1756-2228; DOI 10.3843/GLOWM.411323.

Because the threshold for activating the osmoreceptors for antidiuretic hormone (ADH) and thirst is lowered during pregnancy, the thermostat is reset to lower values of osmolarity. From conception, plasma osmolarity falls by 8–10 mOsm/kg by 10 weeks of gestation, and it stays low until term. The response to water loading or deprivation, as well as the concentration and dilution of urine, occur at the new baseline of osmolarity in a manner comparable to that of non-pregnant people. The placental vasopressinases' 3.4-fold increase in plasma arginine-vasopressin (AVP) clearance is counterbalanced by the posterior pituitary's increased release of the hormone. This keeps maternal circulating levels of arginine and vasopressin constant.

Pregnancy increases both the filtered load of sodium and its reabsorption from the renal tubules. Pregnancy results in a net retention of 900–950 mEq of sodium, which supports the dilated systemic vasculature's increase in plasma volume. Although the exact mechanisms underlying sodium retention are unknown, they most likely involve a balance between progesterone, aldosterone, human placental lactogen, corticosterone, and other anti-natriuretic factors and natriuretic factors like increased GFR, decreased renal vascular resistance, decreased oncotic pressure, decreased serum albumin, vasodilatory prostaglandins, and increased atrial natriuretic peptide. Additionally, relaxin mediates sodium balance. Pregnant women, however, maintain homeostatic balance because the water accumulation balances out the sodium retention.

Throughout pregnancy, there is a constant excretion of potassium, and an increase in tubular reabsorption adjusts to changes in the filtered load. By the end of pregnancy, this causes the body's total potassium stores to increase and be retained by about 300–350 mEq. However, because the extra potassium is being utilized by the mother's and fetus' tissues, the mother's serum potassium level does not increase. The anti-kaliuretic properties of progesterone counteract the kaliuretic effects of aldosterone, which results in the retention of potassium.

The amount of calcium excreted in the urine increases as GFR rises. Because of increased intestinal absorption of calcium, serum ionic calcium levels remain stable despite a decrease in serum levels of calcium and phosphate. To preserve homeostasis and fulfill fetal needs, pregnant women must consume 1200 mg of calcium daily. When a woman is not pregnant, parathyroid hormone is a major factor in the metabolism of calcium and bone, but during pregnancy, vitamin D seems to be a major regulator. The levels of 1,25(OH)2D increase two to three times during pregnancy to guarantee the mineralization of the fetal skeleton and boost intestinal calcium absorption.

To counteract the respiratory alkalosis brought on by increased ventilation during pregnancy, the renal acid–base balance is changed. The loss of respiratory carbon dioxide is balanced by an increase in bicarbonate excretion combined with renal retention of hydrogen ions. Consequently, the serum bicarbonate levels drop by 4–5 mEq/L during the first trimester, reaching values of 20–22 mEq/L. Thus, pregnant women have a limited ability to act as a buffer.

2.6. Physiological Adaptation of the Digestive System to Pregnancy

Supporting maternal and fetal nutrition requires the gastrointestinal and hepatic systems to adapt anatomically and physiologically. The mechanical forces of the growing uterus, which cause the digestive organs to shift, and the hormonal effects of estrogen on the liver and progesterone on the smooth muscle, promote the changes (Table 2.9).

Table 2.9. Alterations in the Gastrointestinal System During Pregnancy

Organ	Alteration	Significance
Mouth	Gingivitis Epulis formation Increased saliva production	Bleeding from gums Interference with chewing Increase risk of periodontal diseases
Esophagus	Decreased lower esophageal sphincter tone decrease tone of hiatus	Heartburn Increase risk of hiatus hernia
Stomach	Decreased tone and motility Delayed gastric emptying Decreased gastric acidity and histamine output Incompetence of pyloric sphincter	Risk of gastroesophageal reflux and vomiting Reflux of biliary material in the stomach Increased risk of vomiting and aspiration with sedatives and anesthetics Improvement of peptic ulcer symptoms
Small and large bowel	Decreased intestinal tone and motility Increased transit time Increased height of duodenal villi Increased activity of brush border enzymes Upward displacement of the cecum and appendix	Increased absorption of nutrients: iron, calcium, amino acids, vitamins and other substances Increased sodium and water absorption with predisposition to flatulence and constipation Difficult diagnosis of appendicitis
Gallbladder	Decreased tone and motility	Alteration of gallbladder function Increased risk of gallstones
Liver	Upward displacement Altered production of enzymes, bilirubin, proteins and lipids	Delayed recognition of hepatomegaly Altered early recognition of liver dysfunction Discomfort due to itching

Source: Vinturache A, Khalil A, Glob. libr. women's med.,ISSN: 1756-2228; DOI 10.3843/GLOWM.411323.

2.6.1. Anatomical Changes

Increased intragastric pressure results from the uterus's displacement of the gastrointestinal tract. Heartburn and reflux are made more likely by the lower tone of the lower esophageal sphincter as well as the decreased motility of the colon. Lower transit times brought on by decreased intestinal and gastric motility also contribute to the bloating and constipation sensations. During pregnancy, the stomach's capacity remains constant (Kelly et al., 2009).

2.6.2. Functional Changes

There is conflicting evidence regarding the relationship between oral health and the risk of pregnancy complications, but recent studies emphasize the connection between oral health and low birth weight and preterm birth. Multiparous pregnant women, have poor dentition, or have periodontal disease are more likely to experience bleeding from their gums due to increased gum vascularization, gingival edema, and a decrease in the thickness of the gingival epithelium. Gingivitis increases with early pregnancy and can affect up to 30–80% of pregnant women by the third trimester. Gingivitis development could be linked to changes in the progesterone and estrogen-stimulated local inflammatory process. Severe and advanced gingivitis may encourage the development of epulis, which affects about 5% of pregnant women in the second and third trimesters. Gingival growths are generally asymptomatic, but they can occasionally bleed and hurt when chewing, which raises the risk of periodontal disease. Salivary changes are linked to pregnancy. Saliva becomes more acidic and has a higher electrolyte content. The microbiome of saliva is altered, and the number of microorganisms is higher. Some women may report increased salivation, even though there is no increase in saliva volume. This could be due to swallowing difficulties, nausea, or vomiting. The percentage of women who develop ptyalism is quite low. The stomach and intestines are among the digestive organs that are displaced as pregnancy progresses by the expanding uterus. Reduced lower esophageal sphincter tone is another significant change. The third trimester is when the pressure drops the most, by 30 to 50%, and reaches its lowest point by 36 weeks of gestation. Esophageal reflux is caused by a decrease in the lower esophageal sphincter's capacity to react to an increase in intragastric pressure. Progesterone is known to cause hypotonia in the stomach and decreased motility, which results in delayed gastric emptying and longer gastrointestinal transit times. These effects are compounded by the mechanical effects of the growing uterus. It's unknown how pregnancy affects the secretion of stomach acid. Under the influence of estrogen and elevated levels of placental histaminases, a decrease in stomach pH has been documented during the first and second trimesters. While the levels of gastrin are normal at this point in the pregnancy, they tend to rise as the third trimester progresses. As pregnancy approaches its end, elevated gastric acidity is linked to elevated levels of gastrin, which is most likely placental in origin during the third trimester.

Serum transaminase and bilirubin levels marginally decrease during pregnancy, while placental production causes an increase in serum alkaline phosphatase levels. Progesterone's effects on intestinal smooth muscle and plasma motilin's inhibition cause the decrease in intestinal tone and motility that occurs during pregnancy. As gestation progresses, the resulting changes in the transit time get bigger. The gallbladder experiences comparable alterations. Progesterone causes a decrease in muscle tone and motility, which, especially in the second and third trimesters, increases gallbladder volume and decreases emptying rate. Gallbladder stones form as a result of a decrease in bile's capacity to solubilize cholesterol and a decrease in water absorption through the mucosa of the gallbladder. Pruritus is caused by the gallbladder's propensity to hold onto bile salts.

The gravid uterus pushes the liver superiorly, but it doesn't change in size. Hepatic blood flow remains relatively constant, averaging between 25 and 35 percent. Pregnancy does not affect liver function. The liver produces different amounts of proteins, lipids, bilirubin, and enzymes when exposed to estrogen and progesterone. The alterations observed in liver function tests follow the same pattern as those observed in liver disease patients (Bacq et al., 1996).

When compared to a non-pregnant state, the majority of routine liver function tests only slightly change during pregnancy (Table 2.10).

Table 2.10. Changes in Liver Function Tests During Pregnancy

Lab Test	Effect of Pregnancy	Time of Change	Significance
Albumin	↓ 20–40%	Second trimester	Hemodilution; decrease proteins for biding, increase concentration of free substances
Globulin	Slight ↑	Third trimester	Facilitate transport of lipids, carbohydrates, iron and hormones to the placenta
Total proteins	↓ by 20%	Second trimester	Mainly related to decrease in albumin; increase in concentration of free proteins
Bilirubin	N	–	–
Aspartate aminotransferase (AST)	Slight ↓ in upper limit; may ↑ during labor	–	Do not change significantly during pregnancy, can be used to assess liver damage during pregnancy
Alanine aminotransferase (ALT)	Slight ↓ in upper limit; may ↑ during labor	–	Do not change significantly during pregnancy, can be used to assess liver damage during pregnancy
Gamma glutamyl transferase (GGT)	Slight ↓ in upper limit		
Alkaline phosphatase	↑ 2 to 4-fold	Third trimester	Increased production by fetus and placenta
Lactate dehydrogenase (LDH)	Slight ↑	Third trimester	Associated with tissue injury

Source: Vinturache A, Khalil A, Glob. libr. women's med. ISSN: 1756-2228; DOI 10.3843/GLOWM.411323.

A Closer Look

Hemodynamic Profile

The hemodynamic profile of an individual refers to the dynamic parameters that characterize the flow and pressure of blood within the cardiovascular system, essential for understanding and managing various medical conditions. This profile encompasses measurements such as cardiac output (CO), stroke volume (SV), heart rate (HR), blood pressure (BP), systemic vascular resistance (SVR), and central venous pressure (CVP). Cardiac output, the volume of blood pumped by the heart per minute, is a critical indicator of cardiac function and overall circulatory health. It is determined by the stroke volume (the amount of blood ejected with each heartbeat) and heart rate. Blood pressure, another vital component, reflects the force exerted by circulating blood on the walls of blood vessels, providing insights into the resistance and compliance of the vascular system.

Systemic vascular resistance represents the resistance to blood flow within the blood vessels, primarily influenced by the tone of the vascular smooth muscle and the diameter of the blood vessels. Central venous pressure measures the pressure in the thoracic vena cava near the right atrium, offering information about venous return and right heart function. Together, these parameters are crucial for assessing the hemodynamic status of patients, especially in critical care settings.

Changes in the hemodynamic profile can indicate various pathological conditions. For instance, a decreased cardiac output may suggest heart failure or hypovolemia, while elevated systemic vascular resistance can indicate hypertension or vasoconstriction. Monitoring these parameters allows clinicians to diagnose, treat, and manage conditions such as shock, heart failure, and sepsis more effectively. Advanced technologies, such as echocardiography, pulmonary artery catheters, and non-invasive cardiac output monitors, provide detailed hemodynamic data, enabling precise and tailored therapeutic interventions. In summary, a thorough understanding of the hemodynamic profile is fundamental to optimizing cardiovascular care and improving patient outcomes in various clinical scenarios.

Summary

- Pregnancy induces a series of profound and multifaceted changes in a woman's body, encompassing physiological, hormonal, and anatomical adaptations.
- During pregnancy, the pregnant mother undergoes significant anatomical and physiological changes to nurture and accommodate the developing fetus.
- Changes in the cardiovascular system in pregnancy are profound and begin early in pregnancy, such that by eight weeks gestation, the cardiac output has already increased by 20%.
- Relaxin, a peptide hormone produced by the corpus luteum, decidua and placenta, plays an important role in the regulation of hemodynamic and water metabolism during pregnancy.
- As a consequence of renal vasodilatation, renal plasma flow and glomerular filtration rate (GFR) both increase, compared to non-pregnant levels, by 40–65 and 50–85%, respectively.
- Arterial under-filling in pregnancy leads to the stimulation of arterial baroreceptors, activating the RAA and the sympathetic nervous systems.
- The nausea symptoms usually resolve by week 20 but about 10–20% of the patients experience symptoms beyond week 20 and some until the end of the pregnancy.
- During pregnancy, there is also an increase in serum levels of deoxycorticosterone, corticosteroid-binding globulin (CBG), adrenocorticotropic hormone (ACTH), cortisol and free cortisol.
- Maternal insulin resistance begins in the second trimester and peaks in the third trimester. This is the result of increasing secretion of diabetogenic hormones such as human placental lactogen, growth hormone, progesterone, cortisol and prolactin.

References

1. Adamopoulos, D. A., Dessypris, A., Xanthopoulos, J., et al. (1982). Gastrin secretion in the menstrual cycle and pregnancy. *Hepato-Gastroenterology*, *29*(1), 24–26.
2. Akinbami, A. A., Ajibola, S. O., Rabiu, K. A., et al. (2013). Hematological profile of normal pregnant women in Lagos, Nigeria. *International Journal of Women's Health*, *5*, 227–232.
3. Akinlaja, O. (2016). Hematological changes in pregnancy: The preparation for intrapartum blood loss. *Obstetrics and Gynecology International Journal*, *4*(3). https://doi.org/10.15406/ogij.2016.04.00109.
4. American College of Obstetricians and Gynecologists (ACOG). (2004). Nausea and vomiting of pregnancy. *Obstetrics & Gynecology, 103*(4), 803–814. Practice Bulletin.
5. American College of Obstetricians and Gynecologists. (2002). ACOG committee opinion: Exercise during pregnancy and the postpartum period. *International Journal of Gynecology and Obstetrics*, *77*(1), 79–81.
6. Angueira, A. R., Ludvik, A. E., Reddy, T. E., Wicksteed, B., et al. (2015). New insights into gestational glucose metabolism: Lessons learned from 21st century approaches. *Diabetes*, *64*(2), 327–334. https://doi.org/10.2337/db14-0588.

7. Bacq, Y., Zarka, O., Brechot, J. F., et al. (1996). Liver function tests in normal pregnancy: A prospective study of 103 pregnant women and 103 matched controls. *Hepatology*, *23*(5), 1030–1034. https://doi.org/10.1002/hep.510230516.

8. Bailey, R. R., & Rolleston, G. L. (1971). Kidney length and ureteric dilatation in the puerperium. *The Journal of Obstetrics and Gynecology of the British Commonwealth*, *78*(1), 55–61. https://doi.org/10.1111/j.1471-0528.1971.tb00389.x.

9. Baldwin, G. R., Moorthi, D. S., Whelton, J. A., et al. (1977). New lung functions and pregnancy. *American Journal of Obstetrics and Gynecology*, *127*(3), 235–239. https://doi.org/10.1016/0002-9378(77)90245-1.

10. Barak, S., Oettinger-Barak, O., Oettinger, M., et al. (2003). Common oral manifestations during pregnancy: A review. *Obstetrical & Gynecological Survey*, *58*(9), 624–628. https://doi.org/10.1097/01.OGX.0000086099.32660.0E.

11. Bedard, E., Dimopoulos, K., & Gatzoulis, M. A. (2009). Has there been any progress made on pregnancy outcomes among women with pulmonary arterial hypertension? *European Heart Journal*, *30*(3), 256–265. https://doi.org/10.1093/eurheartj/ehn607.

12. Beydoun, S. N. (1985). Morphologic changes in the renal tract in pregnancy. *Clinical Obstetrics and Gynecology*, *28*(2), 249–256. https://doi.org/10.1097/00003081-198506000-00005.

13. Blackburn, S. T. (2013). *Maternal, Fetal & Neonatal Physiology: A Clinical Perspective* (4th ed.). Elsevier.

14. Blanchard, D. G., & Shabetai, R. (2009). Cardiac disease. In R. Creasy & R. Resnik (Eds.), *Creasy & Resnik's Maternal-Fetal Medicine: Principles and Practice* (6th ed., pp. 855–877). Saunders Elsevier.

15. Blood-Siegfried, J., & Rende, E. K. (2010). The long-term effects of prenatal nicotine exposure on neurologic development. *Journal of Midwifery & Women's Health*, *55*(2), 143–152. https://doi.org/10.1016/j.jmwh.2009.04.005.

16. Bobrowski, R. A. (2010). Pulmonary physiology in pregnancy. *Clinical Obstetrics and Gynecology*, *53*(2), 285–300. https://doi.org/10.1097/GRF.0b013e3181dbed38.

17. Brewster, L. M., et al. (2010). Ethnic differences in resistance artery contractility of normotensive pregnant women. *American Journal of Physiology-Heart and Circulatory Physiology*, *299*(2), H431–H436. https://doi.org/10.1152/ajpheart.00919.2009.

18. Bridges, E. J., Womble, S., Wallace, M., et al. (2003). Hemodynamic monitoring in high-risk obstetrics patients, I: Expected hemodynamic changes in pregnancy. *Critical Care Nurse*, *23*(4), 53–62.

19. Brizzi, P., Tonolo, G., Esposito, F., et al. (1999). Lipoprotein metabolism during normal pregnancy. *American Journal of Obstetrics and Gynecology*, *181*(2), 430–434. https://doi.org/10.1016/S0002-9378(99)70582-5.

20. Brooks, V. L., Dampney, R. A., & Heesch, C. M. (2010). Pregnancy and the endocrine regulation of the baroreceptor reflex. *American Journal of Physiology-Regulatory, Integrative and Comparative Physiology*, *299*(2), R439–R451. https://doi.org/10.1152/ajpregu.00303.2010.

21. Brown, M. A., Sinosich, M. J., Saunders, D. M., et al. (1986). Potassium regulation and progesterone-aldosterone interrelationships in human pregnancy: A prospective study.

American Journal of Obstetrics and Gynecology, *155*(2), 349–353. https://doi.org/10.1016/0002-9378(86)90704-8.

22. Bucht, H. (1951). Studies on renal function in man: With special reference to glomerular filtration and renal plasma flow in pregnancy. *Scandinavian Journal of Clinical and Laboratory Investigation*, *3*(3), 1–64.
23. Butte, N. F. (2000). Carbohydrate and lipid metabolism in pregnancy: Normal compared with gestational diabetes mellitus. *American Journal of Clinical Nutrition*, *71*, 125S. https://doi.org/10.1093/ajcn/71.5.1255.
24. Capeless, E. L., & Clapp, J. F. (1991). When do cardiovascular parameters return to their preconception values? *American Journal of Obstetrics and Gynecology*, *165*(4 Pt 1), 883–886. https://doi.org/10.1016/0002-9378(91)90453-M.
25. Carbillon, L., Uzan, M., & Uzan, S. (2000). Pregnancy, vascular tone, and maternal hemodynamics: A crucial adaptation. *Obstetrical & Gynecological Survey*, *55*(9), 574–581. https://doi.org/10.1097/00006254-200009000-00025.
26. Carlin, A., & Alfirevic, Z. (2008). Physiological changes of pregnancy and monitoring. *Best Practice & Research Clinical Obstetrics & Gynecology*, *22*(5), 801–823. https://doi.org/10.1016/j.bpobgyn.2008.06.005.
27. Castro, L. C., Hobel, C. J., & Gornbein, J. (1994). Plasma levels of atrial natriuretic peptide in normal and hypertensive pregnancies: A meta-analysis. *American Journal of Obstetrics and Gynecology*, *171*(6), 1642–1651. https://doi.org/10.1016/0002-9378(94)90420-0.
28. Caulin-Glaser, T., & Setaro, J. F. (2004). Pregnancy and cardiovascular disease. In *Medical Complications During Pregnancy* (6th ed.). Saunders Elsevier.
29. Chandra, S., Tripathi, A. K., Mishra, S., et al. (2012). Physiological changes in hematological parameters during pregnancy. *Indian Journal of Hematology and Blood Transfusion*, *28*(3), 144–146. https://doi.org/10.1007/s12288-012-0175-6.
30. Chapman, A. B., Abraham, W. T., Zamudio, S., et al. (1998). Temporal relationships between hormonal and hemodynamic changes in early human pregnancy. *Kidney International*, *54*(6), 2056–2063. https://doi.org/10.1046/j.1523-1755.1998.00188.x.
31. Cheung, K. L., & Lafayette, R. A. (2013). Renal physiology of pregnancy. *Advances in Chronic Kidney Disease*, *20*(3), 209–214. https://doi.org/10.1053/j.ackd.2013.01.012.
32. Christensen, T., Klebe, J. G., & Bertelsen, V., et al. (1989). Changes in renal volume during normal pregnancy. *Acta Obstetricia et Gynecologica Scandinavica*, *68*(6), 541–543. https://doi.org/10.3109/00016348909006261.
33. Clapp, J. F., 3rd. (1991). Exercise and fetal health. *Journal of Developmental Physiology*, *15*(1), 9–14.
34. Clark, P., Brennand, J., Conkie, J. A., et al. (1998). Activated protein C sensitivity, protein C, protein S and coagulation in normal pregnancy. *Thrombosis and Haemostasis*, *79*(6), 1166–1170. https://doi.org/10.1055/s-0037-1614394.
35. Clark, S. M., Costantine, M. M., & Hankins, G. F. (2012). Review of NVP and HG and early pharmacotherapeutic intervention. *Obstetrics and Gynecology International*, *2012*, 252676. https://doi.org/10.1155/2012/252676.

36. Conrad, K. P. (2011a). Emerging role of relaxin in the maternal adaptations to normal pregnancy: Implications for preeclampsia. *Seminars in Nephrology*, *31*(1), 15–32. https://doi.org/10.1016/j.semnephrol.2010.10.003.

37. Conrad, K. P. (2011b). Maternal vasodilation in pregnancy: The emerging role of relaxin. *American Journal of Physiology-Regulatory, Integrative and Comparative Physiology*, *301*(2), R267–R275. https://doi.org/10.1152/ajpregu.00052.2011.

38. Conrad, K. P., & Davison, J. M. (2014). The renal circulation in normal pregnancy and preeclampsia: Is there a place for relaxin? *American Journal of Physiology-Renal Physiology*, *306*(10), F1121–F1135. https://doi.org/10.1152/ajprenal.00569.2013.

39. Cornelis, T., Odutayo, A., Keunen, J., et al. (2011). The kidney in normal pregnancy and preeclampsia. *Seminars in Nephrology*, *31*(1), 4–14. https://doi.org/10.1016/j.semnephrol.2010.10.002.

40. Costantine, M. M. (2014). Physiologic and pharmacokinetic changes in pregnancy. *Frontiers in Pharmacology*, *5*, 65. https://doi.org/10.3389/fphar.2014.00065.

41. Cunningham, F. G., & Leveno, K. J. (2009). *William's Obstetrics* (23rd ed.). McGraw-Hill.

42. Cunningham, F. G., & Leveno, K. J. (2010). Laboratory values in normal pregnancy. In *Protocols for High-Risk Pregnancies: An Evidence-Based Approach* (5th ed.). Blackwell Science Ltd.

43. Curry, R., Swan, L., & Steer, P. J. (2009). Cardiac disease in pregnancy. *Current Opinion in Obstetrics and Gynecology*, *21*(6), 508–513. https://doi.org/10.1097/GCO.0b013e3283326886.

44. Davison, J. M. (1984). Renal hemodynamics and volume homeostasis in pregnancy. *Scandinavian Journal of Clinical and Laboratory Investigation*, *169*, 15–27. https://doi.org/10.3109/00365518409084048.

45. Davison, J. M. (1987). Kidney function in pregnant women. *American Journal of Kidney Diseases*, *9*(4), 248–252. https://doi.org/10.1016/S0272-6386(87)80089-3.

46. Davison, J. M., & Hytten, F. E. (1975). The effect of pregnancy on the renal handling of glucose. *British Journal of Obstetrics and Gynecology*, *82*(5), 374–381. https://doi.org/10.1111/j.1471-0528.1975.tb00506.x.

47. Davison, J. M., Barron, W. M., & Lindheimer, M. D. (1987). Metabolic clearance rates of vasopressin increase markedly in late gestation: Possible cause of polyuria in pregnant women. *Transactions of the Association of American Physicians*, *100*, 91–98.

48. Davison, J. M., Gilmore, E. A., Durr, J., Robertson, G. L., & Lindheimer, M. D. (1984). Altered osmotic thresholds for vasopressin secretion and thirst in human pregnancy. *American Journal of Physiology-Renal Physiology*, *246*(1 Pt 2), F105–109. https://doi.org/10.1152/ajprenal.1984.246.1.F105.

49. Davison, J. M., Sheills, E. A., Barron, W. M., Robinson, A. G., & Lindheimer, M. D. (1989). Changes in the metabolic clearance of vasopressin and in plasma vasopressinase throughout human pregnancy. *Journal of Clinical Investigation*, *83*(4), 1313–1318. https://doi.org/10.1172/JCI114016.

50. Davison, J. M., Shiells, E. A., Philips, P. R., et al. (1988). Serial evaluation of vasopressin release and thirst in human pregnancy: Role of human chorionic gonadotropin in the osmoregulatory changes of gestation. *Journal of Clinical Investigation*, *81*(3), 798–806. https://doi.org/10.1172/JCI113366.

51. De Alvarez, R. R. (1958). Renal glomerulotubular mechanisms during normal pregnancy: I. Glomerular filtration rate, renal plasma flow, and creatinine clearance. *American Journal of Obstetrics and Gynecology*, *75*(5), 931–944.

52. De Boer, K., Ten Cate, J. W., Sturk, A., et al. (1989). Enhanced thrombin generation in normal and hypertensive pregnancy. *American Journal of Obstetrics and Gynecology*, *160*(1), 95–100. https://doi.org/10.1016/0002-9378(89)90151-2.

53. Delivoria-Papadopoulos, M., & McGovern, J. E. (1998). In *Fetal and Neonatal Physiology* (2nd ed.). Saunders Elsevier.

54. Dhariwal, S. K. N. S., Singh, A., & Nema, S. (2016). Evaluation of hematological indices, neutrophils, and platelets in pregnant women attending tertiary care center. *Indian Journal of Pathology and Oncology*, *3*(3), 297–304.

55. Dorr, H. G., Heller, A., Versmold, H. T., et al. (1989). Longitudinal study of progestins, mineralocorticoids, and glucocorticoids throughout human pregnancy. *Journal of Clinical Endocrinology & Metabolism*, *68*, 863. https://doi.org/10.1210/jcem-68-4-863.

56. Dunlop, W. (1981). Serial changes in renal hemodynamics during normal human pregnancy. *British Journal of Obstetrics and Gynaecology*, *88*(1), 1–9. https://doi.org/10.1111/j.1471-0528.1981.tb01048.x.

57. Duong, C., Kidson-Gerber, G., Peters, N., et al. (2015). Trajectory of platelets in pregnancy: Do low-risk women need an intrapartum full blood count prior to epidural? *Australian and New Zealand Journal of Obstetrics and Gynaecology*, *55*(5), 511–514. https://doi.org/10.1111/ajo.12391.

58. Edelstam, G., Lowbeer, C., Kral, G., et al. (2001). New reference values for routine blood samples and human neutrophilic lipocalin during third-trimester pregnancy. *Scandinavian Journal of Clinical and Laboratory Investigation*, *61*(8), 583–592. https://doi.org/10.1080/003655101753354829.

59. Eichinger, S. (2003). D-dimer testing in pregnancy. *Pathophysiology of Haemostasis and Thrombosis*, *33*(5–6), 327–329. https://doi.org/10.1159/000083832.

60. Elkus, R., & Popovich, J. Jr. (1992). Respiratory physiology in pregnancy. *Clinics in Chest Medicine*, *13*(4), 555–565.

61. Elsheikh, A., Creatsas, G., & Mastorakos, G. (2001). The renin-aldosterone system during normal and hypertensive pregnancy. *Archives of Gynecology and Obstetrics, 264*, 182.

62. Erman, A., Neri, A., Sharoni, R., et al. (1992). Enhanced urinary albumin excretion after 35 weeks of gestation and during labor in normal pregnancy. *Scandinavian Journal of Clinical and Laboratory Investigation, 52*(5), 409–413.

63. Everson, G. T. (1992). Gastrointestinal motility in pregnancy. *Gastroenterology Clinics of North America, 21*(4), 751–776.

64. Faundes, A., Bricola-Filho, M., & Pinto e Silva, J. L. (1998). Dilatation of the urinary tract during pregnancy: Proposal of a curve of maximal caliceal diameter by gestational age. *American Journal of Obstetrics and Gynecology, 178*(5), 1082–1086.

65. Faupel-Badger, J. M., Hsieh, C. C., Troisi, R., et al. (2007). Plasma volume expansion in pregnancy: Implications for biomarkers in population studies. *Cancer Epidemiology, Biomarkers & Prevention, 16*(9), 1720–1723.

66. Fogacci, M. F., Vettore, M. V., & Leao, A. T. (2011). The effect of periodontal therapy on preterm low birth weight: A meta-analysis. *Obstetrics & Gynecology, 117*(1), 153–165.

67. Frederiksen, M. C. (2001). Physiologic changes in pregnancy and their effect on drug disposition. *Seminars in Perinatology, 25*(3), 120–123.

68. Freeman, M., Ghidini, A., Spong, C. Y., et al. (2004). Does air travel affect pregnancy outcome? *Archives of Gynecology and Obstetrics, 269*(4), 274–277.

69. Frick, G., Bremme, K., Sjogren, C., et al. (1990). Plasma levels of cholecystokinin and gastrin during the menstrual cycle and pregnancy. *Acta Obstetricia et Gynecologica Scandinavica, 69*(4), 317–320.

70. Fu, Q., & Levine, B. D. (2009). Autonomic circulatory control during pregnancy in humans. *Seminars in Reproductive Medicine, 27*(4), 330–337.

71. Gant, N. F., Worley, R. J., Everett, R. B., & MacDonald, P. C. (1980). Control of vascular responsiveness during human pregnancy. *Kidney International, 18*(2), 253–258.

72. Gardner, M. O., & Doyle, N. M. (2004). Asthma in pregnancy. *Obstetrics and Gynecology Clinics of North America, 31*(2), 385–413, vii.

73. Gei, A. F., & Hankins, G. D. (2001). Cardiac disease and pregnancy. *Obstetrics and Gynecology Clinics of North America, 28*(3), 465–512.

74. Geisinger, M. L., Geurs, N. C., Bain, J. L., et al. (2014). Oral health education and therapy reduces gingivitis during pregnancy. *Journal of Clinical Periodontology, 41*(2), 141–148.

75. George, A., Shamim, S., Johnson, M., et al. (2011). Periodontal treatment during pregnancy and birth outcomes: A meta-analysis of randomized trials. *International Journal of Evidence-Based Healthcare, 9*(2), 122–147.

76. Glinoer, D. (1997). The regulation of thyroid function in pregnancy: Pathways of endocrine adaptation from physiology to pathology. *Endocrine Reviews, 18*, 404.

77. Gonzalez-Campoy, J. M., Romero, J. C., & Knox, F. G. (1989). Escape from the sodium-retaining effects of mineralocorticoids: Role of ANF and intrarenal hormone systems. *Kidney International, 35*(3), 767–777.

78. Gordon, M. C. (2012). *Maternal Physiology in Obstetrics: Normal and Problem Pregnancies* (6th ed.). Saunders, Elsevier.

79. Gustafsson, M. K., Romundstad, P. R., Stafne, S. N., et al. (2018). Alterations in the vitamin D endocrine system during pregnancy: A longitudinal study of 855 healthy Norwegian women. *PLoS ONE, 13*(4), e0195041.

80. Harirah, H. M., Donia, S. E., Nasrallah, F. K., et al. (2005). Effect of gestational age and position on peak expiratory flow rate: A longitudinal study. *Obstetrics & Gynecology, 105*(2), 372–376.

81. Hayashi, M., Ueda, Y., Hoshimoto, K., et al. (2002). Changes in urinary excretion of six biochemical parameters in normotensive pregnancy and preeclampsia. *American Journal of Kidney Diseases, 39*(2), 392–400.

82. Hegewald, M. J., & Crapo, R. O. (2011). Respiratory physiology in pregnancy. *Clinical Chest Medicine, 32*(1), 1–13.

83. Hellgren, M. (2003). Hemostasis during normal pregnancy and puerperium. *Seminars in Thrombosis and Hemostasis, 29*(2), 125–130.

84. Hey, V. M., Cowley, D. J., Ganguli, P. C., et al. (1977). Gastro-oesophageal reflux in late pregnancy. *Anaesthesia, 32*(4), 372–377.

85. Hill, C. C., & Pickinpaugh, J. (2008). Physiologic changes in pregnancy. *Surgical Clinics of North America, 88*(2), 391–401, vii.

86. Hui, C., Lili, M., Libin, C., et al. (2012). Changes in coagulation and hemodynamics during pregnancy: A prospective longitudinal study of 58 cases. *Archives of Gynecology and Obstetrics, 285*(5), 1231–1236.

87. Hytten, F. E., & Paintin, D. B. (1963). Increase in plasma volume during normal pregnancy. *The Journal of Obstetrics and Gynecology of the British Empire, 70*, 402–407.

88. Irani, R. A., & Xia, Y. (2008). The functional role of the renin-angiotensin system in pregnancy and preeclampsia. *Placenta, 29*(9), 763–771.

89. Irani, R. A., & Xia, Y. (2011). Renin angiotensin signaling in normal pregnancy and preeclampsia. *Seminars in Nephrology, 31*(1), 47–58.

90. Jansen, A. J., van Rhenen, D. J., Steegers, E. A., et al. (2005). Postpartum hemorrhage and transfusion of blood and blood components. *Obstetrical & Gynecological Survey, 60*(10), 663–671.

91. Jeyabalan, A., & Conrad, K. P. (2007). Renal function during normal pregnancy and preeclampsia. *Frontiers in Bioscience, 12*, 2425–2437.

92. Jeyabalan, A., & Lain, K. Y. (2007). Anatomic and functional changes of the upper urinary tract during pregnancy. *Urologic Clinics of North America, 34*(1), 1–6.

93. Kametas, N. A., McAuliffe, F., Hancock, J., et al. (2001). Maternal left ventricular mass and diastolic function during pregnancy. *Ultrasound in Obstetrics & Gynecology, 18*(5), 460–466.

94. Kametas, N. A., McAuliffe, F., Krampl, E., et al. (2003). Maternal cardiac function in twin pregnancy. *Obstetrics & Gynecology, 102*(4), 806–815.

95. Kelly, T. F., & T. J. (2009). Gastrointestinal disease in pregnancy. In *Creasy & Resnik's Maternal-Fetal Medicine: Principles and Practice* (6th ed.). Saunders Elsevier.

96. Keser, N. (2006). Echocardiography in pregnant women. *Anadolu Kardiyoloji Dergisi, 6*(2), 169–173.

97. Kline, J. A., Williams, G. W., & Hernandez-Nino, J. (2005). D-dimer concentrations in normal pregnancy: New diagnostic thresholds are needed. *Clinical Chemistry, 51*(5), 825–829.

98. Koch, K. L. (2002). Gastrointestinal factors in nausea and vomiting of pregnancy. *American Journal of Obstetrics and Gynecology, 186*(5 Suppl Understanding), S198–S203.

99. Kovacs, C. S. (n.d.). Calcium metabolism during pregnancy and lactation. In *NCBI Bookshelf*. Retrieved from: http://www.ncbi.nlm.nih.gov/books/NBK279173/ (accessed on 6 September 2024).

100. Krop, M., & Danser, A. H. (2008). Circulating versus tissue renin-angiotensin system: On the origin of (pro)renin. *Current Hypertension Reports, 10*(2), 112–118.

101. Leboulanger, N., Louvet, N., Rigouzzo, A., et al. (2014). Pregnancy is associated with a decrease in pharyngeal but not tracheal or laryngeal cross-sectional area: A pilot study using the acoustic reflection method. *International Journal of Obstetric Anesthesia, 23*(1), 35–39.

102. Lechmanova, M., Kittnar, O., Mlcek, M., et al. (2002). QT dispersion and T-loop morphology in late pregnancy and after delivery. *Physiological Research, 51*(2), 121–129.

103. Lindseth, G., & Bird-Baker, M. Y. (2004). Risk factors for cholelithiasis in pregnancy. *Research in Nursing & Health, 27*(6), 382–391.

104. Linheimer, M. D., Barron, W. M., & Davison, J. M. (1991). Osmotic and volume control of vasopressin release in pregnancy. *American Journal of Kidney Diseases, 17*, 105.

105. Locktich, G. (1997). Clinical biochemistry of pregnancy. *Critical Reviews in Clinical Laboratory Sciences, 34*, 6.

106. Lumbers, E. R., & Pringle, K. G. (2014). Roles of the circulating renin-angiotensin-aldosterone system in human pregnancy. *American Journal of Physiology: Regulatory, Integrative and Comparative Physiology, 306*(2), R91–R101.

107. Luppi, P., Haluszczak, C., Trucco, M., et al. (2002). Normal pregnancy is associated with peripheral leukocyte activation. *American Journal of Reproductive Immunology, 47*(2), 72–81.

108. Magriples, U., Boynton, M. H., Kershaw, T. S., et al. (2013). Blood pressure changes during pregnancy: Impact of race, body mass index, and weight gain. *American Journal of Perinatology, 30*(5), 415–424. https://doi.org/10.1055/s-0032-1326987.

109. Mandal, D., Saha, M. M., & Pal, D. K. (2017). Urological disorders and pregnancy: An overall experience. *Urology Annals, 9*(1), 32–36.

110. Mandel, J., & Weinberger, S. E. (2004). Pulmonary diseases. In *Medical Complications of Pregnancy* (6th ed.). Saunders Elsevier.

111. Mandic-Markovic, V. D., Mikovic, Z. M., Djukic, M. K., et al. (2014). Doppler parameters of the maternal hepatic artery blood flow in normal pregnancy: Maternal hepatic artery blood flow in normal pregnancy. *European Journal of Obstetrics, Gynecology, and Reproductive Biology, 181*, 275–279.

112. Mazaki-Tovi, S., Kanety, H., Pariente, C., et al. (2011). Insulin sensitivity in late gestational and early postpartum period: The role of circulating maternal adipokines. *Gynecological Endocrinology, 27*, 725–731.

113. McAuliffe, F., Kametas, N., Costello, J., et al. (2002). Respiratory function in singleton and twin pregnancy. *BJOG: An International Journal of Obstetrics and Gynecology, 109*(7), 765–769.

114. McLean, K. C., Bernstein, I. M., & Brummel-Ziedins, K. E. (2012). Tissue factor-dependent thrombin generation across pregnancy. *American Journal of Obstetrics and Gynecology, 207*(2), 135.e1–e6.

115. Michimata, T., Sakai, M., Miyazaki, S., Aoki, K., et al. (2003). Decrease of T-helper 2 and T-cytotoxic 2 cells at implantation sites occurs in unexplained recurrent spontaneous abortion with normal chromosomal content. *Human Reproduction, 18*(7), 1523–1528.

116. Mikhail, M. S., & Anyaegbunam, A. (1995). Lower urinary tract dysfunction in pregnancy: A review. *Obstetrical & Gynecological Survey, 50*(9), 675–683.

117. Milman, N. (2006). Iron and pregnancy–A delicate balance. *Annals of Hematology, 85*(9), 559–565.

118. Monga, M. (2009). Maternal cardiovascular, respiratory, and renal adaptation to pregnancy. In *Creasy & Resnik's Maternal-Fetal Medicine: Principles and Practice* (6th ed.). Saunders Elsevier.

119. Moon, R. J., Harvey, N. C., & Cooper, C. (2015). Endocrinology in pregnancy: Influence of maternal vitamin D status on obstetric outcomes and the fetal skeleton. *European Journal of Endocrinology, 173*(2), R69–R83.

120. Morris, S. N., & Johnson, N. R. (2005). Exercise during pregnancy: A critical appraisal of the literature. *The Journal of Reproductive Medicine, 50*(3), 181–188.

121. Muallem, M. M., & Rubeiz, N. G. (2006). Physiological and biological skin changes in pregnancy. *Clinical Dermatology, 24*(2), 80–83.

122. Murphy, V. E., & Gibson, P. G. (2011). Asthma in pregnancy. *Clinical Chest Medicine, 32*(1), 93–110.

123. Nelson-Piercy, C. (2015). *Handbook of Obstetric Medicine* (5th ed.). CRC Press.

124. Newbern, D., & Freemark, M. (2011). Placental hormones and the control of maternal metabolism and fetal growth. *Current Opinion in Endocrinology, Diabetes and Obesity, 18*, 409–416.

125. Niebyl, J. R., & Goodwin, J. M. (2002). Overview of nausea and vomiting of pregnancy with an emphasis on vitamins and ginger. *American Journal of Obstetrics and Gynecology, 186*(5 Suppl Understanding), S253–S255.

126. Odutayo, A., & Hladunewich, M. (2012). Obstetric nephrology: Renal hemodynamic and metabolic physiology in normal pregnancy. *Clinical Journal of the American Society of Nephrology, 7*(12), 2073–2080.

127. Ogueh, O., Clough, A., Hancock, M., et al. (2011). A longitudinal study of the control of renal and uterine hemodynamic changes of pregnancy. *Hypertension in Pregnancy, 30*(3), 243–259.

128. Ouzounian, J. G., & Elkayam, U. (2012). Physiologic changes during normal pregnancy and delivery. *Cardiology Clinics, 30*(3), 317–329.

129. Pacheco, L., Costantine, M. M., & Hankins, G. D. V. (2013). Physiologic changes during pregnancy. In *Clinical Pharmacology During Pregnancy* (pp. 5–14). Academic Press.

130. Parry, E., Shields, R., & Turnbull, A. C. (1970). Transit time in the small intestine in pregnancy. *The Journal of Obstetrics and Gynecology of the British Commonwealth, 77*(10), 900–901.

131. Pelech, A. N. (2004). The physiology of cardiac auscultation. *Pediatric Clinics of North America, 51*(6), 1515–1535, vii–viii.

132. Peña-Rosas, J. P., De-Regil, L. M., Dowswell, T., et al. (2012). Daily oral iron supplementation during pregnancy. *The Cochrane Database of Systematic Reviews, 12*, CD004736.

133. Podymow, T., August, P., & Akbari, A. (2010). Management of renal disease in pregnancy. *Obstetrics and Gynecology Clinics of North America, 37*(2), 195–210.

134. Polyzos, N. P., Polyzos, I. P., Mauri, D., et al. (2009). Effect of periodontal disease treatment during pregnancy on preterm birth incidence: A meta-analysis of randomized trials. *American Journal of Obstetrics and Gynecology, 200*(3), 225–232.

135. Prager, D., & Braunstein, G. (1995). Pituitary disorders during pregnancy. *Endocrinology and Metabolism Clinics of North America, 24*, 1.

136. Quartarone, G. (2013). Gastroesophageal reflux in pregnancy: A systematic review on the benefit of raft-forming agents. *Minerva Gynecological, 65*(5), 541–549.

137. Ramsay, M. (2010). *The Obstetric Hematology Manual.* Cambridge University Press. In Pavord, S., & Hunt, B. (Eds.), Normal hematological changes during pregnancy and the puerperium (pp. 3–12).

138. Rasmussen, P. E., & Nielsen, F. R. (1988). Hydronephrosis during pregnancy: A literature survey. *European Journal of Obstetrics, Gynecology, and Reproductive Biology, 27*(3), 249–259.

139. Regal, J. F., Gilbert, J. S., & Burwick, R. M. (2015). The complement system and adverse pregnancy outcomes. *Molecular Immunology, 67*(1), 56–70.

140. Reyes-Zuniga, M., & Torre-Bouscoulet, L. (2016). Obstructive sleep apnea and perinatal risk. *Revista de Investigación Clínica: Organo del Hospital de Enfermedades de la Nutrición, 68*(6), 281–285.

141. Richani, K., Soto, E., Romero, R., et al. (2005). Normal pregnancy is characterized by systemic activation of the complement system. *Journal of Maternal-Fetal & Neonatal Medicine, 17*(4), 239–245.

142. Richter, J. E. (2005). Review article: The management of heartburn in pregnancy. *Alimentary Pharmacology & Therapeutics, 22*(9), 749–757.

143. Ringholm, L., Pedersen-Bjergaard, U., Thorsteinsson, B., et al. (2011). Atrial natriuretic peptide (ANP) in early pregnancy is associated with development of preeclampsia in type 1 diabetes. *Diabetes Research and Clinical Practice, 93*(3), e106–e109.

144. Roberts, M., Lindheimer, M. D., & Davison, J. M. (1996). Altered glomerular permselectivity to neutral dextrans and heteroporous membrane modeling in human pregnancy. *American Journal of Physiology, 270*(2 Pt 2), F338–F343.

145. Robson, S. C., Hunter, S., Boys, R. J., et al. (1989). Serial study of factors influencing changes in cardiac output during human pregnancy. *American Journal of Physiology, 256*(4 Pt 2), H1060–H1065.

146. Rodger, M., Sheppard, D., Gandara, E., & Tinmouth, A. (2015). Haematological problems in obstetrics. *Best Practice & Research Clinical Obstetrics & Gynecology, 29*(5), 671–684.

147. Roy, C., Saussine, C., Jahn, C., et al. (1995). Fast imaging MR assessment of ureterohydronephrosis during pregnancy. *Magnetic Resonance Imaging, 13*(6), 767–772.

148. Rubler, S., Damani, P. M., & Pinto, E. R. (1977). Cardiac size and performance during pregnancy estimated with echocardiography. *American Journal of Cardiology, 40*(4), 534–540.

149. Ruiz-Extremera, A., Lopez-Garrido, M. A., Barranco, E., et al. (2005). Activity of hepatic enzymes from week sixteen of pregnancy. *American Journal of Obstetrics and Gynecology, 193*(6), 2010–2016.

150. Schrier, R. W. (2010). Systemic arterial vasodilation, vasopressin, and vasopressinase in pregnancy. *Journal of the American Society of Nephrology, 21*(4), 570–572.

151. Sharma, S., Brugnara, C., Betensky, R. A., et al. (2015). Reductions in red blood cell 2,3-diphosphoglycerate concentration during continuous renal replacement therapy. *Clinical Journal of the American Society of Nephrology, 10*(1), 74–79.

152. Shehata, N., Burrows, R., & Kelton, J. G. (1999). Gestational thrombocytopenia. *Clinical Obstetrics and Gynecology, 42*(2), 327–334.

153. Shrotri, K. N., Morrison, I. D., & Shrotri, N. C. (2007). Urological conditions in pregnancy: A

diagnostic and therapeutic challenge. *Journal of Obstetrics and Gynecology, 27*(7), 648–654.

154. Soma-Pillay, P., Catherine, N. P., Tolppanen, H., et al. (2016). Physiological changes in pregnancy. *Cardiovascular Journal of Africa, 27*(2), 89–94.
155. Stephansson, O., Dickman, P. W., Johansson, A., et al. (2000). Maternal hemoglobin concentration during pregnancy and risk of stillbirth. *JAMA, 284*(20), 2611–2617.
156. Sturgiss, S. N., Dunlop, W., & Davison, J. M. (1994). Renal haemodynamics and tubular function in human pregnancy. *Baillière's Clinical Obstetrics and Gynecology, 8*(2), 209–234.
157. Sunitha, M., Chandrasekharappa, S., & Brid, S. V. (2014). Electrocardiographic QRS axis, Q wave, and T-wave changes in the 2nd and 3rd trimester of normal pregnancy. *Journal of Clinical and Diagnostic Research, 8*(9), BC17–BC21.
158. Tan, E. K., & Tan, E. L. (2013). Alterations in physiology and anatomy during pregnancy. *Best Practice & Research Clinical Obstetrics & Gynecology, 27*(6), 791–802.
159. Templeton, A., & Kelman, G. R. (1976). Maternal blood-gases, (PAO2–PaO2), physiological shunt, and VD/VT in normal pregnancy. *British Journal of Anesthesia, 48*, 1001.
160. Thaxter Nesbeth, K. A., Samuels, L. A., Nicholson Daley, C., et al. (2016). Ptyalism in pregnancy–A review of epidemiology and practices. *European Journal of Obstetrics, Gynecology, and Reproductive Biology, 198*, 47–49.
161. Thomsen, J. K., Fogh-Andersen, N., Jaszczak, P., et al. (1993). Atrial natriuretic peptide (ANP) decreases during normal pregnancy as related to hemodynamic changes and volume regulation. *Acta Obstetricia et Gynecologica Scandinavica, 72*(2), 103–110.
162. Tkachenko, O., Shchekochikhin, D., & Schrier, R. W. (2014). Hormones and hemodynamics in pregnancy. *International Journal of Endocrinology and Metabolism, 12*(2), e14098.
163. Torgersen, K. (2006). Complications of the childbearing experience. In S. Nettina (Ed.), *Lippincott Manual for Nursing Practice* (8th ed., pp. 1259–1306). Philadelphia: Lippincott.
164. Torgersen, K. L., & Curran, C. A. (2006). A systematic approach to the physiologic adaptations of pregnancy. *Critical Care Nursing Quarterly, 29*(1), 2–19.
165. Tsai, C. H., & de Leeuw, N. K. (1982). Changes in 2,3-diphosphoglycerate during pregnancy and puerperium in normal women and in beta-thalassemia heterozygous women. *American Journal of Obstetrics and Gynecology, 142*(5), 520–523.
166. Ueland, K., & Hansen, J. M. (1969). Maternal cardiovascular dynamics. II. Posture and uterine contractions. *American Journal of Obstetrics and Gynecology, 103*(1), 1–7.
167. Uppal, A., Uppal, S., Pinto, A., et al. (2010). The effectiveness of periodontal disease treatment during pregnancy in reducing the risk of experiencing preterm birth and low birth weight: A meta-analysis. *Journal of the American Dental Association, 141*(12), 1423–1434.
168. Valera, M. C., Parant, O., Vayssière, C., et al. (2010). Physiologic and pathologic changes of platelets in pregnancy. *Platelets, 21*(8), 587–595.
169. Van Thiel, D. H., Gavaler, J. S., Joshi, S. N., et al. (1977). Heartburn of pregnancy. *Gastroenterology, 72*(4 Pt 1), 666–668.
170. Varga, I., Rigo, J., Jr., Somos, P., et al. (2000). Analysis of maternal circulation and renal function in physiologic pregnancies: Parallel examinations of the changes in the cardiac output and the glomerular filtration rate. *Journal of Maternal-Fetal & Neonatal Medicine, 9*(2), 97–104.

171. Verberg, M. F., Gillot, D. J., Al-Fardan, N., & Grudzinskas, J. G. (2005). Hyperemesis gravidarum: A literature review. *Human Reproduction Update, 11*(5), 527–539.

172. Vinturache, A. E., Gyamfi-Bannerman, C., Hwang, J., et al. (2016). Maternal microbiome–A pathway to preterm birth. *Seminars in Fetal & Neonatal Medicine, 21*(2), 94–99.

173. Whittaker, P. G., Macphail, S., & Lind, T. (1996). Serial hematologic changes and pregnancy outcome. *Obstetrics & Gynecology, 88*(1), 33–39.

174. Whitty, J. E., & Dombrowski, M. P. (2009). Respiratory diseases in pregnancy. In *Creasy & Resnik's Maternal-Fetal Medicine: Principles and Practice* (6th ed., pp. [specific pages]). Saunders Elsevier.

175. Wilson, M., Morganti, A. A., Zervoudakis, I., Letcher, R. L., Romney, B. M., & Von Oeyon, P. (1980). Blood pressure, the renin-aldosterone system, and sex steroids throughout normal pregnancy. *American Journal of Medicine, 68*(1), 97–104.

176. Wise, R. A., Polito, A. J., & Krishnan, V. (2006). Respiratory physiologic changes in pregnancy. *Immunology and Allergy Clinics of North America, 26*(1), 1–12.

177. Woodrow, J. P., Sharpe, C. J., Fudge, N. J., Hoff, A. O., Gagel, R. F., & Kovacs, C. S. (2006). Calcitonin plays a critical role in regulating skeletal mineral metabolism during lactation. *Endocrinology, 147*, 4010–4021.

178. World Health Organization. (2011). Hemoglobin concentrations for the diagnosis of anemia and assessment of severity. *Vitamin and Mineral Nutrition Information System*. Geneva: World Health Organization.

179. Yoshimatsu, J., Matsumoto, H., Goto, K., et al. (2006). Relationship between urinary albumin and serum soluble fms-like tyrosine kinase 1 (sFlt-1) in normal pregnancy. *European Journal of Obstetrics, Gynecology, and Reproductive Biology, 128*(1–2), 204–208.

Chapter 3

PRENATAL CARE

Contents

Introduction

Antenatal care, another name for prenatal care, is a subset of preventive medicine. It is given in the form of medical checkups that include advice on leading a healthy lifestyle and medical information about biological changes, physiological changes in the mother during pregnancy, and prenatal nutrition, including prenatal vitamins. This helps to prevent potential health issues throughout the pregnancy and supports the health of both the mother and the unborn child (Rodreck et al., 2021). Prenatal screening and diagnosis, along with routine care, have contributed to a decrease in the incidence of low birth weight, infections in newborns, miscarriages, maternal deaths, and other avoidable health issues.

Traditional prenatal care in high-income countries generally consists of:

- monthly visits during the first two trimesters (from the 1st week to the 28th week)
- fortnightly visits from the 28th week to the 36th week of pregnancy
- weekly visits after 36th week to the delivery, from the 38th week to the 42nd week
- Assessment of parental needs and family dynamics

The conventional approach to prenatal care emerged in the early 1900s, and the body of research supporting its superiority is fairly thin (Dowswell et al., 2015). Antenatal care is labor-intensive and can be expensive.

Orientation and Directional Terms

Term	Definition	Illustration
Amenorrhea	Amenorrhea is the medical term for the absence of a menstrual period in a female who has reached reproductive age. It can be a symptom of another condition, but it's not a disease itself.	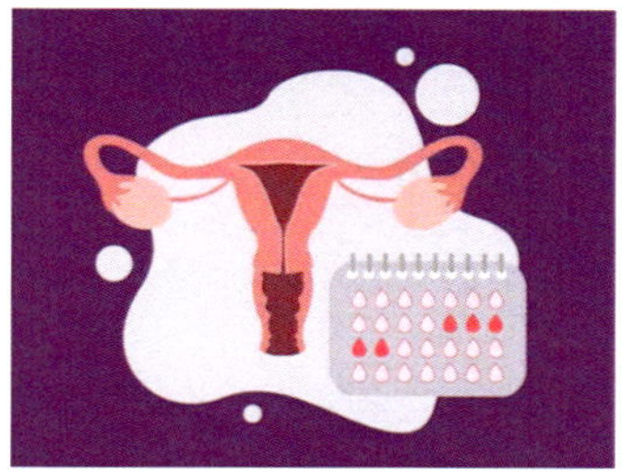
Antenatal care	Antenatal care is a type of preventive healthcare that helps protect the health of pregnant women and their unborn children. It includes medical checkups, tests, scans, and discussions with health professionals.	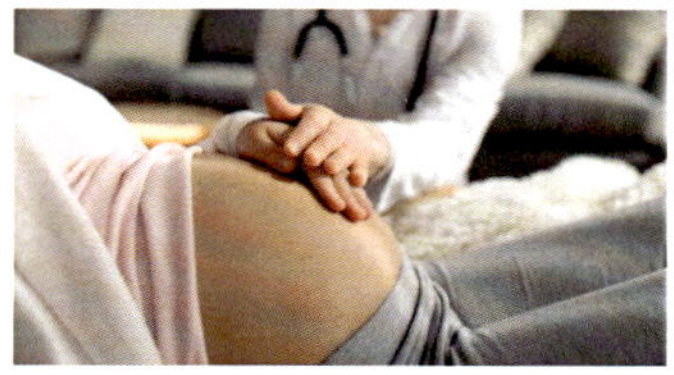
Antiemetics	Antiemetics are drugs that treat or prevent nausea and vomiting. They are commonly used to treat motion sickness, chemotherapy-induced nausea and vomiting, and side effects of general anesthetics and opioid analgesics.	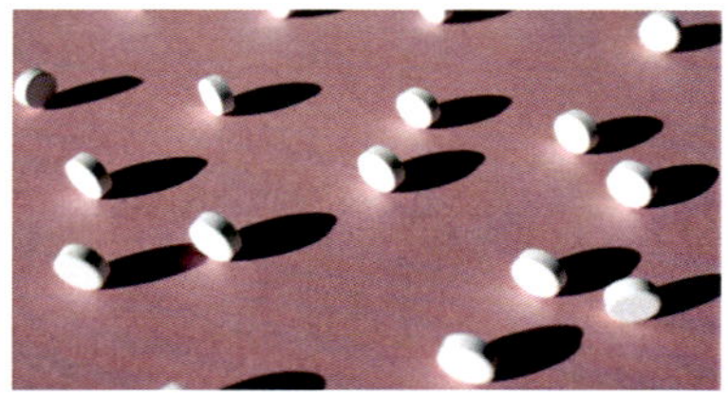
Fatigue	Fatigue is a common complaint during pregnancy, especially in the first and third trimesters. It's a normal sign that your body is adjusting to the changes of pregnancy, such as increased blood volume, hormonal changes, and weight gain.	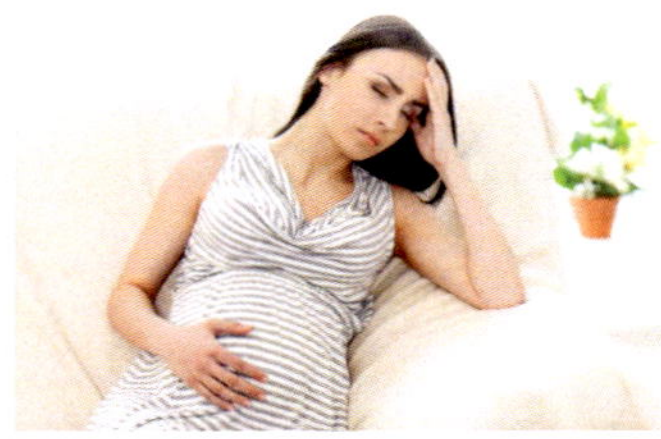
Neonatal infections	Neonatal infections are infections of the neonate (newborn) acquired during prenatal development or within the first four weeks of life.	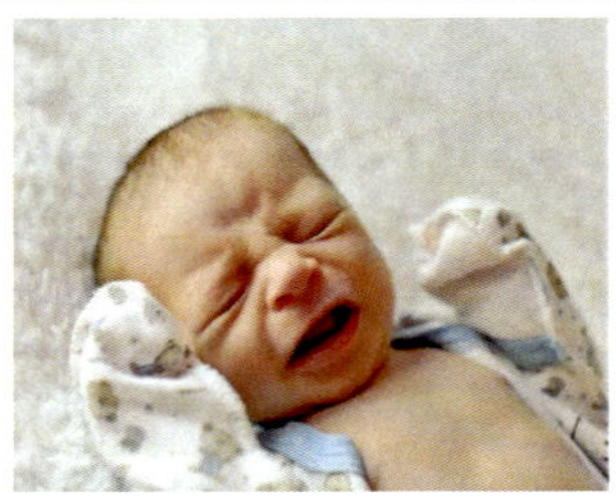
Teratogenic drugs	A teratogenic drug is a substance that can cause birth defects or developmental malformations in a fetus when taken by a pregnant woman.	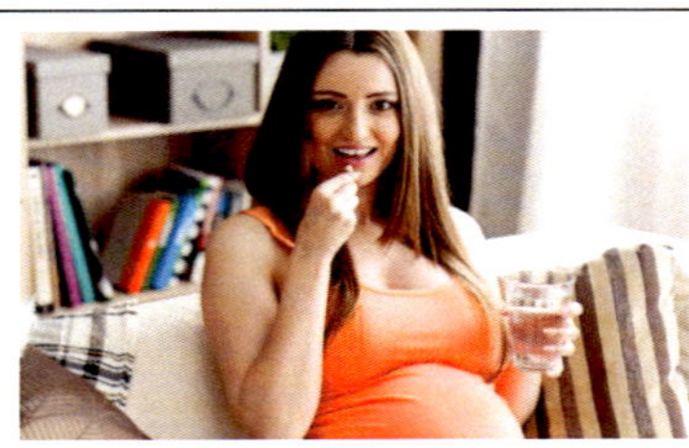

3.1. Diagnosis of Pregnancy

The date of the birth and the presence of a high-risk status are both determined by the medical diagnosis of pregnancy. The diagnosis brings with it a profound sense of accomplishment and fulfillment if the pregnancy was planned. It can cause an equally severe crisis state if it is not anticipated or desired.

Most women make an effort to eat a more nutrient-dense diet, quit drinking and smoking, and cease taking unnecessary medications as soon as their pregnancy is confirmed. Early pregnancy confirmation is crucial because a woman might not take these actions before receiving her pregnancy confirmation. Early diagnosis and therapeutic pregnancy termination are essential if a woman decides she does not want to carry her pregnancy to term. This ensures the safest possible outcome.

To prevent radiation exposure to the fetus, you might recommend that a sexually active woman who is scheduled for diagnostic testing that involves a pelvic x-ray study, such as an intravenous pyelogram for kidney disease, first have a rapid serum pregnancy test to rule out pregnancy as a possibility.

Based on a variety of subjective indicators, the majority of women who visit a medical facility to receive a pregnancy diagnosis have already made this determination. The majority have already verified their own pregnancy with a home pregnancy test.

Official pregnancy diagnoses are made based on the symptoms that the woman reports having and the indicators that a medical professional notices. Traditionally, three categories have been used to categorize these signs and symptoms: positive or documented, probable or objective, and presumptive or subjective (Table 3.1).

Table 3.1. Presumptive, Probable, and Positive Signs of Pregnancy

Time From Implantation (Weeks)	Presumptive Finding	Probable Finding	Positive Finding	Description
1		Serum laboratory tests		Tests of blood serum reveal the presence of human chorionic gonadotropin hormone.
2	Breast changes			Feeling of tenderness, fullness, or tingling; enlargement and darkening of areola
2	Nausea, vomiting			Nausea or vomiting on arising
2	Amenorrhea			Absence of menstruation
3	Frequent urination			Sense of having to void more often than usual
6		Chadwick's sign		Color change of the vagina from pink to violet
6		Goodell's sign		Softening of the cervix
6		Hegar's sign		Softening of the lower uterine segment

6		Evidence on ultrasound of gestational sac		Characteristic ring is evident.
8			Evidence on ultrasound of fetal outline	Fetal outline can be seen and measured by ultrasound.
10–12			Fetal heart audible	Doppler ultrasound reveals heartbeat.
12	Fatigue			General feeling of tiredness
12	Uterine enlargement			Uterus can be palpated over symphysis pubis.
16		Ballottement		When lower uterine segment is tapped on a bimanual examination, the fetus can be felt to rise against abdominal wall.
18	Quickening			Fetal movement felt by woman
20			Fetal movement felt by examiner	Fetal movement can be palpated through abdomen.
20		Braxton Hicks contractions		Periodic uterine tightening occurs.
20		Fetal outline felt by examiner		Fetal outline can be palpated through abdomen.
24	Linea nigra			Line of dark pigment on the abdomen
24	Melasma			Dark pigment on face
24	Striae gravidarum			Red streaks on abdomen

Source: Adele Pillitteri. Maternal & Child Health Nursing: Care of the Childbearing & Childrearing Family. Lippincott Williams & Wilkins. ISBN 978-1-58255-999-5.

3.1.1. Presumptive (Subjective) Signs of Pregnancy

The least suggestive signs of pregnancy are the ones that, when considered separately, could easily point to other medical conditions (Rojas, Wood, & Blakemore, 2007). The woman experiences these findings, which are discussed concerning the body system in which they occur, but an examiner is unable to record them (Figure 3.1).

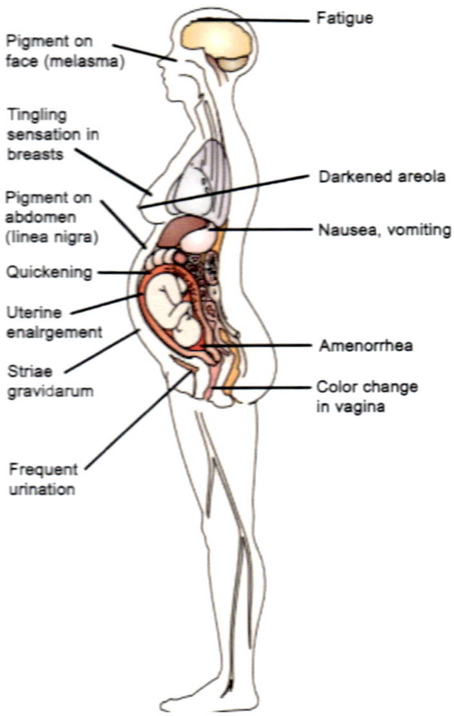

Figure 3.1. *Assessing the client for presumptive signs of pregnancy.*

Source: Adele Pillitteri. Maternal & Child Health Nursing: Care of the Childbearing & Childrearing Family. Lippincott Williams & Wilkins. ISBN 978–1-58255–999–5.

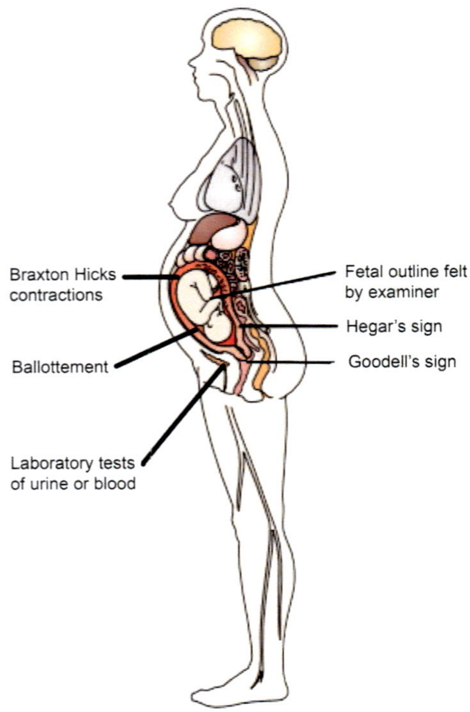

Figure 3.2. *Assessing the client for probable signs of pregnancy.*

Source: Adele Pillitteri. Maternal & Child Health Nursing: Care of the Childbearing & Childrearing Family. Lippincott Williams & Wilkins. ISBN 978–1-58255–999–5.

3.1.2. Probable Signs of Pregnancy

Probable pregnancy symptoms, as opposed to presumed ones, are objective and can be recorded by an examiner. They are not positive or accurate diagnostic findings, despite being more trustworthy than presumed indications (Figure 3.2). They are also talked about in relation to the particular bodily system that experiences them.

3.1.2.1. Laboratory Tests

Pregnancy-related laboratory tests typically involve looking for human chorionic gonadotropin (hCG), a hormone produced by the placenta's chorionic villi, in the pregnant woman's blood or urine. Positive results from these tests are regarded as probable rather than positive signs because all laboratory tests for pregnancy are only 95–98% accurate in diagnosing pregnancy.

Techniques such as radioreceptor assay (RRA), enzyme-linked immunosorbent assay (ELISA), and radioimmunoassay (RIA) are used to conduct these tests. International units are used to measure hCG for these tests. Since there are no trophoblast cells generating hCG in the nonpregnant woman, no units are visible. Traces of hCG can be detected in the serum of a pregnant woman as soon as 24 to 48 hours after implantation. Approximately 50 mIU/mL is the measurable level that they reach 7 to 9 days after conception. Peak levels occur between the 60th and 80th day of gestation, at approximately 100 mIU/mL. Following that, the level of hCG drops once more until it is hardly noticeable in serum or urine at term.

Due to the earlier results of blood serum tests, urine, which was once widely used for pregnancy testing, is now rarely used in medical settings. Home pregnancy tests still rely on urine testing.

3.1.2.2. Home Pregnancy Tests

Over-the-counter pregnancy test kits based on immunologic reactions are available in several varieties. If the guidelines are strictly followed, these tests have a high degree of accuracy (about 97 percent). Because waiting for a doctor's appointment to confirm a pregnancy can be a nervous and stressful time for many women, they are practical to use. The woman administers this kind of test by dipping a reagent strip into her urine stream. Pregnancy is indicated by a change in color on the strip. As little as 35 mIU/mL of hCG can be found with home tests. They take three to five minutes to complete. The majority of manufacturers advise against testing women until the day of the missed menstrual period. Women who suspect they may be pregnant but receive a negative result from a home pregnancy test should be advised to retest the test after a week if they are still experiencing amenorrhea. If symptoms don't go away after two tests, she should visit a doctor because she may have an ovarian tumor, which could be the cause of her amenorrhea. An accurate diagnosis is necessary for this condition. Ladies using psychiatric medications (e.g., anxiety medications) may cause pregnancy tests to come back falsely positive. Oral contraceptive users may also experience false-positive test results; for this type of test to be reliable, the use of oral contraceptives should have stopped five days before the test. False-positive results can also occur in women with hyperthyroidism, proteinuria, and postmenopausal syndrome.

In the past, getting an official pregnancy diagnosis was one of the main reasons women sought out early prenatal care. Because test kits now allow women to diagnose their pregnancies at home, some women may wait to seek prenatal care until their pregnancy seems abnormal or until they are so far along that they feel it is time to start thinking about getting birth insurance. Warn women that in order to protect the outcome of their pregnancy, early and consistent prenatal care is essential. Making plans for prenatal care should come first in the event of a positive pregnancy test (Bernstein & Weinstein, 2007).

3.1.3. Positive Signs of Pregnancy

There are only three documented or positive signs of pregnancy:

- Demonstration of a fetal heart separate from the mother's
- Fetal movements felt by an examiner
- Visualization of the fetus by ultrasound

3.1.3.1. Demonstration of a Fetal Heart Separate from the Mother's Heart

As early as the sixth or seventh week of pregnancy, an ultrasound can reveal the presence of a beating fetal heart. Fetal heart sounds can be identified by ultrasonic monitoring systems as early as the tenth or twelfth week of pregnancy, thanks to the Doppler technique, which converts ultrasonic frequencies to audible frequencies. A heartbeat can be seen on an echocardiogram as early as five weeks.

The fetal heart begins to beat on the 24th day after conception, but it is not audible until approximately 18 to 20 weeks of pregnancy when the abdomen is auscultated with a standard stethoscope. When a woman has a lot of subcutaneous fat on her abdomen or when there is more amniotic fluid than usual, it can be difficult to hear the heartbeat of the fetus (hydramnios). They sound best when the stethoscope is placed over the fetus's back and the position of the fetus is ascertained by palpation. The typical range of a fetal heart rate is 120–160 beats per minute.

3.1.3.2. Fetal Movements Felt by an Examiner

A woman may experience fetal movements as early as weeks 16 to 20 of her pregnancy. Because a woman could confuse the movement of gas through her intestines for fetal movement, those felt by an impartial examiner are thought to be far more reliable. Unless a woman is extremely obese, an examiner can feel fetal movements between weeks 20 and 24 of pregnancy.

3.1.3.3. Visualization of Fetus by Ultrasound

Pregnancy can be diagnosed with high-frequency sound waves directed toward a woman's abdomen. As early as the fourth or sixth week of pregnancy, a woman carrying a child will exhibit a distinctive ring on an oscilloscope screen, signifying the gestational sac. This technique also provides information regarding the location of implantation and the presence of multiple pregnancies. By the eighth week, the fetal outline is visible enough within the sac to measure the length from the crown to the rump to determine the pregnancy's gestational age. For a couple, if they were still unsure that a woman is pregnant, seeing the fetal outline on an ultrasound removes all doubt.

3.2. Routine Screening and Diagnostic Tests

If you are pregnant, a variety of tests are available. These tests can both verify your pregnancy and track the growth of your unborn child inside you. Additionally, there are optional tests available that can reveal whether a pregnancy is impacted by a variety of conditions.

Pregnancy care should include routine check-ups with your doctor or midwife, as well as guidance and information about the tests you and your unborn child may require.

The different kinds of tests available to pregnant women include tests:

- to confirm pregnancy
- to monitor the health of the mother and the baby
- maternal health screening
- for specific medical problems (screening and diagnostic tests).

3.2.1. Tests to Confirm Pregnancy

The first clue that something is pregnant is typically a missed menstrual cycle. Human chorionic gonadotropin (βhCG), a pregnancy hormone, is detected in tests to confirm pregnancy.

The various tests include:

- **Home Test Kit**: these are available from pharmacies. A typical kit includes special paper that is sensitive to the presence of βhCG in urine. It is important to use a home test kit according to the manufacturer's instructions, or false results can occur. Always confirm your results with your doctor. Pregnancy tests taken by your doctor are rarely inaccurate.
- **Urine Test at the Doctor's Office**: the doctor can test your urine for βhCG.

- **Blood test:** a test of the βhCG levels in your blood can be accurate within one week or so of conception.

3.2.2. Prenatal Tests to Monitor the Health of the Mother and the Baby

Meeting with your doctor or midwife regularly to monitor the progress of your pregnancy and the growth of the unborn child is known as pregnancy care. This involves screenings to determine whether there are any possible pregnancy-related issues as well as assessments to determine your health and the health of your unborn child.

Routine prenatal tests may include:

- **Maternal health screening blood tests** at different stages of the pregnancy, such as blood group, iron levels, checks for maternal diabetes, immunity to rubella and other infections.
- **Ultrasound (first trimester)** – a painless, non-invasive scan done within the first 3 months of pregnancy. This can be used to confirm the number of babies and helps to calculate the date you are due to give birth. This is known as your estimated due date.
- **Ultrasound (second trimester)** – this is usually performed between 18 and 20 weeks. It is used to check the baby's development and monitor the size and location of the placenta. The baby's sex can often be determined (if you wish to know), although this may not be 100% accurate.
- **Ultrasound (third trimester)** – in the last 3 months of pregnancy, an ultrasound may be offered to check the baby's growth, fluid levels around the baby and the positioning of the placenta.

3.2.3. Tests for Specific Medical Conditions in Pregnancy

It is not required to get tested for certain medical conditions, such as Down syndrome, genetic disorders known to run in families, or neural tube abnormalities like spina bifida. Before deciding whether to move forward with these tests, a woman may want to talk through her options with her doctors or a genetic counselor.

3.2.4. Screening Tests and Diagnostic Tests in Pregnancy

It is critical to recognize the distinction between diagnostic and screening testing. Although they cannot give a definitive answer, screening tests can provide information about the likelihood that a baby may have a specific health issue. For instance, the results of a screening test could indicate a high or low chance, or they might give an estimate of the chance, like one in 1,000. A diagnostic test provides a more definite result.

3.2.4.1. Routine Screening Tests

Screening tests are used to identify individuals who are more likely to have a health issue. This implies that individuals can receive treatment sooner, which may be more effective, or make well-informed decisions regarding their health.

There are flaws in screening tests. When a person does not have a health condition, some people will be informed that they or their unborn child have a higher chance of having one. Furthermore, some individuals may receive information suggesting that they or their child have a lower likelihood of developing a health condition when, in reality, they do. While screening tests are not able to diagnose conditions, they can estimate the likelihood that a baby is impacted by a variety of conditions. If a screening test indicates a higher likelihood, additional testing can verify that finding.

Examples of routine screening tests include:

- **Combined First-Trimester Screening:** this test combines information from a first-trimester ultrasound (for example, a measurement taken from the back of the baby's neck known as the nuchal translucency) and a blood test from the mother (first-trimester maternal serum screening) to calculate the chance of a group of chromosome differences, including Down syndrome.
- **Second-Trimester Maternal Serum Screening**: this is a maternal blood test that helps to determine the chance of some conditions that may affect the unborn baby, such as chromosome differences (including Down syndrome) or neural tube defects (such as spina bifida).
- **Non-Invasive Prenatal Testing (NIPT, Also Known as Cell-Free DNA Screening)**: is a blood test that looks at the baby's genetic material (DNA), which can be found in the mother's bloodstream. It can provide information about the chance of conditions such as Down syndrome and some other chromosome differences and can be done any time from 10 weeks into the pregnancy. It is more accurate than combined first-trimester screening or second-trimester maternal serum screening, but it is more costly than the screening tests.

3.2.4.2. Diagnostic Tests

Certain pregnancies are known to carry a higher risk of a specific condition. For instance, the mother might be older (we know that the chance of having a baby with a chromosome difference such as Down syndrome increases with age) or there might be a family history of an inherited disorder. In other situations, a pregnancy screening test might have indicated a higher risk of a specific ailment. More precise information regarding the existence of a condition can be obtained through a diagnostic test. Certain diagnostic tests involve taking a sample of placenta or amniotic fluid with a needle, and there is a slight chance of complications, such as miscarriage.

Diagnostic tests include:

- **Ultrasound:** may be used to check the health of the baby in the case of unusual pregnancy symptoms, such as vaginal bleeding or lack of fetal movement.
- **Chorionic Villus Sampling (CVS)**: a test that checks for specific medical conditions by taking a sample of the placenta. The placenta was originally formed from the same cells as the baby, so testing a small sample of the placenta can provide information about the baby. To collect the sample, the doctor inserts a slender needle through the mother's abdomen. The needle is guided with the help of ultrasound. The tissue (known as a chorionic villus sample) is then examined in a laboratory.
- **Amniocentesis**: a doctor inserts a slender needle through the abdomen to withdraw a small amount of amniotic fluid, the fluid that surrounds the baby in the womb. This fluid sample contains some of the baby's cells which have been shed as the baby grows, and these are then examined in the laboratory.

3.2.5. Making Decisions About Diagnostic Testing in Pregnancy

Approximately 20% of pregnant women receive a pregnancy-related concern. A normal pregnancy is the outcome for many women who receive an increased chance result on a screening test since these tests are not able to provide exact information.

The woman and her family, after consulting with her physician or midwife, decide whether to pursue additional testing to determine whether a condition is present.

Diagnostic tests may be considered for a range of reasons. For example, if a diagnostic test confirms the presence of a medical condition:

- Some abnormalities can be surgically corrected while the baby is still in the uterus.
- A woman and her baby may need specialist care before, during and after at the birth.
- Knowing in advance that the baby has a particular condition may provide a family with time to prepare.
- Depending on the condition identified in diagnostic testing, some women or families may decide not to continue a pregnancy and arrange a termination of pregnancy (abortion).

3.2.6. Immunizations in Pregnancy

Immunizations can guard against a variety of infectious diseases for both you and your unborn child. Under the National Immunization Program, the seasonal influenza vaccine—often referred to as the "flu shot"—is advised and financially supported for all expectant mothers. The flu shot protects you and your unborn child for the first six months of life and is safe to receive at any point during pregnancy. Pregnant women can receive the whooping cough combination vaccine, commonly referred to as the "three-in-one dTpa vaccine," for free as early as week twenty. The vaccination protects against tetanus, diphtheria, and whooping cough, commonly known as pertussis. If you are trying to become pregnant, are nursing a child, or are pregnant, you can receive the COVID-19 vaccine.

3.2.7. Best Practice for Health Professionals Talking to Families About Screening and Test Results

Prenatal screening was the subject of research by Down Syndrome Australia, which discovered that 49% of families felt pressured to end their pregnancy by medical professionals, 42% received inaccurate information about the condition, and 45% did not feel they received enough support during their pregnancy.

It is imperative that medical professionals give families time to make an educated decision and accurate, balanced information both before and after prenatal screening and diagnostic testing.

Medical practitioners must also:

- Deliver high chance or confirmed diagnosis results using neutral language (e.g., 'chance' rather than 'risk,' factual delivery of a diagnosis without emotive terms such as 'I'm sorry' or 'bad news').
- Provide up-to-date, evidenced-based information on Down syndrome and other conditions being screened for, both before screening and after results are given.
- Offer referrals to peer support services such as local Down syndrome associations.
- Offer non-directive counseling and support services both before and after a decision is made on whether to continue the pregnancy.
- Give respect for decisions made by families, and not revisit that decision once it has been communicated while making it clear that they have a right to change their mind.

3.3. Common Health Problems During Pregnancy

You may experience heightened emotions and concerns upon discovering your pregnancy. You may be equally as nervous about something going wrong as you are about this new person you are bringing into the world.

Most pregnancies go forward uneventfully. However, about 8% of pregnancies have issues that could harm the mother or the unborn child if they are not treated. Certain complications arise spontaneously and cannot be avoided, while others are related to pre-existing health issues.

Hearing that a complication has been diagnosed by the doctors can be unsettling. Both your own and your baby's health may be causing you concern. You might even experience fear that this was brought on by something you did—or didn't do. These emotions are entirely typical. Knowing that these issues were not caused by anything you did may give you comfort. Furthermore, these issues are manageable. Getting prenatal care from a provider you trust is the best thing you can do for both you and your unborn child. You have a better chance of maintaining both your and your baby's health with early detection and appropriate care.

Pregnancy can cause health issues for some women. These issues may pertain to the health of the fetus, the mother, or both. Health problems can arise even in women who are otherwise healthy before pregnancy. These issues could turn the pregnancy into a high-risk one.

By allowing medical professionals to identify, treat, or manage conditions before they worsen, receiving early and consistent prenatal care can help lower the risk of issues. Identification of pregnancy-related mental health issues like anxiety and depression is another benefit of prenatal care. Some common complications of pregnancy include, but are not limited to, the following.

3.3.1. High Blood Pressure

Reduced artery flow from the heart to the body's organs results in high blood pressure, also known as hypertension. The arteries' pressure rises as a result. This can make it more difficult for blood to get to the placenta during pregnancy, which gives the fetus oxygen and nutrition. Decreased blood flow can cause the fetus to grow more slowly and increase the mother's risk of preterm labor and preeclampsia.

Pregnant women with high blood pressure will need to keep an eye on it and manage it during their pregnancy, possibly with medication. Gestational hypertension is a term used to describe high blood pressure that occurs during pregnancy. Gestational hypertension usually manifests in the second half of pregnancy and resolves postpartum.

3.3.2. Gestational Diabetes

Gestational diabetes occurs when a woman who has never had diabetes before develops high blood sugar during pregnancy.

Normally, when food is broken down by the body, glucose—a type of sugar—is produced. Your body uses glucose as its primary energy source. The glucose enters your bloodstream after digestion and provides your body with energy.

Your pancreas produces the hormone insulin, which helps your body absorb glucose from the blood and use it in its cells. Gestational diabetes is a condition in which the body either produces insufficient insulin or uses it improperly due to hormonal changes brought on by pregnancy. Gestational diabetes is caused by an accumulation of glucose in the blood due to insufficient or improperly used insulin.

Controlling gestational diabetes through adherence to a physician's prescribed treatment plan is the most effective means of mitigating or averting complications linked to elevated blood sugar levels during pregnancy. If left unchecked, it can result in preeclampsia, which raises blood pressure, and having a big baby, which raises the risk of cesarean delivery.

3.3.3. Infections

During pregnancy and/or delivery, infections, including certain STIs, can occur. These infections can cause complications for the pregnant woman, the pregnancy, and the baby after delivery. Certain infections can spread from mother to child through the birth canal during childbirth, while other infections can affect a developing fetus during pregnancy. With the right prenatal, perinatal, and postpartum care, many of these infections can be avoided or treated. Some infections in pregnancy can cause or contribute to:

- Pregnancy loss/miscarriage (before 20 weeks of pregnancy)
- Ectopic pregnancy (when the embryo implants outside of the uterus, usually in a fallopian tube)
- Preterm labor and delivery (before 37 completed weeks of pregnancy)
- Low birth weight
- Birth defects, including blindness, deafness, bone deformities, and intellectual disability
- Stillbirth (at or after 20 weeks of pregnancy)
- Illness in the newborn period (first month of life)
- Newborn death
- Maternal health complications

Consult your healthcare provider about receiving vaccinations against chickenpox, also known as varicella, and rubella, also known as German measles, as well as booster shots before becoming pregnant if you intend to become pregnant. Additionally, you can receive certain vaccinations, like the flu shot, while you are expecting. To improve your chances of a successful pregnancy, discuss any infections you may have, such as STIs, with your doctor before becoming pregnant.

If an infection can be treated with medication, it can be found out early on in pregnancy through testing for STIs and other infections. Alternatively, as soon as possible during your pregnancy, disclose any infections you are aware of to your healthcare provider. The risk to the fetus and baby is reduced with early intervention. You and your healthcare provider can take precautions to safeguard your health and the health of your infant even if the infection cannot be cured.

3.3.4. Preeclampsia

Blood pressure that is dangerously high is a symptom of preeclampsia. If treatment is not received, it may be fatal. After 20 weeks of pregnancy, preeclampsia usually develops in women who have never had high blood pressure before.

Preeclampsia symptoms can include pain beneath the ribs, a strong headache, and vision changes. Many women, though, do not experience symptoms immediately. Usually, the first warning sign is when a woman with high blood pressure shows up for a routine prenatal visit. In those circumstances, in order to distinguish between preeclampsia and high blood pressure, your doctor will perform tests to assess liver and kidney function.

A dangerous medical condition called preeclampsia has the potential to cause preterm delivery and even death. Although the cause is unknown, some women are more susceptible than others. Risk factors include:

- First pregnancies
- Preeclampsia in a previous pregnancy
- Existing conditions such as high blood pressure, diabetes, kidney disease, and systemic lupus erythematosus
- Being 35 years of age or older
- Carrying two or more fetuses
- Obesity

Preeclampsia cannot be avoided, but maintaining good health may help during pregnancy. Experts advise seeing your obstetrician before getting pregnant or very early in the pregnancy if you have risk factors so you and your doctor can talk about ways to lower your risk. For instance, after the first trimester, many women who are at risk for preeclampsia are prescribed low dose aspirin.

The best way to manage preeclampsia is through routine prenatal visits. Your blood pressure will be taken by your doctor during those scheduled visits. If it's high, additional testing can identify the ailment and begin the necessary treatment.

The best course of treatment for preeclampsia is delivery since the condition only goes away after the baby is born. On the other hand, premature birth increases the baby's risk of health issues. The decision regarding your course of treatment will be primarily based on the stage of pregnancy. Hospitalization might be necessary so that your team can keep a close eye on both you and your infant.

Your physician will go over the advantages and disadvantages of going ahead with an early delivery vs extending the pregnancy and attempting to treat the preeclampsia for as long as possible using alternative techniques. The condition will go away after delivery, but you will have a higher chance of developing heart disease in the future. Discuss with your physician the steps you can take to mitigate and control those risks.

3.3.5. Preterm Labor

Labor that starts earlier than 37 weeks of pregnancy is known as preterm labor. The final weeks before a full-term delivery (39 to 40 weeks) are when organs like the brain and lungs finish developing, so any baby born before 37 weeks is usually at risk for health issues.

Preterm labor can result from a number of conditions, such as infections, shortened cervix development, or preterm births in the past.

In certain cases, progesterone, a hormone that is naturally produced during pregnancy, may be used to help prevent preterm birth.

3.3.6. Depression and Anxiety

Studies reveal that anxiety co-occurs in as many as 43% of depressed pregnant and postpartum women, and women reported frequent depressive symptoms following childbirth, making pregnancy-related anxiety and depression among the more common pregnancy complications. The mother's and her child's health may be significantly impacted by these medical conditions. The good news is that these illnesses are medically treatable.

3.3.7. Pregnancy Loss/Miscarriage

A pregnancy lost due to natural causes before 20 weeks of pregnancy is referred to as a miscarriage. Symptoms may include cramping, tissue or fluid leaking from the vagina, or vaginal spotting or bleeding. Vaginal bleeding, however, does not indicate that a miscarriage is occurring or will occur. If a woman notices this symptom at any stage of her pregnancy, she should speak with her doctor.

3.3.8. Stillbirth

A stillbirth occurs when a pregnancy ends after the 20th week of gestation. Medical professionals are unable to determine the cause of the loss in about half of all cases that are reported. However, chromosomal abnormalities, placental issues, low fetal growth, long-term mother health problems, and infection are among the medical conditions that can lead to stillbirth.

3.3.9. Other Complications

Other complications of pregnancy may include the following:

- **Severe, Persistent Nausea and Vomiting:** During pregnancy, nausea and vomiting are common, especially in the first trimester. However, some women have more severe symptoms that persist into the third trimester.

  It is unknown what causes hyperemesis gravidarum, a more severe version of this condition that is pronounced *HEYE-pur-EM-uh-suhss grav-uh-DAR-uhm*. Hyperemesis gravidarum causes persistent nausea in women, as well as weight loss, decreased appetite, dehydration, and dizziness.

  It might be necessary for affected women to stay in a hospital in order to receive nutrition and fluids. While some women experience the symptoms all the way through their pregnancy, others feel better after the 20th week.
- **Iron-Deficiency Anemia:** Because they are producing more blood than usual, pregnant women require more iron than usual. Low iron levels in the body during pregnancy can lead to iron-deficiency anemia, which is linked to low birth weight and preterm delivery. Flushing or feeling lightheaded, having trouble breathing, and turning pale are signs of an iron deficiency. To lessen the risk of iron deficiency anemia, ACOG suggests taking 27 milligrams of iron daily, which is present in most prenatal vitamins. Certain women might require additional iron through supplementation. If you have iron-deficiency anemia, your doctor may screen you for it and suggest iron supplements if necessary.

3.4. Planned Intervention for the Alleviation of Psychological Difficulties During the Perinatal Period

Chalmers has indicated that social support systems, including family education, health care, doctors, and nurses, need to be both present and of high quality. This is because research has shown that expectant mothers' perception of interpersonal support appears to buffer the potential effects of life stress. In order to prevent potential pregnancy complications, social support personnel must conduct a realistic examination of fears and psychological issues during pregnancy. Horsley even goes so far as to say that psychological management of pregnancy is likely to be insufficient if it doesn't start at the first prenatal visit.

3.4.1. Antenatal Classes

Participating in prenatal education classes offers a chance to address psychological issues that arise during pregnancy. The loss of women's customary informal networks of support and the thinning of communication lines between them have had a significant impact on prenatal education. Prenatal classes come in a variety of forms. Some begin early in pregnancy and concentrate mainly on self-care and hygiene; others, held in the final trimester of pregnancy, essentially prepare women for labor; still others, primarily teach mother craft skills. But all of them have one thing in common: they all teach knowledge, skills, and problem-solving techniques.

The Dick-Read method, which originated in England, and the Lamaze method are essentially the two methods that represent the use of psychological or physical, non-pharmaceutical modalities for the prevention of pain during childbirth. This field of study has a pioneering history in prenatal education.

Dick-Read claims that fear, passed down through the generations from mother to daughter, is what initiates the process of anxiety. Anxiety, in turn, causes tension in the uterine's circular muscle fibers, causing stiffness at the cervix opening and, ultimately, the experience of pain. His approach includes teaching pregnancy hygiene, the anatomy and physiology of labor and delivery, breathing and relaxation techniques, and fitness drills. This education is justified by the idea that delivery-related anxiety is eliminated and replaced with a more carefree attitude.

Although the French obstetrician Lamaze (1970) is credited with giving rise to the Lamaze method of childbirth preparation, the technique actually began in the Soviet Union towards the end of the 1950s and is based on Pavlov's theory of conditioning. The principles of Pavlov's theory were applied: verbal stimuli are just as effective as any other form of reinforcement; a stimulus acting on a specific area of the brain irradiates the specialized centers while the surrounding areas become nonresponsive to other incoming stimuli; and conditioned reflexes are formed within the nervous system and become associated by a temporary neurological bond that is subsequently reinforced by repetition. As a result, if an individual experiences fear or pain in response to the stimulation of uterine contractions, it is likely a learned or conditioned response that can be suppressed or substituted with a more positive emotion. In addition, the breathing exercises women use during labor produce such a potent activation that other parts of the cerebral cortex are prevented from reacting to stimuli coming from the uterus, which would be perceived as painful. Lastly, women can be trained to minimize pain, discomfort, and fear in response to verbal cues during labor. Small groups receive instruction in Lamaze training, which includes topics such as anatomy and physiology, breathing exercises, conditioned relaxation, cognitive restructuring, and social support from medical professionals and a "coach."

Katona (1981) charts the development of prenatal education and notes how the focus has shifted over time from the psychosocial aspects of reproduction to labor pain, medication use, and other aspects of labor. Historically, women's experiences have been undervalued and knowledge provision has been overestimated in preventive strategies. The more modern approaches to prenatal education place a greater emphasis on topics like the emotional changes of pregnancy, the underlying mechanisms of pregnancy symptoms, the relationship with the partner, sexuality patterns, the preparation of the other children in the family, enhanced self-esteem and satisfaction, accepting a new role, and a smooth postpartum adjustment, even though the physiological aspects of the reproductive process are undoubtedly useful. Prenatal classes may also be directed towards the partner of the mother. There is now a need for men to be prepared for child care and birthing due to the sharp increase in the number of men attending births. Men want to know how childbirth works, how it might make them and their wives feel, and what to anticipate during the postpartum phase.

Kitzinger (1988) developed a type of childbirth preparation class that is representative of the more modern approach. Having researched childbearing in a variety of cultural contexts, including the Caribbean, the US, and Africa, Kitzinger has created her own "psychosexual approach" to childbirth, accounting for women's emotional states as well as the network of relationships and the specific culture in which they are entangled. Women experience pain differently, according to Kitzinger, because it is always interpreted and situated within a personally and culturally predetermined framework. Prenatal education now addresses a much wider range of consumers and covers a far wider spectrum of ideologies, methods, content, and scope because it is no longer solely focused on pain reduction.

3.4.2. The Effectiveness of Antenatal Classes

It makes sense that there would be special interest in determining how effective prenatal classes are. Numerous factors play a role in determining this effectiveness, including the type and caliber of teachers, the teaching methodology used, the subject matter covered in the classes, and the attendance patterns.

It appears that no research has been done to link the characteristics of teachers or their methods of instruction to how well students apply their newly acquired knowledge in the workplace. Research indicates that the majority of attendees are women who are pregnant for the first time and those who have previously only had unsuccessful pregnancies. These are the characteristics of the attendees. Additionally, several socioeconomic factors and attendance have a strong correlation. The demographics of women who do not attend classes include being younger, being poorer, having dropped out of school earlier, and having a lower likelihood of getting married. The middle classes have been the primary audience for prenatal education. However, since prenatal classes are now regularly provided in more clinics, it is envisaged that lower-class women will also begin to gain from them. Only 12 of the 24 survey countries were able to provide estimates of the percentages of pregnant women attending classes; these estimates range from 10% to 90% of pregnant women, according to the Having a Baby in Europe (1985) study. We are unable to provide estimates for attendance in the United States at this time, but in the late 1960s, very few expectant mothers were using childbirth preparation.

While there is little evidence that traditional classes improve the mechanical aspects of labor and delivery, Katona notes in her review of the literature on prenatal education that measuring the emotional effects has received less attention. Nonetheless, some research indicates that prenatal classes positively impact physiological and psychological outcome variables.

It should be noted that there are significant methodological challenges in conducting a sufficient trial of prenatal childbirth preparation. The study conducted by Timm (1979) in Pittsburgh with 146 very low-income women is the only example of a three-group design that includes non-trained controls, placebo controls, and trained women; random assignment of women stratified for age, race, and parity to each group; and raters' ignorance of women's specific membership. The women who had taken prenatal classes, according to the results, utilized considerably fewer painkillers during labor and delivery.

Results from additional research also show that women who had received prenatal childbirth education were more likely to have spontaneous deliveries and that pain medication was used much less frequently and in smaller doses.

Other obstetrical benefits of prenatal education have also been recognized: trained women had a significant reduction in cesarean sections, postpartum infections, premature births, cases of pregnancy-related toxemia, postpartum hemorrhage, and peritoneal tears compared to controls; additionally, their babies had higher Apgar scores at both the one- and five-minute mark.

Attendees showed more positive views toward pregnancy, labor and delivery, themselves, their partners, and their children, according to the findings of studies looking at how prenatal training affected mothers' attitudes toward the self, the father, the baby, and the entire process. Women had significantly lower recollections of pain in all three studies, and they also typically took less medication, had fewer general anesthesias, and had less than half as many local anesthesias. Happiness during childbirth and less pain are not entirely independent, as the research by Norr, Block, Charles, Meyering, and Meyers and Charles, Norr, Block, Meyering, and Meyers make clear. According to Davenport-Slack and Boylan, Enkin et al., women who had taken prenatal classes reported having a better labor and delivery experience than those who had not as well as Huttel et al.

Women who attended childbirth preparation classes reported feeling less anxious about giving birth, while Zax et al., and Klusman discovered that both before and after the training, the anxiety levels of trained women were significantly lower.

There hasn't been much study done on how successful male preparation programs are. While Felton and Segelman tested men in the final class before the birth, they discovered that they had shifted toward seeing themselves more in control to a greater extent than untrained men. Manion reports that men who had attended prenatal classes participated more in labor and delivery than those who did not. Contrarily, Wente and Crockenberg discovered that fathers who had gone to childbirth education classes did not report having an easier time adjusting compared to controls.

Studies have been conducted on the relationship between information provision, respiration, conditioned relaxation, cognitive restructuring, and social support as potential psychological mechanisms linked to the positive effects of prenatal training. The specific elements of prenatal education that are involved in lowering anxiety and discomfort are outlined in a review by Wideman and Singer: information sharing during labor preparation was found to have a strong positive association with attitudes toward the newborn and the quantity of painkillers used during labor. However, rather than merely describing the objective aspects of the impending event, this relationship seems to be more likely if the information is descriptive/sensory, involving a thorough explanation of the sensations likely to be experienced during the procedure. Controlled breathing can significantly lower autonomic reactivity to a stressful stimulus; however, no research has been done on this topic in relation to getting ready for childbirth. An additional theory regarding respiration is that it could cause the body to secrete endogenous analgesics, which include enkephalins and endorphins, which have been demonstrated to have morphomimetic properties. There hasn't been any research done on these amino acid chains and pregnancy in humans, though. A counterconditioning program of systematic desensitization, in which the progression of contractions is met with a relaxation response, and techniques that contrast tense muscles with a state of relaxation form the basis of the relaxation regimen taught during childbirth preparation training. Lastly, research has looked at social support's ability to mitigate the negative effects of stress. On those studies, we previously reported. Even though social support has been shown to have positive effects, there are still unanswered questions about the mechanisms underlying these findings.

Though many of the results are based on self-report measures and anecdotal reports, methodological issues have been raised again regarding the systematic documentation of the benefits of antenatal education; measurement techniques have not always been satisfactory; findings are not consistently confirmed; attitudinal changes are likely secondary to decreased medication use; observer biases are present; and, generally, it is very difficult to design well-controlled studies.

3.4.3. Controlled Trials of Explicit Social and Psychological Support in the Perinatal Period

Prenatal classes may include general social and psychological support for expectant and new mothers, but it's also possible that this kind of care could be provided as part of routine prenatal care. Provisions like intensive prenatal care, more frequent check-ups, home visits, phone calls, a 24-hour hotline, family-centered care, emotional support, education about health-related behavior and signs of preterm labor, information/feedback sharing, free transportation, etc., could be included in this general support package.

Elbourne, Oakley, and Chalmers (1989) reviewed 14 controlled trials of the kind described above pertaining to increased social and psychological support during pregnancy. Giving social and psychological support was the main goal of six of those studies; in the other eight, this goal was stated explicitly but was not the trial's primary focus. These later studies mostly concentrated on information sharing and feedback, care organization, or getting ready for pregnancy, childbirth, and parenthood.

Overall, the evidence from those trials of increased social and psychological support points to several positive psychological and behavioral effects: mothers who received support were more likely than controls to report feeling "in control" of their pregnancies, to attend antenatal classes, to feel happy, nervous, and worried during their pregnancies, and to be satisfied with the antenatal care they had received. They were also less likely to have negative feelings about the impending birth. Moreover, women who received support were also more likely to report that their labor was worry-free and to have a companion with them. Following delivery, the women who had received more support during their pregnancy were less likely than the controls to feel unhappy, more likely to be nursing their baby when they were discharged from the hospital, and more likely to have their partner help with baby care.

Finally, six weeks after giving birth, the experimental group's mothers were more likely than the controls to continue to breastfeed, to feel "in control," and to have started feeding the infant solid foods. At six weeks postpartum, women in the experimental group were less likely than controls to be feeling physically ill, and their babies were less likely to have concerning health issues. This was a physical manifestation of the positive psychological effects. Lastly, no adverse effects of increased social and psychological support during pregnancy were noted in any of these controlled trials.

Rae Grant cites another recent review of thirty publications detailing supportive prevention programs that span the prenatal and early infancy periods in North America, England, and Australia. It was determined that the programs with the biggest effects were those that included a variety of elements, lasted a long time—between two and five years—started early in pregnancy, and included home visits as a key element. Numerous beneficial effects, both immediate and long-term, were discovered. Better physical health, better nutrition from parents, fewer low birth weight babies, fewer feeding issues, fewer accidents and ER visits, and a lower incidence of child abuse were the short-term effects on children, while better social support networks, increased confidence, better parenting skills, improved parent-child relationships, fewer child abuse incidents, longer intervals between pregnancies, and more frequent, appropriate service use were the short-term effects on parents. Long-term effects of prenatal/pregnancy programming included decreased school aggression and distractibility, decreased delinquency, improved school attitudes, improved social functioning, and higher rates of prosocial attitudes in children. Mothers who had taken part in these programs had greater levels of education, and family employment rates were higher.

Currently underway is a new multicultural controlled supportive prenatal/infancy program, funded by the European Communities and started by the World Health Organization's Regional Office for Europe. Specific supportive intervention techniques are being tested in several Mediterranean countries (Cyprus, Greece, New Yugoslavia, Portugal, Slovenia, and Turkey) to promote the psychosocial development of children. These techniques are administered by primary healthcare workers to mothers at eight different time points, ranging from the last trimester of pregnancy to the child's 24 months of life. The ultimate objective is to encourage the application of the developed intervention strategies across the primary healthcare network in the participating nations.

Although the focus of this paper is pregnancy, it is important to note that continuous human support during labor and delivery can also have significant positive effects on the perinatal stage. In the past, standard birth practices have included women providing continuous social support to one another during labor in a large number of cultures. In studies designed by Sosa, Kennell, Klaus, Robertson, and Urrutia as well as Klaus, Kennell, Robertson, and Sosa, continuous support during labor was implemented. The perinatal complications, such as meconium staining, stillbirths, cesarean sections, forceps deliveries, and oxytocin augmentation, as well as the number of depressed newborns and neonates admitted to neonatal intensive care, were considerably lower in the women who had supportive female companions during labor than in the control group. The women who labored with a companion experienced a significantly shorter labor period than those who did not. Furthermore, compared to unsupported moms, supported mothers behaved differently with their newborns, showing them more affection through stroking, talking, and smiling. The authors come to the conclusion that the companion's presence might explain why the obstetrician performed fewer interventions, but they appear to prefer theories that focused more on the companion's potential effects on the mother. Social support may shorten the labor's duration by reducing anxiety in women who are in labor and preventing an increase in catecholamine concentrations, which would otherwise cause uterine muscle contractions to increase. Based on research on animals, where stress can lower uterine and placental blood flow and subsequently decrease oxygenation to the fetus, the authors hypothesize that social support could lower the number of newborns admitted to intensive care. Replication is necessary, though, in order to investigate the mechanisms by which support affects physiological processes in more detail.

3.5. Psychosocial Effects of the Actual Provision of Prenatal Care

Social circumstances have an impact on women's health, prenatal care utilization, and response to it. Women with less favorable sociodemographic traits typically receive less appropriate prenatal care. Low-risk women typically attend antenatal clinics earlier and more frequently, according to research conducted in various nations with widely disparate prenatal care systems, including the United States, the United Kingdom, and France. These are typically older, married, primiparae, and socioeconomically more affluent women.

The women who need it most, those from socially disadvantaged backgrounds, do not appear to have benefited most from the advancements in prenatal care. One common excuse for nonattendance is a lack of acceptance or access to antenatal clinics. Socially marginalized women frequently exhibit low confidence in the services they receive, feel ashamed of their precarious circumstances, find it difficult to communicate with caregivers, and frequently fail to heed advice. Furthermore, compared to middle-class women, women from lower socioeconomic classes indicate a desire for more information.

Because all pregnancies have the potential to be pathological, the idea that all pregnant women should receive the same care has become increasingly prevalent in prenatal care across many nations. As a result, the opinions of women regarding the procedures and their execution have frequently been ignored in prenatal care research. Throughout the past ten years, researchers—particularly those in the UK—have focused on women's satisfaction with the various aspects of care due to the realization that disgruntled customers make ineffective prenatal attendants.

Pregnant women generally view prenatal care as important, but they do not appear to feel that they personally benefit much from it, and they are unable to articulate why they should attend. According to all the studies, women want more personal care—less waiting time, more visits with the same doctor, improved communication with medical staff, more opportunities to ask questions and get clear answers, and more consideration for their needs and concerns. The women give two explanations for their incapacity to ask questions: either they perceive the doctors as hurried or as intimidating. However, medical professionals often believe that women ask questions because they are anxious, and that the primary goal of responding to them is to allay their fears rather than to impart knowledge. Furthermore, there is evidence to suggest that a portion of the communication breakdown stems from the mismatch between what doctors consider important and what women consider to be threatening. Last but not least, some prenatal care literature may create unrealistic expectations in women, making them anticipate a level of individualized attention that they are unlikely to receive.

There is more data on how women view interventions used during labor and delivery than there are studies that explain how they feel about the various procedures they undergo during pregnancy. Oakley documents the professionals' unwillingness to adequately explain the reasoning behind the various procedures carried out during pregnancy, as well as the ensuing outcomes and the resulting increase in women's anxiety. When it comes to the ultrasound scan's impact, women who are still struggling to accept their pregnancy will benefit the most since it lends the event more realism. However, the closer proximity to the fetus may also make the mother feel more vulnerable to the pregnancy's outcome, which could lead to worry. Regarding amniocentesis, it has been observed that women experience anxiety before the test because they fear it could harm the fetus or result in miscarriage. However, once the results are known, this anxiety subsides for the remainder of the pregnancy. The role that pregnant women have in their own care is a last but crucial point to consider. Most of the time, they merely follow directions and have little to no control over the officially approved care they get. The increasing involvement of women in identifying their health needs, organizing their services, and selecting how they will be used is an area that will require experimentation in the future.

3.6. Drug Use in Pregnancy

Because the physiology of pregnancy affects the pharmacokinetics of medications used and because some medications can harm the fetus, pregnancy is a unique physiological condition when it comes to drug treatment. It is not possible to completely avoid pharmaceutical treatment during pregnancy, and doing so could be harmful as some women have medical conditions that need to be treated intermittently and continuously (e.g., hypertension, epilepsy, and asthma). Additionally, during pregnancy, preexisting medical conditions may worsen or develop new ones (e.g., migraine, headache) that call for medication treatment. One of the traditional issues in medical treatment is the possibility that certain medications taken during pregnancy could harm the fetus. Pregnant women who took thalidomide in the 1960s gave birth to children who had phocomelia. There are numerous other documented instances of teratogenic drug effects. It has been established that fewer than 1% of all congenital abnormalities are brought on by human teratogenic drugs. For this reason, the Food and Drug Administration created a system in 1979 that assesses the teratogenic risk of medications by taking the caliber of data from studies involving both humans and animals into account. The FDA divides all medications used during pregnancy into five groups: A, B, C, D, and X. Pregnancy is strictly prohibited when using category X products, while category A is thought to be the safest option. This gives the clinician therapeutic direction. This section addresses many issues surrounding drug use while pregnant.

3.6.1. Physiological Changes in Pregnancy

Fertilization often occurs in the fallopian tube of the female. The fertilized egg starts dividing right away into a rapidly expanding cluster of cells. The fertilized egg implants into the uterine wall and begins forming the placenta five to seven days after ovulation. By permitting the transfer of oxygen, carbon dioxide, amino acids, fats, vitamins, and minerals from the mother's blood, the placenta sustains and nourishes the fetus. It also permits waste products from the developing infant to be transferred. The baby is referred to as an embryo from the moment of implantation into the uterine wall until roughly the eighth week of life. At this stage, development picks up speed as specialized cells start to form the blood, muscles, bones, nervous system, and essential organs. A fetus is the term for the developing baby after the eighth week of pregnancy. The majority of its internal organs have formed, and its mouth, ears, nose, and eyes have begun to erupt. It measures 2 and a quarter centimeters in length.

Amazing changes in metabolism take place as the fetus and placenta expand and put more and more strain on the mother. Weight gain and a changed body shape are the most noticeable physical changes. Increases in breast tissue, blood volume, and water volume in the form of extracellular and extravascular fluid are the causes of weight gain. Maternal stores are supplemented with increased cellular water, fat, and protein deposition. Pregnancy causes an average weight gain of 12.5 kg. A typical pregnancy gains one kilogram of weight because of protein. Additionally, there is a drop in plasma albumin levels and an increase in fibrinogen levels. Pregnancy causes an increase in total body fat. Plasma lipids rise in the second half of pregnancy, but shortly after delivery, triglycerides, cholesterol, and lipoproteins fall. During pregnancy, the LDL to HDL ratio rises (Moore, 1994). The fetus's developmental stage, as well as the drug's strength and dosage, determine how the drug affects the developing embryo. There is little information available about the effects of medications during the time of conception and implantation. Women who want to get pregnant or who are at risk of getting pregnant are advised to stop taking any unnecessary medications three to six months before getting pregnant. Some medications used between 15 and 21 days after fertilization, early in pregnancy, during the blastogenesis stage of development, have an all-or-nothing effect, either killing the fetus or having no effect at all. The fetus is very resistant to birth defects at this early stage. During the organogenesis period, which lasts from the third to the eighth week after fertilization, the fetus is most susceptible to birth defects. During this time, the development of all major organs begins. Drugs that reach the fetus at this stage have the potential to result in a miscarriage, a visible birth defect, or a permanent, subtle defect that manifests itself later in life. The embryo is referred to as a fetus after the eighth week of gestational age. Development at this point mostly consists of growth and maturation. Drug exposure during this time does not seem to be linked to significant congenital abnormalities, but it may change how normally formed organs and tissues grow and function. The dosage of a drug that reaches the fetus affects its effectiveness as well. The mother's dosage, the drug's distribution in the mother's bloodstream, placental function, the genetic and physiological state of the mother and fetus, and exposure to other medications, chemicals, or environmental dangers all have an impact on this dosage.

3.6.2. Pharmacokinetics in Pregnancy

Pregnant women's medication pharmacokinetics are impacted by the particular physiological changes that occur during pregnancy. A woman's plasma volume rises by 30 to 50% during pregnancy; corresponding increases in cardiac output and glomerular filtration rate also occur. These elements may contribute to subtherapeutic drug levels in pregnant women as well as lower circulating concentrations of some medications (particularly those eliminated by the kidney). Pregnancy also causes an increase in body fat, which expands the volume of drugs that are distributed in a fat-soluble manner. When a pregnant woman's plasma albumin concentration drops, the volume of distribution of highly protein-bound medications rises e.g., anticonvulsants. However, the kidney and liver excrete the unbound drugs more quickly, negating the impact of the increased volume of distribution. Progesterone has the effect of decreasing gastric emptying time, especially in the third trimester, which delays the start of the drug's effects.

Some drugs may bind and become inactive if pregnant women take antacids, iron supplements, or vitamins concurrently. Increased blood flow causes the drug to enter the muscles more quickly, speeding up the rate at which it takes effect and improving systemic drug absorption. Finally, progesterone and estrogen affect the activity of hepatic enzymes, which can either increase or decrease the amount of drugs that are eliminated from the body.

3.6.3. Placental Transfer of Drugs

The placenta, a conceived organ, serves as a functional link between the blood of the fetus and the mother. The placenta maintains the health of the fetus and the mother by performing a variety of metabolic, respiratory, excretory, and endocrine functions. For a medication to have a teratogenic or pharmacological effect on the developing fetus, it needs to diffuse through the placenta from the mother's circulation to the fetal circulation. The drug's chemical characteristics, such as its molecular weight, pH difference, lipid solubility, and protein binding, all affect the rate of transfer. The placenta only allows drugs that are free and unbound to pass through. Fetal albumin rises during pregnancy while maternal plasma albumin falls. The fetus receives the increased concentration of free drugs through the placenta. Weak bases are more likely to cross the placenta in fetal tissue due to its slightly higher acidic pH than in maternal tissue. Drugs that are somewhat lipid soluble can pass through the placental membrane with ease. Medications with a small molecular weight (<500 g/mol) diffuse freely across the placenta. Drugs with a higher molecular weight (between 500–1,000 g/mol) cross the placenta less easily, while a few drugs with a high molecular weight (> 1,000 g/mol) are unable to pass past the placental barrier. Because of the placenta's increased surface area, decreased thickness, and increased maternal and placental blood flow, transplacental drug transfer increases during the third trimester.

3.6.4. Pregnancy and Drug Use

Drugs are a major factor in enhancing human health and wellbeing. However, they must be safe, effective, and used sensibly in order to have the desired effect. Drugs taken by a pregnant woman can reach the fetus and harm it by crossing the placenta, the same route taken by oxygen and nutrients, which are necessary for the fetus's growth and development. As a general rule, drugs should not be used during pregnancy unless absolutely necessary.

While it may be ideal to avoid drugs while pregnant, this is frequently not feasible and can even be harmful because some women have underlying medical conditions that necessitate intermittent and continuous treatment (e.g., hypertension, epilepsy, and asthma). Additionally, during pregnancy, preexisting medical conditions may worsen or develop new ones (e.g., migraine headache) that calls for medication treatment. The mother's and her child's health may suffer if these conditions are not properly managed. Certain medications, such as vitamins, minerals, iron, and dietary supplements, are also necessary for the fetus's and the pregnant woman's health. According to reports, 8% of expectant mothers require medication therapy for a variety of chronic illnesses and pregnancy-related issues. In the first few weeks of pregnancy, many women take medication without even realizing they are pregnant. Pregnant women are prescribed medications in approximately 59% of cases, rather than vitamin or mineral supplements. 13% or so of expectant mothers supplement their diets with herbs. During their pregnancy, over 90% of expectant mothers use prescription or over-the-counter drugs, as well as social drugs like alcohol, tobacco, or illicit substances. One of the traditional issues in medical treatment is the possibility that certain medications taken during pregnancy could harm the fetus.

Results from studies on animals need not be applicable to the human population, and pregnant women are typically excluded from medical trials. As a result, it can be problematic to treat pregnant women with certain medications, and most medical professionals have very strict policies regarding drug use during pregnancy. Clinical research regarding the safety of drugs in pregnancy has faced numerous challenges due to the fear of medication use during pregnancy harming or killing the fetus. Because of these limitations, case reports, epidemiological studies, and animal studies are the actual sources of information about medication safety during pregnancy. These methods make it challenging to assess the risks associated with drug use during pregnancy (Ward, 2001).

According to a 2001 study, over 90% of the drugs approved by the FDA between 1980 and 2000 had insufficient information about their safety or potential risks when taken during pregnancy. Because of this, it can be challenging for pregnant women and medical professionals to decide whether or not to use medications.

The statistics on OTC and prescription drug use during pregnancy show that drug use is widespread, despite the lack of information regarding the safety of drugs during pregnancy. Drug use accounts for two to three percent of all birth defects. Drugs, however, are occasionally necessary for the fetus's and pregnant women's health. It may be advised by a medical professional for pregnant women to take specific vitamins and minerals. Medication is also used to treat edema, nausea and vomiting, aches and pains, and other common pregnancy-related symptoms. Prescription drugs may also be given to treat illnesses unrelated to pregnancy that arise during pregnancy, such as gastrointestinal disorders, upper respiratory infections, and urinary tract infections. Additionally, a pregnant woman may be taking medicine to treat chronic illnesses like epilepsy, hypertension, or psychiatric disorders, or to treat illnesses related to pregnancy like pregnancy-induced hypertension, to induce labor, or to help the fetus that is expected to be delivered prematurely mature lung tissue. Additionally, this patient group might be exposed to any additional substances that could harm the developing fetus. In light of this, it becomes crucial to investigate the pattern of drug use during pregnancy to determine whether or not there is currently enough information to make improvements.

3.6.5. How Drugs Affect the Fetus

Pregnant women's use of drugs can have a variety of effects on the developing fetus. They may directly affect the fetus, resulting in harm or aberrant development that could cause birth defects or even death. They can also change how the placenta functions, usually by narrowing blood vessels and lowering the amount of oxygen and nutrients the fetus receives from the mother. This can lead to an underweight and underdeveloped baby. Additionally, they have the potential to injure the fetus indirectly by reducing its blood supply or inducing preterm labor and delivery by forcing the uterine muscles to contract violently.

3.6.6. FDA Categories for Drug Use in Pregnancy

The Food and Drug Administration created a method in 1979 for assessing a drug's potential for teratogenicity based on the caliber of data from studies involving both humans and animals. It gives the clinician therapeutic direction. Although some medications from categories B, C, and D are also used during pregnancy, category A is thought to be the safest. The only classification that indicates a drug is categorically not recommended for use during pregnancy is Category X (Table 3.2). The FDA's classification of some of the most often used medications during pregnancy is provided in the table below (Table 3.3). Certain medications have been shown to be detrimental to the developing fetus, so it is not advised to use them while pregnant (Table 3.4).

Table 3.2. FDA Categorization of Drugs for Use in Pregnancy

Category	Description
A	Adequate, well-controlled studies in pregnant women have not shown an increased risk of fetal abnormalities.
B	Animal studies have revealed no evidence of harm to the fetus; however, there are no adequate and well-controlled studies in pregnant women. Or
	Animal studies have shown an adverse effect, but adequate and well-controlled studies in pregnant women have failed to demonstrate a risk to the fetus.
C	Animal studies have shown an adverse effect and there are no adequate and well-controlled studies in pregnant women. Or
	No animal studies have been conducted and there are no adequate and well-controlled studies in pregnant women.
D	Studies, adequate well-controlled or observational, in pregnant women have demonstrated a risk to the fetus. However, the benefits of therapy may outweigh the potential risk.
X	Studies, adequate well-controlled or observational, in animals or pregnant women have demonstrated positive evidence of fetal abnormalities. The use of the product is contraindicated in women who are or may become pregnant.

Source: Punam Sachdeva, B. G. Patel, and B. K. Patel. Drug Use in Pregnancy; a Point to Ponder! Indian Journal of Pharmaceutical Sciences. DOI: 10.4103/0250-474X.51941.

Table 3.3. Commonly Used Drugs in Pregnancy and Their Categories

Drugs	Category
Analgesics and Antipyretics	B and C
Acetaminophen	B
Phenacetin	B
Aspirin	C
Antiemetics	B and C
Doxylamine	B
Meclizine	B
Cyclizine	B
Dimenhydrinate	B
Antibiotics	B, C and D
Penicillin, Ampicillin, Amoxycillin,	B
Cloxacillin Cephalosporins	B
Erythromycin	B
Gentamicin	C
Amikacin	C/D
Streptomycin	D
Sulphonamides	B/D

Tetracyclines	D
Amoebicides	B
Metronidazole	
Anthelmentics	B
Piperazine	
Mebendazole	
Antimalarials	C
Antifungals	C
Anti TB Drugs	B and C
Ethambutol	B
INH	C
Rifampicin	C
Pyrazinamide	C
PAS	C
Vitamins	
B,C,D,E,folic acid	A
Hormones	
Thyroxin	A
Androgens	X
Estrogens	X
Progestogens-	
Hydroxyprogestrone	D
Medroxyprogestrone	D
Norethindrone	X
Norgestrel	X
Bronchodilators	C

Source: Punam Sachdeva, B. G. Patel, and B. K. Patel. Drug Use in Pregnancy; a Point to Ponder! Indian Journal of Pharmaceutical Sciences. DOI: 10.4103/0250-474X.51941.

Table 3.4. Medications Contraindicated in Pregnancy

Drug	Comments
Vitamin A and its derivatives including isotretinein, accutane and etretinate.	Significant risk of spontaneous abortion and risk of many significant anomalies
ACE inhibitors	May cause kidney damage in the fetus when used in II and III trimester, decrease in the amount of amniotic fluid and deformities of face, limbs and lungs

Anticoagulants- warfarin	Use during I trimester produces defects like nasal hypoplasia and a depressed nasal bridge; termed as Fetal warfarin Syndrome. Use during II and III trimesters is associated with increased risk of fetal malformations.
- Heparin	Safe but if taken for long time osteoporosis and decrease in number of platelets in pregnant women occurs.
Estrogen and Androgens	Genital tract malformations.
Thyroid preparations-	
Methimazole	Overactive and enlarged Thyroid gland
Carbimazole	Overactive and enlarged Thyroid gland
Radioactive iodine	Underactive Thyroid gland in fetus
Propylthiouracil	Safe.
Anticonvulsants-	
Carbamazepine	Risk of birth defects
Phenytoin, Phenobarbitone	Bleeding problem in the newborn which can be prevented if pregnant woman takes Vit. K by mouth every day for a month before delivery or if the newborn baby is given an injection of Vit. K soon after birth.
	Risk of birth defects.
Trimethadione	Increased risk of miscarriage in the women
Sodium valproate	Increased risk of birth defects in fetus; including a cleft palate and abnormalities of the heart, face, skull, hands or abdominal organs.
Antidepressants- Lithium	Birth defects (mainly of the heart), lethargy, decreased muscle tone, underactivity of Thyroid gland and nephrogenic diabetes insipidus in the new born. Ebstein's anomaly (tricuspid valve malformation) has been reported in a number of fetuses exposed to this drug.
NSAIDs	
Aspirin and other Salicylates	Delay in start of labor, premature closing of ductus arteriosus, jaundice, brain damage in the fetus and bleeding problems in the woman during and after delivery and in the newborn.
Antibiotics- Tetracycline	Slowed bone growth, permanent yellowing of the teeth and increased susceptibility to cavities in the body.
Chloramphenicol	Gray Baby Syndrome.
Ciprofloxacin	Possibility of joint abnormalities (seen in animals)
Kanamycin and Streptomycin	Damage to fetus's ear resulting in deafness (risk of ototoxicity)
Sulfonamides	Jaundice and brain damage in newborn
Antineoplastic agents-	
Busulfan	Birth defects such as less than expected growth before birth, underdevelopment of lower jaw, cleft palate, abnormal development of skull bones, spinal defects, ear defects and club foot.
Chlorambucil	
Cyclophosphamide	

Methotrexate	
Oral Hypoglycemic drugs	A very low level of sugar in the blood of newborn. Inadequate control of diabetes in the pregnant woman
Chlorpropamide	
Tolbutamide	

Source: Punam Sachdeva, B. G. Patel, and B. K. Patel. Drug Use in Pregnancy; a Point to Ponder! Indian Journal of Pharmaceutical Sciences. DOI: 10.4103/0250-474X.51941.

3.6.7. Social Drugs

Other substances that some pregnant women use should not be disregarded, in addition to counseling pregnant women regarding the use of various prescribed and non-prescribed medications during pregnancy. The following substances carry a risk that should be explained to them when they are pregnant.

3.6.7.1. Cigarette Smoking

One of the few known preventable causes of prenatal morbidity and mortality is maternal smoking. A lower birth weight is the most constant result of smoking on the fetus during pregnancy. The heart, brain, and facial birth defects are also more common in children whose parents smoke. The risk of preterm labor, uterine infections, miscarriages, stillbirths, premature births, premature rupture of the membranes, misplaced placenta (placenta previa), and premature placenta detachment (placenta abruptio) is elevated. Premature birth, infant mortality, and spontaneous abortions could all be brought on by variations in uterine and placental oxygenation. As a result, all expectant mothers ought to be made aware of the dangers smoking poses to the developing fetus and motivated to give up the habit.

3.6.7.2. Alcohol

When pregnant women drink, one of the most dangerous outcomes is fetal alcohol syndrome. Fetal alcohol syndrome affects 1 in 2,000 live births worldwide. When a woman consumes alcohol in any form while pregnant, her chance of miscarriage nearly doubles, and her unborn child's birth weight is significantly lower. This syndrome is characterized by small head size, mental retardation, abnormal behavioral development, facial defects, and inadequate growth before or after birth. Low socioeconomic status, smoking, drug abuse, poor nutrition, and genetic predisposition all play a role in the expression of this syndrome.

3.6.7.3. Caffeine

Since caffeine can be found in different amounts in a wide range of drinks, analgesics, diet supplements, and stimulants, it is the most commonly consumed drug when pregnant. There is little to no risk to the fetus from caffeine consumption during pregnancy, according to the evidence. Coffee, tea, some sodas, chocolates, and some medications all contain caffeine, which is a stimulant that easily passes from the mother to the developing fetus. When taken in excess, it may stimulate the fetus, quickening its respiration and heart rate. Additionally, caffeine may reduce iron absorption and blood flow through the placenta, raising the risk of anemia.

3.6.7.4. Illicit Drugs

Using illegal substances like cocaine and opiates while pregnant can lead to major issues and complications for both the developing baby and the fetus. The fetus is likely to grow insufficiently, and preterm birth defects are more prevalent. Cocaine reduces blood flow to the fetus by narrowing blood vessels and crossing the placenta. The fetus's decreased blood and oxygen supply slows the growth of its intestine and bones. Cocaine usage can also lead to difficulties when pregnant. 31% of pregnant women who use cocaine give birth prematurely, and 15% experience premature placental detachment. Additionally, the likelihood of miscarriage rises.

3.6.8. Concerns with OTC Drugs

In India, more drugs are used as self-medication for common complaints and infectious conditions than are prescribed due to the country's easy access to drugs and inadequate health services. As a result, these customers are constantly at risk for negative drug reactions and interactions. While many over-the-counter medications are safe to use while pregnant when taken under a doctor's supervision, some are not. Women who are pregnant, may become pregnant, or are nursing should see a doctor before using over-the-counter medication, as stated on product labels.

One OTC medication that should be avoided during the final three months of pregnancy is aspirin. The FDA warned in 1990 that aspirin use during the final trimester of pregnancy should be avoided unless specifically instructed by a doctor, as it may result in issues for the fetus or complications during delivery. The same caution regarding the use of over-the-counter non-steroidal anti-inflammatory drugs like ibuprofen during the third trimester applies to them as well.

To assess whether herbs and dietary supplements are safe to use during pregnancy, experts emphasize that there is still a lack of knowledge regarding how these substances affect a developing fetus. Therefore, just because a product is over-the-counter and labeled as natural doesn't mean that it's safe to use while pregnant.

3.7. Nutrition During Pregnancy

The Academy of Nutrition and Dietetics recommends the following key components of a healthy lifestyle during pregnancy:

- Appropriate weight gain
- A balanced diet
- Regular exercise
- Appropriate and timely vitamin and mineral supplementation

3.7.1. Dietary and Caloric Recommendations

It takes about 300 extra calories per day to keep a pregnancy healthy. A balanced diet rich in protein, fruits, vegetables, and whole grains should provide these calories. Limiting sweets and fats is a good idea. A nutritious, well-balanced diet can also aid in the reduction of certain pregnancy side effects, like nausea and constipation.

3.7.2. Fluid Intake During Pregnancy

Fluid intake is also an important part of pregnancy nutrition. Follow these recommendations for fluid intake during pregnancy:

- You can take in enough fluids by drinking several glasses of water each day, in addition to the fluids in juices and soups. Talk to your healthcare provider or midwife about restricting your intake of caffeine and artificial sweeteners.
- Avoid all forms of alcohol.

3.7.3. Ideal Foods to Eat During Pregnancy

The following foods are beneficial to your health and fetal development during pregnancy:

- Vegetables: carrots, sweet potatoes, pumpkin, spinach, cooked greens, tomatoes and red sweet peppers (for vitamin A and potassium)
- Fruits: cantaloupe, honeydew, mangoes, prunes, bananas, apricots, oranges, and red or pink grapefruit (for potassium)
- Dairy: fat-free or low-fat yogurt, skim or 1% milk, soymilk (for calcium, potassium, vitamins A and D)
- Grains: ready-to-eat cereals/cooked cereals (for iron and folic acid)
- Proteins: beans and peas; nuts and seeds; lean beef, lamb and pork; salmon, trout, herring, sardines and pollock

3.7.4. Foods to Avoid During Pregnancy

Avoid eating the following foods during pregnancy:

- Unpasteurized milk and foods made with unpasteurized milk (soft cheeses, including feta, queso Blanco and fresco, Camembert, brie or blue-veined cheeses—unless labeled "made with pasteurized milk")
- Hot dogs and luncheon meats (unless they are heated until steaming hot before serving)
- Raw and undercooked seafood, eggs and meat.
- Do not eat sushi made with raw fish (cooked sushi is safe).
- Refrigerated pâté and meat spreads
- Refrigerated smoked seafood

3.7.5. Guidelines for Safe Food Handling

Follow these general food safety guidelines when handling and cooking food:

- **Wash**: Rinse all raw produce thoroughly under running tap water before eating, cutting or cooking.
- **Clean**: Wash your hands, knives, countertops and cutting boards after handling and preparing uncooked foods.
- **Cook**: Cook beef, pork or poultry to a safe internal temperature verified by a food thermometer.
- **Chill**: Promptly refrigerate all perishable food.

3.7.6. Prenatal Vitamin and Mineral Supplements

Before or soon after conception, the majority of medical professionals and midwives will recommend a prenatal supplement to ensure that all of your nutritional requirements are satisfied. Prenatal supplements, however, do not take the place of a balanced diet.

3.7.6.1. The Importance of Folic Acid

For all women of childbearing age, the US Public Health Service advises 400 micrograms (0.04 mg) of folic acid daily. Folic acid is a nutrient found in:

- Some green leafy vegetables
- Most berries, nuts, beans, citrus fruits and fortified breakfast cereals
- Some vitamin supplements.

Neural tube defects are birth defects affecting the brain and spinal cord that can be prevented with the help of folic acid. Incontinence, cerebral disability, and various degrees of paralysis can result from neural tube defects.

Since most neural tube defects occur in the first 28 days after conception, folic acid is most beneficial during this time. Unfortunately, it's possible that you won't become aware of your pregnancy until 28 days. As a result, you should start taking folic acid before getting pregnant and keep doing so all the way through your pregnancy. Your midwife or doctor will advise you on the right dosage of folic acid based on your unique requirements. For instance, in order to prevent neural tube defects, women who take anti-epileptic medications may need to take higher doses of folic acid. When thinking about attempting to become pregnant, they ought to speak with their doctor (Allen, 2000).

A Closer Look

Routine Later Pregnancy Tests

- **Ultrasound for Structural Abnormalities:** An ultrasound examination should be offered at around 20 weeks. This 'anomaly scan' enables the detection of most structural fetal abnormalities, although reported success rates vary widely.
- **Ultrasound Screening for Risk Assessment:** Ultrasound cervical length measurement at around 20 weeks can be used for risk assessment of preterm delivery in otherwise low-risk women. This is currently not recommended for all women in the UK. However, progesterone administration to women who have a short cervix but are otherwise 'low risk' probably halves their risk of preterm delivery.

  Ultrasound measurement of uterine artery resistance can be used as a screening test for intrauterine growth restriction and pre-eclampsia. This is currently not recommended for all women in the UK. However, it identifies women at risk better than history.
- **Other Routine Later Pregnancy Tests**: A full blood count and an antibody assessment are performed at 28 weeks; the FBC is repeated later if treatment for anemia is given. Non-invasive prenatal testing (NIPT) is now recommended in the UK to determine which Rhesus-negative mothers are carrying a Rhesus-positive baby. Unless the fetal status is unknown (e.g., missed test), only those with a positive baby are given anti-D. Glucose tolerance testing is used for all women at increased risk, the most common indications being increased BMI, ethnicity and a first-degree family history of diabetes (Whitworth et al., 2015)

Summary

- Prenatal care is a type of preventive healthcare. It is provided in the form of medical checkups, consisting of recommendations on managing a healthy lifestyle and the provision of medical information such as maternal physiological changes in pregnancy, biological changes, and prenatal nutrition including prenatal vitamins, which prevents potential health problems throughout the course of the pregnancy and promotes the mother and child's health alike.
- The medical diagnosis of pregnancy serves to date when the birth will occur and also helps predict the existence of a high-risk status. If a pregnancy was planned, the diagnosis produces a feeling of intense fulfillment and achievement. If it was not planned or not desired, it can result in an equally extreme crisis state.
- Presumptive signs of pregnancy are those that are least indicative of pregnancy; taken as single entities, they could easily indicate other conditions. These findings, discussed in connection with the body system in which they occur, are experienced by the woman but cannot be documented by an examiner.
- Probable signs of pregnancy are objective so can be documented by an examiner. Although they are more reliable than presumptive signs, they still are not positive or true diagnostic findings. They are also discussed in connection with the body system in which they occur.
- High blood pressure occurs when arteries carrying blood from the heart to the body organs are narrowed. This causes pressure to increase in the arteries.
- Preeclampsia is a condition that causes dangerously high blood pressure. It can be life-threatening if left untreated. Preeclampsia typically happens after 20 weeks of pregnancy, often in women who have no history of high blood pressure.
- The assessment of the effectiveness of prenatal classes is naturally of particular interest. In determining this effectiveness, several factors are involved: the quality and kind of teachers and the teaching method employed, the specific content of the classes, and the characteristics of the attendees.
- Screening tests are used to find people with a higher chance of a health problem. This means they can get earlier, potentially more effective, treatment or make informed decisions about their health.
- Pregnancy is a special physiological condition where drug treatment presents a special concern because the physiology of pregnancy affects the pharmacokinetics of medications used and certain medications can reach the fetus and cause harm. Total avoidance of pharmacological treatment in pregnancy is not possible and may be dangerous because some women enter pregnancy with medical conditions that require ongoing and episodic treatment (e.g., asthma, epilepsy, and hypertension). Also, during pregnancy new medical problems can develop and old ones can be exacerbated (e.g., migraine, headache) requiring pharmacological therapy. The fact that certain drugs given during pregnancy may prove harmful to the unborn child is one of the classical problems in medical treatment.

References

1. Alfirevic, Z., Stampalija, T., & Medley, N. (2015). Fetal and umbilical Doppler ultrasound in normal pregnancy. *The Cochrane Database of Systematic Reviews, 4*(4), CD001450. https://doi.org/10.1002/14651858.CD001450.pub4.
2. Allen, L. H. (2000). Anemia and iron deficiency: Effects on pregnancy outcome. *American Journal of Clinical Nutrition, 71*(5), 1280s–1284s. Retrieved from: https://academic.oup.com/ajcn/article/71/5/1280S/4729385 (accessed on 6 September 2024).
3. Banhidy, F., Lowry, R. B., & Czeizel, A. E. (2005). Risk and benefit of drug use during pregnancy. *International Journal of Medical Sciences, 2*, 100–106.
4. Bernstein, H. B., & Weinstein, M. (2007). Normal pregnancy and prenatal care. In A. H. DeCherney & L. Nathan (Eds.), *Current Diagnosis and Treatment in Obstetrics and Gynecology* (10th ed.). Columbus, OH: McGraw-Hill.
5. Bricker, L., Medley, N., & Pratt, J. J. (2015). Routine ultrasound in late pregnancy (after 24 weeks' gestation). *The Cochrane Database of Systematic Reviews, 6*(6), CD001451. https://doi.org/10.1002/14651858.CD001451.pub4.
6. Brown, H. C., Smith, H. J., Mori, R., & Noma, H. (2015). Giving women their own case notes to carry during pregnancy. *The Cochrane Database of Systematic Reviews, 2015*(10), CD002856. https://doi.org/10.1002/14651858.CD002856.pub3.
7. Carberry, A. E., Gordon, A., Bond, D. M., Hyett, J., Raynes-Greenow, C. H., & Jeffery, H. E. (2014). Customised versus population-based growth charts as a screening tool for detecting small for gestational age infants in low-risk pregnant women. *The Cochrane Database of Systematic Reviews, 5*(5), CD008549. https://doi.org/10.1002/14651858.CD008549.pub3.
8. Catling, C. J., Medley, N., Foureur, M., Ryan, C., Leap, N., Teate, A., & Homer, C. S. (2015). Group versus conventional antenatal care for women. *The Cochrane Database of Systematic Reviews, 2*(2), CD007622. https://doi.org/10.1002/14651858.CD007622.pub3.
9. David, R., Evans, R., & Fraser, H. S. F. (2021). Modelling prenatal care pathways at a central hospital in Zimbabwe. *Health Services Insights, 14*, 11786329211062742. https://doi.org/10.1177/11786329211062742.
10. Dowswell, T., Carroli, G., Duley, L., Gates, S., Gülmezoglu, A. M., Khan-Neelofur, D., & Piaggio, G. (2015). Alternative versus standard packages of antenatal care for low-risk pregnancy. *The Cochrane Database of Systematic Reviews, 2015*(7), CD000934. https://doi.org/10.1002/14651858.CD000934.pub3.
11. Hernandez-Diaz, S., Toh, S., & Cnattingius, S. (2009). Risk of pre-eclampsia in first and subsequent pregnancies: Prospective cohort study. *British Medical Journal, 338*, b2255. Retrieved from: http://www.ncbi.nlm.nih.gov/pmc/articles/PMC3269902/?tool=pubmed (accessed on 6 September 2024).
12. Le Strat, Y., Dubertret, C., & Le Foll, B. (2011). Prevalence and correlates of major depressive episode in pregnant and postpartum women in the United States. *Journal of Affective Disorders, 135*(1–3), 128–138. https://doi.org/10.1016/j.jad.2011.07.004.
13. Leeman, L., & Fontaine, P. (2008). Hypertensive disorders of pregnancy. *American Family Physician, 78*, 93–100.

14. Mbuagbaw, L., Medley, N., Darzi, A. J., Richardson, M., Habiba Garga, K., & Ongolo-Zogo, P. (2015). Health system and community level interventions for improving antenatal care coverage and health outcomes. *The Cochrane Database of Systematic Reviews, 12*(12), CD010994. https://doi.org/10.1002/14651858.CD010994.pub2.

15. McCarter, D. E., & Spaulding, M. S. (2005). Medications in pregnancy and lactation. *American Journal of Maternal Child Nursing, 30*, 10–17.

16. Meis, P. J., Klebanoff, M., Thom, E., Dombrowski, M. P., Sibai, B., Moawad, A. H., et al. (2003). Prevention of recurrent preterm delivery by 17 alpha-hydroxyprogesterone caproate. *New England Journal of Medicine, 348*, 2379–2385.

17. Melton, M. W. (1999). Take two Aspirin or not? Risk of medication use during pregnancy. *Mother Baby Journal, 4*, 25–32.

18. Moore, P. J. (1994). Maternal physiology during pregnancy. In A. H. De Cherney & M. L. Pernoll (Eds.), *Current Obstetrics and Gynecological Diagnosis and Treatment* (8th ed., pp. 146–154). New York: McGraw-Hill.

19. Nabhan, A. F., & Aflaifel, N. (2015). High feedback versus low feedback of prenatal ultrasound for reducing maternal anxiety and improving maternal health behavior in pregnancy. *The Cochrane Database of Systematic Reviews, 2015*(8), CD007208. https://doi.org/10.1002/14651858.CD007208.pub3.

20. Robert Peter, J., Ho, J. J., Valliapan, J., & Sivasangari, S. (2015). Symphysial fundal height (SFH) measurement in pregnancy for detecting abnormal fetal growth. *The Cochrane Database of Systematic Reviews, 2015*(9), CD008136. https://doi.org/10.1002/14651858.CD008136.pub3.

21. Rojas, F., Wood, E., & Blakemore, K. (2007). Preconception counseling and prenatal care. In K. B. Fortner et al. (Eds.), *The Johns Hopkins Manual of Gynecology and Obstetrics*. Philadelphia: Lippincott Williams & Wilkins.

22. Sandall, J., Soltani, H., Gates, S., Shennan, A., & Devane, D. (2016). Midwife-led continuity models versus other models of care for childbearing women. *The Cochrane Database of Systematic Reviews, 2016*(4), CD004667. https://doi.org/10.1002/14651858.CD004667.pub5.

23. Ward, R. W. (2001). Difficulties in the study of adverse fetal and neonatal effects of drug therapy during pregnancy. *Seminars in Perinatology, 25*, 191–195.

24. Whitworth, M., Bricker, L., & Mullan, C. (2015). Ultrasound for fetal assessment in early pregnancy. *The Cochrane Database of Systematic Reviews, 2015*(7), CD007058. https://doi.org/10.1002/14651858.CD007058.pub3.

Chapter

PHYSIOLOGY OF LABOR AND PUERPERIUM

4

Contents

Introduction

The postpartum period begins after the baby is born, signaling the end of pregnancy. During the approximately 6-week period known as the puerperium, special attention is given to the changes taking place in the mother's body. These changes primarily involve the maternal organs returning to their pre-pregnant sizes and functions, hormonal shifts as the placenta is expelled, and the initiation of lactation. It is important to consider contraception early in the puerperium, as well as when to resume sexual activity. While cultural or religious beliefs may influence expectations for new mothers during this time, they do not interfere with the normal physiological processes occurring.

The physiology of labor encompasses a meticulously orchestrated sequence of events aimed at facilitating the safe delivery of a baby. Commencing with uterine contractions, the cervix gradually effaces and dilates, transitioning through latent and active phases. Hormonal surges, particularly oxytocin and prostaglandins, coordinate contractions while softening the cervix. During the second stage, marked by complete cervical dilation, the baby navigates through the birth canal aided by maternal pushing efforts and cardinal movements. The third stage witnesses the expulsion of the placenta, with continued uterine contractions aiding in its detachment and expulsion to minimize postpartum bleeding. Following childbirth, the puerperium heralds a period of remarkable physiological adjustments in the maternal body. Uterine involution initiates, with the uterus gradually contracting to its pre-pregnancy size through the breakdown of excess tissue. Lochia, comprising blood, mucus, and uterine tissue, is expelled over weeks, signaling ongoing uterine healing. Hormonal shifts trigger lactation, with prolactin stimulating milk production and oxytocin facilitating milk ejection while aiding uterine contractions. Cardiovascular and hematologic changes occur, with blood volume decreasing and coagulation returning to pre-pregnancy states. Emotionally, many women experience the transient "baby blues," while others may grapple with postpartum depression, necessitating support and interventions. Musculoskeletal and skin changes include abdominal muscle toning and gradual fading of stretch marks. Overall, comprehending these physiological intricacies is vital in providing tailored care and support during labor and the puerperium, ensuring optimal maternal and neonatal outcomes.

Orientation and Directional Terms

Term	Definition	Illustration
Puerperium	Puerperium is defined as the time from the delivery of the placenta through the first few weeks after delivery. This period is usually considered to be 6 weeks in duration.	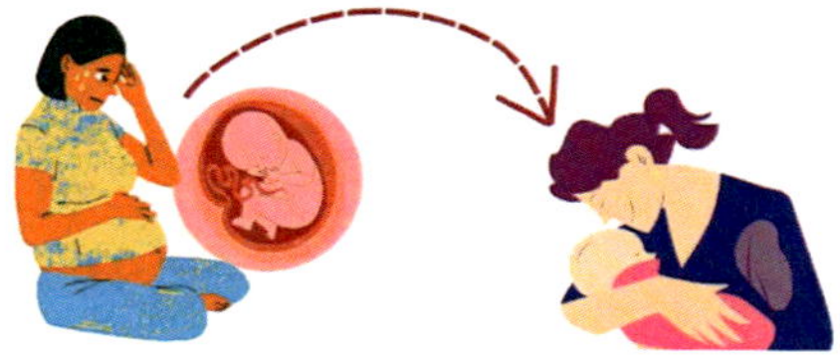
Fetal Heart Rate (FHR)	The average fetal heart rate is between 110 and 160 beats per minute. It can vary by 5 to 25 beats per minute. The fetal heart rate may change as your baby responds to conditions in your uterus. An abnormal fetal heart rate may mean that your baby is not getting enough oxygen or that there are other problems.	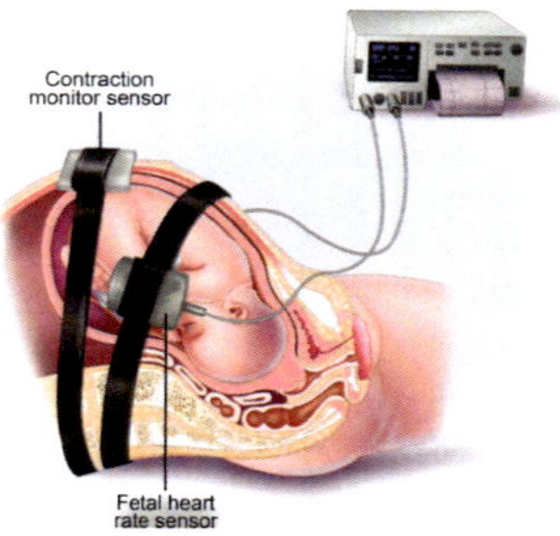
Amniotomy	Amniotomy, also known as artificial rupture of membranes (AROM) and by the lay description "breaking the water," is the intentional rupture of the amniotic sac by an obstetrical provider. This procedure is common during labor management and has been performed by obstetrical providers for at least a few hundred years.	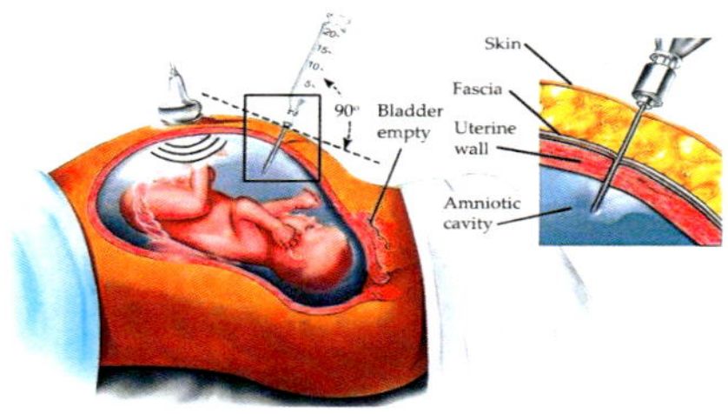
Uterine Distension	The labor in uncomplicated spontaneous delivery is likely triggered by uterine distention, which intensifies with the progression of pregnancy and reaches its peak when fetal size approaches the uterine size.	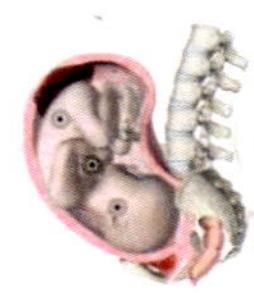
Dehydroepian-drosterone (DHEA)	Dehydroepiandrosterone (DHEA) is a hormone produced by the body's adrenal glands. The body uses DHEA to make androgens and estrogens, the male and female sex hormones. DHEA levels peak at about age 25, then go down steadily as you get older.	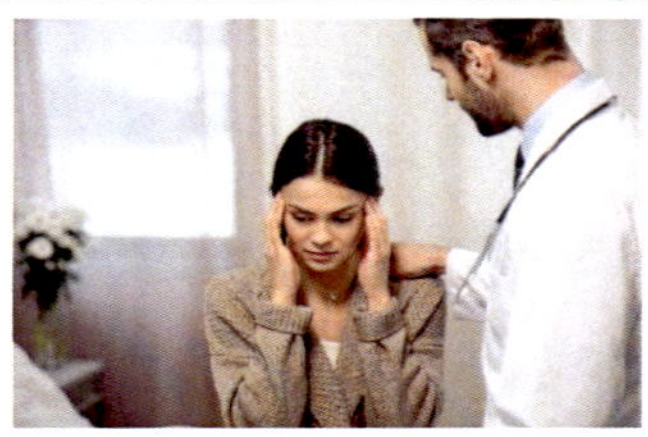

4.1. Mechanism of Labor

The fetus must adjust its head position as it passes through the pelvis during labor in order to successfully negotiate the pelvis. As is the case in 95% of pregnancies, the mechanisms of labor, also referred to as the cardinal movements, are explained in relation to a vertex presentation.

4.1.1. Methods for Cervical Ripening and Induction of Labor

The fetus transitions from the intrauterine to the extrauterine environment during labor. The beginning and continuation of uterine contractions with the intention of causing progressive cervical effacement and dilation is the clinical diagnosis. The precise mechanisms underlying this process are not fully understood at this time. The process of starting uterine contractions before spontaneous labor begins, either medically or surgically, is known as "induction of labor." A successful vaginal birth is less likely if the cervix is unfavorable, as has become more widely known in recent years. There are now several cervical assessment scoring systems available. Bishop created a standardized cervical scoring system and methodically assessed a group of multiparous women for elective induction in 1964. Patients who would be most likely to have a successful induction are identified using the Bishop score. The Bishop score and the length of labor are inversely correlated; a patient with a score higher than 8 has the highest chance of having a vaginal birth. When a bishop score is less than 6, cervical ripening techniques must typically be applied before other techniques.

4.1.1.1. Nonpharmacologic Cervical Ripening

- **Herbal Supplements:** Patients' requests for information about alternative agents for labor induction are not surprising, considering the industry for herbal supplements is growing at a rapid pace. Red raspberry leaves, black haw, black and blue cohosh, and evening primrose oil are among the frequently recommended substances. Even though midwives most frequently use evening primrose oil, it's not known if this oil can cause labor or ripen the cervix. Black haw has been used to help women get ready for labor; it has been described as having a uterine tonic effect. While blue cohosh may induce uterine contractions, black cohosh functions similarly. Once labor has begun, red raspberry leaves are used to intensify contractions in the uterus. Because the quality of the evidence is based on anecdotal case reports and a long history of use by a particular population, the risks and benefits of these agents are still unknown. As of right now, it is only possible to draw the conclusion that there is still no solid evidence supporting the use of herbal remedies for cervical ripening or labor induction (McFarlin et al.,1999).
- **Castor Oil, Hot Baths and Enemas:** Cervical ripening or labor induction has also been associated with the use of castor oil, hot baths, and enemas. These techniques' modes of action are unknown. An analysis of the literature reveals that one shoddy study with 100 participants compared castor oil to no treatment. All of the women who consumed the castor oil reported feeling queasy, even though there didn't seem to be any difference in the outcomes

for the fetus or newborn. At this time, no evidence supports the use of these three modalities as viable methods for cervical ripening or labor induction (Kelly et al., 2002).

- **Sexual Intercourse:** It is generally advised to have sex in order to encourage labor initiation. The stimulation of the breasts and nipples during sexual relations can encourage the release of oxytocin. The lower uterine segment is stimulated upon penetration. Prostaglandins are released locally as a result of this stimulation. It has been demonstrated that female orgasms involve uterine contractions, and prostaglandins, which are found in human semen, cause cervical ripening. There is still uncertainty regarding the role of sexual activity in promoting labor initiation because the one study that included 28 women produced data that was only marginally useful.
- **Breast Stimulation:** It has been demonstrated that nipple stimulation and breast massage help the posterior pituitary gland release oxytocin. The most often recommended method entails giving the breasts a light massage or using warm compresses for an hour, three times a day. Studies have shown that oxytocin release results in an aberrant fetal heart rate (FHR) trace, which is akin to the tracing seen in oxytocin challenge tests in pregnancies at higher risk. Fetal hypoxia and a decrease in placental perfusion could be the cause of this abnormal rate. Two shoddy studies from the 1970s and 1980s showed that there was a difference between the intervention groups, but the shoddy study design implies that there is insufficient data to support breast stimulation as a practical way to induce labor.
- **Acupuncture/Transcutaneous Nerve Stimulation:** In order to prevent or treat disease, very tiny needles are inserted into predetermined locations during an acupuncture treatment. Acupuncture is believed to stimulate channels of qi, or energy (pronounced "Chee") in the Chinese medical system. There are specified locations along each of the twelve meridians that this energy flows along. Each point is given a name and a number and is associated with a specific organ system or function (Beal 1999). Prostaglandin and oxytocin release is believed to be stimulated by transcutaneous nerve stimulation (TENS) and acupuncture in Western medicine. The majority of acupuncture-related research was poorly designed and did not adhere to the strict analysis standards established by the Cochrane reviewers. A well-designed randomized controlled trial (RCT) is needed to evaluate the role of acupuncture and TENS in labor induction (Smith et al., 2002).
- **Mechanical Modalities:** The mechanism of action of all mechanical modalities is the same: a local pressure of some kind triggers prostaglandin release. The risks connected to these techniques include bleeding, ruptured membranes, placental disruption,

and infection (natural osmotic dilators have been linked to endometritis and neonatal sepsis). Hygroscopic dilators expand inside the endocervix and provide controlled mechanical pressure by absorbing endocervical and local tissue fluids. There are two types of osmotic dilation products available: synthetic (Lamicel) and natural (*Laminaria japonicum*). Hygroscopic dilators have two main benefits: they can be used as outpatients and do not require FHR monitoring. In Table 4.1, the method for positioning hygroscopic dilators is explained.

Table 4.1. Technique for Insertion of Hygroscopic Dilators

The perineum and vagina are prepped with antiseptic.
Using a sterile speculum examination to visualize the cervix, the dilator is introduced into the endocervix, allowing the "tails" to fall into the vagina.
Dilators are progressively placed until the endocervix is "full." The number of dilators used is noted in the medical record.
A sterile gauze pad is placed in the vagina to maintain the position of the dilators.

Source: https://www.aafp.org/pubs/afp/issues/2003/0515/p2123.html#references.

Table 4.2. Technique for Placement of Balloon Dilators

The catheter is introduced into the endocervix by direct visualization or blindly by locating the cervix with the examining fingers and guiding the catheter over the hand and fingers through the endocervix and into the potential space between the amniotic membrane and the lower uterine segment.
The balloon reservoir is inflated with 30 to 50 mL of normal saline.
The balloon is retracted so that it rests on the internal OS.

Additional steps that may be taken:
• Apply pressure by adding weights to the catheter end.
    ○ **Constant Pressure:** attach 1 L of intravenous fluids to the catheter end and suspend it from the end of the bed.
    ○ **Intermittent Pressure:** gently tug on the catheter end two to four times per hour.
• Saline infusion[12]: Inflate catheter with 40 mL of sterile water or saline.
Infuse sterile saline at a rate of 40 mL per hour using an infusion pump.
Remove six hours later or at the time of spontaneous expulsion or rupture of membranes (whichever occurs first).
• Prostaglandin E2 infusion[14]

Source: https://www.aafp.org/pubs/afp/issues/2003/0515/p2123.html#references.

As the balloon is filled, balloon devices apply mechanical pressure directly to the cervix. One can use balloon devices specifically made for the purpose or a Foley catheter (26 Fr). Table 4.2 provides a description of the method.

Currently, several RCTs are comparing the administration of laminaria, prostaglandin E_2, or extra-amniotic saline infusion with the use of a balloon device (PGE_2). According to the trial results, all of these techniques are useful for cervical ripening and have similar rates of cesarean delivery in women with unfavorable cervixes.

4.1.1.2. Surgical Methods

- **Stripping of the Membranes:** Phospholipase A_2 and prostaglandin $F_{2\alpha}$ ($PGF_{2\alpha}$) are activated more when the membranes are stripped, and the cervix mechanically dilates to release prostaglandins. The inferior pole of the membranes is separated from the lower uterine segment by passing the examining finger through the internal cervical OS and rotating it in a circular motion to remove the membranes. This procedure carries some risks, such as bleeding, infection, unintentional membrane rupture, and discomfort for the patient. The Cochrane reviewers concluded that while membrane stripping does not appear to provide clinically significant benefits on its own, it does appear to have some benefit when used in conjunction with other treatments, such as lowering the mean amount of oxytocin required and increasing the frequency of normal vaginal deliveries.
- **Amniotomy:** It is postulated that amniotomy either stimulates local prostaglandin production or releases prostaglandins. Umbilical cord prolapse or compression, infection in the mother or newborn, FHR deceleration, placenta previa or low-lying placenta bleeding, and potential fetal harm are among the risks connected to this procedure. Table 4.3 describes the procedure for performing an amniotomy.

Table 4.3. Technique for Performing Amniotomy

A pelvic examination is performed to evaluate the cervix and station of the presenting part.
The fetal heart rate is recorded before and after the procedure.
The presenting part should be well applied to the cervix.
The membranes over the fetal head are removed by the examining finger.
A cervical hook is inserted through the cervical OS by sliding it along the hand and fingers (hook side toward the hand).
The membranes are scratched or hooked to effect rupture.
The nature of the amniotic fluid is recorded (clear, bloody, thick or thin, meconium).

Source: https://www.aafp.org/pubs/afp/issues/2003/0515/p2123.html#references.

Only two well-controlled trials studied the use of amniotomy alone, and the evidence did not support its use for induction of labor.

4.1.2. Uterine Distension

The term "uterine distension" describes the uterus's expansion or stretching, which usually happens during pregnancy but can also happen during certain medical procedures or pathological conditions. Uterine distension is a normal and essential part of pregnancy as the uterus expands to make room for the developing fetus and amniotic fluid. In order to accommodate the growing size of the fetus, the uterine muscles undergo hypertrophy and stretch, growing from the size of a pear to a large, muscular organ that can hold a full-term baby. To assist fetal growth and development, this distension causes several physiological changes, such as changes in blood flow and hormone levels. Uterine distension can also be brought on by pathological diseases like uterine fibroids or adenomyosis, which can result in symptoms like infertility, abnormal bleeding, and pelvic pain. Furthermore, temporary uterine distension can be brought on by medical procedures such as intrauterine device implantation or uterine artery embolization. Comprehending uterine distension plays a pivotal role in obstetrics to oversee fetal growth and health throughout gestation, and in gynecology to accurately diagnose and treat associated disorders.

4.1.3. Cardinal Movements

The forces necessary for fetal descent and the movements the fetus must make to overcome the resistance provided by the mother's bony pelvis and soft tissue—primarily the pelvic floor and levator ani muscle—are described by the mechanics of labor. The pelvic outlet and pelvic inlet form a curved canal with different diameters when they are 90 degrees apart. The birth canal is divided into three sections: the cavity, the outlet, and the inlet. The transverse and more rounded inlet and outlet of the gynecoid pelvis are the widest in dimensions, while the anterior-posterior diameter is the widest. A human fetus's head and shoulders are its critical diameters, and it must rotate to fit through the birth canal. Although they are commonly referred to as the "cardinal movements," the fetal head and shoulders' rotational movements are typically only described as movements in earlier publications. The fetal head often enters the pelvis in a transverse orientation in a gynecoid pelvis, and the flexion of the neck is the first rotational movement in the fetus's long axis. The fetus is then facing the mother's back with its head oriented anteriorly and posteriorly following the second movement, which is a transverse rotation of the occiput anteriorly. Due to its largest anterior-posterior diameter, the pelvic outlet permits the fetal head to exit. The shoulders can now move into the transverse plane and enter the pelvic inlet thanks to this second rotation. The fetal head becomes an extension when the nape of the fetal neck passes beneath the mother's symphysis due to resistance from the soft tissue of the mother. The third rotational movement is the name given to this motion. The external rotation is the fourth movement. Now positioned in the center of the pelvis, the fetal body and shoulders can rotate into the outlet's largest anteroposterior plane. The fetal head turns to face either the mother's left or right thigh during this process.

Understanding the cardinal movements of the fetal head is a relatively recent development in medicine. These are not described in ancient texts, which focus on lie and presentation, however, Soranus mentions that the birth is even more favorable when the fetus descends with its face turned downward. William Smellie in "A Treatise on the Theory and Practice of Midwifery" infers knowledge of the cardinal movements, but does not name them. In Alfred Galabin's "A Manual of Midwifery," the term "cardinal movements" appears and is adopted by later authors such as Munro Kerr. In the German tradition, Spiegelberg from Breslau lists the following 4 "movements" in 1878: flexion, internal rotation, extension, and external rotation, and in Pschyrembel's "Practische Geburtshilfe" from 1947, these 4 movements are called cardinal movements. In the United States, Shears' "Obstetrics, Normal and Operative" talks of "movements of the head" and lists 5 movements, namely flexion, descent, rotation, extension, and external rotation. In "Willams Obstetrics," third edition, J. Whitridge Williams writes that the 3 true cardinal movements are descent, internal rotation, and flexion, whereas extension and external rotation are only accessory movements, and in the 10th edition, editor J. Nicholson opines that the 3 cardinal movements are in fact descent, internal rotation, and extension, whereas flexion and external rotation are now considered accessory movements.

By the 1989 edition, edited by F. Cunningham, the list of cardinal movements had increased to 7. Engagement is called the first movement. Descent is the gradual passage of the fetus through the birth canal and is called the second movement. The next 4 movements are the rotational movements described above and the expulsion of the fetus is called the seventh movement. The 3 extra movements listed in "Williams Obstetrics," refer to fetal descent. Engagement is simply a stage of descent when the largest diameter of the fetal head has passed the pelvic inlet and expulsion is the ultimate result of the descent. One could argue that the descent of the fetal head is an obligate movement without which the fetus cannot be born, as "Williams Obstetrics" and some earlier authors do. However, we would argue that descent is the main purpose of the uterine powers, and the cardinal movements are a description of the rotational movements the fetal head and shoulders must perform to obtain descent.

Although there is no direct clinical value to this descriptive discussion, it is still important to understand the rotational movements. The fetus can only deliver in the occiput anterior (OA) position in a gynecoid pelvis when it makes the four classic rotational movements mentioned above. The pelvic inlet in an anthropoid pelvis has the largest anterior-posterior diameter. The anthropoid pelvis must rotate differently than a gynecoid pelvis, but little is known about the labor mechanics of pelvic forms other than the gynecoid pelvis.

The fetal head's posture and degree of flexion affect the cardinal movements. After the head is born, the third cardinal movement is maximal flexion followed by an extension to a neutral attitude if the internal rotation (second cardinal movement) results in an occiput posterior (OP) position. The fetus in the OP position can never follow the curve of the birth canal as well through extension as the fetus in the OA position can, even at maximum flexion. It is imperative that clinicians comprehend this, as the traction employed during assisted deliveries needs to be different from that of an OA position. Compared to the fetus in the OA position, the fetus in the OP position must continue straight forward for a longer period of time as the head approaches the pelvic floor before upward traction is possible. Anal sphincter tears are much more likely to occur if the clinician overcorrects with downward traction rather than proceeding straight forward. There are more failed deliveries correlated with OP deliveries. This could be due to a number of factors, including the fact that the OP fetus often presents less flexed during delivery than a fetus in an OA position, which may contribute to the underdiagnosis of the condition, and the fact that physicians are not well-versed in the variations in labor mechanics. For ease of delivery, it is beneficial if an OP position can be adjusted to an OA position using a rotating vacuum, forceps, or manual rotation. Although manual rotation is becoming more and more popular, a randomized study lacked sufficient power to demonstrate lower rates of operative deliveries. Reduced risk of operative delivery was observed in another randomized clinical trial following prophylactic manual rotation of the occiput transverse or OP during the early stages of labor. It takes precise diagnostics of the fetal head station, position, and flexion to carry out instrumental or manual rotations successfully.

Early in labor, it is challenging to evaluate the attitude and position of the fetus using clinical examinations, but it is simple to see with ultrasound. Thus, ultrasound can improve knowledge of labor mechanics and support medical professionals in making decisions. In a recent longitudinal ultrasound study of nulliparous women experiencing spontaneous labor, fetal rotation was observed, and it was found that 85% of these women followed the four classical movements, although the length of the internal rotation (second movement) varied depending on the starting position. Fetal position can be compared to a clock face with 12 or 24 divisions, and fetal attitude can be quantified.

The term "head up sign" refers to the position in the pelvic outlet where the head is directed upward and the fetal neck is extended. A fetus just before delivery with its neck extended. Using ultrasound to evaluate the fourth movement is superfluous. Although ultrasound can provide clinically significant information on its own cannot guarantee better results. It's critical to comprehend how to apply the information.

A more thorough grasp of labor mechanics is necessary in order to convert the data obtained from clinical examination and ultrasound into clinical decision making. Unfortunately, most modern textbooks only cover the most superficial aspects of the subject, making it difficult to access this knowledge today. Since there are still many unanswered questions, we think a labor mechanics revival is long overdue. The majority of labor mechanics research is more than 50 years old. To address those questions, ultrasound provides a historically unique opportunity for dynamic, noninvasive studies of the mechanics of labor (Kamel, 2010; Irani & Foster, 2015).

4.2. Mechanisms and Management of Normal Labor

The parameters of normal labor vary depending on the clinical care provider's experience. For some, spontaneous labor that results in a vaginal birth without augmentation or assistance is equivalent to normal labor. This phrase may include high-risk labor like trial of labor after cesarean, induction and augmentation of labor, and interventions like episiotomy and instrumental vaginal delivery in other contexts. The biochemical, hormonal, and mechanical phases of typical spontaneous labor and vaginal delivery will be discussed for this section. We will then go on to discuss how these phases may be influenced at different times by intervention, or by the laboring woman's risk status. Simply, normal labor aims to produce progressive effective uterine contractions, leading to:

- Cervical effacement and dilatation
- Expulsion of the fetus through the birth canal
- Separation and expulsion of the placenta

The more progressive active phase of labor as we know it is preceded by many preparatory steps that make up the complex process of labor. Paracrine and autocrine signaling in the mother and fetus cooperate throughout pregnancy to attain fetal maturity and properly trigger parturition. The necessity of iatrogenic labor induction in cases where spontaneous labor is not possible, such as in cases of fetal death or anencephaly, emphasizes the significance of this collaboration.

4.2.1. Phases of Labor

Four phases of natural parturition have been described:

1. **Quiescence**: This phase involves not only the maintenance of myometrial a

contractility but also that of cervical structural integrity.

- The myometrium increases in vascularity throughout pregnancy, affording essential nutrients and gaseous exchange, not only for the developing fetus but also in anticipation of the extensive energy requirements of labor.
- This phase is controlled by progesterone, relaxin and prostacyclin. Progesterone inhibits contraction associated proteins (CAPs) by increasing the transcription factor zinc finger e-box binding homeobox protein 1 (ZEB1) and connexin 43. ZEB1 and connexin 43 recruit other repressor proteins, such as polypyrimidine tract binding protein-associated splicing factor (PSF) and yeast switch-dependent 3 homolog A/ histone deacetylase corepressor complex (Sin3A/ HDACs). The repressor proteins decrease the number of myometrial gap junctions, thereby maintaining acontractility.

2. **Activation**: The transition from quiescence to active labor.

- This phase is predominantly controlled by the relative increase in the estrogen: progesterone ratio, occurring in a gradually accelerative manner throughout the last few weeks of the third trimester.
- The myometrium becomes more responsive to signaling, and as progesterone decreases, CAPs are no longer inhibited, therefore increasing uterine contractility. This in turn increases PSF and Sin3A/HDACs further.
- Cervical tissue compliance and distensibility increase.

3. **Stimulation**: Including active labor.

- This phase is predominantly mediated by prostaglandins, oxytocin and relaxin.
- Progressive uterine contractions with concurrent cervical effacement and dilatation aim to expel the fetus through the birth canal.
- Placental separation and expulsion.

4. **Involution**: Refers to the recovery of the mother throughout the puerperium

- Oxytocin mediates uterine involution and milk letdown.
- Initiation of inflammatory pathways expediting healing.

4.2.1.1. Hormonal Control of Labor

The hormonal control of labor is a complex interplay of several key hormones that coordinate the onset and progression of childbirth. Central to this process is the hormone oxytocin, which is released from the posterior pituitary gland. Oxytocin stimulates the uterine muscles to contract, initiating and maintaining labor contractions. Its release is regulated through a positive feedback mechanism: as the uterus contracts, stretch receptors in the cervix and uterus send signals to the brain to release more oxytocin, intensifying contractions. Prostaglandins, produced in the fetal membranes and the uterine decidua, also play a crucial role by softening the cervix (cervical ripening) and enhancing uterine contractions. Estrogen levels rise towards the end of pregnancy, increasing the sensitivity of the uterus to oxytocin and upregulating the production of oxytocin receptors on the uterine muscle cells. Additionally, the decrease in progesterone, which has a relaxing effect on the uterus during pregnancy, removes the inhibition on uterine contractions, allowing labor to proceed. These hormonal changes collectively ensure the effective initiation and progression of labor, culminating in the delivery of the baby and the placenta (Figure 4.1).

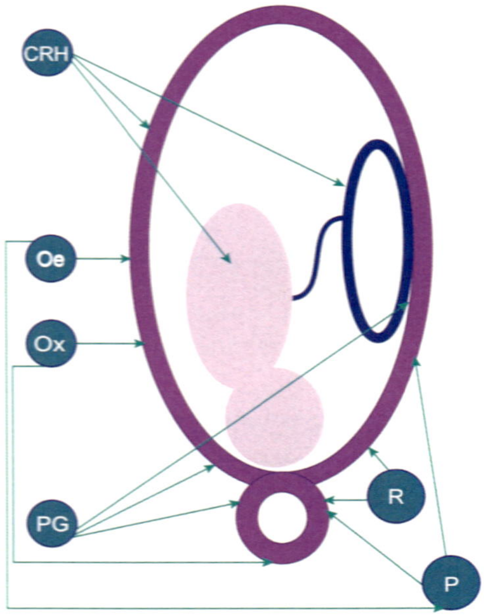

Figure 4.1. *Targets of hormonal control during the initiation and maintenance of labor.*

Source: https://www.nccwebsite.org/content/documents/courses/Normal%20labor.pdf.

4.2.1.2. Corticotropin-Releasing Hormone (CRH)

CRH is a peptide found in the placenta and the hypothalamus. It is known to increase exponentially in the near term but is produced in varying concentrations throughout pregnancy and labor. Elevated CRH levels in the middle of pregnancy are thought to increase the risk of prematurity. It is believed that CRH contributes to the onset of labor by acting on targets in the placenta, myometrial smooth muscle, and fetal adrenal pituitary axis.

Placental CRH increases with the progression of pregnancy, especially during the third trimester. This increase is assumed to play a role in the development of the fetal organs and the fetus's readiness for birth. Increased cortisol production is beneficial to lung development and the generation of surfactant, which is necessary for healthy lung function from birth, in the fetus, which is facilitated by elevated CRH levels.

Additionally, CRH directly influences when labor begins. Prostaglandins and estrogen are produced in greater quantities when CRH levels are high, and these substances are essential for inducing labor. While estrogen upregulates oxytocin receptors in the uterus, increasing its receptivity to oxytocin, prostaglandins promote cervical ripening and amplify uterine contractions. Moreover, CRH can integrate different hormonal pathways to guarantee coordinated labor progression and increase the uterus' sensitivity to other labor-inducing cues.

4.2.1.2.1. Actions and Psychopharmacology

When under stress, parvocellular neurosecretory cells in the paraventricular nucleus of the hypothalamus produce the majority of the hormone CRH, which is then released from these neurons' neurosecretory terminals into the primary capillary plexus of the hypothalamo-hypophyseal portal system at the median eminence. Adrenocorticotropic hormone (ACTH) and other physiologically active substances (β-endorphin) are secreted by corticotropes after the CRH is transported by the portal system to the anterior lobe of the pituitary. The synthesis of cortisol, glucocorticoids, mineralocorticoids, and DHEA is stimulated by ACTH. In addition to increasing subjective feelings of anxiety and decreasing appetite, CRH can also improve attention span.

When compared to healthy individuals, combat veterans with post-traumatic stress disorder (PTSD) have lower blood serum levels of CRH during chronic stress conditions. Chronic stress is thought to increase the HPA axis's negative feedback inhibition, which lowers CRH levels and impairs HPA function. Significantly depressed individuals and suicide victims' cerebrospinal fluid have been shown to have abnormally high levels of CRH.

It has been demonstrated that corticotropin-releasing hormone interacts with both corticotropin-releasing hormone receptor 1 (CRFR1) and receptor 2 (CRFR2) to elicit its effects. CRFR1 expression can be elevated by injecting CRH into the rodent paraventricular nucleus of the hypothalamus (PVN), and this elevated expression can induce behaviors resembling depression. Regarding CRH and the receptors it interacts with, sex differences have also been noted. When compared to male voles, females have higher levels of CRFR1 in the nucleus accumbens, olfactory tubercle, and rostral anteroventral periventricular nucleus (AVPV), while males have higher levels of CRFR2 in the stria terminalis bed nucleus. Pexacerfont, a CRH-1 receptor antagonist, is presently being studied as a potential treatment for generalized anxiety disorder. Although no human trials have been conducted with this compound, another CRH-1 antagonist, antalarmin, has been studied in animal studies for the treatment of anxiety, depression, and other conditions.

4.2.1.2.2. Role in Parturition

The placenta produces CRH, which appears to control how long a pregnancy lasts.

Levels rise towards the end of pregnancy just before birth and current theory suggests three roles of CRH in parturition:

- Increases levels of dehydroepiandrosterone (DHEA) directly by action on the fetal adrenal gland, and indirectly via the mother's pituitary gland. DHEA has a role in preparing for and stimulating cervical contractions.
- Increases prostaglandin availability in uteroplacental tissues. Prostaglandins activate cervical contractions.
- Before parturition, it may have a role in inhibiting contractions, through increasing cAMP levels in the myometrium.

Progesterone inhibits trophoblast CRH in culture and stays elevated during pregnancy. Glucocorticoids and catecholamines, which rise before parturition and lift this progesterone block, stimulate its release.

4.2.1.3. Prostaglandins

Prostaglandins (PG) are essential for the start of labor. By inducing cell apoptosis and remodeling of the cervical extracellular matrix protein, they eventually cause fetal membrane rupture through activation of matrix metalloproteinase (MMP). PGF2⍰, PGHS-2, and PGE2 receptors also help to develop depolarization signals and spread them throughout smooth muscle cells, increasing the responsiveness of the myometrium to contractile agonists. Additionally, PG—more especially, PGF2⍰—contributes to placental separation. In animal studies, it has been shown that lower levels of PGF2⍰ are linked to a higher incidence of retained products of conception, whereas higher levels encourage uterine involution. Additionally, there is a connection between placental abruption and PGE2 use in labor induction.

4.2.1.4. Progesterone

The effects of progesterone include promoting cervical competency and inhibiting myometrial contractility. It reduces prostaglandin synthesis brought on by oxytocin as well as the myometrial response to it. One important factor in helping parturition occur is progesterone withdrawal. Miscarriage is frequently avoided by using progesterone formulations as part of fertility treatment. To increase the number of myometrial gap junctions and soften the cervix and cause an inflammatory response, progesterone antagonists like mifepristone (which is used in the medical management of miscarriage and medical termination of pregnancy) also increase susceptibility to prostaglandins and oxytocin.

4.2.1.5. Estrogen

Estrogen, a crucial steroid hormone, plays a vital role in the regulation of the female reproductive system and is particularly important during pregnancy and labor. As pregnancy progresses, estrogen levels increase significantly, contributing to the preparation of the body for childbirth.

During pregnancy, estrogen is primarily produced by the placenta, with its levels rising steadily throughout gestation. One of the key functions of estrogen is to promote the growth and development of the uterus, allowing it to accommodate the growing fetus. Estrogen also stimulates the blood flow to the uterus, ensuring that the fetus receives an adequate supply of nutrients and oxygen.

In the context of labor, estrogen has several important roles. It enhances the sensitivity of the uterus to oxytocin, a hormone that triggers uterine contractions. Estrogen achieves this by upregulating the expression of oxytocin receptors on the uterine muscle cells, making the uterus more responsive to oxytocin as labor approaches. This increased responsiveness is crucial for the initiation and progression of labor contractions.

Estrogen also stimulates the production of prostaglandins, which are lipid compounds that play a significant role in cervical ripening and the initiation of labor. Prostaglandins help to soften and dilate the cervix, preparing it for the passage of the baby during delivery. Additionally, prostaglandins contribute to the enhancement of uterine contractions, working in concert with oxytocin to facilitate the labor process.

Furthermore, estrogen influences the expression of gap junctions in the uterine muscle. Gap junctions are specialized cell structures that allow for the coordinated contraction of the uterine muscle fibers. By increasing the number of gap junctions, estrogen ensures that uterine contractions are synchronized and effective during labor.

Estrogen is a key hormone in the hormonal control of labor, playing multiple roles in preparing the uterus for childbirth. It increases uterine sensitivity to oxytocin, promotes cervical ripening through prostaglandin production, and enhances the coordination of uterine contractions. These actions collectively ensure the successful initiation and progression of labor, culminating in the delivery of the baby.

4.2.1.6. Oxytocin

Myometrial smooth muscle activation and cervical remodeling are both influenced by oxytocin. The periods of parturition and gestation determine the response to oxytocin, which is indicative of the progesterone: estrogen balance at that particular time. The concentration of oxytocin receptors rises noticeably as term draws near and reaches its peak in the early stages of labor. The decidua and uterine fundus contain the greatest concentration of oxytocin receptors, which are then distributed throughout the lower segment and the cervix. There are direct and indirect effects of oxytocin. It works directly to cause regular, powerful contractions in the myometrium and indirectly to boost prostaglandin synthesis in the decidua.

4.2.1.7. Relaxin

The decidua, placenta, and corpus luteum all produce relaxin. Relaxin levels rise just before delivery, peak at the end of the first trimester, and then decline again. The G protein-coupled receptors that relaxin acts on are the same ones that the luteinizing hormone and folic acid stimulating hormone do. Targeted by relaxin are the decidua, myometrium, endometrium, and cervix. To prepare for labor, it first primarily suppresses uterine contractility and then contributes to the remodeling of cervical connective tissue.

4.2.2. Mechanical Processes of Labor

The fetus must undergo many physical adjustments and movements during the mechanical processes of labor in order to pass through the birth canal and be born. These processes are often described through the "mechanism of labor," which includes several key steps: engagement, descent, flexion, internal rotation, extension, restitution, and external rotation.

- **Engagement:** When the biparietal diameter, the widest portion of the fetal head, enters the pelvic inlet, engagement takes place. This shows that the baby is getting ready to come out of the pelvis by descending into it. Engagement is frequently measured during a vaginal exam or by palpating the fetal head through the abdomen.
- **Descent:** The fetus descends through the birth canal under the influence of gravity, maternal pushing force, and uterine contractions. The process of the fetal head becoming increasingly more embedded in the pelvis starts before labor and lasts through the first and second stages of labor.
- **Flexion:** As the fetal head descends, it encounters resistance from the maternal tissues, causing it to flex. Flexion is the bending of the fetal head forward, so the chin approaches the chest. This positioning reduces the diameter of the presenting part of the head, making it easier for the baby to pass through the birth canal.
- **Internal Rotation:** Internal rotation involves the rotation of the fetal head from its original position (usually transverse) to align with the anteroposterior diameter of the pelvic outlet. This rotation is essential for the head to navigate through the curved pelvic canal. The occiput (back of the head) typically rotates towards the front (anterior) of the mother's pelvis.
- **Extension:** Extension occurs as the fetal head passes under the pubic symphysis and the perineum. The head extends, moving from a flexed to an extended position, allowing the occiput to emerge first, followed by the face and chin. This movement facilitates the delivery of the head through the vaginal opening.
- **Restitution:** Restitution is the slight realignment of the fetal head after it is delivered. As the head emerges, it rotates to align with the shoulders, which are still inside the birth canal and oriented obliquely. This adjustment ensures that the shoulders can navigate the pelvic inlet effectively.
- **External Rotation:** After restitution, the fetal head undergoes external rotation to align with the shoulders, which are rotating internally to anteroposterior alignment. This rotation helps the shoulders fit through the pelvic outlet, with the anterior shoulder usually delivered first, followed by the posterior shoulder.

Each of these mechanical processes is critical for the successful passage of the fetus through the birth canal. They involve intricate coordination between the uterine contractions, the structure of the maternal pelvis, and the movements of the fetus. Understanding these processes helps healthcare providers manage labor effectively and address any complications that may arise, ensuring the safety and well-being of both the mother and the baby during childbirth.

4.2.2.1. Cervix

Fibrous connective tissue, collagen (types I, III, and IV), elastin, vasculature, fibroblasts, and very little smooth muscle make up the cervix. As gestation increases, the percentage of collagen decreases. Increased vascularity, stromal and glandular hypertrophy, and modifications to the cervical extracellular matrix by matrix metalloproteases, proteases, and collagenases all contribute to cervical ripening. Changes in this signaling pathway have been shown in animal studies to delay cervical ripening and decrease immune cell infiltration. Cervical nerve density is maintained or increased at term. Reduced crosslinks between collagen helices and a shift from straight to wavy fibers, along with an increase in hyaluronic acid production and the infiltration of neutrophils and macrophages, further destabilize the cervix's structural integrity.

During pregnancy, the levels of CGRP increase, which aids in vasodilation, vascular remodeling in early pregnancy, uterine quiescence, and cervical ripening. Substance P also plays a crucial role in promoting cervical ripening and inducing uterine contractions.

Increased cervical compliance and cervical response to an increase in intrauterine pressure as a result of progressive uterine contractions is the overall outcome of the alterations described above. To facilitate the delivery of the fetus and placenta, the cervix gradually dilates and becomes effaced, reaching a length of 10 cm. When inducing labor, the cervix can be moved mechanically or chemically. Cervical balloon catheters and vaginal prostaglandins are common techniques.

4.2.2.2. Uterus

The uterus, which is mostly made of smooth muscle, begins to change shape in the first few weeks of pregnancy in order to make room for the developing fetus and get ready for its eventual expulsion. The myometrium produces electrical activity through processes that result in the contractile forces needed for labor, as will be explained in more detail below. Hormonal, metabolic, and mechanical factors govern these processes. The uterus is a myogenic organ—that is, it can contract without nerve stimulation—despite receiving innervation from both the parasympathetic and sympathetic nervous systems. Given the strong contractile forces needed during labor, uterine myocytes are comparatively large. They are joined by gap junctions, which multiply throughout pregnancy and so increase the uterus's ability to contract. The action potential that is produced by the myocyte is what causes uterine contractions. When an action potential is reached, intracellular calcium (Ca^{2+}) levels rise due to the activation of voltage-dependent channels. Repolarization results from the inactivation of L-type Ca^{2+} channels caused by the opening of voltage-dependent potassium (K^{+}) channels, which also causes an outward K+ current. It is believed that as pregnancy progresses, myocyte resting membrane potential becomes more depolarized, which facilitates Ca^{2+} influx and raises the frequency of myometrial contractions. Short-term K+ channel reductions also lengthen myocyte action potentials and improve contractility.

Intracellular Ca^{2+} ions combine with calmodulin to form a complex that activates myosin light-chain kinase (MLCK). This process phosphorylates myosin and causes it to cross-bridge cycle with actin myofilaments, which in turn produces a contraction. This is how current tocolytics, like nifedipine, work: they block voltage-dependent L-type Ca^{2+} channels, which are also known as dihydropyridine receptors, thereby suppressing myometrial contractions. Sarcoplasmic reticula (SR) in myocytes are observed to be proportionately large. The SR have an impact on smooth muscle excitability in addition to storing Ca^{2+}. Uterine contractions are strengthened by the release of Ca^{2+} from SR, which also increases cytosolic Ca^{2+} and supports the actions of oxytocin, vasopressin, and PG. Intracellular pH and metabolites control the release of SR Ca^{2+}. It's interesting to note that uterine contractions during spontaneous labor are caused by Ca^{2+} entry and efflux across the plasma membrane; the SR plays no role in this. When oxytocin binds to a receptor in the cell membrane, it causes the cytosolic Ca^{2+} level to rise, which depolarizes the potential of the mitochondrial membrane and increases contractility. While Ca^{2+} plays a significant role, K^+ conductance is the primary factor influencing myocytes' resting membrane potential. K^+ channel manipulation has an impact on repolarization and action potential duration. K^+ channel activity is linked to uterine quiescence, and KATP is downregulated in the run-up to labor. K^+ current flows outward through TREK-1 K channels in response to myometrial stretching. To accommodate fetal growth and allow for uterine distension, their activity is restricted until close to term when gene expression increases.

It is believed that obese women express a subunit of K^+ voltage-dependent channels at lower levels. The fact that high cholesterol also causes an increase in outward K^+ current may make this worse. Because of both pathways' increased K^+ conductance and purportedly decreased myometrial activity, obese women are more likely to need cesarean sections for childbirth. Although uterine myocytes may naturally have pacemaking activity, no anatomical or histological pacemaking structure has been found as of yet. As labor continues, the frequency and amplitude of contractions increase. Myometrial vessels are compressed and occluded during the process. Therefore, uterine contractions must be phasic to avoid myometrial hypoxia that could prolong and cause fetal asphyxia. Lactic acid accumulates in the myocytes as contractions peak, influencing the Ca^{2+} current and bringing the contraction's intensity down to baseline. The action potential must be reversed and pH must be restored during the ensuing rest interval to prevent hypoxic metabolic changes.

Short cycles of hypoxia are thought to maintain the progressive augmentation of contractions required for labor. This is often referred to as hypoxia-induced force increase (HIFI). Parturition requires significant preparation, not only with respect to myometrial hypertrophy and increases in contractile proteins but also glycogen and free fatty acid storage ahead of the hypoxic challenges of labor. Strict control of Ca^{2+} and pH is necessary for uterine function. Oxidative phosphorylation provides the energy required for contractions, while anaerobic metabolism supports ionic regulation.

Lactate is produced by the myometrium even in the presence of sufficient oxygen and despite transportation out of the myocyte, continues to have an inhibitory effect on contractility. Accumulation of extracellular lactate is thought to contribute to dystocia, and a recent trial has proposed that ingestion of oral bicarbonate may have a therapeutic role in this regard. The changes detailed above are rapidly reversed in involution, where progressive remodeling of the uterine collagen and elastin content occurs. The uterus is back to near pre-pregnancy size in about 6 weeks, due to changes in endocrine levels and removal of mechanical stretch.

4.2.2.3. Perineum and Vagina

The vascularity of the vaginal and perineal muscles increases during pregnancy. To facilitate distension during labor, smooth muscle cells hypertrophy and perineal connective tissue soften. The region between the anus and the vaginal opening is known as the perineum. It is made up of connective tissue, muscle, and skin, and it supports the uterus, bladder, and rectum, among other pelvic organs. The pelvic floor muscles, which are essential for preserving continence and supporting the pelvic organs, attach to the perineal body, a fibromuscular mass located in the center of this region.

The perineum stretches a great deal during childbirth to make room for the baby's passage. A smoother delivery and the avoidance of severe tears are largely dependent on the elasticity and integrity of the perineal tissues. However, if the baby is large or some complications need to be delivered quickly, the perineum is prone to tears or may be surgically incised (episiotomy) to widen the vaginal opening and aid in delivery. In late pregnancy, perineal massage and other appropriate care can help improve tissue elasticity and possibly lower the risk of severe tearing. The vagina is a muscular, tubular structure that connects the cervix of the uterus to the external vaginal opening. Because of its highly elastic walls and mucous membrane lining, which keeps it moist and flexible, it can swell considerably during childbirth. During delivery, the baby passes through the vagina, which acts as the birth canal.

The vagina changes remarkably during labor to make childbirth easier. As the baby passes through the birth canal, the vaginal walls enlarge and contract. The hormone relaxin, which makes the tissues and ligaments in the pelvis more flexible, aids in this process. The descending fetus presses against the vaginal tissues, stimulating them to secrete more lubricant, which lessens friction and makes the baby's passage easier. The lochia, a postpartum discharge consisting of blood, mucus, and uterine tissue, passes through the vagina as the uterus heals and regains its pre-pregnancy size. This discharge lasts for several weeks following childbirth.

4.2.2.3.1. Recovery and Care

The perineum and vaginal tissues must both heal as part of postpartum recovery. Taking good care of the area involves cleaning it up, using sitz baths or cold packs to ease discomfort, and avoiding activities like heavy lifting and vigorous exercise that strain the pelvic floor muscles. Exercises for the pelvic floor, like Kegels, are advised to help heal, strengthen the pelvic muscles, and avoid problems like incontinence.

During childbirth, the vagina and perineum play important roles and undergo significant changes that enable a safe delivery of the baby. The health and wellbeing of the mother depend on her being aware of their roles and knowing how to take care of them both during and after delivery. A more comfortable postpartum recovery and a more seamless delivery process can be achieved with the right support and care (Kamel, 2010; Irani & Foster, 2015).

4.2.2.4. Pelvis

When evaluating the descent of the fetal presenting portion, the ischial spines serve as a landmark. The dimensions of the pelvis are summarized in Table 4.4 and Figure 4.2.

Table 4.4. Dimensions of the Pelvis (cm)

	Boundaries	Transverse	Oblique	Anteroposterior
Inlet	Sacral promontory, linea terminalis, superior rami of the pubic bones, symphysis pubis	12.7 (Longest distance between the bilateral linea terminalis)	11.5 (Iliopectineal eminence -> sacroiliac joint)	10 (Obstetric conjugate: sacral promontory -> symphysis pubis)
Mid	Ischial spines	11.5	11.5 (lower sacroiliac joint -> midpoint of obturator membrane)	11.5 (S3 ->midpoint of pubic symphysis)
Outlet	Base at level of line drawn between the ischial tuberosities, tip of sacrum, subpubic area	10 (between ischial tuberosities)	11.5	12.7 (Pubis -> sacrococcygeal joint)

Source: https://www.nccwebsite.org/content/documents/courses/Normal%20labor.pdf

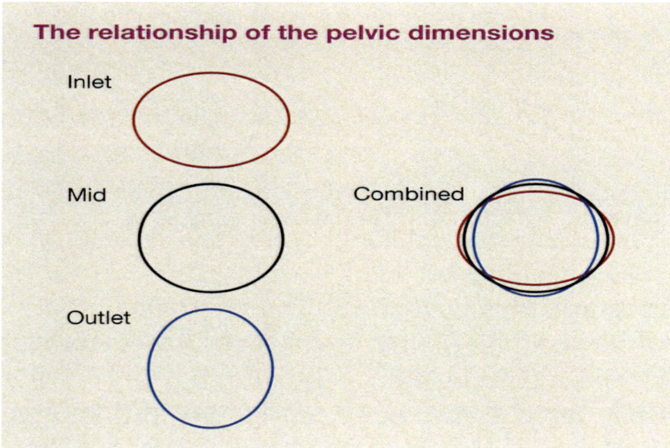

Figure 4.2. *Diagram demonstrating the relationship of the pelvic dimensions, and how they combine to create a passage for fetal descent. The angulation of the birth canal is referred to as the curve of Carus.*

Source: https://www.nccwebsite.org/content/documents/courses/Normal%20labor.pdf.

4.2.2.5. Power

We have already covered the mechanical concepts underlying the production of contractions at the cellular level. In order to exert force on the fetus and the more malleable soft tissues, contractions change the intrauterine pressure. This first causes cervical dilation, which subsequently combines with maternal effort to produce expulsive force.

4.2.2.6. Passage

The cervix needs to ripen and dilate first. It is believed that if a woman remains upright during the first stage of labor, this process will be shortened; however, the specifics of this have not been fully explored. Following are three bony landmarks (Table 4.4) that could pose a challenge to the part of the fetus that is presenting. In this context, maternal position can also be helpful. For example, in cases of shoulder dystocia, McRobert's position can be used to lower the sacral promontory and facilitate delivery. To allow for delivery, the soft tissue of the pelvic floor must also stretch sufficiently. There is disagreement over whether having a high pelvic tone facilitates or hinders the fetal passage. It is believed that it could direct communication in addition to passively extending when necessary. It should come as no surprise that research has shown that as the fetus passes through the pelvis, its perineal muscle force increases. Because of this, women who give birth naturally have been found to have lower levels of pelvic tone than women who have Caesarean sections because of unsuccessful induction.

4.2.2.7. Passenger

A cephalic, fully flexed presentation is ideal because the fetal head's diameter presents the biggest mechanical challenge. In contrast to vaginal breech deliveries, a healthcare provider can be more confident that the remainder of the infant won't present a mechanical challenge if the baby's head is delivered successfully. In this case, there is a relative risk of head entrapment, particularly in preterm deliveries (because of the greater difference in the size of the fetal head compared to the rest of its body).

4.2.2.8. Lie

The lie describes the long axis of the fetus with respect to the long axis of the mother:

- Longitudinal
- Transverse
- Oblique

4.2.2.9. Presentation

Presentation is the term used to describe the fetal part that moves into the maternal pelvis. This has significant mechanical impacts during the second stage of labor (refer to Table 4.5).

- **Cephalic:** Vertex/Occiput, Face, Sinciput, Brow
- **Breech:** This is much less common than cephalic presentation, comprising only 3–4% of term deliveries. Whilst vaginal breech delivery, and indeed is much less common currently, presentation may be further described as frank, complete or footling.

Table 4.5. Diameter of Presenting Part and Important Landmarks of the Fetal Skull

Presenting part of fetal skull	**Diameter**
Occipital (Suboccipitobregmatic)	9.5 cm
Vertex (Occipitofrontal)	11.5 cm
Brow (Mentovertical)	13 cm
Face (Submentobregmatic)	9.5 cm
Other important landmarks	
Biparietal	9.5 cm
Bitemporal	8 cm

Source: https://www.nccwebsite.org/content/documents/courses/Normal%20labor.pdf.

4.2.2.10. Position

The relationship between the fetal presenting part and the mother pelvis is described by position; Figure 4.3 illustrates the cephalic variations of this relationship.

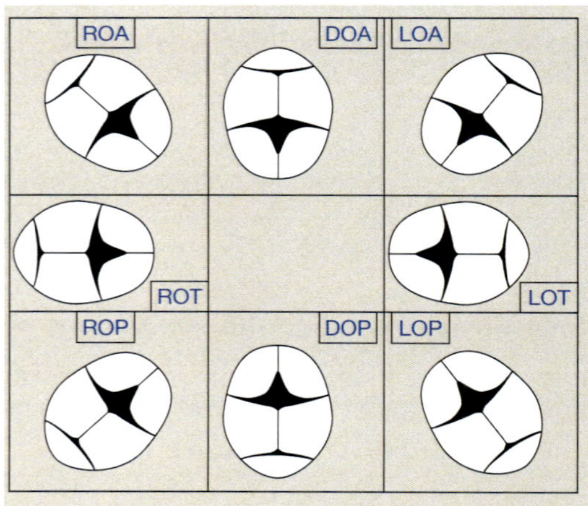

Figure 4.3. *Variations of the fetal head position when the presenting part is cephalic.*

Source: https://www.nccwebsite.org/content/documents/courses/Normal%20labor.pdf.

The diameter of the presenting portion and significant fetal skull landmarks are summarized in Table 4.5. Variations in the fetal head position when the presenting part is cephalic are depicted in Figure 4.3. The descent and delivery of the fetal head during labor is depicted in Figure 4.4.

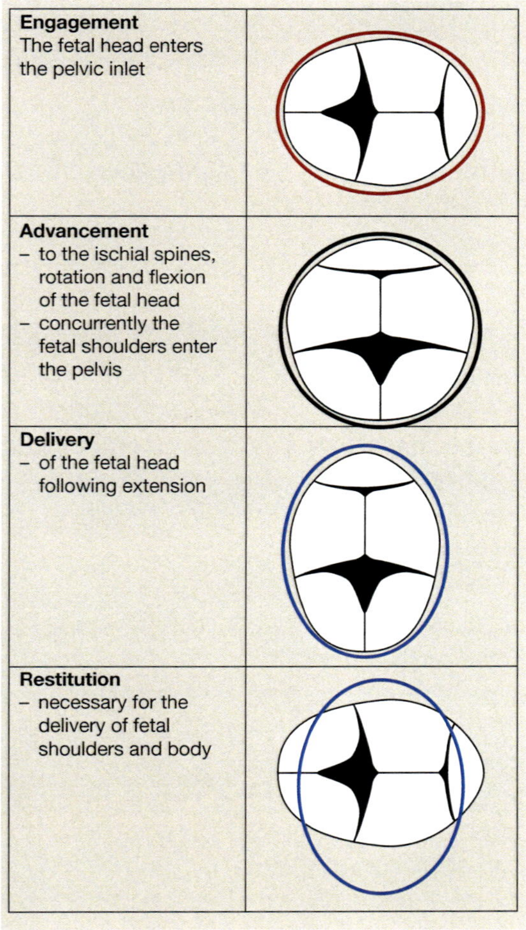

Figure 4.4. *Descent and delivery of the fetal head during labor.*

Source: *https://www.nccwebsite.org/content/documents/courses/Normal%20labor.pdf.*

4.2.3. Management of Normal Labor

For clinical management, labor is divided into three stages:

Stage 1: commencing with preparatory mechanical and biochemical changes as aforementioned, up to the achievement of full cervical dilatation. This stage is further subdivided into:

- **Latent Phase:** up to 4 cm of cervical dilatation.
  - This phase of labor may often be distressing and prolonged, particularly for the nulliparous woman. It has been confirmed that support at this stage reduces maternal anxiety, increases confidence and may be associated with lower rates of epidural use and syntocinon augmentation.

- **Active Phase:** from 4 cm to full cervical dilatation.
  - To guarantee sufficient progress, a vaginal examination should be provided to low-risk women every four hours. According to national guidelines, cervical dilatation at a rate of 1 cm every 2 hours is considered satisfactory progress. If there is a suspicion of slow progress, a second vaginal examination should be performed in two hours, and a delay diagnosis should be made as needed. The partogram should document all findings, including observations made by the mother and the fetus.
  - If there is dystocia or slow progress, a clinical assessment should be sought. Women who have a confirmed delay ought to be moved to a unit under obstetric supervision. At this point, augmentation through oxytocin infusion or amniotomy may be suggested if suitable. Women should be advised that an amniotomy may lengthen labor by about one hour and may make contractions more intense and painful. It should be mentioned that while oxytocin infusion will shorten labor, other outcomes, such as the mode of birth, are unaffected. Women should be made aware that while receiving an oxytocin infusion, they will need ongoing fetal monitoring.
  - At all stages, women should be made aware of all analgesic options available, and in particular, epidural analgesia should be offered prior to commencing an oxytocin infusion.

Stage 2: Encompassing the time between full cervical dilatation and delivery of the fetus. Again, there is further subdivision of this stage.

- Propulsive phase: this refers to passive descent of the fetus, allowing for rotation. Often in the presence of epidural analgesia, and in the absence of fetal or maternal concerns, this phase is limited to 2 h in nulliparous women, and 1 h in multiparous women.
- Expulsive phase: This refers to active pushing, and should be limited to 3 h in the nullipara and 2 h in the multipara. The woman should be guided by her own urge to push, however, guided pushing may be sought if this is not adequately effective. A vaginal examination should be offered hourly to assess descent and fetal position.
- Of note, obstetric review should be sought in the absence of delivery following 2 h of active pushing in nulliparous women, and 1 h of active pushing in multiparous women. At this stage operative vaginal delivery should be considered.
- Perineal trauma is common following vaginal delivery. In order to mitigate this, the "hands on" (perineal guarding and flexion of the infant's head) or "hands poised" technique may be used. Episiotomy should not be performed routinely,

however, it may be indicated if there is suspected fetal distress, or if operative vaginal delivery is performed. A right mediolateral technique is preferred, at an angle between 45 and 60 degrees. Adequate analgesia should be confirmed prior to performing an episiotomy. Postnatally, assessment and repair of perineal trauma should be performed by appropriately trained clinical care providers.

Stage 3: from delivery of the infant to delivery of the placenta and membranes. Active management is recommended, due to the significantly decreased risk of postpartum hemorrhage, and requirement for blood transfusion. However, low risk women may choose to pursue physiological management of the third stage, and should be supported in making an informed decision.

- **Active Management:** routine use of uterotonic drugs, delayed cord clamping and controlled cord traction following signs of placental separation. 10 IU of oxytocin is administered IM following delivery of the anterior shoulder. The cord may be clamped between 1 and 5 min postnatally in the absence of neonatal concern.
- **Physiological Management:** no routine use of pharmacological agents, no cord clamping until the cessation of pulsation, and placental delivery with maternal effort.
- Following delivery, the infant should be dried and stimulated as appropriate and transferred to the mother for skin-to-skin contact.
- Obstetric review should be sought if the third stage is prolonged, at 30 min for active management, and at 1 h for physiological management.

4.2.3.1. Monitoring

Because of the higher rates of intervention without a corresponding decrease in unfavorable outcomes, NICE does not advise continuous monitoring in low-risk women. Because of this, it is advised that low-risk mothers have their fetal heart periodically checked for at least a minute after each contraction. Fetal concerns, such as increasing baseline or audible decelerations, are indicators of escalation to continuous monitoring. A number of maternal concerns, such as persistent abdominal pain, pyrexia or suspected sepsis, proteinuria, dystocia, prolonged contractions lasting more than 60 seconds, or more than five contractions per minute, suggest escalation of monitoring.

4.2.3.2. Particular Circumstances

- **Induction of Labor:** When it has been demonstrated that reducing the length of the pregnancy lowers both maternal and fetal morbidity, induction of labor is indicated in certain situations. While it isn't always regarded as "normal," inducing labor is frequently the most practical way to have a vaginal delivery that is "normal." Exogenous prostaglandin pessaries, or mechanical dilatation devices, are used to start the process in order to promote cervical ripening. Amniotomy then stimulates endogenous prostaglandin release, and when the cervix is "ripe" enough, synthetic oxytocin infusion is started to induce regular, strong contractions. In order to trigger additional prostaglandin release, oxytocin also binds to PG receptors in the decidua and cervix concurrently.

- **Vaginal Birth After Cesarean Section:** Vaginal birth after cesarean section (VBAC, also known as TOLAC) is now regarded as a standard method of delivery in many places due to the rising rates of cesarean sections worldwide. A 2013 review compared VBAC and planned cesarean sections and found that both procedures had advantages and disadvantages. A tiny chance of uterine rupture exists during VBAC, so ongoing monitoring is necessary throughout labor. This raises the number of laboring women who require intervention (Kamel, 2010; Irani & Foster, 2015).

4.3. Intrapartum Surveillance

Intrapartum surveillance involves the continuous monitoring of a woman and her baby during labor and childbirth to assess their well-being and detect any signs of potential complications. This comprehensive approach to monitoring encompasses various methods, including electronic fetal monitoring (EFM) to track the baby's heart rate and uterine contractions, assessments of maternal vital signs such as blood pressure and pulse rate, and evaluations of labor progress through cervical examinations. Additionally, pain management and comfort measures are integrated to ensure the mother's well-being, alongside continuous emotional and physical support. Maternal blood tests may also be conducted periodically to monitor health parameters. The aim of intrapartum surveillance is to identify any deviations from normal progress or signs of distress promptly, enabling healthcare providers to intervene as needed to optimize maternal and fetal outcomes. By ensuring vigilant monitoring throughout labor, intrapartum surveillance plays a vital role in promoting the safety and well-being of both mother and baby during childbirth.

4.3.1. Fetal Surveillance

Fetal surveillance is a crucial aspect of prenatal care aimed at monitoring the well-being and development of the fetus during pregnancy. This surveillance involves various methods and techniques to assess fetal growth, movement, and overall health, as well as to detect any signs of fetal distress or abnormalities. Common methods of fetal surveillance include:

1. **Ultrasound Imaging:** Ultrasound scans provide detailed images of the fetus, allowing healthcare providers to assess fetal growth, development, and anatomy. Ultrasound can also be used to evaluate the placenta, amniotic fluid levels, and fetal movements.
2. **Electronic Fetal Monitoring (EFM):** EFM involves the use of external or internal monitors to track the baby's heart rate and the frequency and duration of uterine contractions during labor. This helps detect signs of fetal distress and guides obstetric management decisions.
3. **Non-Stress Test (NST):** NST is a non-invasive test that measures the baby's heart rate in response to fetal movements. An acceleration in the fetal heart rate with movement indicates a healthy, responsive fetus.
4. **Biophysical Profile (BPP):** BPP combines ultrasound evaluation with fetal heart rate monitoring to assess various parameters such as fetal movement, breathing movements, muscle tone, amniotic fluid volume, and fetal heart rate reactivity.
5. **Doppler Flow Studies:** Doppler ultrasound studies assess blood flow in the umbilical artery, middle cerebral

artery, and other fetal vessels to evaluate placental function and fetal well-being. Abnormal Doppler findings may indicate fetal growth restriction or placental insufficiency.

6. **Kick Counts:** Pregnant women may be advised to monitor fetal movements, commonly referred to as kick counts, to assess fetal activity and well-being. A decrease in fetal movements may indicate fetal distress and warrant further evaluation.

Fetal surveillance is typically performed at regular intervals throughout pregnancy, with the frequency and type of monitoring tailored to individual risk factors and gestational age. The goal of fetal surveillance is to identify any potential concerns early and to facilitate appropriate management to optimize outcomes for both the mother and the baby.

4.3.2. Surveillance of Uterine Activity

Surveillance of uterine activity is a vital component of intrapartum care, particularly during labor, to monitor the progress of contractions and assess the effectiveness of uterine activity in facilitating childbirth. Various methods are employed to monitor uterine contractions, including:

- **Palpation:** Healthcare providers may use palpation, or manual examination of the mother's abdomen, to assess the frequency, duration, and intensity of uterine contractions. Palpation allows for a qualitative assessment of contractions but may not provide precise quantitative measurements.
- **External Uterine Monitoring:** External monitoring involves placing a tocodynamometer (TOCO) on the mother's abdomen to measure uterine contractions. The TOCO sensor detects changes in uterine pressure associated with contractions and provides a graphical representation of contraction patterns.
- **Internal Uterine Monitoring:** In some cases, internal monitoring of uterine contractions may be necessary for more accurate assessment. This involves placing an intrauterine pressure catheter (IUPC) directly into the uterus through the cervix. The IUPC measures the intrauterine pressure generated by contractions, offering more precise quantitative data on contraction frequency, duration, and intensity.

Surveillance of uterine activity allows healthcare providers to assess the progress of labor, monitor the effectiveness of uterine contractions in promoting cervical dilation and fetal descent, and detect any abnormalities or patterns of uterine dysfunction that may require intervention. Continuous monitoring of uterine activity, particularly in conjunction with electronic fetal monitoring, helps ensure the safety and well-being of both the mother and the baby during labor and childbirth.

4.3.3. Post-Partum Pregnancy Risk Assessment Monitoring System

The postpartum period represents a critical phase in maternal healthcare, requiring vigilant monitoring and assessment to identify and manage potential risks to maternal health and well-being. A comprehensive postpartum pregnancy risk assessment and monitoring system encompasses various components aimed at promoting maternal recovery, detecting postpartum complications, and supporting maternal-infant bonding. This system begins with a thorough assessment of the mother's physical and emotional health, including vital signs, uterine involution, vaginal bleeding, pain levels, and emotional well-being. Healthcare providers also evaluate for signs of postpartum complications such as hemorrhage, infection, thromboembolism, and hypertensive disorders. Additionally, monitoring for breastfeeding success, urinary and bowel function, and newborn care practices is integral to ensuring maternal-infant dyad health. The timing and frequency of postpartum assessments depend on maternal risk factors, mode of delivery, and the presence of complications during labor and birth. High-risk mothers, including those with pre-existing medical conditions or pregnancy complications, require closer monitoring and follow-up to mitigate potential postpartum risks. Implementing standardized protocols and guidelines for postpartum risk assessment and monitoring facilitates early detection of complications and ensures timely intervention to prevent adverse outcomes. Moreover, providing education and support to new mothers on postpartum self-care, contraception options, infant care, and emotional well-being promotes maternal empowerment and enhances postpartum recovery. A multidisciplinary approach involving obstetricians, midwives, nurses, lactation consultants, and mental health professionals is essential for the comprehensive management of postpartum risks and the promotion of maternal and infant health during the vulnerable postpartum period. By prioritizing postpartum risk assessment and monitoring, healthcare providers can effectively address maternal health needs, optimize outcomes, and support the transition to motherhood for women and their families.

4.3.4. Maternal Early Warning Systems

Maternal Early Warning Systems (MEWS) are critical tools in obstetric care aimed at promptly identifying and addressing signs of maternal deterioration during pregnancy, labor, and the postpartum period. MEWS utilize a set of predetermined physiological parameters and clinical signs to trigger early intervention when deviations from normal are detected, thus preventing maternal morbidity and mortality. These systems typically include components such as vital signs monitoring (blood pressure, heart rate, respiratory rate, temperature), assessment of urine output, mental status evaluation, and laboratory tests to monitor for signs of organ dysfunction or failure. MEWS are particularly crucial for high-risk pregnancies, including those complicated by hypertensive disorders, hemorrhage, sepsis, thromboembolism, and other medical conditions. Implementation of MEWS involves standardized protocols, staff training, and interdisciplinary collaboration to ensure timely recognition of maternal deterioration and appropriate escalation of care. By facilitating early detection and intervention, MEWS contribute to improved maternal outcomes, reduced morbidity and mortality rates, and enhanced patient safety in obstetric settings. Ongoing research and quality improvement initiatives are essential for refining and optimizing MEWS protocols to further enhance their effectiveness and impact on maternal health (Kamel, 2010; Irani & Foster, 2015).

A Closer Look

Postpartum Checkups

A postpartum checkup is a medical checkup you get after having a baby to make sure you're recovering well from labor and birth. In the United States, too many women experience serious and life-threatening health complications in the days and weeks after giving birth. Research shows that almost 40% of new moms miss their postpartum checkup. Even if you're feeling fine, it's important that you go to all your postpartum checkups. This allows you to share any concerns you have with your care team and allows them to look for warning signs of serious health problems, which can cause long-term health issues and even death, and provide treatment.

If you experienced a miscarriage, stillbirth, or your baby died, a postpartum checkup is especially important. A postpartum checkup may help your healthcare provider or other member of your care team, such as a genetic counselor, learn more about what happened and see if you may be at risk for the same condition in another pregnancy. A genetic counselor is a person who is trained to help you understand about genes, birth defects and other medical conditions that run in families, and how they can affect your health and your baby's health.

A postpartum care plan is a plan that you and your healthcare provider make together. It helps you prepare for your medical care after giving birth. It's best to make a postpartum care plan during pregnancy or at one of your prenatal care checkups. But if you didn't get a chance to, it's never too late. Your postpartum care plan should include:

- **Contact Information for Your Healthcare Provider:** How do you get in touch with your provider if you're worried or have questions?
- **The Dates of All Your Postpartum Checkups:** Get in touch with your provider within 3 weeks of giving birth and schedule a complete checkup within 12 weeks of giving birth. Talk with your provider to make sure this timing is right for you. Find out if your health insurance plan covers all your postpartum checkups. Look at the company's website or call the number on your insurance card.
- **Health Conditions or Pregnancy Complications that Need Treatment After You Have Your Baby:** Your provider can help you manage these conditions or may want to refer you to other providers who specialize in treating certain conditions.
- **Common Physical and Emotional Changes After Pregnancy:** What can you expect after giving birth? What's normal and how do you know when something's more serious? What are signs and symptoms of serious health conditions to look for after giving birth?
- **Postpartum Depression (Also Called PPD) and Other Mental Health Conditions After Pregnancy:** PPD is a kind of depression that some women get after having a baby. It's strong feelings of sadness, anxiety (worry) and tiredness that last for a long time after giving birth. PPD is a medical condition that needs treatment to get better.
- **Your Reproductive Life Plan, Including Birth Control:** A reproductive life plan helps

you think about if and when you want to have more children. For most women, it's best to wait at least 18 months (1½ years) between giving birth and getting pregnant again. Too little time between pregnancies increases your risk of preterm birth (birth before 37 weeks of pregnancy). Talk to your provider about the best birth control options for you. If you want to wait more than 18 months before getting pregnant again, talk to your provider about long-term reversible contraception, such as IUDs and implants. These types of birth control last for several years but can be stopped when you're ready to get pregnant again.

Here's what to expect at your postpartum checkup:

- **Your Provider Checks Your Blood Pressure, Weight, Breasts and Belly:** If you had a Cesarean birth (also called c-section), your provider may want to see you about 2 weeks after you give birth to check on your c-section incision (cut to ensure you're healing well and without any problems.
- **You Get a Pelvic Exam:** Your provider checks your vagina (birth canal), uterus (womb) and cervix. If you had an episiotomy or a tear during birth, your provider checks to see that it's healed. An episiotomy is a cut made at the opening of the vagina to help let the baby out. Your provider can tell you when it's safe to have sex again.
- **Your Provider Checks on Any Health Conditions, Like Diabetes and High Blood Pressure, You had During Pregnancy:** For example, if you have gestational diabetes, your provider may give you a blood glucose test to check your blood sugar. If your provider prescribes any medication and you're breastfeeding, be sure to tell your provider at your visit since some medicines can affect your breast milk.
- **Your provider makes sure your vaccinations are up** to date, including vaccinations for flu and pertussis. By getting vaccinated, you can help keep from getting sick and passing an illness to your baby.

Summary

- The postpartum period commences after the birth of the baby and marks the end of pregnancy. The puerperium is the period of about 6 weeks, when we give special attention to the changes occurring in the mother's body.
- Postpartum care is important because new moms are at risk of serious and sometimes life-threatening health complications.
- Labor is a process through which the fetus moves from the intrauterine to the extrauterine environment. It is a clinical diagnosis defined as the initiation and perpetuation of uterine contractions to produce progressive cervical effacement and dilation.
- Sexual intercourse is commonly recommended for promoting labor initiation. Sexual relations usually involve stimulation of the breasts and nipples, which can promote the release of oxytocin. With penetration, the lower uterine segment is stimulated.
- Breast massage and nipple stimulation have been shown to facilitate the release of oxytocin from the posterior pituitary gland. The most commonly prescribed technique involves gently massaging the breasts or applying warm compresses to the breasts for one hour, three times a day.
- The mechanics of labor describe the forces required for fetal descent and the movements the fetus must perform to overcome the resistance met by the maternal bony pelvis and soft tissue, mainly the levator ani muscle and the pelvic floor.
- CRH is produced in response to stress, predominantly by parvocellular neurosecretory cells within the paraventricular nucleus of the hypothalamus and is released at the median eminence from neurosecretory terminals of these neurons into the primary capillary plexus of the hypothalamo-hypophyseal portal system.
- Oxytocin plays a role in the activation of myometrial smooth muscle, and in cervical remodeling. Response to oxytocin depends on gestation and phase of parturition, reflective of the progesterone: estrogen balance at the time.
- Engagement occurs when the widest part of the fetal head, the biparietal diameter, enters the pelvic inlet. This indicates that the baby is moving down into the pelvis, preparing for birth.
- The cervix is composed of fibrous connective tissue, collagen (types I, III and IV), elastin, vasculature, fibroblasts and minimal smooth muscle.
- The uterus is predominantly composed of smooth muscle and changes shape from the first few weeks of pregnancy to accommodate the growing fetus and prepare for its eventual expulsion.
- Perineal and vaginal muscle vascularity increases throughout pregnancy. Perineal connective tissue softens and smooth muscle cells hypertrophy to enable distension during labor. The perineum is the area between the vaginal opening and the anus.

References

1. Adair, C. D. (2000). Nonpharmacologic approaches to cervical priming and labor induction. *Clinical Obstetrics and Gynecology, 43*, 447–454. https://doi.org/10.1097/00003081-200006000-00007.
2. American College of Obstetricians and Gynecologists. (1999). Induction of labor. *Practice Bulletin No. 10*. Washington, D.C.: ACOG.
3. Beal, M. W. (1999). Acupuncture and acupressure: Applications to women's reproductive health care. *Journal of Nurse-Midwifery, 44*, 217–230. https://doi.org/10.1016/S0091-2182(99)00009-7.
4. Belew, C. (1999). Herbs and the childbearing woman: Guidelines for midwives. *Journal of Nurse-Midwifery, 44*, 231–252. https://doi.org/10.1016/S0091-2182(99)00010-9.
5. Bellew, C., Livi, A., Cataneo, I., Salsi, G., Lenzi, J., & Pilu, G. (2020). Sonographic diagnosis of fetal head deflexion and the risk of cesarean delivery. *American Journal of Obstetrics and Gynecology MFM, 2*, 100217. https://doi.org/10.1016/j.ajogmf.2020.100217.
6. Buhimschi, I., Malinow, A., Saade, G. R., Garfield, R., & Weiner, C. (2003). The forces of labor. *Fetal and Maternal Medicine Review, 14*, 273–307. https://doi.org/10.1017/S0965539503000171.
7. Desseauve, D., Fradet, L., Lacouture, P., & Pierre, F. (2017). Position for labor and birth: State of knowledge and biomechanical perspectives. *European Journal of Obstetrics & Gynecology and Reproductive Biology, 208*, 46–54. https://doi.org/10.1016/j.ejogrb.2016.10.023.
8. Edwards, R. K., & Richards, D. S. (2000). Preinduction cervical assessment. *Clinical Obstetrics and Gynecology, 43*, 440–446. https://doi.org/10.1097/00003081-200006000-00006.
9. Galabin, A. L. (1897). *A Manual of Midwifery* (4th ed.). London, England: J. & A. Churchill.
10. Irani, R. A., & Foster, S. (2015). Overview of the mechanisms of induction of labor. *Seminars in Perinatology, 39*, 426–429. https://doi.org/10.1053/j.semperi.2015.07.007.
11. Kamel, R. M. (2010). The onset of human parturition. *Archives of Gynecology and Obstetrics, 281*, 975–982. https://doi.org/10.1007/s00404-009-1302-7.
12. Kavanagh, J., Kelly, A. J., & Thomas, J. (2002). Sexual intercourse for cervical ripening and induction of labour. *Cochrane Database of Systematic Reviews, 2002*(2), CD003093. https://doi.org/10.1002/14651858.CD003093.
13. Kelly, A. J., Kavanagh, J., & Thomas, J. (2002). Castor oil, bath and/or enema for cervical priming and induction of labour. *Cochrane Database of Systematic Reviews, 2002*(2), CD003099. https://doi.org/10.1002/14651858.CD003099.
14. Ludmir, J., & Sehdev, H. M. (2000). Anatomy and physiology of the uterine cervix. *Clinical Obstetrics and Gynecology, 43*, 433–439. https://doi.org/10.1097/00003081-200006000-00005.
15. McFarlin, B. L., Gibson, M. H., O'Rear, J., & Harman, P. (1999). A national survey of herbal preparation use by nurse-midwives for labor stimulation. *Journal of Nurse-Midwifery, 44*, 205–216. https://doi.org/10.1016/S0091-2182(99)00008-5.
16. Norwitz, E. R., Robinson, J. N., & Repke, J. T. (2002). Labor and delivery. In S. G. Gabbe, J. R. Niebyl, & J. L. Simpson (Eds.), *Obstetrics: Normal and Problem Pregnancies* (4th ed., pp. 353–394). New York: Churchill Livingstone.

17. Schaeffer, O. (1901). *Labor and Operative Obstetrics*. London, England, & Philadelphia, PA: W.B. Saunders & Company.
18. Smith, C. A., & Crowther, C. A. (2002). Acupuncture for induction of labor. *Cochrane Database of Systematic Reviews, 2002*(2), CD002962. https://doi.org/10.1002/14651858.CD002962.

Chapter

COMPLICATIONS OF PREGNANCY

5

Contents

Introduction

Pregnancy complications are health issues that can arise during or be related to pregnancy. Complications that occur during childbirth are known as obstetric labor complications, while those that occur after childbirth are termed puerperal disorders. Although some complications can improve or resolve after pregnancy, others may have lasting effects, result in morbidity, or in severe cases, lead to maternal or fetal mortality.

Pre-eclampsia, anemia, infections, gestational hypertension, and gestational diabetes are common pregnancy complications. These kinds of issues can affect how lab work, imaging, and medical care are monitored and managed during pregnancy.

In the US, 1 in 6 mothers and 1 in 5 mothers in Canada experience severe complications during pregnancy, childbirth, and the puerperium. In the first few months after giving birth, or the puerperium, 87–94% of women report having at least one health issue. 31% of women report long-term health issues, defined as problems that continue beyond six months after giving birth.

Globally, pregnancy, childbirth, and puerperium complications caused 230,600 deaths in 2016, compared to 377,000 in 1990. Maternal bleeding, postpartum infections, including sepsis, hypertensive pregnancy diseases, obstructed labor, and unsafe abortions are the leading causes of maternal death.

Pregnancy-related complications can occasionally result from unusually severe pregnancy symptoms and discomforts, which typically do not seriously impair day-to-day functioning or endanger the health of the expectant mother or fetus. A common mild pregnancy symptom that usually goes away in the second trimester is morning sickness. Hyperemesis gravidarum, on the other hand, is a severe version of this symptom that occasionally calls for medical attention in order to prevent electrolyte imbalances from severe vomiting.

Orientation and Directional Terms

Term	Definition	Illustration
Preterm birth	Preterm birth is the birth of a baby at fewer than 37 weeks gestational age, as opposed to full-term delivery at approximately 40 weeks. Extreme preterm is less than 28 weeks, very early preterm birth is between 28 and 32 weeks, early preterm birth occurs between 32 and 34 weeks, and late preterm birth is between 34 and 36 weeks' gestation.	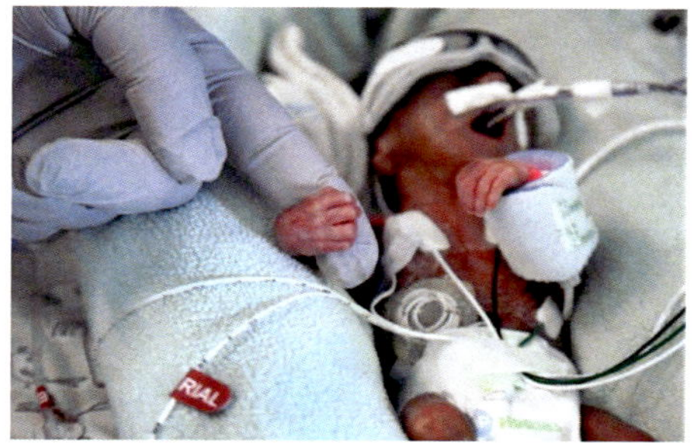
Antiemetics	An antiemetic is a drug that is effective against vomiting and nausea. Antiemetics are typically used to treat motion sickness and the side effects of opioid analgesics, general anesthetics, and chemotherapy directed against cancer. They may be used for severe cases of gastroenteritis, especially if the patient is dehydrated.	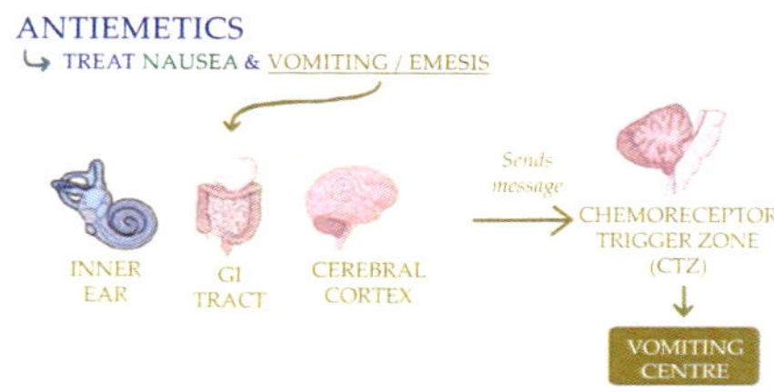
Molar pregnancy	A molar pregnancy shows a uterus filled with small, fluid-filled sacs (tumors). In a molar pregnancy, noncancerous cysts form instead of a healthy placenta.	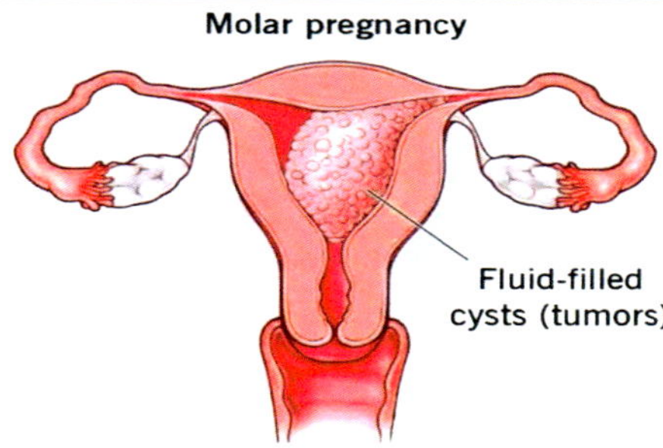
Endometriosis	Endometriosis is a disease in which tissue similar to the lining of the uterus grows outside the uterus. It can cause severe pain in the pelvis and make it harder to get pregnant. Endometriosis can start at a person's first menstrual period and last until menopause.	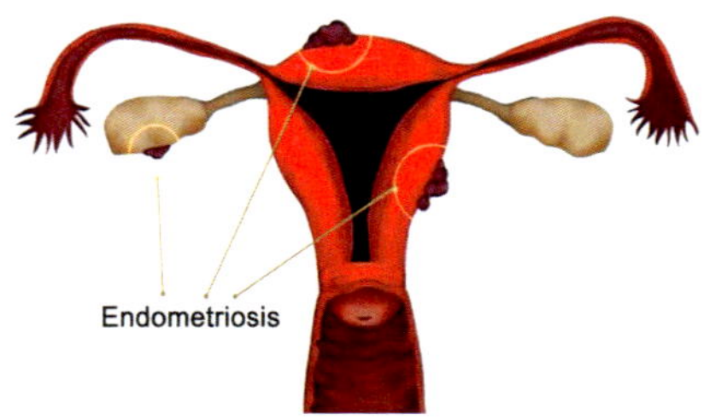
Preeclampsia	Preeclampsia is a type of high blood pressure that some people get during pregnancy. This condition can happen after the 20th week of pregnancy. In some cases, it can happen in the 6 weeks (about 1 and a half months) after giving birth.	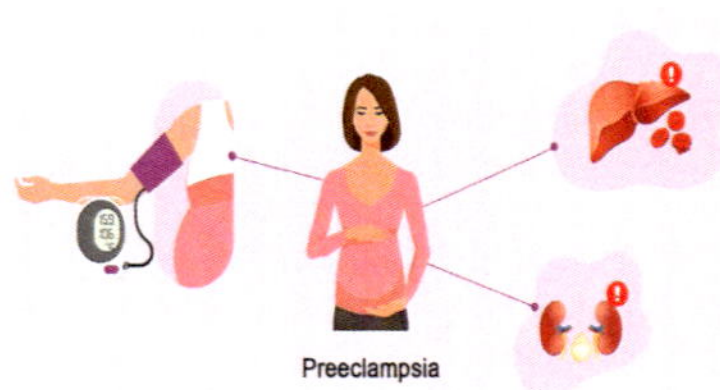

5.1. Hyperemesis Gravidarum

Severe nausea, vomiting, weight loss, and possibly dehydration are the hallmarks of hyperemesis gravidarum (HG), a pregnancy complication. Fainting may also be experienced. It's thought to be worse than morning sickness. Although they may persist the entire pregnancy, symptoms usually improve after the 20th week (Zimmerman et al., 2022).

It is unknown what specifically causes hyperemesis gravidarum. First pregnancy, multiple pregnancies, obesity, a family or prior history of HG, and trophoblastic disorder are risk factors. A December 2023 study that was published in Nature suggested a connection between HG and both elevated sensitivity to that particular hormone and abnormally high levels of the hormone GDF15.

Typically, the signs and symptoms that are observed are used to make the diagnosis. Technically speaking, HG is defined as having more than three vomiting episodes per day to the point where there is a five percent weight loss or three-kilogram weight loss and ketones are found in the urine. It is advisable to rule out other possible causes of the symptoms, such as an overactive thyroid and urinary tract infections.

Treatment consists of a bland diet and drinking plenty of water. Thiamine, electrolyte replacement drinks, and a diet richer in protein are a few possible recommendations. Certain individuals need intravenous fluids. When it comes to drugs, metoclopramide or pyridoxine are recommended. If these don't work, you can try prochlorperazine, dimenhydrinate, ondansetron (marketed under the name Zofran), or corticosteroids. Hospitalization might be necessary because of the severe symptoms that are connected. Psychotherapy could lead to better results. There is not much proof for acupressure.

Although reports of pregnant women vomiting date back to 2,000 BCE, Paul Antoine Dubois provided the first accurate medical description of HG in 1852. According to estimates, HG affects between 0 and 2.0 percent of pregnant women, however, some sources claim that the percentage can reach up to 3 percent. Although once thought to be a frequent cause of pregnancy-related deaths, this is now extremely uncommon with appropriate care. A higher risk of premature birth is associated with those affected, but a lower risk of miscarriage. Because of their HG symptoms, some pregnant women decide to have an abortion.

5.1.1. Signs and Symptoms

When vomiting is severe, it may result in the following:

- Loss of 5% or more of pre-pregnancy body weight
- Dehydration, causing ketosis, and constipation
- Nutritional disorders, such as vitamin B_1 (thiamine) deficiency, vitamin B_6 (pyridoxine) deficiency or vitamin B_{12} (cobalamin) deficiency
- Metabolic imbalances such as metabolic ketoacidosis or thyrotoxicosis
- Physical and emotional stress
- Difficulty with activities of daily living

Hunger, exhaustion, prenatal vitamins (particularly those containing iron), and diet can all exacerbate symptoms. Many women who have HG are highly sensitive to odors in their surroundings, and some smells can make symptoms worse. Sialorrhea gravidarum, or excessive salivation, is another symptom that some women encounter.

Unlike morning sickness, hyperemesis gravidarum usually manifests in the first trimester of pregnancy and lasts much longer.

While the majority of women will see almost total relief from their morning sickness symptoms by the start of their second trimester, some HG patients will continue to have severe symptoms up until and occasionally even after giving birth.

5.1.1.1. Complications

Considering complications in hyperemesis gravidarum involves both the mother and the fetus, as it affects at least two patients.

- **Maternal Complications:** If treatment for severe cases of hyperemesis is not received, complications can include malnutrition, dehydration, and vitamin deficiencies. If left untreated, vitamin-B1 deficiency-related Wernicke encephalopathy can result in death and irreversible disability. Furthermore, there have been case reports of injuries such as pneumothorax and esophageal rupture resulting from frequent and forceful vomiting. Hypokalemia is one example of an electrolyte abnormality that can significantly increase morbidity and mortality. Furthermore, pregnant patients who experience hyperemesis may also experience higher rates of anxiety and depression.
- **Fetal Complications:** Studies on the prevalence of low birth weight and premature babies in the context of pregnancy-related nausea and vomiting provide contradicting results. Studies haven't, however, revealed a link between hyperemesis and newborn or perinatal death. Those who experience hyperemesis do not seem to have a higher frequency of congenital abnormalities.

5.1.2. Causes

Although there are many theories, the precise cause of HG is unknown. It is believed that HG is caused by a variety of factors, some of which may be genetic in nature and many of which may differ amongst women. Women are more likely to get HG if they have family members who have had the condition.

One contributing factor is a negative response to the pregnancy's hormonal shifts, specifically high beta-human chorionic gonadotropin (β-hCG) levels. As β-hCG levels peak in the first trimester and fall thereafter, this theory would also explain why hyperemesis gravidarum is most common during that time (8–12 weeks of gestation). An increase in maternal estrogen levels (which decrease intestinal motility and gastric emptying, causing nausea and vomiting) is another theory regarding the cause of HG.

5.1.3. Diagnosis

It is thought that hyperemesis gravidarum is an excluded diagnosis. In order to diagnose HG in a patient, vomiting that causes severe dehydration and weight loss (at least 5% of the patient's pre-pregnancy weight) is typically required. Typically, a urinalysis is performed, and blood samples may be obtained to look for electrolyte imbalances, ketonuria, and complete blood counts, which can all point to HG or suggest a different diagnosis.

Despite their best efforts to eat, women with hyperemesis gravidarum frequently experience dehydration and weight loss. About five to six weeks into pregnancy is when the nausea and vomiting with hyperemesis usually begin, much like regular morning sickness episodes.

5.1.4. Management

The first line of treatment is oral rehydration and dry, bland food. HG is treated as an emergency because it can lead to severe dehydration and other complications. More intensive treatment, such as the use of antiemetic medications and intravenous rehydration, may be necessary if conservative dietary measures are ineffective. Intravenous nutritional support may be required if oral nutrition is inadequate. Low-molecular-weight heparin or thromboembolic stockings may be used as preventative measures against blood clot formation in women who need to be admitted to the hospital.

5.1.4.1. Intravenous Fluids

Intravenous IV hydration often involves adding electrolytes because ongoing vomiting can lead to an electrolyte deficiency. Similarly, it is important to supplement lost thiamine (vitamin B1) to prevent Wernicke's encephalopathy. Malnutrition can deplete A and B vitamins within two weeks, so prolonged malnutrition should prompt evaluation and supplementation. Monitoring and supplementing electrolyte levels is also crucial, especially for sodium and potassium.

Following the completion of IV rehydration, patients usually start to tolerate small, frequent meals that are bland in nature. Following rehydration, the goal of treatment is to control symptoms so that eating can resume normally. Nevertheless, there may be cycles of hydration and dehydration, necessitating ongoing attention. Peripherally inserted central catheters (PICC) are a type of home care that can provide nutrition and hydration. Compared to prolonged or recurrent hospital stays, home treatment is frequently less expensive and lowers the risk of contracting an infection while in the hospital.

5.1.4.2. Medications

Several antiemetics, such as phenothiazines (like promethazine), antihistamines (like diphenhydramine), and pyridoxine/doxylamine, are safe and effective during pregnancy. It's unclear which one works better than the other in terms of effectiveness when it comes to treating nausea or vomiting. Medication for hyperemesis gravidarum is suggested based on limited data from published clinical trials. Some have questioned the efficacy of pyridoxine/doxylamine, a combination of vitamin B6 and doxylamine, in treating HG, despite its effectiveness in treating pregnancy nausea and vomiting.

Although there is a lack of high-quality data and some concerns about a possible association with cleft palate, ondansetron may be helpful. Additionally used and generally well tolerated is metoclopramide. There is insufficient evidence to support the use of corticosteroids; however, there is some evidence that using them during pregnancy may slightly raise the infant's risk of cleft lip and palate and may also suppress fetal adrenal activity. After 12 weeks, hydrocortisone and prednisolone, which are inactivated in the placenta, can be used to treat hyperemesis gravidarum.

5.2. Anemia in Pregnancy

Anemia is a disorder where the red blood cell or hemoglobin content of the blood is below normal. A reduction in the amount of hemoglobin or total red blood cells (RBCs) in the blood during pregnancy is known as anemia. Anemia during pregnancy is a very common condition that carries a number of health risks for both the mother and the unborn child. While anemia during pregnancy can be harmful, in healthy pregnancies, the rise in red blood cell mass is less than the rise in plasma volume, resulting in physiologic (or dilutional) anemia, which is characterized by a slight drop in hemoglobin concentration. Generally non-specific, maternal signs and symptoms can include pallor, fatigue, dyspnea, palpitations, and dizziness. Anemia has many well-known effects on mothers, such as increased risk of maternal mortality, decreased physical and mental function, decreased peripartum blood reserves, and increased risk of peripartum blood product transfusion (Figure 5.1).

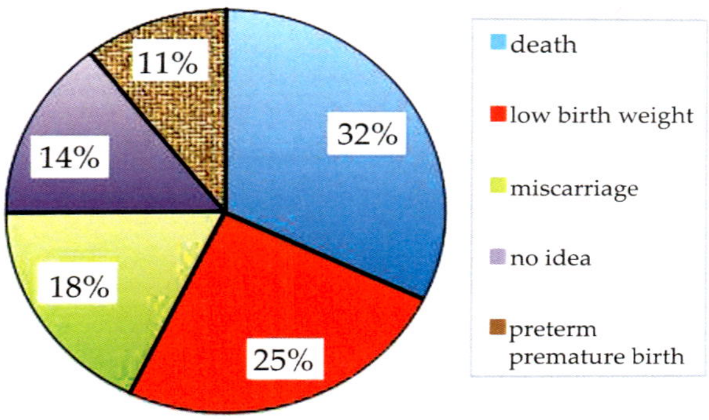

Figure 5.1. *Perceived effects of anemia in pregnancy.*

Source: https://www.researchgate.net/figure/Perceived-effects-of-anemia-in-pregnancy_fig2_259493929.

5.2.1. Types of Anemia During Pregnancy

Several types of anemia can develop during pregnancy. These include:

- Iron-deficiency anemia
- Folate-deficiency anemia
- Vitamin B12 deficiency

Here's why these types of anemia may develop:

- **Iron-Deficiency Anemia:** When the body doesn't have enough iron to make enough hemoglobin, anemia of this kind develops. Hemoglobin is a protein in red blood cells. It transports oxygen throughout the body from the lungs.

  Anemia due to iron deficiency prevents the blood from supplying enough oxygen to all of the body's tissues. The most frequent cause of anemia in pregnancy is iron deficiency.
- **Folate-Deficiency Anemia:** The vitamin folate, a form of B vitamin, is naturally occurring in some foods, such as green leafy vegetables. The body requires folate to create new cells, including healthy red blood cells.

  Women require more folate during pregnancy. However, occasionally their diet falls short of what they need. When that occurs, the body is unable to produce enough healthy red blood cells to carry oxygen to all of the body's tissues. Folic acid supplements are synthetic forms of folate.

  Low birth weight and neural tube abnormalities (spina bifida) are two birth defects that can be directly linked to folate deficiency.
- **Vitamin B12 Deficiency:** For the body to produce healthy red blood cells, vitamin B12 is required. A pregnant woman's body cannot create enough healthy red blood cells if she does not consume enough vitamin B12. Avoiding meat, poultry, dairy products, and eggs increases the risk of vitamin B12 deficiency in women. This can result in preterm labor and birth defects like abnormalities of the neural tube.

5.2.2. Signs and Symptoms

Early signs of anemia, such as weakness, lightheadedness, fatigue, and mild dyspnea with exertion, are typically nonexistent or nonspecific. Pallor and tachycardia or hypotension, if the anemia is severe, are possible additional symptoms and indicators.

Anemia increases the risk of:

- Preterm delivery
- Low birth weight
- Postpartum maternal infections

5.2.3. Causes

To put it simply, blood loss, increased red blood cell destruction, or decreased red blood cell production are the main causes of anemia. Anemia can be acquired (i.e., conditions like iron deficiency anemia or anemia as a result of an infection) or congenital (i.e., illnesses like sickle cell anemia and thalassemia). Physiologic and non-physiologic causes make up the two main groups of causes of anemia during pregnancy.

5.2.4. Risks of Anemia in Pregnancy

Severe or untreated iron-deficiency anemia during pregnancy can increase your risk of having:

- A preterm or low-birth-weight baby
- A blood transfusion (if you lose a significant amount of blood during delivery)
- Postpartum depression
- A baby with anemia
- A child with developmental delays

Untreated folate deficiency can increase your risk of having a:

- Preterm or low-birth-weight baby
- Baby with a serious birth defect of the spine or brain (neural tube defects)

Untreated vitamin B12 deficiency can also raise your risk of having a baby with neural tube defects.

5.2.5. Tests for Anemia

You will receive a blood test at your initial prenatal visit so your doctor can determine whether you have anemia.

- Hemoglobin test measures the amount of hemoglobin -- an iron-rich protein in red blood cells that carries oxygen from the lungs to tissues in the body.
- Hematocrit test measures the percentage of red blood cells in a sample of blood.

If your hemoglobin or hematocrit levels are below the normal range, it is possible that you have iron-deficiency anemia. Your doctor may conduct additional blood tests to confirm whether iron deficiency is the cause of your anemia or if there is another underlying reason.

Your doctor will probably advise getting another blood test in the second or third trimester to check for anemia, even if you don't have it at the start of your pregnancy.

5.2.6. Prevention

Anemia is a fairly typical pregnancy side effect. Blood dilution can result in a mild form of anemia. In every pregnancy, there is a comparatively greater increase in blood plasma than in total red cell mass. This leads to blood dilution and physiologic anemia. These adjustments are made to make sure the fetus receives enough blood and to get the body ready for the anticipated blood loss that occurs during delivery.

More severe types of anemia may result from vitamin or iron deficiencies, among other things.

5.2.6.1. Prevention of Iron Deficiency Anemia

The most frequent cause of non-physiologic anemia is iron deficiency. You can avoid iron deficiency anemia by taking an extra 27–30 mg of iron orally every day. This dosage usually matches the iron content of prenatal vitamins that contain iron. To find out if you require any additional supplements, speak with your doctor. To detect iron deficiency anemia early in pregnancy, complete routine laboratory tests.

Eating foods high in iron can also help prevent iron deficiency anemia. This comprises eggs, meat, fish, dried beans, dark green leafy vegetables, and fortified grains.

This may be only applicable to select individuals.

- **Vitamin B12:** Women who consume strictly vegan diets are advised to take Vitamin B12 supplements; this helps prevent anemia due to low Vitamin B12 levels.
- **Folic Acid:** Folic acid supplement recommended for women with a history of documented folate deficiency. Folic acid supplementation is also recommended for the prevention of neural tube defects in the fetus.

5.2.7. Treatment

To treat iron deficiency anemia in pregnant women, it is recommended to take iron supplementation at doses higher than what is found in prenatal supplements. The usual doses of oral iron typically range from 40 mg to 200 mg of elemental iron per day. It is important to consult with your healthcare provider to determine the appropriate dosage for your specific condition, as taking more iron than necessary might increase the risk of adverse effects.

Although iron supplements are simple to take, there is a chance that they will cause gastrointestinal side effects, such as nausea, diarrhea, or constipation. Other options include longer intervals between oral doses, liquid iron supplements, or intravenous iron if taking an oral iron supplement is intolerable. If a pregnant woman has severe iron deficiency anemia in the second or third trimester of her pregnancy, intravenous iron may also be used.

Supplementation can also be used to treat anemias resulting from other deficiencies, such as those in folic acid or vitamin B12; the dosage will depend on the severity of the deficiency.

Different types of anemias, including those that are inherited or acquired before pregnancy, will also need to be consistently managed throughout pregnancy.

Treatment should target the underlying disease or condition affecting the patient.

- The majority of obstetric anemia cases can be treated based on their etiology if diagnosed in time. Oral iron supplementation is the gold standard for the treatment of iron deficiency anemia and intravenous iron can be used when oral iron is not effective or tolerated from the second trimester of pregnancy onwards.
- Treatment of postpartum hemorrhage is multifactorial and includes medical management, surgical management along with blood product support.

5.3. Ectopic Pregnancy

A pregnancy complication known as ectopic pregnancy occurs when the embryo attaches itself outside of the uterus. Abdominal pain and vaginal bleeding are the classic signs and symptoms, but less than half of the affected women experience both. One could characterize the pain as sharp, dull, or cramping. If there has been bleeding into the abdomen, pain may also radiate to the shoulder. Severe bleeding may cause shock, fainting, or a rapid heartbeat. Except in extremely rare cases, the fetus cannot survive.

Less than 2% of pregnancies worldwide are affected by ectopic pregnancies. Risk factors for ectopic pregnancy include pelvic inflammatory disease, smoking, endometriosis, prior tubal surgery, infertility history, and the use of assisted reproductive technology. Those who have had a previous ectopic pregnancy are at a higher risk of having another one. Most ectopic pregnancies occur in the fallopian tube, but implantation can also happen in other areas such as the cervix, ovaries, cesarean scar, or abdomen. Detection of ectopic pregnancy is typically done through blood tests for human chorionic gonadotropin (hCG) and ultrasound, possibly requiring multiple tests. Other conditions that can cause similar symptoms include miscarriage, ovarian torsion, and acute appendicitis.

By screening for and treating chlamydia infections, risk factors like these can be reduced. The standard treatment for ectopic pregnancy involves either removing the embryo from the fallopian tube or removing the fallopian tube entirely, though some ectopic pregnancies will miscarry without treatment. In certain situations, methotrexate medication is just as effective as surgery. In particular, it functions best when the ectopic's size is small and the beta-HCG is low. If the woman's vital signs are unstable, there is a fetal heartbeat, or the tube has burst, surgery like a salpingectomy is still usually advised. A laparoscopy or a larger incision known as a laparotomy may be used for the procedure. Treatment lowers maternal mortality and morbidity (Figure 5.2).

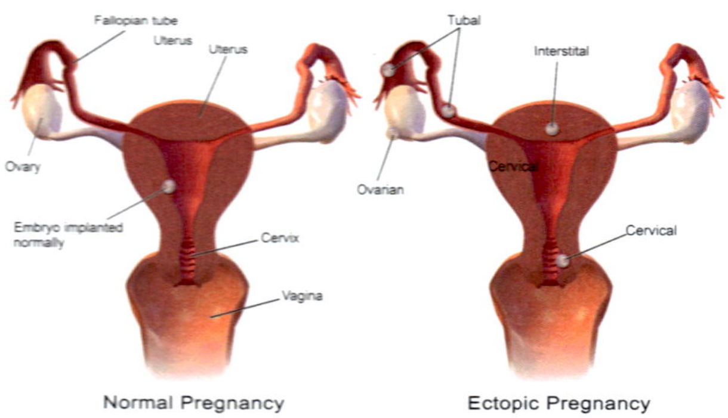

Figure 5.2. *Normal pregnancy vs. ectopic pregnancy.*

Source: By BruceBlaus – Own work, CC BY-SA 4.0, https://commons.wikimedia.org/w/index.php?curid=44897672.

In developed nations, the incidence of ectopic pregnancy ranges from 11 to 20 per 1,000 live births, with a possible 4 percent among women utilizing assisted reproductive technology. At roughly 6–13% of all first-trimester deaths among women, it is the most common cause of death. Results have improved in the developed world, but poverty is still a common occurrence in the developing world. In the developed world, the risk of dying is between zero and three percent, whereas in the developing world, it is between one and three percent. Al-Zahrawi wrote the first recorded account of an ectopic pregnancy in the eleventh century. The word "ectopic" means "out of place."

5.3.1. Signs and Symptoms

One-third of ectopic pregnancy patients show no medical symptoms, and up to 10% have none at all. The symptoms often have low specificity and can be confused with those of other gastrointestinal and genitourinary conditions, including urinary tract infections, appendicitis, salpingitis, ruptured corpus luteum cysts, miscarriages, and ovarian torsion. The last regular menstrual period can occur anywhere between four and eight weeks before the clinical manifestation of an ectopic pregnancy, with a mean of seven and a half weeks. Communities lacking access to modern diagnostic tools tend to have later presentations more frequently.

Increased hCG, variable vaginal bleeding, abrupt lower abdominal pain, pelvic pain, tender cervix, adnexal mass, or adnexal tenderness are among the warning signs and symptoms of an ectopic pregnancy. If an ultrasound or hCG assessment is not performed, severe vaginal bleeding could result in an incorrect miscarriage diagnosis. Three additional uncommon signs of an ectopic pregnancy are vomiting, diarrhea, and nausea.

Symptoms like tenderness, peritonism, hypovolemic shock, and abdominal distension can result from the rupture of an ectopic pregnancy. When lying flat, a person with a ruptured ectopic pregnancy may feel pain. They may also prefer to keep their posture upright because intrapelvic blood flow can cause the abdominal cavity to swell and exacerbate the pain.

- **Complications:** Rupture with internal bleeding is the most frequent consequence, and it can result in hypovolemic shock. Impaired fallopian tubes can make it more difficult to conceive in the future. It's possible that the woman's other fallopian tube is functional enough for pregnancy. Future conception is still feasible following the removal of one damaged fallopian tube. In vitro fertilization is still an option for women who want to get pregnant if both are removed.

5.3.2. Causes

Ectopic pregnancies are associated with a variety of risk factors. But in as many as one-third to one-half of cases, no risk factors are discernible. Pelvic inflammatory disease, infertility, using an IUD, having previously been exposed to diethylstilbestrol (DES), tubal surgery, intrauterine surgery (e.g., D&C), smoking, endometriosis, and tubal ligation are risk factors. It doesn't seem that having an induced abortion before increases the risk. Although there is no increased risk of an ectopic pregnancy when using an IUD, the likelihood of an ectopic pregnancy is higher than that of an intrauterine pregnancy. After chlamydia infection, there is little chance of an ectopic pregnancy. It's unclear exactly how chlamydia raises the risk of an ectopic pregnancy, but some research points to the infection's potential impact on fallopian tube structure.

5.3.2.1. Tube Damage

When the egg is implanted in the fallopian tubes, it results in tubal pregnancy. The fertilized egg is transported to the uterus by hair-like cilia that are found on the inside surface of the fallopian tubes. There is a theory that cilia damage in the fallopian tubes is likely to cause an ectopic pregnancy because fallopian cilia are occasionally observed to be reduced in number after an ectopic pregnancy. Smoking increases a woman's risk of developing an ectopic pregnancy in the fallopian tubes. Smoking increases the chance of cilia being harmed or destroyed. The time it takes for the fertilized egg to enter the uterus will lengthen as cilia become less functional. The fertilized egg will hatch from the non-adhesive zona pellucida and implant itself inside the fallopian tube, resulting in ectopic pregnancy, if it does not reach the uterus in time.

It is common for women with pelvic inflammatory disease (PID) to become pregnant erratically. This is the outcome of cilia damage brought on by the accumulation of scar tissue in the fallopian tubes. On the other hand, fertilization of the egg would be naturally impossible and neither a normal pregnancy nor an ectopic pregnancy could occur if both tubes were completely blocked, preventing sperm and egg from physically meeting. Ectopic cervical pregnancy or ectopic tubal pregnancy can result from intrauterine adhesions (IUA) in Asherman's syndrome if the adhesions partially obstruct the ostia's ability to access the tubes. Usually following D&C, intrauterine surgery results in Asherman's syndrome. Ectopic pregnancy can also result from endometrial, pelvic, or genital tuberculosis, which is another cause of Asherman's syndrome. This is because infection can cause tubal adhesions in addition to intrauterine adhesions.

Ectopic pregnancy can be predisposed to by tubal ligation. Ectopic pregnancy is a possible side effect of tubal reversal, or the reversal of tubal sterilization. This is greater in cases where more invasive techniques for tubal ligation—such as partial tube removal or tubal cautery—have been employed in contrast to less invasive techniques like tubal clipping. The likelihood of another tubal pregnancy rising to roughly 10% is increased by a history of one. Even if the other tube seems normal, removing the afflicted tube does not lessen this risk. Early ultrasound diagnosis is the most effective way to treat this.

5.3.2.2. Endometriosis

A condition known as endometriosis occurs when cells that normally line the inside of the uterus, known as the endometrium, start to proliferate outside of it. An ectopic pregnancy results when an embryo attaches to one of these lesions. The 2015 European Society of Human Reproduction and Embryology (ESHRE) annual congress featured the presentation of findings from a 30-year study on reproductive and pregnancy outcomes, involving over 14,000 women of childbearing age. Within the study group, 39% had endometriosis confirmed by surgery. The endometriosis subgroup was associated with a 270% increased risk of an ectopic pregnancy and a 76% increased risk of miscarriage when compared to their peers. The increased pelvic inflammation and structural and functional alterations in the uterine lining were linked to the elevated endometriosis risks.

5.3.2.3. Other

Age is thought to be a variable that could substitute for other risk factors, even though some research has indicated that patients may be more susceptible to an ectopic pregnancy as they age. Some people believe that vaginal douching increases the risk of ectopic pregnancies. DES daughters, or women exposed to DES in utero, are also more likely to experience an ectopic pregnancy. However, the United States has not used DES since 1971. Additionally, it has been proposed that pathologic nitric oxide generation via elevated iNOS production may impact embryo transport by reducing tubal ciliary beats and smooth muscle contractions, potentially leading to ectopic pregnancy. Ectopic pregnancy risk factors may include a low socioeconomic status.

5.3.3. Differential Diagnosis

As most of the signs and symptoms described above are not specific you should always think of other causes of the women's complaints:

- Abortion (spontaneous or induced)
- PID
- Bleeding corpus luteal cyst
- Torsion of an ovarian cyst.

And of course, any other causes of an acute abdomen which can also present in pregnancy such for example, an appendicitis.

5.3.3.1. Necessary Diagnostics

It depends on whether there is time to carry out diagnostic testing, as was previously indicated. As previously stated, the best course of action is to operate on a patient in an appropriately equipped facility as soon as possible if you believe she has a ruptured ectopic pregnancy and she is in shock. If a pregnancy test is available, there might still be time to do so; however, historically, a negative urine pregnancy test did not always rule out an ectopic pregnancy. The reason for this is that different qualitative urine pregnancy tests had different thresholds, with some only reporting a positive result at 750 IU of β-hCG/ml of urine. A negative pregnancy test typically rules out an ectopic pregnancy, but false-negative results are still possible with modern tests that have a much better threshold of at least 75 IU/ml. It is advisable for you to verify the pregnancy test threshold level. When in doubt, perform a laparotomy even if the urine pregnancy test comes out negative because there may still be other reasons why surgery is necessary.

You will be able to run diagnostic tests once the patient is (relatively) stable. A skilled healthcare provider can perform a transvaginal ultrasound and measure the woman's blood β-hCG levels to make the best diagnosis of an ectopic pregnancy.

As a result, additional tools are required to assist in the diagnosis. Initially, admit a woman to the ward if you think she may be experiencing an ectopic pregnancy. Don't just leave her there after admittance; instead, monitor her closely and take regular checks on her pulse and blood pressure. After drawing blood to determine her hemoglobin level and for cross-matching, set up an IV line and administer fluids to her. Find out if there is a donor available for her if blood is not readily available at your hospital or health center. Next, take a pregnancy test with urine. The likelihood that she is experiencing an ectopic pregnancy increases if the test results are positive.

Do an ultrasound if possible; as was previously mentioned, a transvaginal ultrasound is the ideal procedure. Demonstrating fluid in the Douglas pouch is the most effective way to identify an ectopic pregnancy and determine whether the tubal pregnancy has ruptured. However, a transabdominal ultrasound may also be used to diagnose an ectopic.

An investigation carried out in a reputable hospital in Accra, Ghana, demonstrated the influence of abdominal ultrasonography on the identification of an unruptured ectopic pregnancy. Abdominal ultrasound was introduced into the hospital, and as a result, the percentage of unruptured ectopic pregnancies that were diagnosed increased from 0.3 to 8.5 percent. This represents a significant improvement, even though it still accounts for only 10% of unruptured ectopic pregnancies that are diagnosed. Nevertheless, a different study carried out in Cameroun in 2000 demonstrated that abdominal ultrasonography was an ineffective method for identifying an ectopic pregnancy. It was mentioned that doing an abdominal ultrasound can take longer than expected because, frequently, the procedure is carried out in a medical facility by an untrained healthcare provider. Therefore, it may be challenging and time-consuming to identify an ectopic pregnancy with a transabdominal ultrasound, especially for a novice or unskilled healthcare provider.

On the other hand, an ectopic pregnancy is unlikely but not ruled out if an intrauterine pregnancy is clearly visible on an ultrasound. It is extremely uncommon for there to be a combination of an intrauterine and extrauterine pregnancy. An ectopic pregnancy is highly likely to be diagnosed when there is no intrauterine pregnancy, the woman has a positive pregnancy test, and fluid is visible in the Douglas pouch along with a pelvic mass.

When β-hCG measurement, ultrasound, and sometimes urine pregnancy tests are unavailable, culdocentesis—a condition in which free fluid (or blood) is produced vaginally from the Douglas pouch—is an additional means of diagnosing a ruptured ectopic pregnancy. The test is an essential diagnostic tool, particularly in low-resource settings, because it is not very difficult to learn or administer. Culdocentesis will be positive in over 90% of women whose ectopic pregnancy ruptured. If the test is successful, you will have drawn at least 0.5 milliliters of non-clotting blood from the Douglas pouch. Certain proteins in the peritoneal cavity of a patient prevent blood from clotting easily, which makes blood from there difficult to clot. Clots can still occur, though, particularly in women who have a history of ruptured ectopic pregnancy. Non-clotting blood is aspirated in over 60% of unruptured ectopic pregnancies. In conclusion, bloody fluid that does not clot or fluid that contains some clots indicates abdominal bleeding and may indicate a ruptured ectopic pregnancy.

5.3.3.2. Technique of Performing a Culdocentesis

Perform a thorough bimanual vaginal examination to identify the position of the uterus and any tubo-ovarian masses. Next, conduct a speculum examination to visualize the cervix. Using a tenaculum, gently grasp the cervix and pull it anteriorly to visualize the posterior fornix. Clean the area with an antiseptic, such as betadine. Insert a long needle (16 or 18 gauge) attached to a syringe through the posterior vaginal fornix while maintaining traction on the tenaculum and applying continuous suction with the syringe. The needle only needs to be inserted a few millimeters, and if blood is present, aspiration should be straightforward. Complications are expected to be minimal.

5.3.4. Treatment/ Management

5.3.4.1. Expectant Management

Serum hCG levels and additional TVS exams are typically performed on women with PULs until a definitive diagnosis is made. After two weeks, low-risk PUL cases that seem to be failing pregnancies can get a telephone consultation and a urine pregnancy test. In order to determine viability, low-risk PUL cases that are most likely intrauterine pregnancies might undergo another TVS in two weeks. High-risk PUL cases need to be evaluated further, either with a follow-up hCG measurement or a TVS within 48 hours.

5.3.4.2. Medical

An ectopic pregnancy can be effectively treated with methotrexate as an alternative to surgery. Methotrexate was established as a treatment option in the 1980s. When administered early in the pregnancy, methotrexate stops the growth of the developing embryo, which may then be naturally absorbed by the woman's body or pass during her menstrual cycle. People with liver, kidney, or blood conditions, as well as those with an ectopic embryonic mass exceeding 3.5 cm, are not suitable candidates for this treatment.

Additionally, it might result in a severe abnormality in any pregnancy that survives or the unintentional termination of an undetected intrauterine pregnancy. Methotrexate should therefore only be given if hCG has been serially monitored and has increased by less than 35% over the course of 48 hours, essentially ruling out a viable intrauterine pregnancy.

The data from randomized clinical trials in women with CSP regarding the efficacy, drawbacks, and adverse effects of methotrexate in treating nontubal ectopic pregnancy is inconclusive when compared to surgery (uterine arterial embolization or uterine arterial chemoembolization).

Methotrexate (MTX) is administered in the US using a multidose protocol that includes four intramuscular doses and an intramuscular injection of folinic acid to protect cells from the drug's effects and minimize side effects. The single-dose protocol is adhered to in France; however, the failure rate associated with a single dose is higher.

5.3.4.3. Surgery

If bleeding has already started, surgery might be required. On the other hand, in a stable patient with scant evidence of a blood clot, deciding whether to proceed with surgical intervention can be challenging.

Surgeons typically use laparoscopy or laparotomy to access the pelvis for the treatment of ectopic pregnancy. They can choose between two procedures: salpingostomy, where only the pregnancy is removed, or salpingectomy, where the affected fallopian tube is also removed. The first successful surgery for ectopic pregnancy was performed by Robert Lawson Tait in 1883. It is estimated that between 0.5 and 11% of pregnancies in unknown locations eventually require surgery. The recurrence rates for ectopic pregnancy after salpingectomy and salpingostomy are similar at 5% and 8%, respectively. Both procedures also have similar rates of intrauterine pregnancy success, at 56% and 61%.

In cases where a woman's abdominal bleeding is severe, autotransfusion of her own blood as it was drained during surgery may be helpful.

5.3.5. Prognosis

In Western countries, the prognosis for mothers with treated ectopic pregnancies is excellent; maternal death is uncommon, but all fetuses die or are aborted. For example, in the UK, 32,100 ectopic pregnancies between 2003 and 2005 resulted in 10 maternal deaths (i.e., 1 in 3,210 women with an ectopic pregnancy died). The UK Confidential Enquiry into Maternal Deaths, which took place between 2006 and 2008, discovered that ectopic pregnancy accounts for 6 maternal deaths (or 0.26 per 100,000 pregnancies).

In less developed regions, particularly in Africa, the mortality rate is considerable, with ectopic pregnancies being a significant contributor to fatalities among women of reproductive age. The likelihood of experiencing another ectopic pregnancy in subsequent pregnancies for women with a history of the condition is approximately 10%.

5.3.5.1. Future Fertility

A history of infertility is the most significant factor influencing fertility after an ectopic pregnancy. The choice of treatment has little bearing on outcomes; a 2013 randomized study found that rates of intrauterine pregnancy following ectopic pregnancy treatment were roughly 64% with radical surgery, 67% with medication, and 70% with conservative surgery two years later. In contrast, over 90% of women under 40 who have been pregnant over the course of two years are part of the general population.

Future fertility treatments are unaffected by methotrexate. There is no difference in the quantity of oocytes that were extracted before and following methotrexate treatment.

The likelihood of another ovarian ectopic pregnancy or infertility is minimal in cases of ovarian ectopic pregnancy. Massage doesn't seem to increase fertility after an ectopic pregnancy.

5.4. Hypertensive Disease of Pregnancy

Preeclampsia, preeclampsia superimposed on chronic hypertension, gestational hypertension, and chronic hypertension are among the high blood pressure conditions that make up hypertensive disease of pregnancy, also referred to as maternal hypertensive disorder.

About 20.7 million women had maternal hypertensive disorders in 2013. Hypertensive diseases complicate about 10% of pregnancies worldwide. About 8–13% of pregnancies in the US result in hypertensive disease of pregnancy. The developing world has seen an increase in rates. Compared to 37,000 deaths in 1990, they caused 29,000 deaths in 2013. They account for 16% of pregnancy-related deaths, along with puerperal infections (2 percent) and postpartum hemorrhage (13 percent) (Figure 5.3).

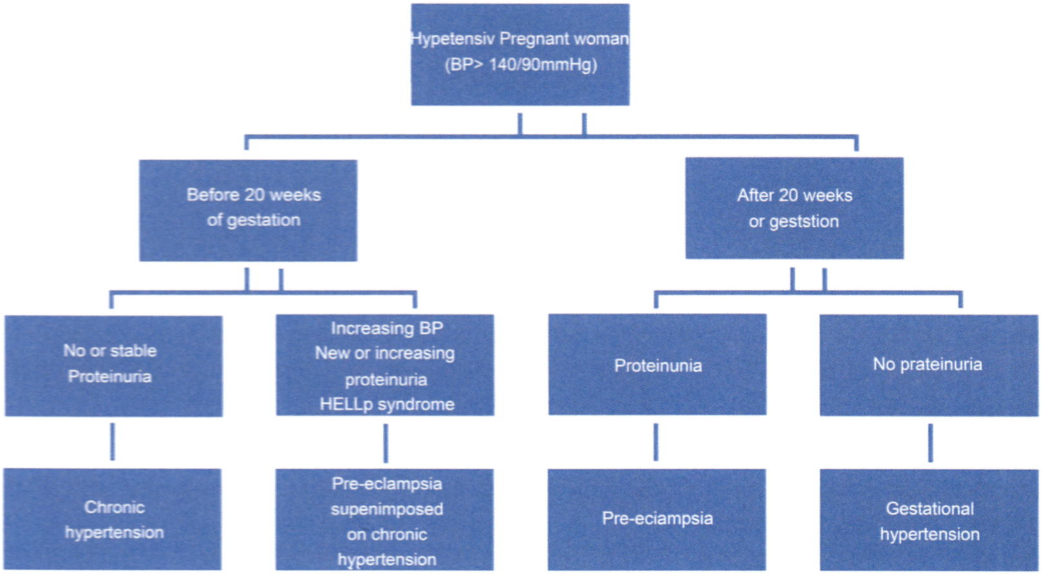

Figure 5.3. *Differentiation of the hypertensive disorders of pregnancy.*

Source: https://www.researchgate.net/figure/Differentiation-of-the-hypertensive-disorders-of-pregnancy-11_fig1_291071599.

5.4.1. Signs and Symptoms

Even though many high-blood-pressure pregnant women give birth to healthy, problem-free babies, high blood pressure can be harmful to both the mother and the unborn child. Compared to women with normal blood pressure, those with pre-existing or chronically high blood pressure are more likely to experience specific pregnancy complications. On the other hand, some pregnant women experience elevated blood pressure (sometimes referred to as gestational hypertension).

An uncontrolled high blood pressure condition before and during pregnancy increases the risk of complications for both the expectant mother and her unborn child. It is linked to a higher risk of maternal complications, including gestational diabetes, placental abruption (a condition in which the placenta separates from the uterine wall), and preeclampsia. Additionally, these women are more likely to experience unfavorable birth outcomes, such as premature delivery, small-for-gestational-age infants, and infant deaths.

5.4.2. Risk Factors

Some women have a greater risk of developing hypertension during pregnancy. These are:

- Women with chronic hypertension (high blood pressure before becoming pregnant).
- Women who developed high blood pressure or preeclampsia during a previous pregnancy, especially if these conditions occurred early in the pregnancy.
- Women who are obese before pregnancy.

- Pregnant women under the age of 15 or over the age of 30.
- Women who are pregnant with more than one baby.
- Women with diabetes, kidney disease, rheumatoid arthritis, lupus, or scleroderma.

5.4.3. Diagnosis

Preeclampsia cannot be diagnosed or predicted by a single test. Elevated blood pressure and protein in the urine (proteinuria) are important indicators. Preeclampsia also appears to be accompanied by other symptoms such as ongoing headaches, light sensitivity or blurred vision, and stomach pain.

All of these feelings can be brought on by other conditions, and they can also happen during a healthy pregnancy. Frequent visits are planned to measure blood pressure and the amount of protein in the urine, order and examine blood tests that look for preeclamptic symptoms, and keep a closer eye on the development of the fetus.

5.4.3.1. Classification

A classification of hypertensive disorders of pregnancy uses 4 categories as recommended by the U.S. National High Blood Pressure Education Program Working Group on High Blood Pressure in Pregnancy:

- Chronic hypertension;
- Preeclampsia-eclampsia;
- Preeclampsia superimposed on chronic hypertension;
- Gestational hypertension (transient hypertension of pregnancy or chronic hypertension identified in the latter half of pregnancy).

Because it is more accurate, this terminology is preferred over the more commonly used but outdated term pregnancy-induced hypertension (PIH). The relationship between pregnancy and the onset or first detection of hypertension is the only thing that the new terminology represents; for the majority of medical purposes, the question of causality—though pathogenetically fascinating—is not crucial. Instead of treating HELLP syndrome as a separate condition, this classification views it as a subtype of preeclampsia.

5.4.3.1.1. Chronic Hypertension

A pregnant woman with chronic hypertension has high blood pressure if it was present prior to conception, detected early in the pregnancy, or continues to be a major problem after the pregnancy has ended. It is not caused by pregnancy itself and affects approximately 5% of pregnancies. It can be a primary disorder of essential hypertension or a secondary condition to another one.

At least two separate blood pressure readings taken at least four hours apart with a systolic blood pressure of at least 140 mmHg, a diastolic blood pressure of at least 90 mmHg, or both, identified prior to pregnancy, before 20 weeks gestation, or continuing for at least 12 weeks after giving birth are generally considered the diagnostic criteria for chronic hypertension. The usefulness of lowering the diagnostic thresholds for chronic hypertension, which are more in line with current guidelines for the diagnosis of adult hypertension from the American College of Cardiology and the American Heart Association, is up for debate. Although there is disagreement over the most suitable cutoffs for this definition, chronic hypertension in pregnancy is currently classified as mild if blood pressure is less than 159 mmHg systolic and 109 mmHg diastolic and as severe if it is greater than 160 mmHg systolic or 110 mmHg diastolic. It is crucial to correctly diagnose chronic hypertension as soon as possible, ideally before becoming pregnant, and to start treatment to lower the blood pressure of the parents, as the illness can worsen and lead to other health problems. This is frequently challenging since a lot of people who are fertile might not go to the doctor on a regular basis and might first seek prenatal care in the second trimester of their pregnancy.

5.4.3.1.2. Pre-Eclampsia and Eclampsia

Preeclampsia is a medical condition that typically appears after 20 weeks of pregnancy and is characterized by proteinuria and recently elevated blood pressure (> 140/90 mmHg).

Fetal complications, such as low birth weight, preterm birth, and stillbirth, are primarily caused by preeclampsia. Preeclamptic women are advised to give birth after 37 weeks of pregnancy in order to reduce the chance of serious complications.

Preeclampsia can also be diagnosed if a woman has both increased blood pressure and 1 or more signs of significant organ damage. Signs of significant organ damage include:

- Severely elevated blood pressure (blood pressure > 160/110)
- Thrombocytopenia
- Increased or rapidly elevating levels of creatinine in the blood
- Increased liver enzymes
- Pulmonary edema
- New or persistent headaches that do not respond to pain medication
- Blurred or altered vision

A woman is diagnosed with preeclampsia with severe features if she exhibits any of these indicators of substantial organ damage. Even in cases where the patient does not have proteinuria, this diagnosis can be made. To reduce the likelihood of serious complications, women with severe features of preeclampsia are advised to deliver the baby after 34 weeks of gestation.

Seizures are another way that preeclampsia manifests in a pregnant woman. In this instance, eclampsia would be the diagnosis given to the patient.

There is no proven way to prevent preeclampsia/eclampsia. Most women who develop signs of preeclampsia, however, are closely monitored to lessen or avoid related problems. The only way to "cure" preeclampsia/eclampsia is to deliver or abort the baby.

5.4.3.2.3. Preeclampsia Superimposed on Chronic Hypertension

When a pregnant woman with chronic hypertension experiences pre-eclampsia, it is usually diagnosed when she shows new symptoms of proteinuria, which are usually defined as ≥30 mg/dL (1+ in the dipstick) in at least two random urine specimens collected ≥4 h apart (but within a 7-day interval) or 0.3 g in a 24-hour period. Superimposed pre-eclampsia, like ordinary pre-eclampsia, can also occur with severe features, which include thrombocytopenia (platelet count <100,000/microL), impaired liver function, new-onset or worsening renal insufficiency, pulmonary edema, and persistent cerebral or visual disturbances. These symptoms can occur even after antihypertensive therapy has been increased. Therefore, when a sudden increase in previously well-controlled blood pressure is accompanied by severe pre-eclampsia features, superimposed pre-eclampsia can be diagnosed without proteinuria.

5.4.3.2.4. Gestational Hypertension

The term "gestational hypertension" refers to a provisional diagnosis of newly elevated blood pressure in a pregnant woman that typically appears after 20 weeks of pregnancy and does not yet exhibit proteinuria or other preeclamptic features. Preeclampsia develops in as many as 50% of patients with gestational hypertension.

After giving birth, gestational hypertension usually goes away within 12 weeks. In this instance, the diagnosis of transient pregnancy-related hypertension will replace the original diagnosis of gestational hypertension. Chronic hypertension will replace gestational hypertension as the new diagnosis if the elevated blood pressure does not go down by 12 weeks after delivery.

5.4.4. Treatment of Severe-Range Hypertension and Hypertensive Emergencies in Pregnancy

Blood pressure readings higher than 160/110 mm Hg are classified as severe-range hypertension. Three criteria are used to classify a hypertensive emergency of pregnancy: (1) an abrupt rise in blood pressure that is greater than or equal to 160/110 mm Hg; (2) the emergence of symptoms resembling severe preeclampsia; and (3) signs of end-organ damage. Severe hypertension has been linked to damage to the central nervous system; from 2003 to 2005, cerebral hemorrhage or infarction accounted for two-thirds of maternal deaths. In order to quickly lower blood pressure, pregnant women with severe hypertension that manifests itself within 15 minutes or less should start antihypertensive medication within 30 to 60 minutes. Intravenous (IV) labetalol and hydralazine are considered first-line agents for the treatment of acute-onset, severe hypertension in pregnant and postpartum women. For over 65 years, IV hydralazine has been used as an acute treatment for severe hypertension, and ACOG recommends it. Oral nifedipine with immediate release is another option. For the treatment of acute, severe hypertension, current ACOG guidelines advise using immediate-release oral nifedipine as a first-line substitute for labetalol when IV access is not available. Treatment options for severe pregnancy-induced hypertension complicated by pulmonary edema include IV nitroglycerin. (Cotton et al., 1986) (Table 5.1).

Table 5.1. Antihypertensive Medications for Pregnant Women with Severe Hypertension

Agent	Dose	Side Effects
Labetalol (IV)	5–20 mg (increase every 10–15 min to max ag 220 mg/d)	Hypotension, increased liver enzyme levels, persistent fetal bradycardia, and neonatal hypoglycemia
		Avoid in asthma because of risk of bronchospasm and congestive heart failure
Hydralazine (IV)	5–10 mg (increase every 20 min to max dosage 30 mg/d)	Severe headache, peripheral edema, flushing, reflex bradycardia, hypotension.
		Avoid use in isolation because of reflex tachycardia
Immediate-release nifedipine (PO)	5–10 mg (increase every 30 min to max dosage 50 mg/d)	First-line alternative to labetalol only in the absence of IV access for treatment of acute, severe hypertension

Source: https://www.ncbi.nlm.nih.gov/pmc/articles/PMC7720658/table/T3/?report=objectonly.

Mother and obstetric care should be expedited if blood pressure doesn't go down or if the baseline reading is higher than or equal to 180/120 mm Hg. Additionally, it is strongly advised to begin accelerated management by a maternal fetal medicine specialist or a critical care specialist if the blood pressure is higher than 240/150 mm Hg or if there is any indication of end-organ damage.

Even though IV magnesium sulfate lowers blood pressure, it is not advised as an antihypertensive medication. Since magnesium has been shown to be more effective than phenytoin, diazepam, and nimodipine in reducing the risk of eclampsia and is the drug of choice to prevent eclampsia in both intrapartum and postpartum women, it continues to be the most commonly prescribed seizure prophylaxis in pregnant women with acute-onset severe hypertension. Currently, an intravenous loading dose of 4–6 g is the recommended dosage, followed by a maintenance dose of 1–2 g/h. Because of the possibility of synergistic hypotension, it is best to avoid using nifedipine in combination with magnesium sulfate (Euser and Cipolla, 2009).

Delivery is always the final treatment for women with preeclampsia who have significantly elevated blood pressure that is not responding to medication. Giving birth is always good for the mother, but depending on the fetus's gestational age, it could be bad for it. Maternal fetal medicine specialists and neonatologists must collaborate to make decisions that balance the risks of preterm birth with the possible benefit of removing the fetus from the preeclamptic environment where it is at risk for intrauterine growth restriction and stillbirth. Prolonged observation is often appropriate for women with a preterm fetus who have gestational hypertension or preeclampsia without severe features. On the other hand, the HYPITAT trial discovered that women who underwent induction of labor and had preeclampsia and gestational hypertension without severe features after 36 weeks experienced a significant reduction in adverse maternal outcomes, such as HELLP syndrome, eclampsia, pulmonary edema, and placental abruption. Neonatal complications did not significantly differ between expectant management and labor induction.

5.5. Placenta Previa

When the placenta attaches inside the uterus but lies over or close to the cervical opening, it is known as placenta previa. In the latter half of pregnancy, vaginal bleeding is one of the symptoms. Bright red in color, the bleeding usually has no pain associated with it. Placenta accreta, extremely low blood pressure, and postpartum hemorrhage are possible complications. Fetal growth restriction is one possible reason for the baby's complications.

Older age at pregnancy, smoking, history of cesarean section, induction of labor, or pregnancy termination are risk factors. Ultrasound is used for diagnosis. It falls under the category of pregnancy complication (Figure 5.4).

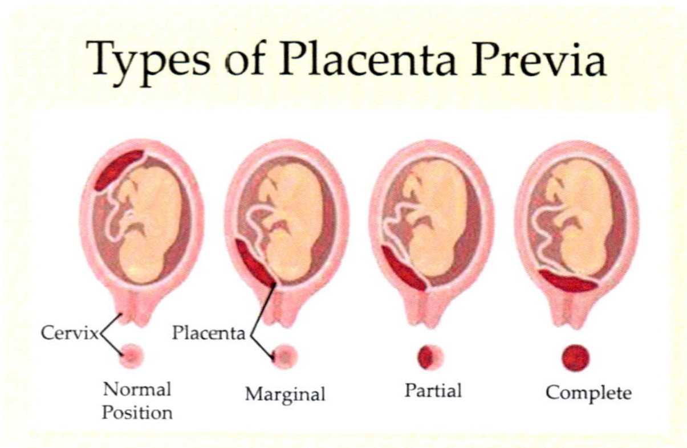

Figure 5.4. *Types of placenta previa.*

Source: https://www.cryo-cell.com/blog/october-2023/placenta-previa-types-signs-risks.

Recommendations for patients who are less than 36 weeks pregnant and only slightly bleeding could include staying in bed and refraining from sexual activity. A cesarean section is typically advised for pregnant women who are 36 weeks along or who are bleeding significantly. Corticosteroids may be administered to pregnant women under 36 weeks to expedite the development of the fetus's lungs. Early pregnancy cases might clear up on their own.

About 0.5 percent of pregnancies are impacted by placenta previa. However, 10% of pregnancies are affected after four cesarean sections. Over the course of the late 20th and early 21st centuries, disease rates have increased. Paul Portal was the first to describe the ailment in 1685.

5.5.1. Signs and Symptoms

Women who have placenta previa frequently exhibit bright red, painless vaginal bleeding. This can happen as early as the late mid-trimester, but it usually happens at 32 weeks of gestation. 51.6% of women with placenta previa experience bleeding prior to delivery. Usually beginning slowly, this bleeding may get worse as the placental separation area grows. If bleeding persists after 24 weeks of gestation, placenta previa should be suspected. About 22% of those affected experience bleeding after delivery.

5.5.2. Cause

Placenta previa's precise cause is unknown. It is thought to be connected to aberrant endometrial vascularization brought on by atrophy or scarring from prior infections, surgeries, or trauma. These elements might lessen the lower segment's differential growth, which would prevent the placenta from shifting upward as pregnancy progresses.

5.5.2.1. Risk Factors

The following have been identified as risk factors for placenta previa:

- Previous placenta previa (recurrence rate 4–8%), cesarean delivery, myomectomy or endometrium damage caused by D&C.
- Women who are younger than 20 are at higher risk and women older than 35 are at increasing risk as they get older.
- Women who have had previous pregnancies (multiparity), especially a large number of closely spaced pregnancies, are at higher risk due to uterine damage.
- Smoking during pregnancy; cocaine use during pregnancy
- Women with a large placenta from twins or erythroblastosis are at higher risk.
- Race is a controversial risk factor, with some studies finding that people from Asia and Africa are at higher risk et al finding no difference.
- Placental pathology (velamentous insertion, succenturiate lobes, bipartite i.e., bilobed placenta etc.)
- Baby is in an unusual position: breech (buttocks first) or transverse (lying horizontally across the womb).

5.5.3. Diagnosis

A history of antepartum hemorrhage may be found. Upon abdominal examination, the uterus is typically found to be soft, relaxed, and non-tender. Due to the placenta's aberrant position, Leopold's maneuvers may result in the fetus lying transversely or in an oblique or breech position. Around 35% of cases have malpresentation. In cases of placenta previa that are known to exist, vaginal exams are avoided.

5.5.3.1. Confirmatory

An ultrasound can confirm the presence of previa. Because transvaginal ultrasound is more accurate than transabdominal ultrasound, it can be used to measure the distance between the placenta and the cervical os. Because of this, the placenta previa's traditional classification is no longer valid.

False positives may be due to the following reasons:

- Overfilled bladder compressing lower uterine segment
- Myometrial contraction simulating placental tissue in an abnormally low location
- Early pregnancy low position, which in the third trimester may be entirely normal due to differential growth of the uterus.

In such cases, repeat scanning is done after an interval of 15–30 minutes.

In regions of the world without access to ultrasound, a surgical theater examination is frequently used to confirm the diagnosis. It's crucial to time examinations in theaters correctly. Up until the 36th week, the woman can be managed non-operatively if her bleeding is not severe. The baby has the same chance of surviving at this point as at full term.

5.5.4. Treatment

The patient is scheduled for an elective cesarean section delivery at 36 to 37 weeks after being diagnosed with placenta previa. On the other hand, some placenta previa patients experience complications and need an early cesarean section due to urgency.

Vital signs should be taken and electronic fetal monitoring should be started for patients who have a history of placenta previa and vaginal bleeding. Two large-bore intravenous lines with a full blood count, type, and screen, along with the drawing of coags, should be given to the patient. It is recommended to cross-match two to four units of blood if she exhibits significant bleeding.

Regardless of gestational age, patients experiencing excessive or continuous vaginal bleeding should have a cesarean section. If the bleeding stops, expectant mothers with gestational ages under 36 weeks may proceed with expectant management. Cesarean delivery is advised if the gestational age is 36 weeks or higher. If the patient meets the requirements, they should be admitted and given steroids to promote fetal lung maturity and magnesium sulfate for fetal neuroprotection. It is common practice to mandate bed rest, reduced activity, and avoid sexual activity, even though there is no obvious benefit. If the fetus is found to be healthy and the vaginal bleeding stops for more than 48 hours, the patient may be released for outpatient care or kept under observation while in the hospital. The stability of the patient, the frequency of bleeding episodes, the patient's proximity to the hospital, and compliance all play a role in outpatient management.

5.5.4.1. Delivery

It is best to have a cesarean section under carefully monitored circumstances. During prenatal care, the patient and the doctor should talk about the diagnosis, any potential complications, the plan for a cesarean section, and the possibility of a hysterectomy if the patient experiences uncontrollable postpartum hemorrhage (PAS). These patients should be reported to the blood bank, anesthesiologist, pediatricians, nurses, and surgeons. Urology, general surgery, and interventional radiology ought to be involved as well if PAS is a concern. In order to enable the different units to be aware of the patient in the event that the patient presents earlier in an emergency setting, communication between the teams regarding the anticipated date of surgery, scheduled procedures such as uterine artery embolization, and updated imaging studies is necessary.

Two large bore IV lines should be in place for the patient, and their blood should be cross-matched. Interventional radiology may also place uterine artery catheters prior to the procedure as a precaution. For non-urgent cases, a combination of spinal and epidural anesthesia is advised at the time of delivery. The patient can switch to general anesthesia if a hysterectomy is required. Because there is less blood loss during surgery and less need for blood transfusions, regional anesthesia is thought to be preferable to general anesthesia. Postpartum hemorrhage may worsen as a result of uterine relaxation brought on by inhaled anesthetics. In the event of a postpartum hemorrhage during the procedure, the uterus's blood supply can be reduced by inflating the catheters.

For the best exposure during surgery, it is recommended to make a vertical skin incision. In some cases, a high vertical uterine incision may be necessary if the placenta covers the lower uterine segment or if it is not fully developed. After the baby is delivered, the placenta will detach on its own and the incision can be closed. Sometimes there may be bleeding after the placenta detaches due to the lower uterine segment not contracting properly, which can be treated with various methods such as massage, medications, or surgical procedures. In severe cases, a hysterectomy may be required. If the placenta does not detach completely, the patient may have placenta accreta spectrum (PAS) and a cesarean hysterectomy may be necessary. In cases where PAS is suspected, it is important to perform a cesarean section without disturbing the placenta.

If a patient wants to become fertile, conservative management is an option for them with PAS. In order to allow for the safer removal or self-resorption of the remaining placental tissue, the placenta may be left in place until the placental bed devascularizes. Excellent fertility rates after conservative treatment have been reported in a number of studies. However, placenta accreta recurs frequently, with a 17–29% incidence rate. It is necessary to talk to the patient about both an emergency cesarean hysterectomy and a potential second hysterectomy procedure. A third of women receiving conservative treatment will continue to bleed vaginally, putting them at risk for infection, delayed hysterectomy, or blood transfusions. Because there is insufficient or no trophoblastic proliferation for methotrexate to take effect at term, there is no conclusive evidence of its benefits.

Compared to women with normal placentation, patients with a low-lying placenta—one that is more than 2 cm from the cervical OS—may be eligible for a labor trial, but they also face a higher risk of postpartum hemorrhage and an emergency cesarean section. Regarding the best method of delivery for marginal placenta previa, there is no agreement. As an example, Jansen et al., demonstrated that a labor trial should be advised if the distance between the placenta's edge and the internal os is more than 10 mm. (Jansen et al 2019).

5.6. Preterm Labor

The start of labor before 37 weeks of gestation is known as preterm labor. This represents the largest percentage of perinatal death that occurs after preterm birth and roughly 5–18% of births globally. Survivors of preterm birth also face serious long-term health consequences. Preterm labor, premature preterm rupture of membranes (PPROM), or medically indicated preterm delivery for reasons pertaining to the mother or the newborn can all result in preterm birth. The severity of prematurity determines the newborn and long-term risks, which are inversely correlated with the gestational age at birth. There are four categories for gestation at birth: near term (34–36 weeks), moderate prematurity (32–34 weeks), severe prematurity (28–32 weeks), and extreme prematurity (<28 weeks). As gestational age and birth weight decrease, there is a noticeable increase in neonatal mortality.

5.6.1. Signs of Premature Labor

Signs and symptoms of preterm labor include (Figure 5.5):

- Regular or frequent sensations of abdominal tightening (contractions)
- Constant low, dull backache
- A sensation of pelvic or lower abdominal pressure
- Mild abdominal cramps
- Vaginal spotting or light bleeding
- Preterm rupture of membranes — in a gush or a continuous trickle of fluid after the membrane around the baby breaks or tears
- A change in the type of vaginal discharge — watery, mucus-like or bloody

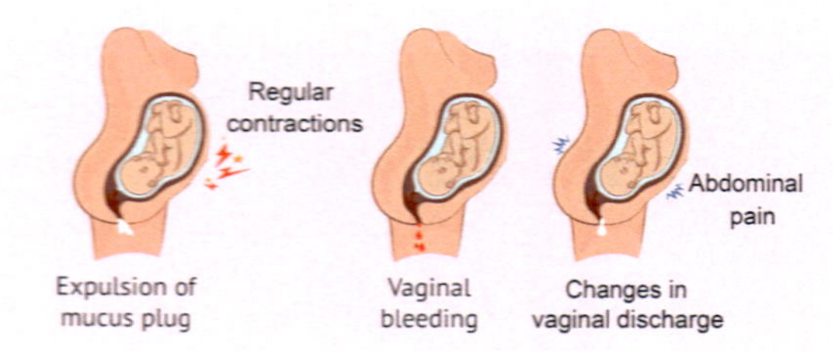

Figure 5.5. *Symptoms of preterm labor.*

Source: https://www.invitra.com/en/preterm-delivery/symptoms-preterm-birth-preterm-birth/.

5.6.2. Pathophysiology

Labor is primarily caused by three factors: activation of the decidua and membranes, prolonged uterine contractions, and cervical changes. Preterm labor differs from term labor in that the former is the result of a pathological process, while the latter is the result of a normal physiological process. Some of the processes leading up to preterm labor are acute, while others may take several weeks.

Intrauterine inflammation, often referred to as chorioamnionitis, is a major pathological event in preterm labor. It is characterized by systemic inflammation and elevated fetal plasma interleukin-6, usually in response to a trigger like chorioamnionitis. The fetal hypothalamus sends a signal that causes the CRH to be secreted, which in turn causes the fetal adrenal glands to produce more cortisol and activate the parturition pathway. Cytokines and prostaglandins are released when inflammatory cells invade the cervical stroma, promoting cervical ripening. The structures of the collagen and glycosaminoglycans that make up cervical tissue are impacted by these modifications. Progesterone inhibits collagen degradation while estrogen promotes it. Progesterone is therefore used to stop or postpone ripening. The formation of gap junctions and the upregulation of connexin 43 proteins, which aid in parturition, are both regulated by these hormones.

Furthermore, contractions are a necessary component of labor. Neural control is thought to be responsible for the transition from uncoordinated myometrial contractions to coordinated uterine contractions. The circadian rhythm of these contractions is dependent on oxytocin.

Fetal fibronectin detection in cervicovaginal secretions is used to measure the extracellular matrix degradation, which is a part of the parturition process. When it is found between

22 and 37 weeks of gestation, there is a higher chance of preterm labor and a disruption of the decidual-chorionic interface. Research suggests that apoptosis is a key element causing the aforementioned process.

5.6.3. History and Physical

As previously stated, history, symptoms, and physical examination are the main methods used to diagnose preterm labor. A thorough medical history pertaining to current and previous obstetrical complications can be instructive. Fetal biometry should be done if an early gestational age ultrasound is not available. When evaluating a patient who is in labor, it is crucial to consider the mother's vital signs, the fetal heart rate, and the frequency, duration, and intensity of the uterine contractions.

To evaluate firmness, abdominal tenderness, fetal size, and position, a physical examination is performed. Cervical dilatation and effacement in the absence of symptoms can be detected by a cervical exam. Regular contractions before the term gestational age linked to cervical change, pelvic pressure, menstrual-like cramps, watery vaginal discharge, and lower back pain are signs of preterm labor. While lower back pain can also occur during a normal pregnancy, if it manifests prior to term, there is a known correlation between it and the likelihood of preterm labor.

Preterm birth is highly likely for the patient if cervical dilatation is measured at less than 34 weeks and is at least 2 or 3 cm. Another sign, as determined by transvaginal ultrasound, is a short cervix. A cervical length of 35 to 48 mm is typical. A short cervical length is defined as less than 25 mm between weeks 16 and 24 of gestation. Notably, cervical effacement from active labor can be distinguished from that from cervical insufficiency with the use of a transvaginal ultrasound.

5.6.4. Treatment/Management

The gestational age at which the mother arrives at the hospital determines how the management is carried out. If the mother exhibits preterm labor at 34 weeks or older, she is admitted. Following a four to six-hour observation period, if there are no signs of progressive cervical dilation and effacement, fetal well-being is noted on a reactive non-stress test, and pregnancy complications have been ruled out, she can be sent home with instructions to follow up in one to two weeks, and to return if there are any new preterm labor symptoms or concerns about her pregnancy. Mothers who exhibit preterm labor symptoms and signs at 34 weeks or less are admitted to the hospital. Tocolytic medications are used to block labor for up to 48 hours in preterm labor with intact membranes. Guidelines regarding tocolytic medications: normally, between 22 and 34 weeks of gestation, and only in the absence of contraindications, should tocolytics be taken into consideration.

The classes of these drugs include:

- **Calcium Channel Blockers:** Nifedipine is preferred as it has fewer side effects than other drugs
- **Beta Adrenergic:** The most commonly used beta-2 agonist is terbutaline
- **COX Inhibitors**: indomethacin is safest if given no longer than the recommended 48 hours due to the risk of PDA closure
- Nitric oxide donors.
- Weaker tocolytic drugs
  - o Atosiban (oxytocin-vasopressin receptor antagonist) – not available in the United States
  - o Magnesium sulfate – of note, this is one of the most commonly used drugs in preterm labor. Mothers on this medication should have monitoring for the following: Deep tendon reflexes,

vital signs, magnesium levels, urine output, and respiratory depression

- o Glyceryl trinitrate

Preeclampsia with severe features, intrauterine fetal death, lethal fetal anomaly, chorioamnionitis, hemorrhage, and significant maternal cardiac disease are among the conditions that preclude the use of tocolytic drugs. Pregnancy cannot usually be prolonged for additional intrauterine growth and maturation once the membranes have ruptured. Nonetheless, the following forms of appropriate therapy should lower neonatal morbidity and mortality:

- Transferring the mother to a hospital with advanced obstetric and neonatal capabilities for care
- Administering appropriate antibiotics in labor to prevent GBS
- Antenatal administration of steroids to the mother to reduce morbidity and mortality of the fetus secondary to respiratory distress
- Intraventricular hemorrhage
- Necrotizing enterocolitis
- PDA
- Administration of magnesium sulfate in preterm labor before 32 weeks for neuroprotection

The doctor has to reevaluate the patient for amniotic infection, fetal compromise, potential abruption, and whether the cervix is still changing if contractions continue even after receiving appropriate tocolytic therapy. Preterm labor induction may be required in some cases. Intraamniotic infection, oligohydramnios, fetal growth restriction, placental abruption, and elevated blood pressure as a result of preeclampsia or eclampsia are a few examples of these situations. Fetal heart tracings are used in these situations to monitor the fetus in a manner similar to that of term fetuses. Monitoring has been demonstrated to lower neonatal seizures and intrapartum mortality. The patient's status should also be communicated to the neonatal care team so that the right staff and supplies are on hand in case they are needed. It is noteworthy that delayed cord clamping, or DCC, has been found to benefit preterm infants after birth. Higher initial hematocrits, high diastolic blood pressures, higher circulating blood volumes, and a lower rate of resuscitation are all associated with DCC.

5.6.5. Complications

- **Maternal Complications:** For unknown reasons, preterm labor has been linked to a higher risk of cardiovascular death and morbidity, usually years after delivery.
- **Infant Complications:** Impaired neurodevelopmental outcomes, such as reduced cognitive abilities, motor deficits, cerebral palsy, and loss of vision and hearing, are linked to preterm labor and delivery. As gestational age decreases, these risks rise. Preterm labor is also associated with behavioral problems like anxiety, depression, ADHD, and autism spectrum disorders.
- **Neonatal Complications:** Necrotizing enterocolitis, intraventricular hemorrhage, bronchopulmonary dysplasia, immature retinopathy, weak growth, and congenital abnormalities are a few of these.

The rate of complications in preterm births has dropped with improved obstetric and neonatal care. With patient-specific follow-up and education, the disability and long-term effects have improved (Feng et al., 2018).

A Closer Look

Medical Complications of Twins, Triplets and Multiples

Because there is a wider range of potential complications with multiple births, prenatal care is always more important. That being said, it is entirely possible to give birth to twins, triplets, or multiples in good health with routine examinations and ongoing care. It is necessary to maintain active vigilance and to be aware of potential complications so that the expectant mother can receive treatment as soon as symptoms manifest.

- Gestational Diabetes: Gestational diabetes is a temporary form of diabetes that can affect pregnant women. It occurs when the body is unable to produce enough insulin to regulate blood sugar levels during pregnancy. Approximately 2–9% of pregnant women may experience gestational diabetes. Common symptoms include frequent urination, constant thirst, and elevated levels of sugar in the blood and/or urine.

  The healthcare provider will typically test for gestational diabetes during the 24th to 28th week of pregnancy. Treatment typically involves a specific diet and exercise regimen. Close monitoring of both the mother and babies is essential, and insulin therapy may be recommended in certain instances.

  Cesarean section is generally preferred for delivering triplets, although in some cases, vaginal delivery may be considered. If there is a breach, fetal distress, or the gestational period is less than 32 weeks, twins may need to have a Cesarean section. Numerous complications could occur, so a full team of medical professionals and complete neonatal support should be present during the delivery.

- **Preeclampsia:** This condition is also referred to as pregnancy-induced hypertension (PIH) or toxicity. 50% of pregnant women who are carrying twins or triplets are likely to experience the condition. High blood pressure, water retention, protein in the urine, headaches, exhaustion, blurred vision, nausea, vomiting, dyspnea, bruising easily, and upper right abdominal pain are some of the symptoms.

  Preeclampsia is typically screened for in the twentieth week of pregnancy. Treatment options might include the pregnant woman being placed on bed rest, having more frequent prenatal checkups, eating less salt, drinking more water, and adding extra protein to her diet.

- **Preterm Delivery/Cesarean Section: A**lthough a typical pregnancy lasts 40 weeks, twins and triplets frequently arrive before week 37. Preterm babies frequently need intensive care to survive because they have not developed enough to do so on their own. When there are several births, vaginal delivery is the exception rather than the rule. When delivering twins, the mother might be able to give birth normally if the lower fetus is in the head first position, which is when the head is facing downward.

Cesarean section is almost always used to deliver triplets. If there is a breach, fetal distress, or the gestational period is less than 32 weeks, twins may need to have a Cesarean section. Numerous complications could occur, so a full team of medical professionals and complete neonatal support should be present during the delivery.

- **Umbilical Cord Entanglement:** For the babies, the umbilical cord serves as a lifeline. The umbilical cord connects the fetus to the placenta, where it receives the blood and nourishment required for healthy growth and development. However, there is a chance that complications could arise from umbilical cord entanglement or compression in monochorionic and monoamniotic twins who share a single amniotic sac in addition to the same placenta.

  When tangled up or knotted, the umbilical cord cannot perform at its best. An inadequate supply of blood and nutrients puts the fetus at risk of developing improperly. In rare circumstances, it might even tangle around the baby's neck and result in demise. An ultrasound can be used to diagnose problems with the umbilical cord.

- **Intrauterine Growth Restriction:** The term "poor fetal growth" is used to describe intrauterine growth restriction (IUGR). Numerous factors, such as inadequate nutrition during pregnancy, drug, alcohol, or cigarette use, complications related to the umbilical cord, gestational diabetes in the mother, and low levels of amniotic fluid accessible to the fetuses, can contribute to this condition. By measuring the fetus during an ultrasound and comparing its development to normal gestational age-based development, the condition is diagnosed.

  A Doppler ultrasound may be suggested by the medical professional in certain situations where IUGR is suspected. The fetuses will be closely monitored as a result of the detection. To achieve an early delivery, labor may be induced if the gestation period exceeds 34 weeks. A Cesarean section is more likely as a result of the condition.

- **Amn**iotic Fluid Problems: The watery substance surrounding the fetus in the amniotic sac is known as the amniotic fluid. Its presence insulates and buffers the developing embryo against physical trauma. It is also crucial for the growth of numerous organs. The fetus's kidneys and lungs produce amniotic fluid. Roughly 7% of pregnancies may experience issues with this fluid.

  A condition called hydramnios occurs when there is an excessive amount of amniotic fluid surrounding the fetus. The symptoms include abdominal pain, uterine contractions, and the uterus growing quickly. The term "oligohydramnios" refers to a condition in which there is very little amniotic fluid surrounding the umbilical cord. A possible sign of an amniotic sac rupture is the leaking of amniotic fluid. It can also be found via ultrasonography.

Summary

- Complications that occur primarily during childbirth are termed obstetric labor complications, and problems that occur primarily after childbirth are termed puerperal disorders.
- Hyperemesis gravidarum (HG) is a pregnancy complication that is characterized by severe nausea, vomiting, weight loss, and possibly dehydration.
- Diagnosis is usually made based on the observed signs and symptoms. HG has been technically defined as more than three episodes of vomiting per day such that weight loss of 5% or three kilograms has occurred and ketones are present in the urine.
- Gestational trophoblastic disease (GTD) is a term used for a group of pregnancy-related tumors. These tumors are rare, and they appear when cells in the womb start to proliferate uncontrollably.
- Anemia is a condition in which blood has a lower-than-normal amount of red blood cells or hemoglobin. Anemia in pregnancy is a decrease in the total red blood cells (RBCs) or hemoglobin in the blood during pregnancy.
- Folate is the vitamin found naturally in certain foods like green leafy vegetables A type of B vitamin, the body needs folate to produce new cells, including healthy red blood cells.
- Ectopic pregnancy is a complication of pregnancy in which the embryo attaches outside the uterus. Signs and symptoms classically include abdominal pain and vaginal bleeding, but fewer than 50% of affected women have both of these symptoms.
- Endometriosis is a disease in which cells similar to those of the endometrium, the tissue covering the inside of the uterus, grow outside the uterus.
- Hypertensive disease of pregnancy, also known as maternal hypertensive disorder, is a group of high blood pressure disorders that include preeclampsia superimposed on chronic hypertension, gestational hypertension, and chronic hypertension.
- Chronic hypertension is a type of high blood pressure in a pregnant woman that is pre-existing before conception, diagnosed early in pregnancy, or persists significantly after the end of pregnancy.
- Preeclampsia is a medical condition which usually develops after 20 weeks of gestation and traditionally involves both newly increased blood pressure (blood pressure $> 140/90$ mmHg) and proteinuria.
- Placenta previa is when the placenta attaches inside the uterus but in a position near or over the cervical opening. Symptoms include vaginal bleeding in the second half of pregnancy.
- Preterm labor is parturition that occurs when birth occurs between 20 0/7 weeks of gestation and 36 6/7 weeks. It further categorizes into early and late preterm.
- Three main components contribute to labor: cervical changes, persistent uterine contractions, and activation of the decidua and membranes.

References

1. Cotton, D. B., Jones, M. M., Longmire, S., et al. (1986). Role of intravenous nitroglycerin in the treatment of severe pregnancy-induced hypertension complicated by pulmonary edema. *American Journal of Obstetrics and Gynecology, 154*(1), 91–93. https://doi.org/10.1016/S0002-9378(86)80014-7.
2. Erick, M., Cox, J. T., & Mogensen, K. M. (2018). ACOG Practice Bulletin 189: Nausea and vomiting of pregnancy. *Obstetrics & Gynecology, 131*(5), 935. https://doi.org/10.1097/AOG.0000000000002622.
3. Euser, A. G., & Cipolla, M. J. (2009). Magnesium sulfate for the treatment of eclampsia: A brief review. *Stroke, 40*(4), 1169–1175. https://doi.org/10.1161/STROKEAHA.108.542406.
4. Feng, Y., Li, X. Y., Xiao, J., Li, W., Liu, J., Zeng, X., Chen, X., Chen, K. Y., Fan, L., Kang, Q. L., & Chen, S. H. (2018). Risk factors and pregnancy outcomes: Complete versus incomplete placenta previa in mid-pregnancy. *Current Medical Science, 38*(4), 597–601. https://doi.org/10.1007/s11596-018-2023-5.
5. Findeklee, S., & Costa, S. D. (2015). Placenta accreta and total placenta previa in the 19th week of pregnancy. *Geburtshilfe und Frauenheilkunde, 75*(8), 839–843. https://doi.org/10.1055/s-0035-1545017.
6. Haas, D. M., Imperiale, T. F., Kirkpatrick, P. R., Klein, R. W., Zollinger, T. W., & Golichowski, A. M. (2009). Tocolytic therapy: A meta-analysis and decision analysis. *Obstetrics & Gynecology, 113*(3), 585–594. https://doi.org/10.1097/AOG.0b013e3181951a79.
7. Iams, J. D., Cebrik, D., Lynch, C., Behrendt, N., & Das, A. (2011). The rate of cervical change and the phenotype of spontaneous preterm birth. *American Journal of Obstetrics and Gynecology, 205*(2), 130.e1–130.e6. https://doi.org/10.1016/j.ajog.2011.04.032.
8. Jansen, C., de Mooij, Y. M., Blomaard, C. M., Derks, J. B., van Leeuwen, E., Limpens, J., Schuit, E., Mol, B. W., & Pajkrt, E. (2019). Vaginal delivery in women with a low-lying placenta: A systematic review and meta-analysis. *BJOG: An International Journal of Obstetrics & Gynecology, 126*(9), 1118–1126. https://doi.org/10.1111/1471-0528.15692.
9. Lacasse, A., Rey, E., Ferreira, E., Morin, C., & Bérard, A. (2008). Nausea and vomiting of pregnancy: What about quality of life? *BJOG: An International Journal of Obstetrics & Gynecology, 115*(12), 1484–1493. https://doi.org/10.1111/j.1471-0528.2008.01852.x.
10. Lacasse, A., Rey, E., Ferreira, E., Morin, C., & Bérard, A. (2009). Epidemiology of nausea and vomiting of pregnancy: Prevalence, severity, determinants, and the importance of race/ethnicity. *BMC Pregnancy and Childbirth, 9*, 26. https://doi.org/10.1186/1471-2393-9-26.
11. Lurain, J. R. (2010). Gestational trophoblastic disease I: Epidemiology, pathology, clinical presentation and diagnosis of gestational trophoblastic disease, and management of hydatidiform mole. *American Journal of Obstetrics and Gynecology, 203*(6), 531–539. https://doi.org/10.1016/j.ajog.2010.06.043.
12. Magee, L. A., Pels, A., Helewa, M., Rey, E., & von Dadelszen, P., Committee SHG. (2014). Diagnosis, evaluation, and management of the hypertensive disorders of pregnancy: Executive summary. *Journal of Obstetrics and Gynecology Canada, 36*, 416–441, 575–576. https://doi.org/10.1016/S1701-2163(15)30303-4.

13. McParlin, C., O'Donnell, A., Robson, S. C., Beyer, F., Moloney, E., Bryant, A., Bradley, J., Muirhead, C. R., Nelson-Piercy, C., Newbury-Birch, D., Norman, J., Shaw, C., Simpson, E., Swallow, B., Yates, L., & Vale, L. (2016). Treatments for hyperemesis gravidarum and nausea and vomiting in pregnancy: A systematic review. *JAMA, 316*(13), 1392–1401. https://doi.org/10.1001/jama.2016.13972.

14. O'Hara, S., Zelesco, M., & Sun, Z. (2013). Cervical length for predicting preterm birth and a comparison of ultrasonic measurement techniques. *Australasian Journal of Ultrasound in Medicine, 16*(3), 124–134. https://doi.org/10.1002/j.2205-0140.2013.tb00098.x.

15. Orabona, R., Sciatti, E., Vizzardi, E., et al. (2017). Endothelial dysfunction and vascular stiffness in women with previous pregnancy complicated by early or late pre-eclampsia. *Ultrasound in Obstetrics & Gynecology, 49*, 116–123. https://doi.org/10.1002/uog.17489.

16. Riveros-Perez, E., & Wood, C. (2018). Retrospective analysis of obstetric and anesthetic management of patients with placenta accreta spectrum disorders. *International Journal of Gynaecology and Obstetrics, 140*(3), 370–374. https://doi.org/10.1002/ijgo.12453.

17. Werntoft, E., & Dykes, A. K. (2001). Effect of acupressure on nausea and vomiting during pregnancy: A randomized, placebo-controlled, pilot study. *Journal of Reproductive Medicine, 46*(9), 835–839.

18. Yusuf, S., Hawken, S., Ounpuu, S., et al. (2004). Effect of potentially modifiable risk factors associated with myocardial infarction in 52 countries (the INTERHEART study): Case-control study. *The Lancet, 364*, 937–952. https://doi.org/10.1016/S0140-6736(04)17018-9.

19. Zimmerman, C. F., Ilstad-Minnihan, A. B., Bruggeman, B. S., Bruggeman, B. J., Dayton, K. J., Joseph, N., et al. (2022). Thyroid storm caused by hyperemesis gravidarum. *AACE Clinical Case Reports, 8*(3), 124–127. https://doi.org/10.1016/j.aacecr.2022.01.003.

Chapter

MEDICAL DISEASES COMPLICATING PREGNANCY

6

Contents

Introduction

The occurrence of medical issues during pregnancy is on the rise due to a combination of demographic changes, lifestyle choices, and advances in medical technology. Despite a decrease in overall maternal mortality rates, conditions such as venous thromboembolism, epilepsy, and autoimmune diseases continue to pose risks to pregnant women. It is essential for all healthcare providers to have a basic understanding of these medical issues in order to provide proper care. This includes taking preventive measures before pregnancy, managing conditions throughout pregnancy, and promptly treating any illnesses that may arise. Many medications and diagnostic tests are safe to use during pregnancy, and a multidisciplinary approach to care is recommended.

Orientation and Directional Terms

Term	Definition	Illustration
Ovary	The ovaries are two almond-shaped structures that sit on either side of the uterus, connected to the uterine tubes.	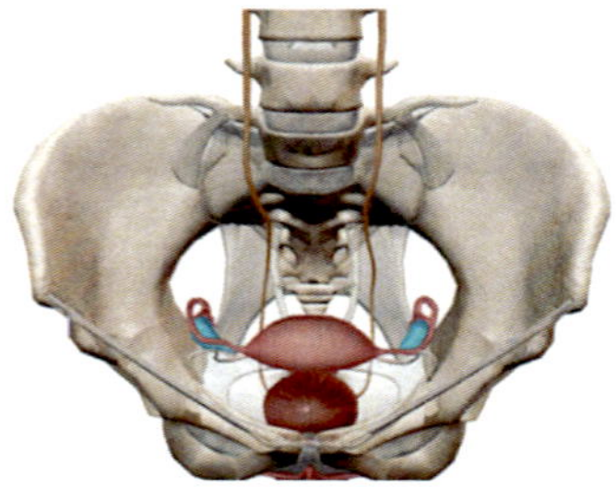
Cervix	The lower part of the uterus constricts into a segment called the cervix, which leads to the vagina.	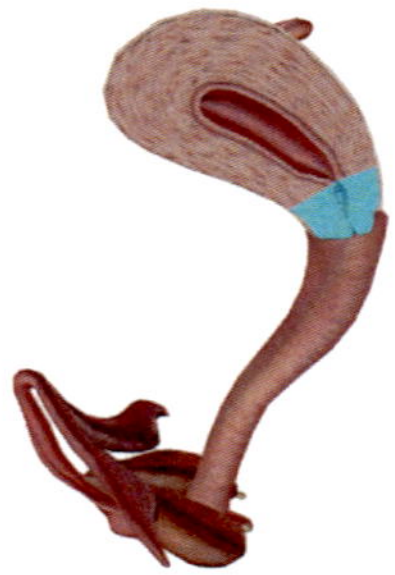
Vagina	The vagina extends down from the cervix, the lower part of the uterus, to the vestibule, which is part of the vulva and the external genitalia. It sits behind the bladder and in front of the rectum.	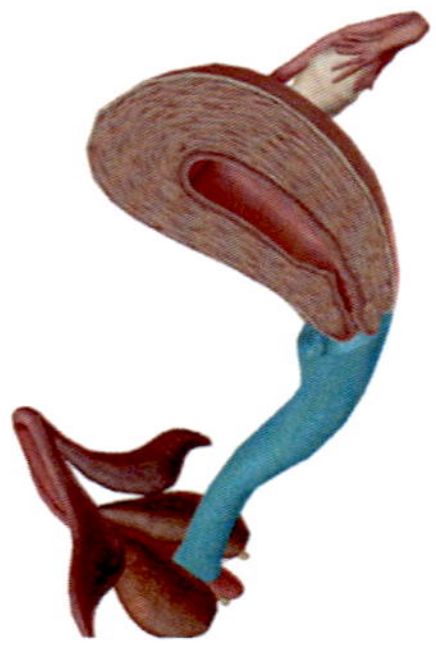
Vulva	The external genitalia (vulva) of the female reproductive system include the mons pubis, the labia majora and labia minora, the clitoris and prepuce (clitoral hood), the vestibule of the vagina, urethral orifice, and the greater vestibular glands.	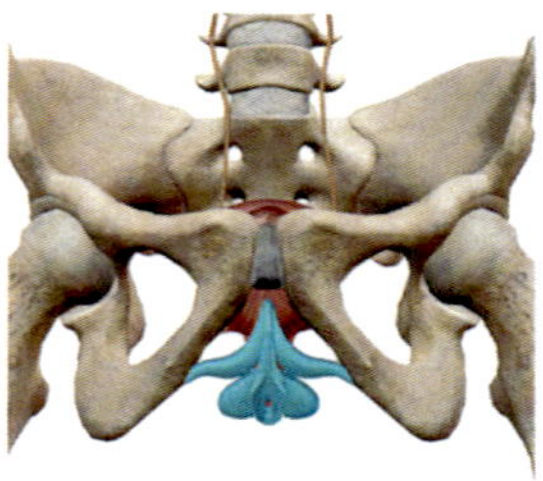
Embryo	A developing human during weeks 3–8.	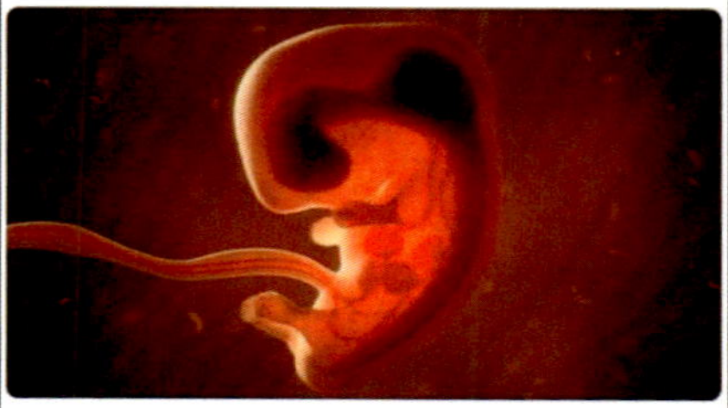

6.1. Diseases of the Cardiovascular System

Pregnancy-related cardiac disease includes a wide range of pathologies. Numerous cardiac conditions that occur during pregnancy are being studied, and there are still many that need to be learned more about. A few of these illnesses could be the pregnant woman's pre-existing conditions made worse, or they might be a brand-new illness that arises as a result of the intricate hormonal fluctuations and pregnancy's physiology. Pre-existing conditions such as diabetes mellitus, congenital heart disease, and hypertension can put pregnant women at risk for cardiovascular disease. All things considered, cardiac disease during pregnancy is a major cause of morbidity and mortality and has been reported to occur in 1–4% of pregnancies. Even though these pregnancies carry a high risk, most of these cases can be successfully treated if routine care includes early detection and careful follow-up.

6.1.1. Etiology

Pregnancy-related cardiovascular diseases have a variety of etiologies, depending on the underlying pathology. Some common cardiovascular diseases that occur during pregnancy are summarized below, along with some theories as to why they may occur.

- **Cardiomyopathy:** The etiology of this disease process is the subject of multiple theories. Hemodynamic instability, microchimerism, autoimmune causes, viral myocarditis, and other theories are among the most popular ones. It is crucial to remember that the risk factors for cardiomyopathy that are present in non-pregnant people still exist during pregnancy and the weeks that follow, and the heart may even be more vulnerable to these exposures. These include abussing alcohol, abussing drugs like cocaine and methamphetamines, and abussing doxorubicin.
- **Coronary Artery Disease:** Pregnant women and non-pregnant women share a similar etiology for ischemic heart disease. These people are susceptible to ischemic heart disease due to risk factors such as diabetes mellitus, obesity, smoking, immobility, hypertension, hyperlipidemia, and hypertriglyceridemia.
- **Pregnancy-Associated Myocardial Infarction:** There are similar risk factors for pregnancy-related MI as there are for coronary artery disease. Preeclampsia and eclampsia are two pregnancy conditions that have been linked to myocardial infarction, according to theory.
- **Valvular Disease:** It is unclear if pregnancy plays a particular role in the genesis of newly diagnosed valvular disorders, despite the fact that the hemodynamics of pregnancy can make some valvular diseases worse.

6.1.2. Epidemiology

Uncertainty exists regarding the prevalence of cardiac illness in women. Whether there is a higher frequency of people in developed vs. less developed nations. The best available data suggest that at least 0.2% of pregnancies result in cardiac disease complications (Ashrafi & Curtis, 2017). According to reports from the European Society of Gynecology (ESG) in 2011, this frequency may reach 4%. This figure would increase even more if hypertensive disease was taken into account, since it has been estimated that up to 8% of pregnancies result in hypertensive disorders.

6.1.3. Pathophysiology

The physiological changes that occur during pregnancy, particularly in relation to the heart, play a key role in the development of certain diseases. It is believed that these changes can begin as early as 5 weeks into pregnancy, and can vary from one woman to another. The attachment of the placenta to the uterine walls triggers the release of hormones, leading to changes in maternal physiology. These changes are typically hemodynamic and counter-regulatory, but ultimately aim to maintain the new mean arterial pressure of pregnancy while supporting the health of both the mother and the baby.

- **Cardiac Output:** Increases in cardiac output are estimated to be between 20 and 50 percent. These results appear during the first five weeks of pregnancy and continue to rise until the late gestational age; an increased stroke volume of roughly 25% during the first trimester is typically responsible for these findings. Pregnant women with pre-existing cardiac conditions may experience such dramatic effects, especially later in pregnancy, due in part to this significant increase in cardiac output. People who suffer from illnesses like cardiomyopathy might not be able to recover from this stress in a sufficient amount of time, which could lead to complications like fluid overload or pulmonary edema.
- **Heart Rate:** In the first trimester of pregnancy, there is a 15–30% increase in heart rate in addition to an increase in stroke volume, which both add to an increase in cardiac output.
- **Systemic Vascular Resistance:** During pregnancy, systemic vascular resistance lowers. This change could be as high as 30%, according to estimates. The mother's vasculature is less responsive to angiotensin II and norepinephrine, among other hormonal changes. Additionally, the mother female releases prostaglandins and nitric oxide, two vasodilators, at a faster rate.
- **Blood Pressure:** Early in pregnancy, there is a slight drop in blood pressure. Generally, early in pregnancy, diastolic blood pressure lowers more frequently than systolic blood pressure. Usually, by the end of the pregnancy, this value returns to normal or even rises.

Certain decompensated states of pregnancy, such as cardiomyopathy, congenital heart diseases, and valvular disease, are thought to be caused by a confluence of the aforementioned physiological and hormonal changes.

However, it is undeniable that the mother heart undergoes unique structural changes, and that these changes may contribute to the dysfunction of some of these underlying conditions. An enlargement of both ventricles and atria by the end of pregnancy is a common consequence of the increase in volume during pregnancy. By the third trimester, left ventricular mass can increase by as much as 50%, and increases in septal thickness are also associated with an increase in eccentric hypertrophy. Since many of the changes that occur to the mother heart are frequently observed to be reversed 6 to 8 months postpartum, there is some degree of cardiac remodeling present in the mother heart. It is understandable why such drastic changes would contribute to the exacerbation of disease processes for processes such as peripartum cardiomyopathy. The precise reason why these females are significantly more susceptible to this disease process than others has not, however, been determined by specific studies.

Table 6.1. Classification of Maternal Risks Based on the Type of Cardiovascular Abnormality; Adapted from Thorne et al.

Category	Maternal Risk Factors
Class I: No detectable increase in maternal mortality and no or mild increase in morbidity)	Uncomplicated small or mild: pulmonary stenosis, VSD, PDA, mitral valve prolapse Successfully repaired simple lesions, such as secundum ASD, VSD, PDA, total anomalous pulmonary, and venous drainage
Class II: Small increase in maternal mortality and moderate increase in morbidity	Unoperated ASD Repaired tetralogy of Fallot Most arrhythmias
Classes II-III	Mild left ventricular impairment Hypertrophic cardiomyopathy Native or tissue valve disease not considered class IV Marfan syndrome (or other aortopathy, such as, EDS type IV, FTAA or LDS) without aortic dilatation Repaired coarctation Heart transplantation
Class III: Significantly increased in risk of maternal mortality or severe morbidity	Mechanical valve Systemic right ventricle: CCTGA, TGA Post-Fontan repair Cyanotic heart disease Other complex congenital heart disease Marfan syndrome with aorta 40–45 mm
Class IV: Extremely high risk of maternal mortality or severe morbidity	Pulmonary hypertension of any cause Severe systemic ventricular impairment e-LVEF <30% or NYHA III-IV Previous peripartum cardiomyopathy with any residual ventricular impairment Severe left heart obstruction Marfan syndrome with aorta >45 mm

Source: Sahu AK, Harsha MM, Rathoor S. (2022). Cardiovascular Diseases in Pregnancy – A Brief Overview. Curr Cardiol Rev.;18(1), e250821195824. doi: 10.2174/1573403X17666210825103653. PMID: 34525935; PMCID: PMC9241116.

† VSD, Ventricular septal defect; PDA, Patent ductus arteriosus; ASD, Atrial septal defect; EDS, Ehlers Danlos syndrome; CCTGA, congenitally corrected transposition of the great arteries; TGA, Transposition of the great arteries; LDS, Loeys-Dietz syndrome; FTAA, Familial thoracic aortic aneurysm; LVEF, Left ventricular ejection fraction; NYHA, New York Heart Association (NYHA) Classification.

Thus, possible explanations for the resulting peripartum cardiomyopathy include concurrent myocarditis, an autoimmune phenomenon, or familial linkage. The chamber and valvular enlargement, in addition to a possible volume overloaded state, can lead to morbidity and mortality in the case of pre-existing valvular disorders such as mitral stenosis, mitral regurgitation, aortic stenosis, and others. These ailments can all lead to a state of fluid overload and put patients at risk for hypoperfusion and respiratory compromise (Table 6.1).

6.1.4. Evaluation

When evaluating cardiac disease in expectant mothers, a more involved workup is frequently necessary. Basic laboratory tests like CBC, CMP, and urinalysis can provide the first indications of potential underlying processes. A higher than normal white blood cell count can be used to screen for inflammatory heart conditions like myocarditis or myocardial infarction. Regular serum creatinine measurements can assist the physician in determining whether the patient has experienced hypo-perfusion episodes recently. Liver enzyme levels may be used to diagnose congestive hepatopathy, just as they would in non-pregnant patients. Protein levels in the urine may be able to help diagnose pre-eclampsia. Certain lab tests, like brain natriuretic peptide (BNP) double during pregnancy, may be useful. Nevertheless, BNP levels have been found to be higher in those with overt peripartum cardiomyopathy than in those without it.

An ECG may also be performed and may show different results, comparable to those of nonpregnant individuals with cardiovascular disease. Pregnancy-related normal cardiac changes result in a mild left axis deviation and left heart rotation. Pregnancy causes dilation of all the heart's chambers, as was previously mentioned, which puts pregnant women at risk for dysrhythmias. Atrioventricular premature beats, supraventricular tachycardias, and ventricular premature beats are a few of the most prevalent dysrhythmias observed during pregnancy. Ventricular tachyarrhythmias are much less common but can still occur. A patient undergoing ischemic changes should exhibit ECG abnormalities such as ST elevations or depressions, T-wave inversions, or Q-wave formation, all of which are indicative of an ischemic burden. Unspecific alterations to the T-waves or ST-segment occur in as many as 14% of pregnancies.

When assessing a pregnant patient experiencing cardiac insults, an echocardiogram is necessary. Physiologic findings could include dilatation of the valves, tricuspid regurgitation, aortic regurgitation, and mitral regurgitation. A clinician will need to assess the clinical manifestations of these processes as well as the extent of echocardiographic findings in order to determine their significance. There is no set threshold that has been established as "normal" or "abnormal" for any of these in pregnancy. Exaggerated septal thickening, end-diastolic posterior wall thickening, and the ensuing eccentric hypertrophy may be seen in cardiomyopathy findings. If the end-diastolic dimension is greater than 2.7 cm/m^2, the peripartum cardiomyopathy can be diagnosed by echocardiography if the ejection fraction is less than 45% and/or the M-mode shortening is less than 30%. In cases of myocardial ischemia or infarction, there may be anomalies in the localized wall motion. Pericardial effusion can also be visible during pregnancy and, in small amounts, can be physiologic; however, echocardiography should be used to evaluate tamponade if the patient is displaying symptoms of hypotension, JVD, or pulsus paradoxus.

6.1.5. Treatment/Management

It is not recommended to follow any empirical regimens to prevent cardiac disease during pregnancy. People with a history of heart disease should be given extra attention and should stick to their previous treatment plan. If such regimens include teratogenic drugs, these drugs should be replaced by a qualified healthcare provider. The best course of action for treating cardiac disease during pregnancy depends on the specific disease process and calls for a customized strategy. The following lists a few common cardiac conditions along with the appropriate treatment plans that are suggested for them:

- **Ventricular Dysfunction of Pregnancy:** Many women who have had heart failure in the past start pregnant. Depending on their level of function, these people might have known about these before getting pregnant or not. Pregnancy-related physiologic changes can be difficult for these patients to adjust to. By the time the second trimester arrives and these pregnancy-related physiological changes (increased heart rate, increased circulating volume) take full effect, these expectant patients may suffer a significant worsening of their underlying condition. Other heart failure medications can be resumed in addition to angiotensin-converting enzyme inhibitors and angiotensin receptor blockers. Renal dysplasia, renal failure, oligohydramnios, and intrauterine growth retardation are among the known teratogenic effects of ACEs and ARBs, which are frequently the cornerstone of treatment for heart failure with reduced ejection fraction. An equivalent result can be obtained by combining nitrates with hydralazine. It is acceptable to keep taking beta-blockers, with a preference for cardio-selective ones like metoprolol. If diuretics are necessary, they can be taken as prescribed.
- **Peripartum Cardiomyopathy:** Treatment for this dilated cardiomyopathy, which manifests in the final four weeks of pregnancy or up to five months after giving birth, will be comparable to that for patients with ventricular dysfunction during pregnancy. An exception is if peripartum cardiomyopathy is diagnosed; after delivery, ACE inhibitors or ARB therapy may resume.
- **Mitral Stenosis:** Pregnant patients with obstructive mitral stenosis have a high morbidity and mortality rate (Silversides, Colman, Sermer, and Siu, 2003). Although no medication has been demonstrated to reverse this disease in these individuals, beta-blockers continue to be the recommended treatment. It is believed that beta-blockers reduce the trans-mitral gradient. Diuretics can also help with the symptoms of heart failure.
- **Aortic Stenosis:** Even though pregnancy-related aortic stenosis is less common, treating it can be more difficult. Similar to aortic stenosis in non-pregnant people, there are no mainstay treatments or medications that can reverse the disease. Beta-blockers are not as good at lowering trans-valvular gradient as mitral stenosis is. Patients who are pregnant should not use ace inhibitors. Diuretic therapy carries a risk of decreased

cardiac output and reduced diastolic filling, which makes caution necessary.

- **Tachyarrhythmias:** Treatment for tachyarrhythmias must be tailored to the individual. However, adenosine, verapamil, digoxin, flecainide, and beta blockers seem to be safe to use in pregnant women with tachyarrhythmias. Because amiodarone tends to induce hypothyroidism in fetuses, it is best to avoid using it.
- **Spontaneous Coronary Artery Dissection (SCAD):** This is not the usual reason for acute MI. Pregnant women experience an increased incidence of it. Any pregnant woman who presents with symptoms suggestive of acute coronary syndrome should be evaluated for spontaneous coronary artery dissection. Usually, the left anterior descending artery or the left main artery are affected by this dissection. It is thought that SCAD results from hemodynamic changes that weaken the arterial wall and from the hormonal changes associated with pregnancy. It is further postulated that this involves infiltrates of inflammation. Coronary angiography can be used to make a diagnosis. However, because management is so uncommon, it has not been standardized. Numerous management techniques have been applied. These consist of medical supervision, coronary artery bypass grafting (CABG), and heart transplantation. If more than one artery has been severely damaged, if PCI has failed, or if the left main stem has been severed, CABG might be the best course of action.
- Acute coronary syndrome Although ACS and MI are rare in pregnant women, they are becoming more frequent due to the rising average age at which women are becoming pregnant. Growing older facilitates the development of ACS risk factors. Diabetes mellitus, hyperlipidemia, and hypertension are some of these risk factors. Pregnant mothers should avoid fluoroscopy exposure, but since acute coronary syndromes have a high death rate, PCI should be tried with the mother covered by a lead. Thrombolysis is another option, but because of the documented cases of subchorionic hematomas, spontaneous abortion, bleeding in the uterus, and maternal hemorrhage, it needs to be administered closely monitored. Due to the prolonged need for dual antiplatelet therapy, drug-eluting stents should be avoided if at all possible. Combining dual antiplatelet therapy with cesarean section deliveries is becoming more common. (Roth and Elkayam, 2008). A list of commonly used drugs and their pregnancy category class are listed below.

o Morphine (Risk Category C)

o Beta-blockers (Category B: metoprolol; Category C: atenolol)

o Calcium channel blockers: (Category C)

o Angiotensin receptor blockers (ARBs) (Category D in the second and third trimesters and Category C in the first trimester) and angiotensin-converting enzyme (ACE) inhibitors.

o Unfractionated heparin (Category C)

o Low-molecular-weight heparin (Category B)

o Aspirin (Category C)

o Glycoprotein IIb/IIIa inhibitors (Category B: eptifibatide, tirofiban; Category C: abciximab)

- Depending on the severity, patients

who arrive with blood pressure higher than 160/100 should receive antihypertensive medication under close observation in the clinic or possibly in the hospital (Phipps et al., 2016).

Some common anti-hypertensive agents which have been shown to be safe in pregnancy include:

- o Methyldopa (oral)
- o Labetalol (oral/IV)
- o Nifedipine (oral)
- o Hydralazine (oral/IV)
- o Nicardipine (IV

6.1.6. Differential Diagnosis

Pregnancy-related cardiac illnesses must be assessed as either entirely new conditions or aggravating existing ones. Any cardiac disease process that is found during pregnancy needs to have any underlying pathology ruled out. These consist of hypertensive obstructive cardiomyopathy, restrictive cardiomyopathy, dilated cardiomyopathy, ischemic heart disease, and prior valvular disorders.

6.1.7. Deterrence and Patient Education

From the beginning, patients should be informed about their cardiac conditions and allowed to participate in the decision-making process. Drawing attention to the risks to both the patient and the fetus is crucial. Moms should be counseled about the risk factors linked to pregnancy-related cardiac disease as soon as they become pregnant. Among these risk factors are myocarditis, drug and alcohol abuse, diabetes mellitus, hypertension, pre-existing heart disease, and familial heart disease in pregnancy.

6.1.8. Enhancing Healthcare Team Outcomes

To provide coordinated and efficient care, a team of professionals must collaborate on every pregnancy. In patients with heart disease who are pregnant, this degree of cohesion is even more critical. In order to differentiate between normal and abnormal pregnancy states—which can be challenging to do in the case of cardiac disease because pregnant women frequently show signs of cardiac disease during a healthy pregnancy—physicians are essential. When it comes to pregnant patients with heart disease, nurses play a critical role in the healthcare system. When these patients are admitted to the hospital, their nurses need to be aware of the intricate dynamics of pregnancy, particularly when interventions might be required. It is crucial to identify disease states early on in order to shield these patients from worse outcomes. In the treatment of female patients with cardiac disease who are pregnant, pharmacists play a special role. Many substances and medicines that are frequently used at other times may be harmful to expectant mothers and/or their unborn children. The special responsibility of knowing about these drugs, their interactions, and when to make recommendations for changes falls on pharmacists. Lynch et al., emphasized how important it is for doctors and pharmacists to communicate in order to provide the best possible pregnancy outcomes. An integral component of the healthcare system is the interprofessional team. In order to manage the pregnant patient through a safe pregnancy for both the mother and the child, the need for balanced coordination of care only grows.

6.2. Maternal Infections During Pregnancy

Achieving pregnancy is a common goal for many women, as it is a normal and healthy state. Nonetheless, certain infections may become more contagious in pregnant women. These infections may also worsen during pregnancy. Pregnant women are susceptible to serious illness from even mild infections.

Certain infections that arise during pregnancy are mainly dangerous for the expectant mother. Other infections may be passed from mother to child during delivery or through the placenta. The infant is also susceptible to health issues when this happens. Certain infections that arise during pregnancy have the potential to cause birth defects, premature labor, or miscarriage. For the mother, they might even pose a threat to her life. The fact that drugs used to treat infections can have major adverse effects, particularly for the unborn child, further complicates matters. In order to reduce risks to the mother and the unborn child, it is crucial to try to prevent infections during pregnancy.

6.2.1. Reason for Pregnant Women Susceptible to Infection

Every system in your body is impacted by pregnancy. You may be more susceptible to infections and life-threatening consequences due to changes in hormone levels and immune system performance. You and your child are particularly vulnerable during labor and delivery.

6.2.1.1. Changes in Immunity

The body's immune system protects it from dangerous invaders. It combats pathogens, cancerous cells, and organ transplants alike. An intricate network of participants collaborates to locate and eradicate foreign encroachment.

Your immune system adapts during pregnancy to shield you and your unborn child from illness. Your immune system is suppressed in some areas and enhanced in others. This establishes a balance that can shield the infant from infection without endangering the mother's health. These modifications also aid in shielding your child from the defenses of your body. Though technically your body ought to reject the baby as "foreign," it doesn't. Like after receiving an organ transplant, your body recognizes your baby as both "foreign" and "self." This prevents the baby from being attacked by your immune system. Even with these defenses, you're more vulnerable to infections that don't typically result in disease. Your immune system has to function harder during pregnancy because it is supporting two people. You become more prone to certain infections as a result.

6.2.1.2. Changes in Body Systems

Hormonal changes can raise your risk of infection in addition to immune function changes. The urinary tract, which consists of the following, is frequently impacted by these changes in hormone levels.

- the kidneys, which are organs that produce urine
- ureters, which are tubes that carry urine from the kidneys to the bladder
- bladder, which is where urine is stored
- urethra, which is a tube that transports urine out of the body

The ureters are under increased pressure during pregnancy due to the uterus's growth. Concurrently, the body produces more progesterone, a hormone that relaxes the muscles in the bladder and ureters. Urine may thus remain in the bladder for an extended period of time. Your chance of getting a urinary tract infection rises as a result. Additionally, hormonal changes increase your risk of developing candidiasis, a type of yeast infection. Having more estrogen in your reproductive system puts you at risk for yeast infections.

Furthermore, variations in lung fluid content can increase your risk of developing lung infections like pneumonia. Pregnancy causes your lungs to retain more fluid, which puts additional pressure on your abdomen and lungs. This causes the fluid to accumulate in the lungs and makes it more difficult for your body to eliminate. The excess fluid weakens your body's defenses against infection and promotes bacterial growth.

6.2.2. Risks for Mother and Baby

6.2.2.1. Risks for Mother

Pregnancy-related infections can cause issues mainly for the mother. These consist of postpartum infections, vaginitis, and urinary tract infections.

6.2.2.2. Risks for Baby

The baby is especially troubled by other infections. Toxoplasmosis, parvovirus, and cytomegalovirus, for instance, can all be passed from mother to child. Should this transpire, there might be dire repercussions. For an inherited cytomegalovirus infection, there is currently no proven cure. There exist antibiotics that have the potential to effectively treat toxoplasmosis. Intrauterine blood transfusions can be used to treat parvovirus infection, despite the lack of antibiotics for it.

6.2.2.3. Risks for Both Mother and Baby

Some infections are particularly harmful to both mother and baby. These include:

- syphilis
- listeriosis
- hepatitis
- HIV
- group B *streptococcus* (GBS)

If the infection is identified early on, antibiotics can effectively treat both syphilis and listeria in both the mother and the child. Vaccines are now available to help prevent hepatitis A and B infections, even though there are no known treatments for viral hepatitis.

6.2.2.4. HIV Infection

HIV infection during pregnancy is a dangerous condition that could be fatal. New multidrug combinations, however, now considerably increase life expectancy and enhance the quality of life for HIV-positive individuals. These medication therapies have been remarkably successful in lowering the rate of HIV infection transmission from pregnant women to their offspring, when combined with cesarean delivery performed prior to the onset of labor.

6.2.2.5. Group B Streptococcus

Every woman is tested for GBS by doctors at the end of her pregnancy. Group B streptococcus is a common bacterium that causes this infection. Approximately one in four women have a GBS infection, according to the Centers for Disease Control and Prevention. Because the bacterium may be in the mother's rectum or vagina, vaginal deliveries are the most common way that this infection is spread. The infection can result in internal inflammation and stillbirth in expectant mothers. GBS infections in newborns can lead to serious, possibly fatal infections. Meningitis, pneumonia, and sepsis are a few of these. If such infections are not treated, the baby may be born with birth defects such as chronic mental impairments, learning disabilities, or loss of hearing or vision.

6.2.3. The Importance of Knowledge and Ongoing Care

Throughout your pregnancy, your doctor-patient relationship is essential. You can help prevent transmission by being aware of the increased risk of infection during pregnancy as well as the possible risks to both you and your unborn child. Understanding the various kinds of infections that might occur also makes it easier for you to identify the signs. If you fall ill, getting a timely diagnosis and efficient care can help you avoid complications. During your pregnancy, make sure to discuss any worries or inquiries you have with your doctor.

6.2.4. Prevention

Pregnancy infections can be avoided. Minimal, daily safety measures can significantly lower the risk of injury to both you and your child. You should try to avoid infections while you're pregnant.

- Hands should be frequently cleaned with soap and water. This is especially crucial after using the restroom, chopping vegetables and meat, and engaging in kid-centered play.
- Make sure to thoroughly cook meats. It is always best to reheat undercooked meats, like hot dogs and deli meats, until they are thoroughly cooked.
- Don't consume unpasteurized, or raw, dairy products.
- Don't share eating utensils, cups, and food with other people.
- Avoid changing cat litter and stay away from wild or pet rodents.
- Practice safe sex and get tested for sexually transmitted infections.
- Make sure your vaccinations are up-to-date.

Make sure to schedule an appointment with your doctor immediately if you are feeling unwell or suspect that you have come into contact with a contagious illness. Early diagnosis and treatment of any infections can greatly improve the health outcomes for both you and your baby.

6.3. Diabetes in Pregnancy

There are unique difficulties for both the mother and the fetus when a pregnant woman with diabetes has diabetes. Pre-existing diabetes in a pregnant woman can lead to early labor, birth defects, and larger-than-average babies. Therefore, about three months prior to deciding to become pregnant, doctors advise diabetics to keep their blood sugar levels within a normal range. Planning ahead is crucial if one wishes to become pregnant when they already have type 1 or type 2 diabetes, as strict blood glucose control is required before becoming pregnant.

6.3.1. Physiology

Type 1 and Type 2 pre-gestational diabetes can be distinguished based on the physiological mechanism involved. Type 2 diabetes mellitus is linked to obesity and is caused by a combination of insulin resistance and insufficient insulin production. Type 1 diabetes mellitus is an autoimmune disease that results in the destruction of insulin-producing cells in the pancreas. Human placental lactogen (HPL), a hormone with counter-regulatory effects that raise blood glucose levels, is produced by the placenta during pregnancy. When combined with diabetes mellitus, these physiological changes in mothers can result in dangerously elevated blood glucose levels. This is important because, in comparison to non-pregnant states, the effects of inadequate glycemic control are more severe during pregnancy.

6.3.2. Risks for the Fetus

The negative impacts of pregestational diabetes are primarily due to elevated levels of blood sugar and insulin in the first trimester of pregnancy, unlike gestational diabetes which can cause complications in the later stages. These high levels during the crucial period of fetal development can result in congenital abnormalities such as abnormal heart and central nervous system development. Conditions like sacral agenesis, holoprosencephaly, and limb deficiencies have been associated with diabetes. Heart defects like truncus arteriosus, atrioventricular septal defect, and single ventricle complex are also more likely with pregestational diabetes. However, tight control of blood sugar can help prevent these complications. In addition, children of mothers with pregestational diabetes may have mild neurological and cognitive deficits, such as ADHD symptoms, impaired motor skills, and memory issues.

Pre-existing diabetes in the mother can result in complications for the newborn such as neonatal jaundice, hypoglycemia, and macrosomia. However, pregestational diabetes does not increase the risk of chromosomal abnormalities like Down Syndrome. Miscarriages may occur due to abnormal early development in pregnancy. Poorly controlled blood glucose levels can lead to underdeveloped lungs in the infant and respiratory issues. Hypoglycemia may occur after birth if the mother had high blood sugar near delivery, causing the baby to produce extra insulin. A hyperglycemic maternal environment may also increase the risk of future health issues like obesity, insulin resistance, type 2 diabetes, and metabolic syndrome in the newborn.

6.3.3. Diabetes Pregnancy Management

Pregnant women should have their blood glucose levels closely monitored. Due to strict blood sugar control and the additional glucose required for the developing fetus, less insulin treatment is needed during the first few weeks of pregnancy. In order to avoid hypoglycemia at this point, basal and bolus insulin may need to be decreased. To keep things under control, blood sugar should be tested frequently. The body produces more hormones as the fetus grows and the pregnancy progresses, potentially leading to insulin resistance and an increased need for insulin. Blood sugar levels must stay within normal limits during this period because the baby will need to produce more insulin to compensate for its mother's elevated blood sugar, which could result in fetal macrosomia. Insulin must be lowered once more during delivery, which is analogous to exercise, to prevent hyperglycemia. Insulin demand gradually returns to normal levels after the baby is delivered and in the days that follow because the placenta no longer produces the hormones that required more insulin.

Effective management of diabetes mellitus can be achieved through proper meal planning, incorporating more physical activity into your routine, and ensuring insulin treatment is administered correctly. For women with diabetes during pregnancy, here are some helpful tips for controlling the condition:

- Reduce the amount of sweets consumed, eat three small meals and one to three snacks each day, observe regular mealtimes, and consume a diet rich in fruits, vegetables, and whole grains that is balanced in fiber.
- Increased physical activity – walking, swimming/aquaerobics, etc.
- Keep an eye on your blood sugar levels; your doctor might advise checking your blood sugar more frequently than usual.
- After eating, blood sugar levels should be below 120 mg/dL (6.7 mmol/L), below 140 mg/dL (7.8 mmol/L) an hour later, and below 95 mg/dL (5.3 mmol/L) when you wake up.
- Maintain accurate records of your blood sugar readings and provide them to the medical team for review and treatment modification each time you check your blood sugar. A perinatal diabetes management team may recommend strategies to meet targets if blood sugar levels are higher than expected.
- To meet their blood sugar goals during

pregnancy, many women may require additional insulin. The unborn child is not harmed by insulin.

All type 1 diabetic women who are pregnant or intend to become pregnant are now advised to consider closed-loop insulin systems. This recommendation comes from the National Institute of Health and Care Excellence.

6.3.4. Breastfeeding

In general, even when a mother has diabetes mellitus, breastfeeding is beneficial for the child. In fact, breastfeeding may reduce the child's chance of acquiring type 2 diabetes mellitus in the future. Breastfeeding aids in the infant's maintenance of a healthy body weight as well. Nonetheless, it has been shown that the composition of breastmilk from mothers with diabetes differs from that of mothers without the disease, with higher levels of insulin and glucose and lower levels of polyunsaturated fatty acids. While there is evidence supporting the benefits of breastfeeding for children of diabetic mothers, consuming diabetic breast milk has also been dose-dependently associated with delayed language development.

Pregnant women with diabetes may occasionally be advised to express and freeze their colostrum in case their blood sugar levels are too low to support nursing the unborn child. Pregnant women with diabetes who express and store their breast milk before the baby is born are not shown to benefit from doing so.

6.3.5. Classification

In honor of Priscilla White, the White classification (White P. 1949) who initiated studies on the impact of diabetes kinds on perinatal results, is frequently utilized to evaluate the risk to both the mother and the fetus. It makes a distinction between diabetes that predated pregnancy (pregestational diabetes) and gestational diabetes (type A). These two groups are further separated based on the risks and management that go along with them.

There are 2 classes of gestational diabetes (diabetes which begins during pregnancy):

- Class A_1: gestational diabetes; diet controlled
- Class A_2: gestational diabetes; medication controlled

The second group of diabetes which existed before pregnancy can be split up into these classes:

- Class B: onset at age 20 or older or with a duration of less than 10 years
- Class C: onset at age 10–19 or duration of 10–19 years
- Class D: onset before age 10 or duration greater than 20 years
- Class E: overt diabetes mellitus with calcified pelvic vessels
- Class F: diabetic nephropathy
- Class R: proliferative retinopathy
- Class RF: retinopathy and nephropathy
- Class H: ischemic heart disease
- Class T: prior kidney transplant

The first three subtypes are associated with higher risks due to an early age of onset or a long-standing disease.

6.3.6. Prevention

While there are no guarantees when it comes to preventing gestational diabetes, it is best to establish as many healthy habits as possible before becoming pregnant. Making these healthy decisions may also lower your chance of developing type 2 diabetes later in life or of developing gestational diabetes again if you have already experienced it.

- **Eat Healthy Foods:** Select foods that are rich in fiber and low in fat and calories, with an emphasis on fruits, vegetables, and whole grains. Aim for diversity in your choices to reach your objectives while still enjoying delicious and nutritious meals. Pay attention to portion sizes.

- **Keep Active:** Being physically active both before and during pregnancy can help lower your risk of gestational diabetes. For most days of the week, try to get in 30 minutes of moderate exercise. Go for a daily brisk walk. Get on your bike. Do laps in the pool. Short bursts of activity add up, like when you park farther away from the store to run errands or take a quick stroll break.
- **Start Pregnancy at a Healthy Weight:** If you intend to become pregnant, shedding excess weight before becoming pregnant could lead to a healthier pregnancy. Concentrate on implementing long-term dietary adjustments that will support you during your pregnancy, like increasing your intake of fruits and vegetables.
- **Don't Gain More Weight Than Recommended:** It's normal and healthy for pregnant women to gain some weight. However, gaining too much weight too soon can make gestational diabetes more likely. Find out from your doctor how much weight gain is appropriate for you.

6.4. Tumors of the Uterus and Adnexa

One of the most typical pregnancy complications is adnexal masses. For the safety of both mothers and newborns, proper management of adnexal mass is crucial. The prevalence of adnexal masses has increased over time as a result of the widespread use of ultrasonography (US) technologies; these masses are typically diagnosed as coincidental findings during routine prenatal exams. Even though the majority of adnexal masses are benign or functional, ovarian cancer can complicate certain pregnancies. Pregnancy does not appear to have a detrimental effect on mother survival when compared to non-pregnant patients, despite a number of physiological changes, including hormonal and metabolic changes (de Haan, Verheecke, Van Calsteren, et al., 2018). However, because these patients belong to a subgroup with ambiguous symptoms that frequently overlap with pregnancy symptoms, early diagnosis—which is crucial for appropriate management—may prove challenging. Through US, the risk of malignancy from an adnexal mass is only partially predictable in women who are not pregnant. A number of ultrasonography characteristics may indicate whether an ovarian mass is benign or malignant, but histology confirmation is occasionally necessary. Furthermore, a portion of adnexal masses are still unintentionally found during cesarean sections. For ovarian masses larger than 6 cm in diameter, or when symptomatic and in the second trimester, surgical management has been advised in order to reduce the risk of miscarriage, torsion, rupture, and delayed diagnosis of malignancy. Furthermore, because of the possibility of miscarriage and congenital malformation, chemotherapy during pregnancy determines large interrogative.

6.4.1. Epidemiology

Although ovarian cancer during pregnancy is a rare occurrence, given the increasing frequency of delaying childbearing to a later reproductive age, its prevalence is expected to increase.

Adnexal masses, with an incidence of approximately 1–5.3%, are among the most frequent pregnancy complications. About 5% of adnexal masses during pregnancy are malignant; the majority are benign or functional. Globally, ovarian cancer continues to be the most lethal kind of gynecologic tumor. The average lifetime risk for ovarian cancer is 1 in 78 women, or 1.3%. The highest incidence of epithelial ovarian cancers (about 16.5 cases per 100,000 women) is found in white women. Women of reproductive age still receive ovarian cancer diagnoses, despite the fact that women over 60 account for a disproportionate number of these cases. Malignancy complicates about 1 in 1000 pregnancies, and the incidence of ovarian cancer is estimated to be 2.8–11 per 100,000 pregnancies. But the majority of ovarian masses discovered during pregnancy are benign or represent stage I illness. For instance, simple functional cysts and corpus luteum of pregnancy are highly prevalent during pregnancy, with an incidence ranging from 11 to 41%. They are primarily hormone-dependent and will usually go away on their own by 20 weeks. Mature cyst teratoma, along with serous and mucinous cystoadenomas and endometriomas, is the most common diagnosis among hystotypes that continue past the second half of pregnancy. The most frequent ovarian cancers during pregnancy are germ cell tumors, stromal tumors, and borderline tumors. Instead, 35% of all ovarian cancers discovered during pregnancy are epithelial cell cancers. Furthermore, compared to women who are not pregnant, borderline ovarian tumors (BOTs) exhibit more aggressive features during pregnancy.

6.4.2. Diagnosis

Imaging in pregnancy presents a challenge as clinicians must consider the well-being of both the mother and fetus. The three identities of the mother, fetus, and tumor all play a role in this complex interaction, with the mother's desire to continue the pregnancy being a key factor to consider. Currently, ultrasound (US) and magnetic resonance imaging (MRI) are the preferred imaging methods during pregnancy due to their lack of ionizing radiation. Ultrasound is commonly used for routine check-ups and initial abdominal evaluations as it is safe and cost-effective with no adverse effects on the mother or fetus. However, there are concerns about the use of Color Doppler in the first trimester due to potential theoretical risks for the embryo.

When an ovarian mass is detected during pregnancy, appropriate follow-up care should be provided. Any discoveries must be accurately measured, reported, and any suspicious features must be identified. Particularly during the first trimester, US is crucial in distinguishing between benign and malignant masses. Transabdominal (TA) and transvaginal (TV) examinations are important components of sonographic evaluation; however, transvaginal examination is the ideal method for studying the pelvis. TV US has advanced over the years in the investigation of the anatomy of the female pelvis because it enables imaging at a higher frequency, offering greater discriminating power and resolution. The uterus gradually obscures the pelvic organs and retroperitoneal space as a pregnancy progresses, decreasing the uterus's sensitivity in identifying malignancies and adnexal masses. Color Doppler can provide additional information and be used to evaluate vascular flow both inside and outside of the mass. Outside of pregnancy, simple descriptors or rules from the International Ovarian Tumor Analysis (IOTA) are frequently used to identify specific tumor features and predict malignancy. While their applicability in pregnancy has not been established, their guidelines can be used to raise doubts regarding a specific adnexal mass. Pregnancy can cause Doppler indices to fluctuate quickly, so this criterion needs to be used with caution. MRI is the second-line modality after US for the diagnosis and staging of gynecologic adnexal masses during pregnancy when a sonographic diagnosis is unsatisfactory. It provides better tissue contrast, bigger imaging fields of view, and no radiation; it is very accurate in characterizing adnexal lesions. Furthermore, according to the American College of Radiology, MRIs up to 3 T are safe and have no negative effects on the organogenesis or embryo. Computed tomography (CT) is typically avoided during pregnancy due to its radiation use. Its application is strictly restricted to circumstances in which US or MRI cannot provide the necessary information.

Written informed consent from the patient is required. Just like in the case of women who are not pregnant, tumor markers have a limited role. The most researched tumor marker, Ca125, is elevated in most cases of epithelial ovarian cancer but has limited use because it is also elevated in other benign conditions like endometriosis and fibroids. Moreover, Ca125's usefulness as a tumor marker in pregnant women is further limited because of its physiologically higher levels during the first trimester of pregnancy. In any case, Ca125 levels above normal could raise the suspicion of ovarian cancer in a suspect with an ovarian mass and serve as a baseline for further investigation. As the most prevalent ovarian tumor in women of reproductive age, germ cell tumors also occur during pregnancy. Alpha-fetoprotein (AFP), lactate dehydrogenase (LDH), and human chorionic gonadotropin (hCG) are molecules that are typically elevated during pregnancy, which renders their use even more meaningless as markers for germ cell tumors. Other molecules that are used as makers—like Ca 19-9, human epididymis protein 4 (HE4), anti-mullerian hormone (AMH), and inhibin B—are not anticipated to increase during pregnancy and may even be utilized in certain situations to support a diagnosis. Imaging is useful for determining whether or not there are peritoneal implants and metastases, as well as for evaluating the extent of disease prior to surgery. The possibility that adnexal masses could develop morphologic changes associated with pregnancy and mistakenly represent cancer is another issue brought up by pregnancy status.

6.4.3. Complications

These days, ovarian masses are more frequently discovered by accident during standard US scans. Nonetheless, a portion of adnexal masses continue to manifest as an acute incident due to rupture, torsion, or peritoneal hemorrhage. Adnexal mass complications during pregnancy are comparable to those experienced by non-pregnant individuals. Pregnancy has a number of implications when it comes to surgery, but in an emergency, surgery shouldn't be put off.

6.4.3.1. Adnexal Torsion

A rotation of the ovarian peduncle around its own axis is known as adnexal torsion (AT), an emergent condition that may cause ischemia and ultimately ovarian necrosis. Although the actual frequency of ovarian torsion is unknown, it appears to be higher during pregnancy, most likely as a result of the adnexa being displaced from the pelvis. Because of this, the first and early second trimesters, when the adnexa are displaced, appear to be the times when it occurs more frequently. The risk of AT may be higher in pregnancies conceived through assisted reproductive technologies, especially when there is ovarian hyperstimulation.

According to studies (Schmeler et al., 2005), the incidence of pregnant women with an adnexal mass is approximately 5%, and it is 20% more common for larger masses (> 6 cm). Koo et al., demonstrated in 2011 that surgery to prevent torsion is not warranted, even for masses larger than 6 cm, in the absence of symptoms and complications. Torsion symptoms can be hard to distinguish from common pregnancy-related symptoms because they are similar to those experienced by non-pregnant women and include pain, nausea, and vomiting.

Also, an objective exam frequently reveals no peritoneal symptoms.

6.4.3.2. Rupture

Although the risk of rupture is low, it is still a relatively common reason for surgery during pregnancy, occurring in less than 1% of cases.

6.4.3.3. Obstetric Outcome

Adnexal masses may be linked to a poor obstetric outcome due to a mechanical effect, depending on their size and location. Preterm delivery and an increased risk of miscarriage have been associated with them. Large adnexal masses may occasionally predispose a woman to labor dystocia, particularly if they are near the lower uterine segment. Furthermore, there may be a significant obstetric risk associated with prenatal surgical treatment of these lesions, whether it is done as part of a planned regimen or an emergency.

6.4.3.4. Malignancy

With an estimated incidence ranging from 0.02% to 1%, cancer during pregnancy is a rare occurrence. With an incidence of 1:12.500 to 1:25.000 pregnancies, ovarian cancer is the second most common gynecological cancer in pregnancy, despite being extremely rare. According to published series, the percentage of adnexal masses in pregnancy that correspond to malignant tumors ranges from 0% to 10% (Sayar, Lhomme, and Verschraegen, 2005). A growth rate greater than 0.35 cm/week (10 times greater risk of malignancy) and the size of the lesion (different cut-offs have been proposed) are also significant factors (Cavaco-Gomes, Moreira, Rocha, Mota, Paiva, and Costa, 2016). Germ cell tumors and epithelial tumors are the most common malignant ovarian tumors in younger age groups; during pregnancy, the latter may even be more common than the former (Fruscio, de Haan, Van Calsteren, Verheecke, and Amant, 2017). In contrast to women who are not pregnant, most ovarian tumors are detected in their early stages (80% in stage 1 of FIGO), with a significant percentage of tumors that are borderline. A multidisciplinary team of experts is needed to decide when to perform chemotherapy and staging surgery.

6.4.4. Management

While observation may promote tumor spread and result in unfavorable sequelae like rupture or torsion, surgical intervention carries risks for both the mother and her fetus. When the patient exhibits no symptoms and the ultrasonographic characteristics point to a benign etiology, observation makes sense. When there is a high suspicion of malignancy or when there is mass persistence, enlargement, rupture, torsion, bleeding, or other symptoms, surgical intervention (laparotomy or laparoscopy) is typically recommended. When masses present with acute symptoms, surgical management is the best course of action. Reduced hospital stay, opioid demand, postoperative pain, and uterine manipulation and irritation are the benefits of laparoscopy over laparotomy. Additionally, it permits postoperative ambulation sooner, which lowers the chance of thromboembolic episodes. The effects of pneumoperitoneum using CO_2 in causing fetal acidosis, however, are still debatable and need more research. Even with benign masses, cyst aspiration is not always therapeutic, so it should not be considered. Furthermore, there is a chance that cancer cells may leak or seed into the peritoneal cavity, changing the prognosis and stage. Aspiration is not advised in cytology due to its low sensitivity (25–82%) in identifying malignancies, making it an inadequate diagnostic modality.

Masses found in the first trimester of asymptomatic patients should be evaluated with ultrasound to check for signs of cancer. If cancer is suspected, surgery should be done in the second trimester to avoid the risk of miscarriage if done earlier or premature delivery if done later. If ultrasound does not show signs of cancer, the mass should be monitored and checked again during the fetal anatomy scan at 18–22 weeks. MRI may be used if ultrasound is not sufficient for evaluation. For masses found in the second trimester, a similar plan can be followed with a reevaluation at 32–36 weeks. Masses found in the third trimester without signs of cancer can be managed during cesarean section or 6 weeks after delivery.

On the other hand, adnexal mass management guidelines for women of reproductive age who are not pregnant are categorized based on the risks associated with US features. Surgery must be performed right away for high-risk masses with characteristics of malignancy or any adnexal mass accompanied by ascites and/or signs of metastatic disease suggestive of ovarian cancer. Rather than being surgically removed, intermediate- and low-risk masses are typically closely monitored.

During pregnancy, adnexal masses are frequently seen. Although there is always a chance of malignancy, they are usually benign or functional. The diagnosis is crucial to the management process. When US is inconclusive, MRI can be used safely to estimate the risk of malignancy. US is a very useful tool for this purpose. Surgery is required in the event of an acute event in any trimester; however, if possible, the procedure should be planned for the second trimester. Because laparoscopy has fewer complications and requires less recovery time than laparotomy, it is safer and advised. When applying it, one should exercise caution if there is a suspicion of cancer. It is imperative to perform appropriate staging whenever there is a suspect of clearly invasive ovarian cancer. Whether for benign or low-risk tumors, surgery that preserves fertility should be an option. Chemotherapy may be considered during the second and third trimesters if necessary. Furthermore, a multidisciplinary approach is necessary for the optimal management of adnexal masses during pregnancy, and patients must be sent to referral centers.

6.5. Surgical Emergencies During Pregnancy

Up to 2% of pregnancies are affected by the more than 8,000 urgent non-obstetrical surgical procedures that are carried out annually (Augustin and Majerovic, 2007). The risks and benefits of the diagnostic process and treatment for the pregnant patient must be considered, as well as the effects on the developing fetus. The typical physiological and anatomical changes that occur during pregnancy can make it challenging to interpret signs that are typically used in the early diagnosis of emergency conditions, which complicates care. The high rate of complications in this patient population is partly caused by the delay in diagnosis and treatment of surgical abdomen in pregnant patients due to fear of needless tests and procedures. Emergency surgical conditions can prevent needless complications for mothers and fetal loss by implementing measures such as increased suspicion, systematic evaluation, serial physical examination, clinical awareness, and attention to detail.

6.5.1. Normal Physiologic and Anatomic Changes in Pregnancy

Nearly all organ systems are impacted by the physiological alterations that occur during a mother's adaptation to pregnancy. The "physiologic anemia of pregnancy" is caused by a nearly 50% increase in plasma volume during pregnancy but only a 20% increase in red cell mass. A baseline hematocrit between 31 and 33% is not unusual. The pregnant patient can tolerate a substantial blood loss before experiencing overt signs of shock because of the increased plasma volume. Heart rate starts to rise in the second trimester. As the fetus develops, uterine blood flow also rises and by term, accounts for 20% of cardiac output. This system is very sensitive to external stimuli like maternal intravascular volume loss and catecholamines, and it is also highly regulated. Reduced uterine flow may serve as compensation for maternal hemorrhage. Fetal distress may indicate maternal hypovolemia prior to the manifestation of maternal tachycardia or hypotension.

During pregnancy, an increase in tidal volume brought on by rising progesterone levels causes an increase in oxygen consumption and resting ventilation. A respiratory alkalosis with a pCO_2 of about 30 mm Hg and a metabolic compensation with bicarbonate levels in the range of 19–20 mEq/L are the outcomes of this. Pregnant patients are more likely to experience gastroesophageal reflux and have an increased risk of aspiration with general anesthesia, as well as decreased gastrointestinal motility and a decrease in resting lower esophageal pressure. Hematologically, there is a relative leukocytosis in addition to the drop in hemoglobin levels brought on by the physiologic anemia. The white cell count typically ranges from 12,000/mm^3 to 15,000/mm^3 and can go as high as 25,000/mm^3, which frequently makes the infection diagnosis more difficult. Pregnant patients who exhibit relative hypercoagulability are known to have a higher risk of thromboembolic complications.

Anatomically, at about 12 weeks of gestation, the uterus transforms into an intra-abdominal organ. The uterus can be felt at the umbilicus at 20 weeks, and by 36 weeks, it has reached the costal margin. The uterus's growth can make invasive procedures more difficult, like laparoscopic surgery's port placement. Maternal organs are displaced upwards with uterine enlargement; in the latter stages of pregnancy, most of the gastrointestinal tract may be located above the inferior costal margins. Additionally, the diaphragm may be raised by up to 4 cm. Finally, as the pregnancy goes on, uterine compression of the vena cava reduces venous return, which causes the cardiac output to drop by 30%. The "supine hypotensive syndrome" can be lessened by placing pillows under the patient's right side to elevate it slightly or by placing the patient in the left lateral decubitus position, which displaces the uterus from the vena cava.

Pregnancy causes a decrease in ureteral tone and peristalsis, resulting in a dilated ureter and hydronephrosis. This is mainly because the growing uterus puts pressure on the ureters, particularly on the right side. These changes increase the risk of infection or kidney stones.

6.5.2. Radiological Issues in the Pregnant Patient

The impact of ionizing radiation on the developing fetus is the main worry when it comes to imaging during pregnancy. Radiation poses a risk for birth defects, mental retardation, microcephaly, growth retardation, and childhood cancers. Studies on animals and observations of radiation-exposed human populations, mainly from Hiroshima and Nagasaki, have provided information about the effects of radiation on fetal development (Delongchamp et al., 1997; Cullings et al., 2006). Although <5 rad exposure has not been linked to an increase in fetal abnormalities or pregnancy loss, according to the American College of Obstetricians and Gynecologists, the clinically significant fetal dose for teratogenesis is most likely between 10 and 20 rads. Always keep in mind the idea that a "pregnant patient should not be penalized for being pregnant" when choosing the right workup for any pregnant patient.

A standard "PanScan," which includes CT imaging of the head, neck, chest, abdomen, and pelvis, typically produces less than 5 rads. With just 0–3 rads, an abdominal CT scan can be done to assess abdominal pathology. Ultrasound is not known to be harmful to the developing fetus and is helpful in diagnosing cholecystitis, appendicitis, and free fluid following abdominal trauma. MRI is becoming a more helpful test for assessing pregnant patients' abdomens.

It is possible to considerably lower the radiation exposure during endoscopic retrograde cholangiopancreatography (ERCP) to less than 5 rads. Pregnant patients were exposed to radiation during ERCP in a number of series, ranging from 0 to 18 rads, without experiencing any short-term complications for the unborn child or the mother. A strong correlation has been observed between radiation exposure and the duration of fluoroscopy time. To reduce exposure, it is advised to take precautions like utilizing lead shielding (placed underneath the pregnant patient), increasing the patient's distance from the X-ray source, and shortening the fluoroscopy times. It has been described how pregnant patients can undergo radiation-free ERCP. After ERCP, non-invasive methods such as magnetic resonance cholangiopancreatography (MRCP), choledochoscopy, and endoscopic ultrasound have all been utilized to verify biliary system clearance.

6.5.3. Laparoscopy in Pregnancy

A new diagnostic and therapeutic tool in the treatment of pregnant patients experiencing abdominal pain is laparoscopy. In all trimesters, laparoscopy is well tolerated by the mother and the fetus with few side effects. While a 2012 meta-analysis comprising 11 studies discovered weak indications that a higher rate of fetal loss was linked to laparoscopic appendectomy as opposed to open appendectomy (Wilasrusmee et al., 2012), a more recent Nationwide Inpatient Sample study involving 20,000 patients discovered that open surgery was associated with a three times higher risk of an unfavorable obstetrical outcome (Sachs et al., 2017). As long as the laparoscopic technique seems safe for trochar insertion given the body habitus and stage of pregnancy, that is our preferred method. It is advised to insert the Veress needle into Palmer's point, an alternative site, or open trochar placement (Hasson technique) to prevent uterine injury during entry. In the left upper quadrant, 3 cm below the costal margin in the midclavicular line, is where Palmer's point is located. After the second trimester, laparoscopy becomes technically challenging, and an open incision can be made vertically or over the point of maximum tenderness. During the procedure, the surgeon should refrain from manipulating the uterus. For all viable pregnancies 24 weeks or older, immediate preoperative and postoperative fetal monitoring should be implemented.

6.5.4. Acute Abdomen in the Pregnant Patient

Non-obstetrical abdominal surgery is needed during pregnancy for about 1 in 635 women (Kort et al., 1993). The expanding uterus, which displaces other intra-abdominal organs and makes physical exams challenging, the high frequency of nausea, vomiting, and abdominal pain that are commonly experienced by normal obstetric patients, and the general reluctance to operate unnecessarily on a gravid patient are some of the factors that make making the diagnosis difficult. The most frequent non-obstetrical emergencies requiring surgery during pregnancy are acute appendicitis and cholecystitis.

6.5.4.1. Appendicitis

Around 70% of female cases of appendicitis occur in women under the age of 35; consequently, the peaks of appendicitis and childbearing occur at the same age. The incidence of appendicitis is one in 750–1500 deliveries; however, it does not appear to rise during pregnancy. Two thirds of gastrointestinal tract surgeries performed during pregnancy are due to appendicitis; the remaining 24% are related to trauma and biliary surgery. Unfortunately, pregnant patients have a more difficult time getting an appendicitis diagnosis than non-pregnant patients.

A number of factors make diagnosis challenging. The diagnosis of appendicitis can be complicated by potential obstetric complications, as well as by alterations in the anatomy and physiology of the mother. Patients experiencing ovarian accidents, septic abortions, spontaneous abortions, or ectopic pregnancies may exhibit symptoms and signs of appendicitis during the first trimester. Diagnosis confusion can occur in late pregnancy due to chorioamnionitis, abruptio placentae, or leiomyoma infarction. The shifting of the appendix's location is a second factor. The appendix is pushed posteriorly, laterally, and upwards as the uterus grows. 90% of appendices are at least two centimeters above the iliac crest and three centimeters lateral to McBurney's point by the eighth month. Even though the umbilicus is still the source of the initial visceral pain, the posterior displacement of the appendix in late pregnancy removes the possibility of the localized peritonitis that is typically seen% in patients who are not pregnant. Weingold recorded the variations in the physical characteristics associated with appendicitis and gestational age. In the first trimester, 100% of patients had rebound tenderness, compared to 43% in the third trimester. In the first trimester, rectal tenderness was detected in 67% of cases of appendicitis, while it was not detected in any third trimester cases. In first trimester appendicitis cases, the incidence of right lower quadrant tenderness was 100%, whereas in third trimester cases, it was 14%. In 60% of third trimester cases of appendicitis, but not in first trimester cases, there was tenderness in the right upper quadrant. The higher incidence of perforated appendices in late pregnancy—30% in the first trimester and 70% in the third—is most likely due to these changes.

Surgery shouldn't be put off once the diagnosis is suspected because the risk of perforation rises with time, rising from 20% during the first 24 hours of symptoms to 70% within 48. In cases where the diagnosis is uncertain, the surgeon ought to perform a midline incision to enhance visibility to the left adnexa. An essential procedure during the first trimester is diagnostic laparoscopy. A transverse incision, centered on the midclavicular line, is made 1 to 3 cm below the umbilicus when the diagnosis is evident in the first trimester. As the uterus grows later in pregnancy, the transverse incision is moved more cephalad and laterally because it is centered on the point of maximum tenderness. The incision's length is roughly equal to the surgeon's hand's width. The direction of the muscle fibers determines the incision or split of the aponeurosis and muscles. To facilitate better retraction, the anterior rectus sheath is sliced, but not the enclosed muscle. It is necessary to carefully avoid or ligate the inferior epigastric artery, which is located on the posterior rectus sheath. The appendix is usually visible at the site of incision in first-trimester women.

Anatomical landmarks that are useful are the ileocecal junction and anterior cecal taenia. Since there may be necrotic, friable tissue involved, extensive exploration should be avoided. A series of clamps, cuts, and ligations are performed on the mesoappendix using hemostats, Metzenbaum scissors, and 00 polyglycolic sutures. This step typically moves from a distance to a close proximity. This is not always the case with retrocecal appendices. After crushing and clamping the free appendix at its base and distally, a single 00 plain catgut ligature is inserted into the groove. If additional ligature is required for control, it is used. The knife and clamp are taken out of the field, and the appendix is removed in close proximity to the clamp. The results are most likely unaffected by the application of electrocautery or phenol and alcohol on the stump. However, phenol can scorch normal bowel upon contact if it is not neutralized with alcohol. Z-type sutures or 000 silk purse string are used to invert the stump. The reperitonealization (inversion) and security of the appendiceal artery's intramural branch (ligation) are the benefits of this technique.

Saline irrigation is used to the appendiceal bed, and purulent debris is cleared out. Antibiotics in the irrigant may help to stop the formation of an abscess. The customary method of closing the abdominal wall is used. When there is significant contamination, the skin is kept open to allow for a later closure. Prophylactic intravenous antibiotics are advised for pregnant patients, even though they are not always necessary for uncomplicated cases of appendicitis in non-pregnant patients. An acceptable option would be a gram-negative, anaerobic, second- or third-generation cephalosporin. The patient should receive antibiotics until their temperature drops to less than 37.4°C for a full 48 hours.

30–70% of cases of appendicitis complicating pregnancy result in a perforation. During pregnancy, different intraoperative management is required for perforations resulting in abscess formation. Expectant management with observation and intravenous antibiotics may be recommended for nonpregnant patients with a fixed periappendiceal mass. An appendectomy is carried out afterwards. But pregnant women are less able to control the infection, and endotoxins pose a serious risk to the developing fetus. Pregnancy always warrants surgical management.

To prevent additional contamination of the peritoneum, a retroperitoneal approach is taken when treating an abscess located near the tip of the appendix. An incision is made just beside the ilium crest, exposing the peritoneum and entering the abscess from the lateral and retroperitoneal sides. Cultures are taken and the abscess is carefully dissected, avoiding disruption of any adhesions that may be containing it. If accessible, an appendectomy is performed during the procedure. A closed-suction drainage is inserted through a separate incision, and the wound is irrigated with antibiotic solution. The fascia is closed with nylon sutures and the skin is left open for later closure. The drainage system is left in place for up to 48 hours before being removed gradually over a period of 2 to 4 days.

Pregnant women may occasionally exhibit diffuse peritoneal symptoms. Rapid surgical exploration is recommended when diffuse peritonitis and fever are present; the cause is frequently an appendix rupture. In order to provide more exposure for the diagnosis and treatment of intra-abdominal abscesses, a midline abdominal incision is made. An incision in the upper midline is necessary for exposure following 20 weeks of gestation. Most of the time, the appendix is examined and removed. Rubber drains with soft surfaces are used to empty specific pus accumulations. Prophylactic drains are not advised because their purpose is defeated by their quick walling off. An enormous volume of diluted antibiotic solution is used to irrigate the abdominal cavity. The Smead-Jones technique is used to apply permanent sutures to close the fascia. The skin and subcutaneous fat are packed with gauze that has been moistened with saline to prevent wound infection. Three or four days after surgery, if there is no infection, the skin is closed while the patient is under local anesthesia. The dressing is changed three to four times a day.

Intravenous systemic antibiotics should be administered for a minimum of five days. Once the patient has been afebrile for twenty-four hours, the antibiotic course can be ended. Throughout the first few days following surgery, the head of the bed should be raised by 15 to

30 degrees. While drainage toward the pelvis is encouraged, subphrenic abscess is not prevented by doing this. Relatively speaking, complications are 5–10% in cases of early, nonperforated appendicitis and 30%–50% in cases where a perforation has occurred. Although uncommon, maternal death rates range from 0.1 to 0.5%. The main side effects include peritonitis, abscesses, and wound infections. Fever that doesn't go down suggests more abscess formation. Rectal examinations can identify pelvic abscesses that are developing. Vaginal exams should only be performed in order to identify any potential obstetric complications (e.g., premature labor). Preterm delivery is always dangerous; it happens in 27% of cases with a perforation and 40.5% of cases without one.

6.4.5.2. Gallbladder Disease

The second most frequent non-obstetric surgical issue is biliary tract disease. Pregnant women are more likely to develop gallstones and biliary sludge due to weight gain and hormonal changes. During fasting and postprandially, the gallbladder's volume increases due to weaker contractions and decreased emptying. Biliary stasis plays a role in the sequestration of cholesterol crystals, which may result in the formation of sludge and stones. Progesterone hinders gallbladder emptying, while estrogen raises bile lithogenicity. The risk of sludge formation appears to be increased by increasing parity and lower gallbladder ejection fractions. Gallstone formation ranges from 3% to 12%, while biliary sludge formation has been reported to occur up to 31% of the time. In all, 1 in 1000 pregnancies will result in biliary colic symptoms. In the next two years, about one-third of biliary colic patients will not have any more bouts. Regretfully, recurrence of symptoms occurs in about 80% of pregnant women who present with symptoms, with 20–40% of cases occurring before delivery. Frequently, this recurrence is more serious than the original presentation. For acute cholecystitis, gallstone pancreatitis, and obstructive jaundice, surgery is recommended. Data now suggest that pregnant patients with symptomatic cholelithiasis should undergo cholecystectomy early due to the increase in the rate of recurrent hospitalizations, preterm deliveries, spontaneous abortions, and fetal morbidity associated with non-operative management, whereas previously the non-operative management with delayed cholecystectomy of symptomatic cholelithiasis was encouraged. Moreover, there is a 15% chance of gallstone pancreatitis when symptomatic cholelithiasis is managed non-operatively. A increasing amount of research indicates that laparoscopy can be carried out safely throughout all trimesters, contrary to the previous belief that the second trimester was the best time for cholecystectomy because it was associated with a lower risk of spontaneous abortions and preterm labor.

6.4.5.3. Cholangitis

Despite the rarity of choledocholithiasis in pregnancy—roughly 1 in 1200 births—therapeutic intervention is nearly always required. In both pregnant and non-pregnant patients with choledocholithiasis, the presence of fever, leukocytosis, stomach pain, hyperbilirubinemia, and elevated alkaline phosphatase, with or without shock, suggests the diagnosis of cholangitis. It has been shown that for cholangitis, Charcot's original triad is 95% specific but only 26% sensitive. Nowadays, endoscopic treatment is the preferred course of action for pregnant patients with choledocholithiasis, especially in cases where cholangitis is present. Baillie et al., published the first study on therapeutic ERCP during pregnancy in 1990. For ERCP, both general anesthesia and conscious sedation have been utilized with comparable safety. Under the obstetrician's supervision, maternal fetal monitoring should be used during the procedure. When ERCP is either not available or does not work, percutaneous transhepatic cholangiography with drainage can be performed.

6.4.5.4. Acute Pancreatitis

About 1 in 1,000–5,000 pregnancies are complicated by acute pancreatitis, which typically develops late in the third trimester or in the early postpartum phase. The most frequent cause, accounting for 67%–100% of cases, is cholelithiasis, which is followed by hyperlipidemia and ethanol consumption. The medical treatment for pancreatitis in non-pregnant women is the same and includes analgesics, bowel rest, and fluid and electrolyte resuscitation. An intensive care unit is the best place to manage these patients. As was previously mentioned for choledocholithiasis, if the determined etiology was biliary, a prompt cholecystectomy should be performed when the patient improves during the same hospitalization due to the high recurrence of gallstone-related symptoms.

6.4.5.5. Intestinal Obstruction

With an incidence of 1 in 1,500 pregnancies, acute intestinal obstruction ranks as the third most frequent non-obstetric abdominal emergency. In 60–70% of cases, adhesions are the cause. Appendicitis, volvulus, intussusception, hernia, and neoplasm are some additional causes. Notably, in up to 25% of cases of gestational obstruction, volvulus can be the cause of obstruction; in patients who are not pregnant, this percentage is only 5%. It is important to distinguish between gestational bowel obstruction and hyperemesis gravidarum, as the former may present with abdominal examination findings and cause a delay in diagnosis. The treatment of intestinal blockage in pregnancy is similar to that for the general public. Most patients will resolve with medical management that includes hydration, bowel rest, and nasogastric decompression. Both open and laparoscopic surgical techniques are appropriate. When gestational age increases, the mortality rate for patients with gestational intestinal obstruction rises relative to non-pregnant patients. It is best to refrain from manipulating the uterus excessively. In all cases that are still viable and older than 24 weeks, fetal monitoring should be used.

When a potential surgical diagnosis is made, clinical judgment is frequently overshadowed by pregnant patients' concerns about the potential harm to the fetus. In this population, limiting the amount of time spent exposed to radiation and avoiding needless surgery is crucial, but postponing diagnosis and treatment can also have negative effects on the mother and fetus. Because pregnancy causes normal physiologic and anatomic changes, getting the right diagnosis in a pregnant patient can be difficult. Depending on one's practice setting, availability and time constraints may make it difficult to use reduced radiation imaging techniques like MRIs or radiation-free ERCPs, which may limit the amount of radiation that the fetus is exposed to. Depending on the surgeon's comfort level with the length of the pregnancy, minimally invasive surgery may be done safely. Should a patient experience a general surgical emergency while pregnant, prompt diagnosis and treatment should be provided to avoid ever penalizing the patient for her pregnancy.

6.6. Liver Diseases in Pregnancy

Caring for liver disease in pregnant women is a complex task that requires a multidisciplinary approach. The hepatologist must be able to navigate the physiological and anatomical changes that occur during pregnancy, as well as the intricate relationship between the mother and the fetus. Additionally, the rarity of liver disease in pregnancy presents its own set of challenges. It is essential to carefully weigh the potential impacts on both the mother and the fetus when considering diagnostic and treatment options.

6.6.1. Function

6.6.1.1. The Liver During Normal Pregnancy

Pregnancy causes the liver, like other organs, to go through a number of physiological and anatomical changes. It can be easier to distinguish between pathological and physiological changes if one is aware of these changes. These modifications fall roughly into the following categories:

- **Physical Findings:** The liver appears largely unaltered on a gross examination during pregnancy, but skin conditions like palmer erythema and spider angiomata (vascular spiders) can be observed. In the later stages of pregnancy, these physical manifestations are particularly noticeable, particularly in women of Caucasian descent. It should be mentioned that the expanding uterus may make it difficult to understand these findings.
- **Laboratory Findings:** With a few notable exceptions, the majority of liver biochemical tests are within normal ranges during pregnancy. Because placental alkaline phosphate levels are higher in the third trimester, serum alkaline phosphate (ALP) rises noticeably—up to four times the normal level. Since serum gamma-glutamyl transpeptidase levels are normally slightly decreased during normal pregnancy, a conjugate increase in these levels along with serum alkaline phosphate usually indicates a pathological process. Serum levels of other liver biochemical tests, including total and free bilirubin, aspartate aminotransferase (AST), and alanine transferase (ALT), usually stay within normal ranges, and any elevated value should be investigated further. Moreover, a well-known pregnancy phenomenon called hemodilution causes a drop in serum albumin levels, which gets worse as the pregnancy goes on. Ceruloplasmin, fibrinogen, total cholesterol, and triglycerides are a few other laboratory results that are markedly elevated during pregnancy.
- **Radiographic Findings:** Pregnancy-related ultrasonography examinations typically show a normal biliary tree. The only noteworthy ultrasonographic results are the larger gallbladder volume during fasting and the residual volume following contraction.

6.6.2. Issues of Concern

6.6.2.1. Approach to Hepatobiliary Disease in Pregnancy

Treatment for liver diseases related to pregnancy requires a methodical approach, just like for other liver diseases. A thorough history, a clinical examination, and laboratory and radiographic testing are all part of a basic workup. The history should cover the duration of the pregnancy, intravenous drug use, transfusions, previous pregnancies and the liver problems they caused, as well as the use of oral contraceptives. Clinical findings such as nausea, vomiting, jaundice, generalized pruritus, polyuria, polydipsia in the absence of diabetes, and abdominal pain should be evaluated, even though they are not specific to pregnancy. In general, there are three types of liver diseases that can occur during pregnancy: those specific to the condition, those unrelated to the condition, and those that existed before the pregnancy.

6.6.2.2. Liver Disease Unique to Pregnancy

Multi-organ diseases like HELLP syndrome or liver-specific conditions like acute fatty liver of pregnancy are examples of liver diseases that are only observed during pregnancy. The most prevalent liver conditions that are specific to pregnancy are listed below:

6.6.2.2.1. Hyperemesis Gravidarum

A type of morning sickness known as hyperemesis gravidarum (HG) typically affects the first trimester and is characterized by extreme nausea and vomiting in the patient. Up to 10.5% of pregnant women may have it. While there isn't a consensus definition, the main indicators of HG are uncontrollably high levels of nausea and vomiting, weight loss (more than 5% of pre-pregnancy weight), and ketonuria. Although the precise etiology of Helicobacter pylori infection, age under 20, obesity, diabetes mellitus, nulliparity, hormonal changes during pregnancy, and abnormal gastrointestinal motility have all been linked to Helicobacter HG. HG is diagnosed clinically, and hospitalization is frequently necessary. Elevation of ALT and AST is the main liver manifestation. In the case of ALT, the levels typically range from less than 250 international units/L to as high as 1,000 international units/L. Because human chorionic gonadotropin stimulates the thyroid, up to 60% of patients may experience transient hyperthyroidism. Bowel rest, antiemetics, intravenous fluids, and, if necessary, correcting electrolyte imbalances are the standard treatment protocols. If vomiting has lasted for an extended amount of time, it may be necessary to administer thiamine. Although they are uncommon, complications can include central pontine myelinolysis, spontaneous pneumomediastinum, retinal hemorrhage, esophageal rupture, and Wernicke encephalopathy. Future pregnancies usually do not experience a recurrence of this condition.

6.6.2.2.2. Intrahepatic Cholestasis of Pregnancy

A cholestatic illness of the second or third trimester that is reversible is called intrahepatic cholestasis of pregnancy (ICP). It can begin as early as the second or third month of pregnancy, even though it usually shows symptoms in the third trimester. The disease is present in up to 1.5% of pregnancies in the United States, though its prevalence varies geographically. Although the pathogenesis of ICP is unclear, it is most likely complex. Changes in hormone levels, the use of oral contraceptives at high doses (high estrogen causes cholestasis), regional variations, and genetic predisposition are all possible causes of changes in the way sex steroids are transported across the hepatic and canalicular membranes as well as intracranial pressure. ICP has been linked to at least ten distinct MDR3 mutations, with the ABCB4 variant being linked to a severe form of the disease. In Asian or Black women, ICP is uncommon.

The presence of pruritus and abnormal LFTs characterize ICP, which is an exclusion diagnosis. The primary symptom of ICP is pruritus; jaundice is uncommon but usually appears two weeks after the onset of pruritus. Usually more prevalent on the palms and soles, pruritus is worse at night. Abdominal pain and encephalopathy are not common in patients with ICP, and if they are, they should prompt additional testing to rule out other liver disease causes. The concentration of total and fasting serum bile acid has increased in ICP, which is one of the main laboratory findings. This might be the only laboratory abnormality in certain circumstances. Additional abnormalities in the laboratory include elevated serum concentrations of direct and total bilirubin, ALP, and ALT (which rarely exceed 250 International Units/L; however, viral hepatitis must be ruled out). The ratio of cholic acid to chenodeoxycholic acid is usually greater than 42%, which is indicative of

ICP, even though it is not routinely performed. This is because both chenodeoxycholic acid and cholic acid are elevated. Steatorrhea is common, and vitamin K malabsorption—which can be made worse by cholestyramine therapy—may result in a prolonged prothrombin time. In every suspected case of ICP, ultrasonography should be performed to rule out biliary obstruction. Although a liver biopsy is not usually required, focal and irregular cholestasis is a characteristic.

ICP usually goes away 4–6 weeks after delivery and is safe for the mother; however, it can return in subsequent pregnancies. On the other hand, adverse fetal outcomes have been linked to preterm, respiratory distress syndrome, and intrauterine death. 38 weeks is the recommended delivery age, or 36 weeks if the cholestasis is severe. In order to reduce the risk of post-partum hemorrhage, vitamin K should be administered at least six hours before delivery. Ursodeoxycholic acid (10–20 mg/kg/day) is one of the treatment options; it alters the bile acid pool, reduces pruritus, and enhances both the fetal outcome and liver biochemical tests. If the first course of treatment is unsuccessful, other options like hydroxyzine and cholestyramine can be tried, but they are less successful than ursodeoxycholic acid. Ursodiol improves the fetal outcome. Alternative conditions like primary biliary cholangitis and familial cholestatic disorder (MDR3 mutations are also present in progressive familial intrahepatic cholestasis) should be considered if pruritus and alkaline phosphatase elevation do not go away after pregnancy. If present, a cholestatic reaction to a postpartum trial of low doses of estrogen therapy is predictive of poor tolerance to oral contraceptives.

6.6.2.2.3. HELLP Syndrome

HELLP syndrome is a rare and severe form of preeclampsia, characterized by high blood pressure after 20 weeks of pregnancy along with proteinuria or organ dysfunction. The cause of HELLP is not fully understood, but is believed to involve abnormal placental blood vessel development and damage to maternal vascular endothelial cells, leading to poor blood flow to organs. Preeclampsia causes widespread blood vessel constriction, resulting in increased vascular resistance and reactions to vasoconstrictors. Damage to blood vessel lining leads to blood clotting in the liver, causing liver cell death and bleeding in zone 1. Zone 3 liver damage and bleeding, seen in severe preeclampsia, is due to shock. Mild preeclampsia may show slight increases in liver enzyme levels and signs of blood clotting issues, with low platelet count. Jaundice is rare in preeclampsia, but if present, is typically due to terminal hemolytic causes with total bilirubin levels generally staying below 6 mg/dL.

HELLP syndrome can present in a wide range of clinical ways. The patient may show up with no symptoms at all or with symptoms like nausea, vomiting, jaundice, abdominal pain in the right upper quadrant, or confusion. Significant laboratory results include intravascular hemolysis, schistocytes on peripheral smear, low platelet count, and elevated LFTs (typically ALT). Serum aminotransferases are over ten times higher than normal, and hemolysis may be the cause of unconjugated hyperbilirubinemia. Since HELLP syndrome has a prognostic value, diagnostic criteria such as Tennessee or Mississippi classifications should be used for diagnosis and grading. The maternal mortality rate from HELLP is as low as 5%, while the fetus death rate can reach up to 30%. Prematurity continues to be the most frequent risk linked to fetal outcomes, similar to ICP. The gestation age affects how HELLP is treated. The foundation still lies in the early delivery of the fetus, but supportive management with anti-hypertensive medications and magnesium sulfate administration should be taken into consideration with regard to the mother. Before attempting to deliver the fetus, treatment with steroids for 24 to 48 hours should be considered if the gestation age is less than 34 weeks.

6.6.2.2.4. Acute Fatty Liver of Pregnancy

Pregnancy-related acute fatty liver disease (AFLP) is an uncommon but dangerous liver condition. The hepatocytes' microvascular fatty infiltration is the cause. Long-chain 3-hydroxy acyl-CoA dehydrogenase (LCHAD) in the fetus in the context of the mother having heterozygosity for LCHAD has been linked to the pathophysiology of AFLP. This causes the fatty acid in the fetal mitochondria to be improperly beta-oxidized. It is still unknown, though, how AFLP in a heterozygous mother results from LCHAD in the fetus. Liver biopsy is not frequently performed, and the diagnosis of AFLP is made clinically.

Common clinical signs of liver disease include abdominal pain, jaundice, nausea, and vomiting. Possible diagnoses to consider are viral hepatitis, drug-induced liver injury, HELLP syndrome, hemolytic uremic syndrome, and thrombotic thrombocytopenic purpura. AFLP and HELLP syndrome share similarities in symptoms, but AFLP is characterized by symptoms like encephalopathy, hyperammonemia, coagulopathy, hypoglycemia, hypoalbuminemia, and renal insufficiency that are not typically seen in HELLP syndrome. Hyperbilirubinemia in AFLP is mostly conjugated, while in HELLP syndrome it is unconjugated due to hemolysis. Other symptoms like vomiting, weakness, lactic acidosis, hypoglycemia, and metabolic acidosis are attributed to defective energy supply in mitochondrial cytopathy. Elevated serum uric acid levels are a result of tissue destruction and lactic acidosis. Laboratory findings may include normal GGT levels, but elevated levels can indicate viral hepatitis. Increased white cell count, platelet count, PT, and PTT, as well as low fibrinogen levels, may also be present. Severe bleeding is common, but DIC is only present in a small percentage of cases. Radiological imaging may show signs of fatty liver, but a lack of fatty liver does not rule out the diagnosis. Liver biopsy, typically performed transjugularly, may reveal microvesicular and macrovesicular steatosis, ballooned hepatocytes with dense central nuclei, cholestasis, and signs of inflammation and necrosis in liver cells.

Acute fatty liver of pregnancy (AFLP) is a serious obstetric emergency that requires immediate delivery of the fetus regardless of gestational age. The method of delivery – cesarean or vaginal – will depend on the condition of both the fetus and the mother. It is important to address any hypoglycemia or coagulopathy present before delivery. Children born to mothers with AFLP may be at risk for various health complications, including hypoglycemia, dilated cardiomyopathy, progressive neuromyopathy, and sudden infant death syndrome. AFLP can have a high mortality rate for both the fetus and the mother if not identified and addressed promptly. It is important for the mother to be aware of the slightly increased risk of AFLP recurrence in future pregnancies.

6.6.2.3. Liver Disease Unrelated to Pregnancy

Pregnant women, like anyone else, can develop liver diseases that are common in the general population. However, some liver diseases during pregnancy have more severe outcomes compared to the general population, with a higher risk of mortality and morbidity. This is especially evident in conditions like hepatitis E.

6.6.2.3.1. Viral Hepatitis

Pregnant individuals share the same levels of Hepatitis A, B, and C prevalence, incidence, and outcomes as the general population. If there is a risk of perinatal transmission, the newborn should receive immunoprophylaxis at the time of delivery, particularly if there is an acute hepatitis B infection. Immunoglobulin and immunization should be given to pregnant women who have been in close contact with people who have the hepatitis A or B virus as soon as possible. Hepatitis B treatment guidelines during pregnancy are the same as those outside of pregnancy. If the HBV viral load is more than 200,000 International Units/mL, mothers who are not already receiving treatment may be offered antiviral therapy with tenofovir disoproxil fumarate at 28 to 30 weeks of gestation in order to lower the risk of hepatitis B infection transmission to the unborn child. There is very little chance of hepatitis C being passed from mother to child. Any of these situations should not be treated with a routine C-section. Usually a self-limiting infection, hepatitis E can have negative effects during pregnancy. Hepatitis E has a 30% maternal death rate and a 50% fetal death rate if it develops during the third trimester. It is also linked to fulminant liver failure. Hepatitis E can be transmitted from mother to fetus and may be the cause of acute hepatitis in a newborn. Hepatitis E infection is most frequently found in endemic regions, such as northern Africa and sub-continental nations; however, zoonotic transmission and increased travel to endemic areas have been linked to a recent increase in the non-endemic region. Women who are expecting in the third trimester should be advised about the risks involved in visiting endemic areas. Hepatitis E is typically treated with supportive care. Pregnant women have been reported to have Herpes simplex virus (HSV) type II, most likely as a result of the compromised cell-mediated immunity that is common during pregnancy. Serum aminotransferases (anicteric hepatitis) can have marked elevations that resemble AFLP but do not cause jaundice. There could be herpes lesions on the cervix or vulva. Imaging studies may reveal several low-density necrosis areas. A liver biopsy reveals extensive hepatocellular necrosis along with intranuclear Cowdry A inclusions. The preferred treatment is acyclovir, and the death rate is significant.

6.6.2.3.2. Vascular Liver Disease

The elevated serum estradiol level during pregnancy causes the procoagulant factors to rise and the anticoagulant factors to fall. Moreover, pregnancy has been linked to a drop in aPTT, PT, and thrombin time. Pregnancy-related changes raise the risk of thrombosis, which may result in conditions like Budd-Chiari syndrome (BCS) or portal vein thrombosis. While pregnancy is a risk factor, other thrombotic risk factors, such as factor V Leiden mutation and protein S deficiency, are more frequently associated with BCS. A pregnant patient with BCS should have a thorough workup to rule out other thrombotic conditions. Low molecular weight heparin is typically used as treatment because oral anticoagulants should not be used due to their teratogenicity. In the case of severe BCS, other invasive treatments like TIPS, thrombolysis, or percutaneous transluminal angioplasty may be explored.

6.6.2.3.3. Biliary Tract Disease

Gallstones are more common during pregnancy because, during a typical pregnancy, the gallbladder's motility slows down and its volume increases. While biliary sludge and gallstones are typically resolved postpartum in asymptomatic pregnant women, 0.8% of them may experience acute cholecystitis within a year after giving birth. Pregnancy can also cause acute cholecystitis. Intravenous fluids and antibiotics are part of the initial management. Cholecystectomy is typically done postpartum. However, patients who do not respond to conservative treatment should have a laparoscopic cholecystectomy as soon as possible. Other conditions like gallstone pancreatitis and choledocholithiasis/cholangitis should be treated as usual. Beginning in the second trimester, sphincterotomy and ERCP procedures are possible.

6.6.2.4. Preexisting Liver Disease During Pregnancy

Since most patients with chronic liver disease are either past childbearing age or in a pathological anovulatory state, it is rare to see pregnant patients in a clinical setting. Nonetheless, the following circumstances come up regularly:

6.6.2.4.1. Cirrhosis

There have been reports of cirrhotic patients becoming pregnant without any negative effects on their liver; however, it is common to see cirrhosis complications in pregnant cirrhotic patients, including ascites, hepatic encephalopathy/coma, and declining liver function, including worsening jaundice. Because pregnancy increases the effective circulatory volume, a pregnant woman's preexisting portal hypertension remains highly susceptible to worsening. Upper endoscopy should be performed either before or during the second trimester of pregnancy in a cirrhotic pregnant woman in order to assess and potentially treat varices. Although reports of variceal bleeding during pregnancy have been made, it is still unknown whether or not pregnant patients are more likely to experience this condition than non-pregnant patients. Preventive measures for managing portal hypertension in a cirrhotic pregnant woman include nonselective beta-blockers, which are safe to use throughout pregnancy, or banding varices before or during pregnancy. The newborn should be monitored for side effects from the beta-blocker administration, such as bradycardia and low blood sugar. Poor fetal outcomes are typically linked to the presence of ascites in pregnant women. Unless otherwise noted, vaginal delivery is the usual method of delivery for a pregnant woman with cirrhosis. Every expectant mother who has chronic liver disease ought to be treated in a high-risk pregnancy unit, ideally near a liver transplant center, with advice from a hepatologist and an obstetrician.

6.6.2.4.2. Autoimmune Hepatitis

Since younger women are more likely to suffer from autoimmune hepatitis, it is important to understand how to manage pregnancy in someone with autoimmune hepatitis. Elevated levels of ALT and serum gamma globulin concentration are indicative of autoimmune hepatitis. It is linked to infertility (anovulation) and can manifest as either acute or chronic liver failure, or as asymptomatic liver failure; however, after autoimmune hepatitis is successfully treated, most women regain their fertility. Azathioprine and prednisone are the typical treatments. Since the activity of autoimmune hepatitis typically decreases during pregnancy, a successful prenatal treatment of autoimmune hepatitis usually results in a smooth pregnancy. During pregnancy, autoimmune hepatitis can be treated with prednisone alone. Even though azathioprine is classified as a category D medication, it is still safe to use at a reduced dosage while pregnant. A relative barrier to azathioprine and its metabolites is the placenta. Breastfeeding is permitted despite the use of azathioprine or corticosteroids by mothers. Autoimmune hepatitis remains linked to an increased risk of preterm birth, maternal death, and fetal loss even with appropriate treatment.

6.6.2.4.3. Wilson Disease

Similar to the majority of liver diseases, Wilson's disease is linked to infertility, which usually goes away with treatment. A chelating medication, such as zinc, trientine, or D-penicillamine, is typically used to treat Wilson's disease. The importance of continuing treatment for Wilson disease patients during pregnancy cannot be overstated, as untreated Wilson disease is linked to poor outcomes for both the mother and the fetus, including preterm birth, stillbirth, and miscarriages. Zinc is the least dangerous chelating agent to use while pregnant, with varying degrees of teratogenicity. In order to reduce the teratogenic risk, chelating agent doses are typically decreased in the first and third trimesters. Trientine or D-penicillamine can still be used, but at a higher dose and with a higher risk of teratogenic effects. This is especially true for D-penicillamine, as there is a chance of transient goiter hypothyroidism in the fetus. It is not advisable for mothers taking D-penicillamine to breastfeed.

6.6.3. Clinical Significance

Because managing liver disease during pregnancy can be extremely complex, a multispecialist approach is necessary. Finding the underlying cause is crucial because it will determine the best course of action. Because many liver diseases that are specific to pregnancy overlap, a thorough understanding and a wide differential diagnosis are necessary for timely and appropriate management.

6.6.4. Other Issues

6.6.4.1. Liver Transplantation and Consultation with a Hepatologist

Although safe pregnancies have been reported in women who have had liver transplants, waiting a year or more is advised before trying to conceive. This is done to give immunosuppressive medications enough time to stabilize their profiles after a liver transplant. Patients who experience renal dysfunction while undergoing liver transplantation are linked to unfavorable outcomes for the mother and fetus. It is recommended that pregnant women in this population undergo heightened surveillance for both opportunistic and general infections. It is best to refrain from breastfeeding when using immunosuppressive drugs. While reports of liver transplants during pregnancy (in conditions like HELLP or AFLP) exist, these procedures are extremely risky and typically involve pregnancy termination as the mother's survival and support come first.

It is advised to see a hepatologist as soon as possible to manage liver disease during pregnancy. Women with liver disease who are expecting should be informed about the risks and potential complications of pregnancy. The patient should also receive thorough counseling regarding the method of delivery and potential risks of pregnancy in the future.

6.6.5. Enhancing Healthcare Team Outcomes

A multispecialty approach involving gastrointestinal nurses with specialized training and other specially trained providers is necessary to manage liver disease in pregnancy. Since there are many reasons why liver dysfunction can occur during pregnancy, it's critical to consult a gastroenterologist and internist as soon as possible. There are two lives at risk, so the patient needs to be closely watched. Using an interprofessional approach will yield optimal results (Phipps et al., 2016).

6.7. Diseases of the Urinary System

Pregnancy causes major changes to the anatomy of the urinary tract. Renal calyces dilation, ureteral dilatation, and urinary stasis are all caused by hormonal and mechanical factors, and these changes increase the risk of urinary tract infections (UTIs) in expectant mothers. Smooth muscle is relaxed by progesterone, and the gravid uterus compresses the bladder, reducing its volume. Urinary stasis, increased residual urine in the bladder, and vesicoureteral reflux could be observed. A pregnancy-related UTI is more likely as a result of any of these changes.

Pregnancy-related UTIs usually have a predictable natural history, beginning with asymptomatic bacteriuria (ASB), which can develop into symptomatic infections like cystitis or pyelonephritis if treatment is not received. Reduced urethral tone and altered bladder dynamics from pregnancy-related changes facilitate the ascending infection from the lower urinary tract that is a common pattern of UTI spread during pregnancy. In order to effectively identify, diagnose, and treat UTIs during pregnancy, healthcare providers must have a thorough understanding of these factors. This will help to avoid complications and ensure the best possible outcomes for both the mother and the fetus.

6.7.1. Etiology

Pregnancy-related UTIs can result from a number of factors, but they are mostly related to the physiological and anatomical changes that take place during the gestational period. One important contributing factor is the shift in hormones, specifically the rise in progesterone levels, which causes the smooth muscle tissue in the urinary tract, including the bladder and ureters, to relax. Bacteria can more easily move from the urethra to the bladder and possibly the kidneys as a result of this relaxation, which also changes bladder dynamics and lowers ureteral tone.

Furthermore, the growing uterus can mechanically obstruct the ureters and urinary flow, increasing the risk of UTIs in expectant mothers. Hormonal fluctuations may also have an impact on the vaginal flora, which could lead to an increase in uropathogenic colonization. Furthermore, physiological immune system alterations during pregnancy, such as a reduction in cell-mediated immunity, may make it more difficult for the body to successfully fight bacterial infections. These elements work together to foster an environment that is favorable to the development of UTIs during pregnancy, underscoring the significance of taking preventative and therapeutic action to protect the health of both the mother and the fetus.

6.7.2. Pathophysiology

The same uropathogens that frequently cause UTI in patients who are not pregnant also cause UTI in pregnant women. Escherichia coli is the most frequently isolated organism. An analysis conducted 18 years later discovered *E. coli* is thought to be the cause of pyelonephritis in between 60 and 82.5% of pregnant patients. Additional bacteria that could be observed are Streptococcus, Enterococcus species, Proteus (5%), Klebsiella pneumonia (11%), and Staphylococcus.

Although they are uncommon pathogens, *Gardnerella vaginalis* and Ureaplasma can still cause isolation, particularly in women who have underlying renal disease. In the third trimester of pregnancy, Group B Streptococcus (GBS) is frequently isolated from urine cultures and may even be more prevalent than *E. coli*.

6.7.3. History and Physical

Because ASB patients do not exhibit symptoms, it is critical to screen for the condition as early in pregnancy as possible. These patients might have a history of recurrent urinary tract infections or may have had ASB during a previous pregnancy. Although there is no set recommendation for how frequently pregnant patients with sickle cell trait should be screened for UTIs, it makes sense to screen them more frequently during pregnancy. It can be harmful to screen patients with diabetes or spinal cord injuries more frequently.

The symptoms of cystitis are the same as those that non-pregnant people experience. Urinary frequency (82%), burning or pain during urination (dysuria in 55% of cases), and urgency are possible symptoms. There may be tenderness and suprapubic pain (73%). Only 26% of women with symptoms have a positive urine culture result, meaning that there is a high rate of false positives for these symptoms alone.

Patients with pyelonephritis also display symptoms similar to those of the illness in non-pregnant individuals. Colitis, chills, and a fever of 38.0°C or higher are possible symptoms. When nonspecific symptoms like nausea, vomiting, anorexia, and malaise are reported, the differential diagnosis is frequently wide at first. Acute intraabdominal conditions like pancreatitis, cholecystitis, and appendicitis, as well as pregnancy-related issues like placental abruption and preterm labor, are included in the differential diagnosis.

With uterine monitoring, patients can either report or show contractions. This uterine activity is frequently brought on by an infection-induced irritability of the smooth muscle. Cervical dilation should be evaluated in patients if contractions are detected or felt. Patients should be closely watched because they may go into preterm labor. There could be sepsis signs and symptoms, such as tachycardia and hypotension. Patients like these need to be evaluated and treated right away. A thorough physical examination is necessary, with special attention to vital signs and evaluation of the heart and lungs. Tenderness may also be found on an abdominal examination, and pyelonephritis frequently manifests as costovertebral tenderness. It is crucial to perform a genitourinary examination at the time of admission in order to determine cervical dilation and screen for cervical infection. It is advisable to keep an eye out for contractions or any other abnormalities during the hospital stay, even if there are no immediate concerns about pregnancy complications.

6.7.4. Evaluation

A clean catch urinalysis and urine culture are part of the evaluation process for a pregnant patient who is suspected of having a UTI. There are a few important things to keep in mind when collecting urine samples while pregnant. Patients who are well hydrated may excrete diluted urine, which would reduce the accuracy of some assessed parameters. Contamination can lead to hematuria, especially when samples are taken from patients who are in labor or have recently given birth. Small amounts of protein may typically be eliminated due to decreased protein reabsorption. Proteinaceous material in pregnant women's urine may also be a result of contamination, as can happen with mucous vaginal discharge.

Generally not helpful, urine dipstick screening during pregnancy yields a high false positive result for infection. Nitrites were found in symptomatic patients with a specificity of 98.6%, a negative predictive value of 81.9%, and a positive predictive value of 86.6%, indicating their significant presence. Furthermore, some historical symptoms, such as hematuria (specificity of 93%) and dysuria (specificity of 88%), were less reliable in ruling out UTIs but proved to be effective in predicting UTIs confirmed by culture. Contagious urine cultures are also very common during pregnancy. A higher chance of urine culture contamination is linked to a higher BMI. Pregnant women's urine cultures frequently show the growth of skin flora, and repeating the culture is useless. It's interesting to note that obtaining a midstream urine specimen without perineal cleaning reduces contamination more than having the patient perform perineal cleaning, also referred to as a clean catch. The risk of developing pyelonephritis is minimal following a negative screening urine culture.

Laboratory testing should include a complete blood count (CBC), electrolytes, and serum creatinine when pyelonephritis is suspected in pregnancy. If pancreatitis is thought to be the cause of the patient's symptoms, then tailored studies, such as those involving lipase and amylase, should be included as appropriate. Blood cultures and lactic acid should be obtained if sepsis is suspected. It is best to obtain all cultures as soon as possible and prior to beginning antibiotic treatment. Fetal heart rate and contraction monitoring ought to take place once the fetus is viable. In the unlikely event that complications related to pregnancy arise, consideration should be given to obtaining GBS and cervical cultures at admission. Renal ultrasonography is occasionally necessary to check for potential renal abscesses.

6.7.5. Management

Antibiotics are the treatment of choice for urinary tract infections. Practitioners frequently prescribe trimethoprim/sulfamethoxazole, nitrofurantoin, or cephalexin. When no other options are available, trimethoprim/sulfamethoxazole and nitrofurantoin are only used during the first trimester. Antibiotics must be taken during pregnancy by women who have experienced multiple bladder infections or kidney infections in order to prevent further urinary tract infections.

6.7.6. Differential Diagnosis

The differential diagnosis of UTIs during pregnancy includes a number of conditions that can exhibit similar symptoms, so a thorough assessment is necessary to guarantee a precise diagnosis and suitable treatment. Pregnancy-related physiological changes, such as increased frequency of urination due to pressure on the bladder from the growing uterus, may also be responsible for symptoms such as suprapubic pain, urgency, and dysuria in pregnant women. Furthermore, symptoms of UTIs during pregnancy can be mimicked by illnesses like pelvic inflammatory disease, vaginal infections, and sexually transmitted infections. More precisely, pregnancy-related problems like preterm labor, chorioamnionitis, or placental abruption are included in the differential diagnosis of pyelonephritis, along with acute intraabdominal illnesses like appendicitis, pancreatitis, cholecystitis, and kidney stones.

6.7.7. Prognosis

The timely and efficient diagnosis and treatment of pregnant patients with UTIs determines their prognosis. The health of the mother and fetus may be severely impacted by major complications like pyelonephritis, preterm birth, low birth weight, and maternal sepsis that can result from untreated or insufficiently treated UTIs during pregnancy. However, most pregnant patients with UTIs have a good prognosis with proper management, which includes prompt antibiotic administration and careful observation.

When asymptomatic bacteria (ASB) started to be routinely tested for in the 1960s and 1970s, the incidence of pyelonephritis in pregnancy dropped from 20% to 35% to 1% to 4%. However, since many of these studies were conducted more than 30 years ago, it is unclear if ASB treatment reduced the rates of low birth weight and preterm birth. As a result, new research has called into question the necessity of screening for and treating ASB during pregnancy, concluding that doing so may not reduce the risk of preterm birth and low birth weight babies. The overuse of antibiotics by pregnant women is another significant issue to be aware of. Compared to other continents, Europe and Asia have been found to have higher rates of this. The frequent use of antibiotics to treat ASB during pregnancy may lead to a rise in *E. coli* and other extended-spectrum beta-lactamase-producing (ESBL) bacteria. *Klebsiella pneumonia* and *E. coli*.

6.7.8. Complications

Acute respiratory distress syndrome (ARDS), anemia, disseminated intravascular coagulopathy, preterm labor and contractions, and renal abscess are among the complications that can arise from UTIs during pregnancy. Admission to the intensive care unit (ICU) might be necessary. Research shows that blood bacteria are present in 7.5% of pyelonephritis patients, sepsis is present in 13.3%, and septic shock is present in 1.9% of cases. Preterm premature rupture of membranes (PPROM) is a common complication of UTI in pregnancy, accounting for 6.3% of cases. Other complications include preterm delivery (11%) and birth weights <2800 g (8.2%). 7% of patients have reported delivery within 72 hours.

As many as 10% of pregnant patients receiving treatment for pyelonephritis experience pulmonary complications. This can appear as ARDS or pulmonary edema and is caused by endotoxin-mediated alveolar damage. Monitoring urine output and oxygen status is important, and patients may need to be admitted to the intensive care unit (ICU) for respiratory support. Anemia caused by endotoxin release usually goes away on its own after treatment. With up to 25% of patients experiencing this complication, it is the most frequent side effect of pyelonephritis. Uterine contractions may also result from endotoxin release, and patients should be closely watched for PPROM, preterm labor, and preterm delivery.

6.7.9. Deterrence and Patient Education

To protect the developing fetus's health as well as the mother's, it is imperative to prevent and deter urinary tract infections during pregnancy. Promoting good hygiene habits, such as regular hand washing and taking care of the perineum, can help reduce the risk of bacterial colonization and ascending infection. Urinary stasis can be avoided and the risk of UTIs reduced by encouraging pregnant women to drink enough water and go to the bathroom on a regular basis. During prenatal visits, screening for asymptomatic bacteriuria is another preventive measure. Positive cases should be treated right away to stop the infection from progressing to symptoms. Pregnant people who are able to identify UTI symptoms and seek prompt medical attention and treatment are greatly enhanced by education. Pregnancy-related UTI incidence can be further decreased by putting evidence-based recommendations for antibiotic prophylaxis into practice in high-risk populations. Healthcare providers can lessen the incidence of UTIs during pregnancy and support the best possible outcomes for both the mother and the fetus by emphasizing preventive measures and patient education.

6.7.10. Enhancing Healthcare Team Outcomes

Pregnant patients with UTIs require comprehensive care from a variety of health professionals, including physicians, nurses, pharmacists, and advanced care practitioners. This entails providing a prompt and precise diagnosis, initiating treatment appropriately, educating patients, keeping an eye out for complications, and making follow-up care easier. Nurses monitor and educate patients, pharmacists make sure medications are used safely, and doctors and advanced practitioners oversee diagnosis and treatment. The prevention, diagnosis, and treatment of UTIs in pregnancy should be handled by the interprofessional healthcare team using evidence-based practices. This entails putting screening procedures in place for asymptomatic bacteriuria, prescribing antibiotics in accordance with the principles of antimicrobial stewardship, and encouraging patient education regarding hygiene and preventive care. Creating uniform procedures and guidelines for the treatment of urinary tract infections can guarantee uniformity and enhance results.

For patient-centered care and outcomes related to UTIs in pregnancy to be optimized, effective interprofessional communication is essential. To make sure that pertinent information is shared, treatment plans are coordinated, and patient preferences are taken into consideration, clinicians should communicate in an open, courteous, and clear manner. Collaborating seamlessly is made possible by electronic communication platforms, case conferences, and interdisciplinary team meetings. Care coordination is the methodical arrangement and integration of medical services to address the unique requirements of pregnant patients suffering from urinary tract infections. In order to guarantee continuity of care and enable seamless transitions between care settings, the interprofessional team needs to collaborate. This entails scheduling consultations, lab work, referrals, and appointments in addition to offering thorough assistance all the way through the care continuum. Patient-centered care can be prioritized to improve team performance, safety, and outcomes, which will ultimately improve the overall quality of care for pregnant patients with UTIs (Phipps et al., 2016).

A Closer Look

High Blood Pressure and Pregnancy

Pregnancy-related high blood pressure can cause fetal growth retardation and placental problems. Severe hypertension can result in deadly seizures, strokes, and even death in the mother and fetus if treatment is not received. In order to keep an eye on your health and the development of your fetus, your doctor may do more frequent testing, including kidney function tests, growth ultrasounds, and pregnancy tests, if you have high blood pressure.

- **Chronic Hypertension:** It is likely that you will need to continue taking your antihypertensive medication if you had high blood pressure before becoming pregnant. In order to help you manage your pregnancy-related hypertension, your doctor might prescribe a safer antihypertensive medication.
- **Gestational Hyperte**nsion: Pregnancy in young women is the most common cause of gestational hypertension. If you had blood pressure issues during a previous pregnancy or if you are carrying twins, you are more likely to develop gestational hypertension. Pregnancy-induced elevated blood pressure is a characteristic of pre-eclampsia (formerly known as toxemia). Urine containing protein is typically present with this condition, which can also result in swelling from fluid retention. You might require bed rest if you have pre-eclampsia. When you experience a seizure brought on by pre-eclampsia, you are diagnosed with eclampsia, the most severe form of this illness. Your physician may prescribe medication, hospitalization, and frequently even delivery to treat eclampsia or pre-eclampsia.

Summary

- Cardiac disease of pregnancy encompasses a broad arena of pathologies. Some of these diseases may be exacerbations of pre-existing conditions that the pregnant woman may already have, or they may develop a new disease process that presents because of the complex hormonal changes and physiology of pregnancy. Pre-existing conditions that can predispose pregnant women to cardiovascular disease include hypertension, diabetes mellitus, and congenital heart disease.
- Evaluation of cardiac disease in pregnant females will often require advanced workup. Initial basic workup with labs such as CBC, CMP, and urinalysis can give necessary clues to underlying processes that may be occurring.
- Pregnancy is a normal and healthy state that many women aspire to at some point in their lives. However, pregnancy can make women more susceptible to certain infections. Pregnancy may also make these infections more severe. Even mild infections can lead to serious illness in pregnant women.
- Pregnancy affects every system in your body. Changes in hormone levels and immune system function can make you more vulnerable to infections and serious complications. Labor and delivery are especially susceptible times for both you and your baby.
- For pregnant women with diabetes, some particular challenges exist for both mother and fetus. If the pregnant woman has diabetes as a pre-existing disorder, it can cause early labor, birth defects, and larger than average infants.
- Adnexal masses are one of the most common complications during pregnancy. Correct management of adnexal mass is of paramount importance both for maternal and neonatal safety.
- Pregnancy is associated with reduced ureteral tone and peristalsis, which can lead to a dilated ureter and hydronephrosis. This is due in part to mechanical compression on the ureters as the uterus enlarges, with the rate of right-sided hydronephrosis significantly higher than the left side. These changes can lead to infection or urolithiasis.
- The key concern regarding imaging during pregnancy is the effect of ionizing radiation on the growing fetus. The risks of radiation include fetal death, growth retardation, microcephaly, malformations, mental retardation and childhood cancers.
- Managing liver disease during pregnancy is quite challenging and requires a multispecialty approach. Physiological and anatomical changes during pregnancy, the complex interaction between the mother and the fetus, and the rarity of liver disease in pregnancy itself are some of the many challenges that a hepatologist faces while managing liver disease during pregnancy.
- The anatomy of the urinary tract undergoes significant changes during pregnancy, with hormonal and mechanical factors contributing to ureteral dilation of the renal calyces, and urinary stasis, all of which predispose pregnant patients to urinary tract infections (UTIs).

References

1. Ashrafi, R., & Curtis, S. L. (2017). Heart disease and pregnancy. *Cardiology Therapy, 6*(2), 157–173. https://doi.org/10.1007/s40119-017-0082-4.
2. Augustin, G., & Majerovic, M. (2007). Non-obstetrical acute abdomen during pregnancy. *European Journal of Obstetrics & Gynecology and Reproductive Biology, 131*, 4–12. https://doi.org/10.1016/j.ejogrb.2006.07.052.
3. Baillie, J., Cairns, S. R., Putman, W. S., & Cotton, P. B. (1990). Endoscopic management of choledocholithiasis during pregnancy. *Surgical Gynecology & Obstetrics, 171*, 1–4.
4. Cavaco-Gomes, J., Moreira, C. J., Rocha, A., Mota, R., Paiva, V., & Costa, A. (2016). Investigation and management of adnexal masses in pregnancy. *Scientifica (Cairo)*, 3012802. https://doi.org/10.1155/2016/3012802.
5. de Haan, J., Verheecke, M., Van Calsteren, K., et al. (2018). Oncological management and obstetric and neonatal outcomes for women diagnosed with cancer during pregnancy: A 20-year international cohort study of 1170 patients. *Lancet Oncology, 19*, 337–346. https://doi.org/10.1016/S1470-2045(17)30707-4.
6. Fruscio, R., de Haan, J., Van Calsteren, K., Verheecke, M. M., & Amant, F. (2017). Ovarian cancer in pregnancy. *Best Practice & Research Clinical Obstetrics & Gynaecology, 41*, 108–117. https://doi.org/10.1016/j.bpobgyn.2016.09.008.
7. Hancock, H. (1848). Disease of the appendix caeci cured by operation. *The Lancet, 2*, 381.
8. Koo, Y. J., Kim, T. J., Lee, J. E., et al. (2011). Risk of torsion and malignancy by adnexal mass size in pregnant women. *Acta Obstetricia et Gynecologica Scandinavica, 90*, 358–361. https://doi.org/10.1111/j.1600-0412.2011.01014.x.
9. Kort, B., Katz, V. L., & Watson, W. J. (1993). The effect of nonobstetric operation during pregnancy. *Surgical Gynecology & Obstetrics, 177*, 371–376.
10. Lynch, M. M., Amoozegar, J. B., McClure, E. M., Squiers, L. B., Broussard, C. S., Lind, J. N., Polen, K. N., Frey, M. T., Gilboa, S. M., & Biermann, J. (2017). Improving safe use of medications during pregnancy: The roles of patients, physicians, and pharmacists. *Qualitative Health Research, 27*(13), 2071–2080. https://doi.org/10.1177/1049732317705371.
11. Phipps, E., Prasanna, H. R., Brima, W., & Jim, B. (2016). Preeclampsia: Updates in pathogenesis, definitions, and guidelines. *Clinical Journal of the American Society of Nephrology, 11*(6), 1102–1113. https://doi.org/10.2215/CJN.09040915.
12. Regitz-Zagrosek, V., Blomstrom Lundqvist, C., Borghi, C., Cifkova, R., Ferreira, R., Foidart, J. M., Gibbs, J. S., Gohlke-Baerwolf, C., Gorenek, B., Iung, B., Kirby, M., Maas, A. H., Morais, J., Nihoyannopoulos, P., Pieper, P. G., Presbitero, P., Roos-Hesselink, J. W., Schaufelberger, M., Seeland, U., & Torracca, L. (2011). ESC guidelines on the management of cardiovascular diseases during pregnancy: The Task Force on the Management of Cardiovascular Diseases during Pregnancy of the European Society of Cardiology (ESC). *European Heart Journal, 32*(24), 3147–3197. https://doi.org/10.1093/eurheartj/ehr218.
13. Roth, A., & Elkayam, U. (2008). Acute myocardial infarction associated with pregnancy. *Journal of the American College of Cardiology, 52*(3), 171–180. https://doi.org/10.1016/j.jacc.2008.04.021.

14. Sachs, A., Guglielminotti, J., Miller, R., Landau, R., Smiley, R., & Li, G. (2017). Risk factors and risk stratification for adverse obstetrical outcomes after appendectomy or cholecystectomy during pregnancy. *JAMA Surgery*, E1–E6. https://doi.org/10.1001/jamasurg.2017.1426.

15. Sayar, H., Lhomme, C., & Verschraegen, C. F. (2005). Malignant adnexal masses in pregnancy. *Obstetrics & Gynecology Clinics of North America, 32*, 569–593. https://doi.org/10.1016/j.ogc.2005.06.005.

16. Schmeler, K. M., Mayo-Smith, W. W., Peipert, J. F., et al. (2005). Adnexal masses in pregnancy: Surgery compared with observation. *Obstetrics & Gynecology, 105*(5), 1098–1103. https://doi.org/10.1097/01.AOG.0000154060.62927.7d.

17. Silversides, C. K., Colman, J. M., Sermer, M., & Siu, S. C. (2003). Cardiac risk in pregnant women with rheumatic mitral stenosis. *American Journal of Cardiology, 91*(11), 1382–1385. https://doi.org/10.1016/S0002-9149(03)00352-4.

18. Thorne, S., MacGregor, A., & Nelson-Piercy, C. (2006). Risks of contraception and pregnancy in heart disease. *Heart, 92*(10), 1520–1525. https://doi.org/10.1136/hrt.2006.095240.

19. Weingold, A. B. (1983). Appendicitis in pregnancy. *Clinical Obstetrics and Gynecology, 21*, 801.

20. White, P. (1949). Pregnancy complicating diabetes. *American Journal of Medicine, 7*(5), 609–616. https://doi.org/10.1016/0002-9343(49)90382-4.

21. Wilasrusmee, C., Sukrat, B., McEvoy, M., Attia, J., & Thakkinstian, A. (2012). Systematic review and meta-analysis of safety of laparoscopic versus open appendicectomy for suspected appendicitis in pregnancy. *British Journal of Surgery, 99*, 1470–1478. https://doi.org/10.1002/bjs.8889.

Chapter 7

THE NEWBORN INFANT

Contents

Introduction

A newborn infant, also known as a neonate, is a child that is within the first 28 days of life, which is a crucial time marked by quick physiological changes and developmental leaps. Breathing, circulation, and temperature regulation all require major adjustments as the newborn leaves the reliant intrauterine environment and enters the outside world. As the infant draws its first breaths, its respiratory system must start working on its own, and in order to reroute blood flow, the circulatory system must close the ductus arteriosus and foramen ovale. Newborns usually weigh between 2.5 and 4 kg and have a length of approximately 50 cm, although these measurements can vary greatly. Newborns' limited vision allows them to see objects up to 8 to 12 inches away, and they are especially drawn to faces and patterns with high contrast. Their sense of hearing is complete, so they can identify their mother's voice, which comforts them and strengthens their relationship. A variety of reflexes, including the grasp, rooting, and Moro reflexes, are also displayed by newborns. These reflexes are essential for their survival and show a healthy nervous system.

Another crucial component of newborn care is feeding. Because breast milk provides antibodies that help protect against infections and is tailored to the infant's needs, breastfeeding is highly recommended for its nutritional and immunological benefits. Due to their small stomach capacity and quick digestion, newborns require frequent feedings. Newborns have irregular sleep patterns, sleeping 16 to 18 hours a day in between wakeful intervals for interaction and feeding. A newborn's skin is sensitive and can develop conditions like jaundice, which is caused by high bilirubin levels and manifests as a yellowish tint on the skin. The majority of cases are benign and go away on their own. Newborns also need close observation of their surroundings and physical state because they are vulnerable to hypothermia and dehydration. During this time, routine pediatric examinations are crucial for tracking growth and developmental milestones as well as for administering vaccinations that offer protection against a range of illnesses. During the neonatal stage, attachment and bonding are essential for the development of the mind and emotions. Establishing a secure attachment between an infant and caregivers is crucial for their future social and emotional well-being. This can be achieved through skin-to-skin contact, responsive caregiving, and consistent affection.

Orientation and Directional Terms

Term	Definition	Illustration
Neonate	Neonates are obligate nose breathers and have narrow nasal passages, which account for a baseline airway resistance they must overcome.	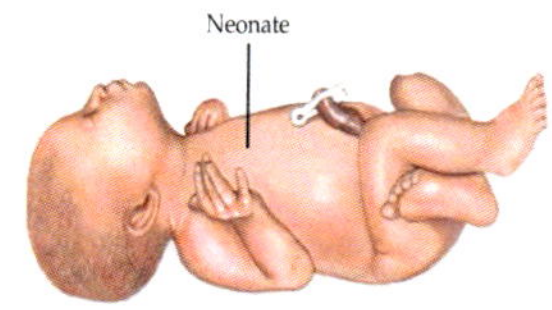
Fontanelles	Fontanelles allow for stretching and deformation of the neurocranium both during birth and later as the brain expands faster than the surrounding bone can grow.	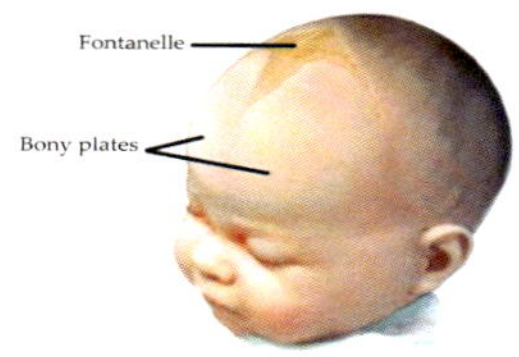
Respiratory distress syndrome	Occurs in babies born early (premature) whose lungs are not fully developed. The earlier the infant is born, the more likely it is for them to have RDS and need extra oxygen and help breathing.	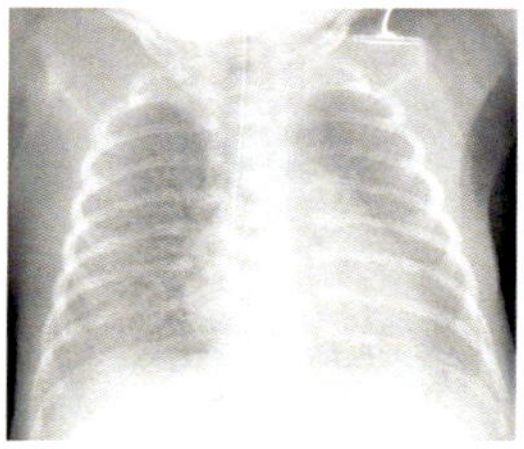
Polycythemia	A laboratory finding in which the hematocrit and/or hemoglobin concentration are increased in the blood.	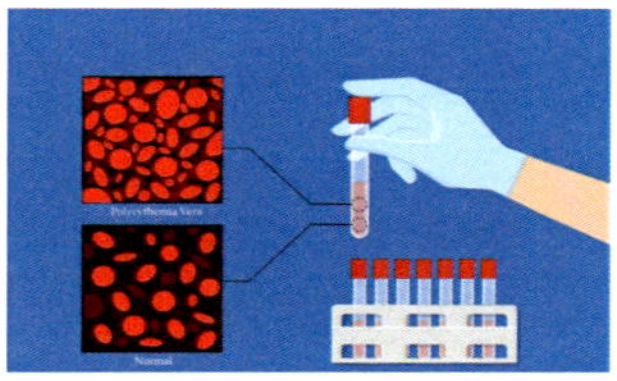
Phenylketonuria	Phenylketonuria is an inherited disorder that increases the levels of a substance called phenylalanine in the blood.	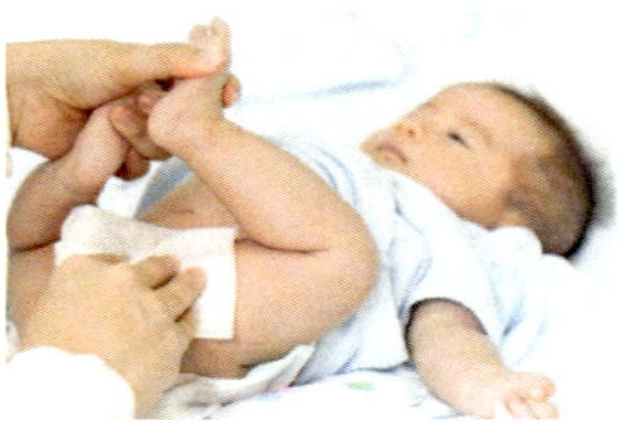

7.1. Examination of the Newborn

A baby or infant is a human being's very young offspring. Other organisms' juveniles can also be referred to by these terms. In common parlance, an infant as young as a few hours, days, or even a month is referred to as a newborn. Within the medical domain, an infant within the first 28 days of life is referred to as a newborn or neonate (derived from the Latin neonatus, newborn); this classification encompasses premature, full-term, and postmature infants. Premature babies are those born before 37 weeks of pregnancy, full term babies are those born between 39 and 40 weeks, late term babies are those born through 41 weeks, and post term babies are those born after 42 weeks. The offspring is referred to as a fetus prior to birth. Although definitions can differ and include children as young as two years old, the term "infant" is commonly used to refer to very young children under the age of one. A human child is referred to as a toddler when they learn to walk.

7.1.1. Physical Characteristics

A newborn's shoulders and hips are wide, the abdomen protrudes slightly, and the arms and legs are relatively long with respect to the rest of their body.

7.1.1.1. Head

A newborn's cranium is enormous in relation to their face, and their head is very large in relation to their body. A newborn's skull makes up around 1/4 of the entire body length, whereas an adult human skull makes up around 1/7. A full-term infant's normal head circumference at birth is 33–36 cm. Fontanels are soft patches on a newborn's skull that remain after many areas have not yet hardened into bone. The two biggest are the smaller, triangular-shaped posterior fontanel, which is situated at the back of the head, and the larger, diamond-shaped anterior fontanel, which is situated at the top front portion of the head. These bones will naturally fuse together later in the child's life. A protein known as noggin is the cause of an infant's delayed fusion of the skull. The baby's skull reshapes during labor and delivery in order to fit through the birth canal, which can result in an abnormally large or malformed head when the child is born. It usually takes a few days or weeks for it to naturally return to normal. Certain exercises that doctors occasionally recommend could help with the process.

7.1.1.2. Hair

A fine, downy body hair known as lanugo is present on certain newborns. Premature babies' backs, shoulders, foreheads, ears, and faces may be especially noticeable. In a few weeks, Lanugo vanishes. Some newborns, especially those who are Caucasian, may have very fine hair or may even be bald. Other babies may have full heads of hair when they are born. Even though the parents don't have fair skin, the fine hair may be blonde. The color and texture of an infant's hair can change; thick, dark hair may reappear much sparser and lighter, curly hair may become straight, and red hair may turn blond. Additionally, the area around the eyes may be puffy, and the scalp may experience temporary swelling or bruises, particularly in newborns without hair.

7.1.1.3. Length

A newborn's total body length in developed nations ranges from 35 to 50.6 cm (14 to 20.0 in), though premature babies may be significantly smaller. A baby's length can be determined by laying them down and measuring the distance between the top of their head and the bottom of their heel with a measuring tape.

7.1.1.4. Weight

A full-term newborn's average birth weight in developed nations is roughly 3.4 kg (7+1/2 lb), and it usually falls between 2.7 and 4.6 kg (6.0–10.1 lb). A term neonate's body weight drops by 3–7% during the first 5–7 days after birth. This is mostly due to the fluid that first fills the lungs being reabsorbed and urined, as well as the fact that breastfeeding frequently takes a few days to start working. Healthy term neonates should gain 10–20 grams/kg/day after the first week.

7.1.1.5. Skin

Newborns typically have grayish to dusky blue skin right after birth. The skin tone of the newborn returns to normal as soon as they start breathing, which usually happens in a minute or two. A white substance called vernix caseosa, which is thought to function as an antibacterial barrier, covers newborns and leaves them wet with blood streaks. Along with these birthmarks, the newborn may also have peeling skin, especially on the hands, feet, ankles, and wrists, or Mongolian spots.

7.1.1.6. Umbilical Cord

A newborn's umbilical cord has a bluish-white hue. The umbilical cord is often severed 1–2 inches after delivery. In roughly three weeks, the umbilical stub will dry out, shrivel, turn dark, and fall off on its own. When it heals, this will eventually turn into a belly button. There are three vessels in the umbilical cord: two arteries and one vein. One vein returns blood to the baby while the other two arteries transport blood from the baby to the placenta.

7.1.1.7. Genitals

A newborn's genitalia are reddened and enlarged, and the scrotum of male infants is disproportionately large. Even in male infants, the breasts may enlarge. This is a transient condition brought on by maternal hormones that occur naturally. It is possible for both males and females to secrete a milky or bloody substance from the vagina, as well as milk (also known as witch's milk) from the nipples. Either way, this is regarded as typical and will go away in due course.

7.1.2. Care and Feeding

Babies use their cries as a basic, instinctual means of communication. A crying baby could be attempting to communicate a number of emotions, such as loneliness, overstimulation, hunger, discomfort, or want. Because they are altricial, infants must rely entirely on their mothers or other adult caregivers for a considerable amount of time. All of the major infant health organizations advise breastfeeding as the preferred method of childrearing. Bottle feeding is done with expressed breast milk or baby formula if breastfeeding is not possible or desired. Babies are born with two natural behaviors: they root, or find their way to the nipple, and they suck, which enables them to take milk from the nipples of the breasts or the baby bottle. Although it is uncommon—especially in developed nations—hiring a wet nurse to nurse the baby is sometimes possible.

Consuming enough food from an early age is essential to a baby's development. The first 1,000 days of life lay the groundwork for lifetime neurodevelopment, growth, and optimal health. Infants should only be fed breast milk or an unadulterated milk substitute from birth to six months of age. As an infant's diet develops, finger foods, along with small amounts of fruit, vegetables, and meat, may be introduced. Food supplements can be added to infants as they grow. Many parents decide to supplement their child's breast milk or formula with commercially prepared baby foods, while others modify their regular meals to meet their child's nutritional needs. While lower-fat milk should wait until the child is two to three years old, whole cow's milk can be used as early as one year. The process of weaning involves substituting solid foods for breast milk and removing breast milk from the infant's diet. Diapers are worn by infants in developed nations until they are potty trained. An important developmental stage in an infant or baby's transition from diapers to training pants is the switch from diapers to pants. Compared to adults, children require more sleep—up to 18 hours for newborns, though this amount decreases with age. Babies are carried in the arms, held in slings or baby carriers, or moved in strollers or baby carriages until they can walk. The majority of developed nations have laws mandating child safety seats for infants riding in cars.

7.1.2.1. Benefits of Touch

Negative touch (poking, pinching, or tickling)

as well as positive touch (stroking or cuddling) have both been used in experiments with infants as young as four months old. Compared to the infants who were touched negatively, the ones who experienced positive touch cried less, spoke more, and smiled more. Negative touch on infants has also been associated with emotional and behavioral issues in later life. It has been found that cultures with higher levels of positive physical touching have lower rates of adult physical violence.

7.1.2.2. Language Development

It is recommended that caregivers observe their infant's facial expressions and mimic them. Infants can feel effective and recognize their own actions more readily when they can mimic and empathize with their facial expressions (see mirror neurons). Since they are more readable forms of expression, exaggeratedly replicated gestures and facial expressions are advised. You should also pick up on and repeat the baby's babble. The earliest basic conversations are started by mimicking each other's sounds. Words in a sentence are easier to identify when spoken with emphasis and in a melodic tone. On the other hand, using simplified baby talk (e.g., Did you injure yourself? should read, "Did you ouch?" Parents who respond promptly to their infants' babble—even if they are still unable to understand them—help their child acquire language more quickly. This was verified by researchers who observed how mothers behaved with their 8-month-old babies before testing the infants' vocabulary at 15 months of age. The realization that they can influence their parents by babbling is one of an infant's first significant developmental milestones (development of intentional communication). Parents who engage in babbling with their infants can help to foster this. As a result, babies turn to their parents more frequently, which further encourages language development.

According to earlier research, parents who, for instance, smile at their child or touch them whenever the child looks at them and babbles, are encouraging their speech. Additionally, it is beneficial if parents react to what they believe their infant is saying (by offering a ball or making a comment when the infant stares at the ball and babbles, for instance). Thus, a baby can learn the name of an object by responding to sounds made when it looks at it (object-directed vocalizations). Babies pick up on the idea that sounds and objects are related in this way. But language development only occurs when parents respond favorably (e.g., grinning) in reaction to the baby's babbling. In the absence of any correlation with the infant's utterances, a high response rate does not result in language promotion. Instead, trying to distract an infant's attention with something else is bad for language development.

7.1.2.3. Nutritional Needs of a Newborn

It is widely acknowledged that the best nutrition for newborns and infants comes from human breast milk. In addition to its nutritional advantages, breastfeeding promotes the baby's overall health and development. For sick or premature babies, breast milk serves as medicine. Every drop counts when it comes to your baby's health! The World Health Organization states that breastfeeding exclusively for the first six months of a baby's life is the best method of feeding them. After that, babies should continue to be breastfed for at least two years and be given complementary foods. Numerous studies have demonstrated the advantages of giving human milk to newborns and early infants, including increased intelligence, decreased gastrointestinal disorders, and better feeding tolerance. Additionally, there are significant health advantages for the mother. The uterus contracts back to its original size more quickly when breastfeeding is started as soon as possible after delivery. Additionally, breastfeeding lowers the risk of ovarian and breast cancers.

7.1.2.4. Sleep

After analyzing 146 studies on infant sleep behavior, a 2018 review identified a number of factors that are related to both the length of sleep and the frequency of night awakenings. On the other hand, studies have shown that frequent awakenings prevent SIDS. Baby sleep is not linear; it varies according to age and developmental milestones. The National Sleep Foundation recommends a general number of hours of sleep, which typically decreases as one gets older.

7.1.2.5. Maternal Sensitivity

In the relationship with the baby and for the child's healthy emotional development, maternal sensitivity is especially important. This entails paying close attention to the ways the infant expresses themselves behaviorally, interpreting their actions appropriately and not based on one's own emotions, responding to the situation right away, and determining the best course of action based on the needs that have been expressed and the context. Responding in a timely, appropriate, and sympathetic manner fosters a secure attachment. Infants exhibit an innate behavior of seeking proximity to their mother or another primary caregiver in order to fulfill their basic needs, which subsequently cultivates an attachment. Babies cry and move their bodies in protest when they are taken away from their mothers.

7.1.2.6. Other

Babies find wearing to be soothing. According to a 2013 study, babies who were carried by their mothers while they were out and about considerably calmed down, whereas babies who were placed in cradles cried and kicked more frequently and had an elevated heart rate (indicating stress). Being held still in the arm had an effect that was halfway between being carried around and being put down. The fact that carrying (e. g., in a baby sling) has previously been demonstrated in a randomized study to increase infant contentment and decrease crying. All of the major infant health organizations advise breastfeeding as a method of infant feeding. For domestic flights, many airlines won't allow boarding for any baby younger than seven days, and for international flights, older than fourteen days. Infants can travel internationally on Asiana Airlines as early as seven days of age. Babies younger than 14 days old are not permitted to board any flights operated by Garuda Indonesia. Infants who are younger than seven days old can travel on Delta Air Lines provided they have a letter of medical clearance from their doctor. An infant under the age of eight days is not permitted to travel on SkyWest.

7.1.3. Behavior

A newborn baby's behavior is the result of an intricate and fascinating interaction between reflexes, sensory perception, and early developmental processes. Caregivers can better meet the needs of the infant and encourage healthy development by being aware of these behaviors.

7.1.3.1. Reflexive Behaviors

Newborns exhibit a range of innate reflexes that are essential for survival and neurological assessment. Some of the most prominent reflexes include:

1. **Moro Reflex**: It happens when a baby is startled by a loud sound or sudden movement and is also referred to as the startle reflex. In response, the baby flings out their arms, arches their back, and then brings them back together.
2. **Rooting Reflex**: When a newborn

needs to start feeding, this reflex helps it locate the breast or bottle. A baby will turn their head toward contact and open their mouth when their cheek is stroked. Sucking Reflex: This reflex, which is activated when the baby's roof of the mouth is touched, allows the baby to suckle and is essential for feeding.

3. **Sucking Reflex**: Triggered when the roof of the baby's mouth is touched, this reflex enables the infant to suck and is crucial for feeding.
4. **Grasp Reflex**: A newborn will grasp anything firmly when it is placed in their palm. When the sole of the foot is touched, the toes curl as a result of this reflex.

7.1.3.2. Sensory Responses

Newborns have limited but rapidly developing sensory capabilities:

1. **Vision**: A newborn's vision is quite blurry, but they can see objects and faces 8 to 12 inches away. They are particularly attracted to high-contrast patterns and human faces.
2. **Hearing**: Hearing is well developed at birth. Newborns can recognize and are calmed by familiar sounds, such as their mother's voice.
3. **Smell and Taste**: These senses are also well-developed. Newborns can recognize their mother's scent and show a preference for sweet tastes, such as breast milk.
4. **Touch**: The sense of touch is highly developed, and newborns respond positively to gentle stroking and cuddling. This sense is crucial for bonding and comfort.

7.1.3.3. Crying and Sleeping Patterns

A newborn's main way of communicating is through crying. It may signal a number of needs, including the need for a diaper change, hunger, discomfort, or fatigue. Caretakers eventually pick up on the differences between various cries and know how to react. Newborns sleep a lot—usually 16 to 18 hours every day—but not all at once. They sleep in shorter stretches of time and wake up frequently to eat and socialize. Both physical and mental development depend on this pattern.

7.1.3.4. Feeding Behavior

As a result of their small stomach capacity and the quick digestion of formula or breast milk, newborns often feed every two to three hours. Feeding is a time for comfort and bonding in addition to providing nourishment.

7.1.3.5. Social Interactions

Despite their limited capabilities, newborns are social beings. They show a preference for human faces and voices and engage in early forms of communication, such as making eye contact and cooing. These interactions are foundational for emotional and social development.

7.1.3.6. Adaptation and Learning

Newborns adjust to their surroundings quite quickly. They get a sense of security from being able to identify their caregivers and their go-to routines. Caregiving that is responsive and consistent promotes the general development of newborns and makes them feel safe. In conclusion, a newborn baby's behavior includes a variety of reflexes, sensory reactions, and early social interactions. These behaviors lay the groundwork for the infant's early growth and learning and are essential for survival, bonding, and development. A healthy and happy start to life can be encouraged by being aware of these behaviors and reacting to them with compassion and understanding.

7.1.3.7. Emotional Development

The main tenet of attachment theory is ethology and evolution; in times of fear or distress, a baby or child will seek out and attach itself to a specific attachment figure in order to survive. The development of attachments is thought to lay the groundwork for an infant or child's ability to form and maintain relationships throughout their life. Despite their frequent association, love and affection are not the same as attachment. It is common for attachment and attachment behaviors to emerge between the ages of three and six months. When it comes to social interactions, infants get attached to adults who are responsive and sensitive, and who provide consistent care for a while. Parental reactions cause attachment patterns to form, which then result in "internal working models" that influence a person's emotions, ideas, and expectations in subsequent relationships. There are several attachment "styles," some more problematic than others, including "secure," "anxious-ambivalent," "anxious-avoidant," and (all 'organized'). Severe disorders may result from either a severe disruption of attachment or from a lack of attachment. Infants form unique bonds with their fathers, siblings, mothers, and other caregivers who are not related to them. In addition to dyadic attachment relationships, the development of an infant's mental health depends on the quality of the triadic relationships between the mother, father, and child.

7.1.3.8. Response to sounds

Babies react to sounds such as the hissing of a snake, adult voices that are angry, the crackling sound of a fire, thunder, and the cries of other babies. Their eyes blinking, their heart rate dropping, and their increased turning to face the parent or speakers are all signs that they were paying closer attention. It's thought that this is an evolutionary reaction to danger. During their first year of life, babies' ability to precisely locate sounds is refined.

7.1.4. Health Issues

The severity and impact of health problems in newborns can vary greatly, from common conditions that are easily treated to more serious complications that call for intensive medical care. Comprehending these health concerns is essential for prompt identification and handling, guaranteeing the baby's welfare. Jaundice, which is caused by elevated bilirubin levels in the blood and manifests as yellowing of the skin and eyes, is one of the most common health problems in newborns. If left untreated, severe cases of jaundice can cause neurological damage, but mild cases usually go away on their own or with phototherapy. Respiratory distress is another prevalent ailment that is frequently observed in premature infants with underdeveloped lungs. This may show up as a brief tachypnea or more serious problems like respiratory distress syndrome (RDS), which calls for the use of mechanical ventilation or oxygen therapy. For newborns, infections are a serious concern because of their developing immune systems. If newborn sepsis, a serious bloodstream infection, is not treated with antibiotics right away, it may be fatal. Careful observation and management are also necessary for other infections, such as urinary tract infections and conjunctivitis. Congenital anomalies are defects in structure or function that exist from birth and can vary in severity. Neural tube defects, cleft lip or palate, and congenital cardiac defects are common examples. To effectively manage these conditions, early diagnosis through prenatal screening and postnatal examinations is essential.

Newborns frequently experience digestive problems, such as gastroesophageal reflux disease (GERD), which can be uncomfortable and interfere with feeding. More severe cases, especially in premature infants, can result in conditions like necrotizing enterocolitis, a serious intestinal disease. Timely medical attention is imperative in order to avoid complications. The act of premature birth itself presents many health risks. Preterm babies are those who are born before 37 weeks of pregnancy and are more likely to experience feeding problems, developmental delays, and underdeveloped organs. To address these issues, long-term care and follow-up are frequently necessary. Another problem that can impact newborns is hypoglycemia, or low blood sugar; this is especially true for preterm infants, babies whose mothers have diabetes, and babies who have growth limitations. Lethargy, jitteriness, and poor feeding are examples of symptoms that need to be treated right away to avoid worsening complications. Additionally, newborns may experience hematological issues like anemia, which are frequently brought on by insufficient red blood cell synthesis or excessive red blood cell destruction. It is also possible to have polycythemia, which is characterized by an unusually high concentration of red blood cells and may require medical attention. Despite their rarity, metabolic disorders must be detected early. If left untreated, diseases like hypothyroidism and phenylketonuria (PKU) can cause serious developmental problems. Programs for newborn screening aid in the early detection of these conditions, allowing for prompt intervention. Finally, problems with nutrition and feeding, such as lactation problems and formula intolerance, are frequent. Growth and development depend on getting enough nutrition, and it might be necessary to use alternate feeding techniques or lactation support.

7.1.4.1. Diseases

The infant is undergoing many adaptations to extrauterine life, and its physiological systems, such as the immune system, are far from fully developed. Potential diseases of concern during the neonatal period include:

- Neonatal jaundice
- Infant respiratory distress syndrome
- Neonatal lupus erythematosus
- Neonatal conjunctivitis
- Neonatal tetanus
- Neonatal sepsis
- Neonatal bowel obstruction
- Benign neonatal seizures
- Neonatal diabetes mellitus
- Neonatal alloimmune thrombocytopenia
- Neonatal herpes simplex
- Neonatal hemochromatosis
- Neonatal meningitis
- Neonatal hepatitis
- Neonatal hypoglycemia

7.1.4.2. Mortality

Infant mortality refers to the death of an infant within the first year of life, typically measured as the number of deaths per 1,000 live births (infant mortality rate). Common causes of infant mortality include dehydration, infection, congenital abnormalities, and SIDS. This measurement is crucial for evaluating the quality of healthcare in a country, as it reflects the overall health of infants, children, and pregnant women, as well as access to medical services, socioeconomic conditions, and public health practices.

Countries with higher national wealth tend to have lower infant mortality rates due to their advanced healthcare systems, with examples being Canada, the United Kingdom, the United States, and Japan. In contrast, countries like Mexico, which allocate less budget to healthcare, tend to have higher infant mortality rates due to poorer overall population health. In the U.S., minority groups tend to have higher infant mortality rates, with non-Hispanic black women experiencing a rate of 13.63 per 1,000 live births compared to non-Hispanic white women whose rate is much lower at 5.76 per 1,000 live births. The average infant mortality rate in the U.S. is 6.8 per 1,000 live births.

7.1.5. Babyhood

The first two years of life are commonly referred to as babyhood, which is the time span from infancy to toddlerhood. This developmental stage is characterized by swift physical, cognitive, and emotional advancement, setting the groundwork for subsequent development and education. Comprehending the developmental milestones and obstacles associated with infancy is essential to ensuring that babies receive the right kind of attention and stimulation.

- **Physical Development:** Babyhood is a time of rapid growth. By the time they turn one year old, babies typically triple their birth weight and gain roughly 50% of their original length. Babies acquire motor skills in a predictable order: rolling over, sitting up, crawling, and eventually walking come first, followed by control over their heads and necks. Additionally, there is a notable advancement in fine motor skills, which include holding objects and coordinating hand movements. During this phase, nutrition is very important. For the first six months, the baby gets the nutrients they need from breastfeeding or formula, and then they gradually start eating solid foods.
- **Cognitive Development:** Babies have amazing cognitive development during this time. Babies explore and experiment with their senses to learn about and engage with the world around them. During this time, object permanence emerges, a fundamental cognitive milestone that involves the understanding that objects exist even when they are out of sight. By the end of the second year, babbling and cooing give way to the first words and simple sentences in language development. Along with improving their memory and problem-solving abilities, babies also grow more inquisitive and skilled at picking up knowledge through play and imitation.
- **Emotional and Social Development:** Developing socially and emotionally is a fundamental aspect of infancy. The foundation of emotional security is attachment to primary caregivers. Babies display a spectrum of emotions, including fear, frustration, and joy. They also start to learn how to control their emotions. Other family members and peers are included in social interactions in addition to primary caregivers. Babies acquire social norms and behaviors through watching and imitating those in their environment. A secure attachment is fostered and healthy emotional development is promoted by responsive caregiving, which is defined by constant affection, attention, and reassurance.
- **Communication:** Communication abilities develop in infancy. Babies learn to communicate primarily through crying at first, but they also quickly pick up on making sounds, gestures, and facial expressions. Talking starts when a person babbles and then uses words that are familiar to them. Many toddlers can comprehend and use simple phrases by the end of this stage, as well as follow simple instructions and have basic conversations. It is crucial to

promote language development in the infant by reading, talking, and singing to them.

- **Challenges and Health Considerations:** Parenting is not without its difficulties. Common health issues include minor illnesses like colds and ear infections, as well as teething, which can be uncomfortable and interfere with sleep. Frequent pediatric examinations are essential for tracking immunizations, growth, and development. Babies often struggle to establish a regular sleep schedule due to their unpredictable sleep patterns. These problems can be lessened by creating a relaxing nighttime routine and making sure the sleeping environment is secure (Remien and Majmundar, 2023).

7.2. Physiology of the Newborn

A newborn's physiology is distinct and intricate since it varies over the course of minutes, hours, days, and months. Human physiology is normally stable and predictable once we reach adulthood; any deviation from this can result in pathology and disease. Nonetheless, the quick and constantly evolving physiology of a newborn is crucial for their adaptation to the world outside the womb. A newborn's physiology is always changing to accommodate life outside the womb. It's critical to take notice of these modifications and make sure that the right development occurs when it should. When an infant takes its first breath, for example, it is crucial that the intrauterine cardiovascular shunts in its body close and are remodeled. Failing to do so may result in physiological imbalances, including insufficient oxygen delivery to the brain. Furthermore, it's critical to recognize the nutrients that the newborn is deficient in and needs to be supplemented. An infant born with low vitamin K deficiency, for example, is susceptible to hemorrhagic disease. All newborns should receive vitamin K prophylaxis in order to avoid this.

7.2.1. Organ Systems Involved

7.2.1.1. Cardiovascular System

The ductus venosus, foramen ovale, and ductus arteriosus are among the shunts involved in intrauterine fetal circulation, which must be understood in order to comprehend the changes in the newborn's cardiovascular physiology. First, the placenta oxygenates the mother's blood before it passes through to the fetus through the umbilical vein. The ductus venosus transports the oxygenated blood from the umbilical vein to the inferior vena cava (IVC), avoiding the hepatic circulation. Blood enters the right atrium from the IVC. The foramen ovale is then used to transfer oxygenated blood from the right atrium to the left atrium. From the left atrium, blood flows to the left ventricle, the coronary arteries, and the aorta. A tiny quantity of blood leaves the right atrium and enters the right ventricle, pulmonary artery, and finally the lungs instead of passing through the foramen ovale. But most blood is diverted from the pulmonary artery via the ductus arteriosus and goes straight to the aorta, avoiding the lungs. Blood that has been oxygenated is subsequently sent from the aorta to the systemic circulation.

7.2.1.1.1. Changes in Fetal Circulation at Birth

Decreased Pulmonary Vascular Resistance and Increased Systemic Vascular Resistance

- An increase in systemic circulation is made possible by the removal of the low-resistance circuit that results from cutting the umbilical cord. The newborn's lungs fill with fluid when it takes its first breath, and oxygen seeps into the blood vessels that encircle the alveoli. When the pulmonary arteries relax, blood can enter the lungs and the pulmonary resistance decreases.

Closure of the Ductus Arteriosus

- The ductus arteriosus remains patent during pregnancy when there is an abundance of prostaglandins, low oxygen tension, carbon monoxide, and nitric oxide. The ductus arteriosus starts to functionally close once the baby starts breathing, and this process may take several days. Prostaglandins are reduced as a result of the rise in oxygen and fall in pulmonary arterial resistance, which helps the ductus arteriosus close. As a result of the placenta's separation, prostaglandin synthesis is also reduced, which aids in the ductus arteriosus' closure.

Closure of the Foramen Ovale

- Left atrial pressure rises when a newborn breathes for the first time due to decreased pulmonary vasculature resistance. The foramen ovale closes when the left atrial pressure surpasses the right atrial pressure.

Closure of the Ductus Venosus (DV)

- Permanent closure of the DV takes approximately one to three months, with the remnant consisting of connective tissue forming the ligamentum venosum of the liver.

Maternal-fetal circulation is no longer needed after birth, so the umbilical vein's remnant forms the liver's round ligament.

7.2.1.2. Pulmonary System

The lungs must be carefully coordinated to clear fetal lung fluid, secrete surfactants, and start regular breathing in order to adapt to the external environment. The fetal lung fluid secreted by the airway epithelium during intrauterine life fills the lungs and is necessary for healthy lung development. The proper and prompt clearance of lung fluid is the most crucial step in the fetal transition to extrauterine air breathing. Osmotic gradients produced by the active solute transport of alveolar epithelial cells facilitate the majority of fluid clearance. Changes in sodium channel expression during development and changes in hormones linked to labor control this process. A newborn's rapid onset of vigorous breathing is caused by a variety of factors, including changes in the blood's levels of oxygen and carbon monoxide, diffuse tactile and cold stimuli, and clamping of the umbilical cord, which eliminates prostaglandin secretion, which suppresses breathing. The majority of full-term babies will successfully start breathing if there isn't any severe hypoxia. Particular hormonal adjustments start prior to birth and are essential for the removal of fetal lung fluid upon delivery. An increase in cortisol, thyroid hormones, and catecholamines inhibits the active chloride-mediated secretion of fetal lung fluid. These hormones activate the type II cells of the airway epithelium's basal Na-K-ATPase, which permits sodium from the fetal lung fluid to be pumped into the interstitium along with water and other electrolytes, clearing the airways of fluid. When a baby breathes deeply and under pressure at birth, their lungs expand physiologically normal, pushing lung fluid from the airways into the distal airspace. The newborn keeps expelling lung fluid after inflation. A further aid in the clearance of fetal lung fluid in newborns delivered vaginally is the thoracic squeeze, which compresses the lungs' fluid and permits additional fluid clearance (Jain & Eaton, 2006).

Breathing is typically a laborious task for a newborn. Newborns breathe at a higher rate (30 to 60) breaths per minute) because they use accessory muscles, intercostal retractions, and grunting to counteract the high surface tension.

In addition, perfusion-ventilation differences and compensating for high metabolic rate are factors. Significantly, the infant's breathing effort is increased due to the existence of circulatory shunts. Respiratory effort decreases as the fluid exits the lung alveoli. Babies may have apnea episodes that last less than five seconds because of immature central drive responses. Newborns are expected to experience apneic episodes, even though this is rare in adults.

7.2.1.3. Hematological System

Red blood cells, white blood cells, and platelets are the two main types of blood cells that make up plasma. The liver makes blood while the fetus is growing, and the bone marrow takes over the primary role of blood cell production (hematopoiesis) from the liver after birth. Hemoglobin (Hb), which is carried by red blood cells, carries iron and oxygen from the lungs to the body's tissues and organs. Hemoglobin comes in various forms; the two that are relevant to this conversation are HbF and HbA. The main hemoglobin that the fetus produces is called HbF, and its function is to carry oxygen to areas with low oxygen levels. Because of its strong affinity for oxygen, HbF can effectively extract oxygen from mother hemoglobin and transfer it across the placenta. HbF is crucial not only for intrauterine development but also during the neonatal period because it affects the tissues' ability to receive oxygen. Adult hemoglobin, or HbA, takes the place of HbF at six months of age. Due to immature hepatocyte function and a lack of enteric bacteria that produce vitamin K, infants are deficient in vitamin K. Because vitamin K is necessary for the synthesis of proteins C and S as well as clotting factors II, VII, IX, and X, people who are deficient in it are more susceptible to bleeding from any source. Because of this vitamin K deficiency, every newborn receives a prophylactic shot of vitamin K to guard against hemorrhagic disease.

7.2.1.4. Metabolism and Thermoregulation

The cold extrauterine environment causes the newborn's temperature to drop quickly after birth. The newborn increases heat production through non-shivering thermogenesis (NST), which involves the lipolysis of brown adipose tissue, which is found around the kidneys and back muscles, in order to combat this temperature change. By using uncoupled protein to oxidize fatty acids in the mitochondria, uncoupled protein synthesizes ATP, generating heat. A hypoxic neonate cannot generate enough heat to raise its body temperature because thermogenesis requires adequate oxygenation. Because their skeletal muscle mass is still developing, infants usually do not use shivering thermogenesis—an increase in skeletal muscle activity and limb movements—to raise their body temperature until around six months. Because of the high metabolic rate of activity required to maintain breathing, feeding, and thermogenesis, newborns are usually tachycardic (120 to 160 beats per minute).

7.2.2. Testing

7.2.2.1. Newborn Screening

The Department of Health and Human Services (HHS) in the United States has developed a list of disorders known as the Recommended Uniform Screening Panel (RUSP), which advises states to screen every newborn. Filter papers and a few drops of the newborn's heel blood are used in the majority of these tests to diagnose the condition. Between 36 and 72 hours of life is the ideal window of time to screen for these disorders.

- Metabolic disorders
  - Organic acid metabolism disorders
  - Fatty acid oxidation disorders
  - Amino acid disorders (e.g.,

homocystinuria, phenylketonuria, maple syrup urine disease)

- Endocrine disorders
  - o Congenital adrenal hyperplasia (CAH)
  - o Primary congenital hypothyroidism
- Hemoglobin disorders
  - o Sickle cell anemia
  - o Beta thalassemia
- Other
  - o Glycogen storage disease type II (Pompe)
  - o Critical congenital heart disease
  - o Cystic fibrosis (CF)
  - o Classic galactosemia
  - o Hearing loss
  - o Severe combined immunodeficiencies (SCID)
  - o X-linked adrenoleukodystrophy (XLA)
  - o Spinal muscular atrophy (SMA)
  - o Biotinidase deficiency
  - o Mucopolysaccharidosis type I and II

7.2.3. Pathophysiology

7.2.3.1. Cardiovascular System

One of the most prevalent congenital defects is congenital heart disease (CHD) (Blue GM, et al., 2012). Approximately 80% of cases of CHD are caused by multifactorial factors, which result from different combinations of genetic and environmental factors. The remaining 20% are linked to chromosomal abnormalities or teratogens. Among patients with congenital heart disease, the two most prevalent syndromes are velocardiofacial syndrome and down syndrome.

There are two main categories of CHDs; cyanotic and acyanotic.

- Cyanotic – right-to-left shunts
  - o Tetralogy of Fallot
  - o Transposition of the great vessels
  - o Tricuspid atresia
  - o Total anomalous pulmonary venous return (TAPVR)
  - o Truncus arteriosus
- Acyanotic – further classified into:
  - o Left-to-right shunts
    - – Atrial septal defect (ASD)
    - – Ventricular septal defect (VSD)
    - – Patent ductus arteriosus (PDA)
- Outflow obstruction
  - – Pulmonary stenosis
  - – Aortic stenosis
  - – Coarctation of the aorta

The size of the shunt and the volume of blood being shunted in shunt cases influence the severity of the symptoms. Small acyanotic (left-to-right) shunts are usually benign and don't need to be surgically corrected. Bigger left-to-right shunts, however, will eventually require surgery to prevent pulmonary arterial hypertension and the heart's ongoing volume overload. Eisenmenger syndrome can result from a left-to-right shunt evolving and reversing blood flow from the right to the left if these shunts are not corrected. Blood that has been deoxygenated can escape the lungs and return to the body without gaining oxygen thanks to right-to-left (cyanotic) shunts. These shunts are more severe, and the condition is usually cyanotic from birth.

7.2.3.2. Pulmonary

It is commonly recognized that a necessary adaptation for getting ready for birth and life outside of the uterus is the proper development of the fetal lung and surfactant secretion. The synthesis of surfactant starts around weeks 22–28 of pregnancy. A mixture of lipids and proteins that are present in the fluid that lines the lung's alveolar surface is known as pulmonary surfactant. Preventing alveolar collapse at low lung volumes is the main function of surfactants. The volume of fetal lung fluid decreases as delivery gets closer because fetal lung fluid secretion stops. One can classify a newborn's pulmonary pathophysiology according to the time and/or mode of birth. Because they lack enough surfactant to reduce surface tension, preterm babies, for instance, have immature lungs that are difficult to ventilate.

- Preterm (birth before 37 weeks gestation)
    - o Neonatal respiratory distress syndrome (NRDS)
        - Cause: Deficiency of pulmonary surfactant
        - Clinical features: tachypnea, hypoxia, cyanosis, decreased breath sounds
        - Complications: bronchopulmonary dysplasia, pneumothorax
    - Apnea of prematurity (AOP)
        - Causes: immature medullary respiratory center and/or weak airway or breathing muscles
        - Clinical features: cessation of breathing for > 20 seconds and typically accompanied by bradycardia
- Cesarean section
    - Transient tachypnea of the newborn (TTN)
        - Cause: delayed resorption of fetal lung fluid
        - Clinical features: tachypnea, diffuse crackles on auscultation

7.2.3.3. Endocrine

The endocrine system is typically adequately developed at birth, and no immediate endocrine abnormalities occur. However, there are particular circumstances in which abnormalities may be seen at birth.

- Hermaphroditism and the masculinization of the female sexual organs can result from an androgenic hormone treatment during pregnancy or from the development of an androgenic tumor in a pregnant woman carrying a female child.
- Since elevated insulin levels promote fetal growth and heighten birth weight, poorly managed type 2 diabetes mellitus in mothers is the most common cause of large for gestational age (LGA) babies. On the other hand, because of insufficient insulin secretion, babies born to mothers with uncontrolled type 1 diabetes mellitus are usually small for gestational age and have a high death rate if they do not survive to full term. 75% of these deaths are attributable to respiratory distress syndrome if the patient does not survive.
- A baby born to a woman who is hyperthyroid or receives excessive thyroid hormone treatment is more likely to have transient hypothyroidism. A fetus may experience mental retardation and poor bone growth if it is born without thyroid hormone secretion, a condition known as cretin dwarfism. On the other hand, if the

mother underwent a thyroidectomy prior to becoming pregnant, her pituitary gland might secrete too much thyrotropin during the pregnancy, which could cause the baby to be born temporarily hyperthyroid.

7.2.3.4. Neonatal Jaundice

Bilirubin produced in the fetus can pass through the placenta to the mother and be eliminated through her liver. After birth, newborns rely on their own liver to eliminate excess bilirubin, but the liver is not fully functional for the first week of life, leading to a build-up of bilirubin in the body. About 60% of full-term and 80% of premature babies experience physiologic jaundice in the first 1–2 weeks after birth, causing yellowing of the skin, eyes, and mucous membranes. This type of jaundice typically appears after the first day of life, with a peak bilirubin concentration below 15 mg/dL, and usually resolves without treatment. Pathologic jaundice, on the other hand, occurs within the first 24 hours of life, with a peak bilirubin concentration exceeding 15 mg/dL, and can persist beyond one week in term babies and two weeks in premature infants. Potential causes of pathologic jaundice include infections, blood disorders, high red blood cell count, trauma, metabolic issues, and genetic conditions like Crigler-Najjar syndrome.

7.2.4. Clinical Significance

Throughout the formation and birth of a human being, numerous problems may potentially arise. Below is a summary of some of the most common and clinically relevant issues that may exist at birth.

- Cephalohematoma
- Caput succedaneum
- Transient head molding
- Bulging fontanelles (increased intracranial pressure)
- Brachial plexus injuries/facial nerve palsy
- Subgaleal hemorrhage
- Clavicle fracture
- Conjunctivitis
- Torticollis
- Club foot
- Hip dysplasia
- Neural tube defects
- Cleft lip/palate
- Choanal atresia
- Hirschsprung disease

7.2.4.1. Vitamin K Deficiency Bleeding

Since vitamin K is not produced by the newborn's gut, does not cross the placenta, and is not found in breast milk, all newborns are vitamin K deficient. Baby clotting factors that are dependent on vitamin K are deficient in this lack of vitamin K, which puts them at risk of bleeding and potentially fatal hemorrhage. To avoid this, a vitamin K injection should be administered from birth. Infants who do not receive this injection run the risk of bleeding internally, subgaleally, or in their gastrointestinal tract.

7.2.4.2. Metabolism and Thermoregulation

Preterm babies are particularly at a disadvantage when it comes to thermoregulation because their brown adipose tissue has not developed sufficiently to allow for an appropriate heat response. Important actions should be performed to support infants' thermoregulation, especially those who are preterm. Initially, the newborn needs to be dried multiple times with warm cloths as soon as they are delivered. The baby should be put in a bed warmer that heats the air around the baby and the bed via convection. Furthermore, an incubator—a crib-like device with a plastic dome covering it—would be especially helpful for some preterm babies in order to raise the humidity and decrease chilly outside airflow (Asakura, 2004).

7.2.4.3. Newborn Nutrition

The majority of the fetus's energy prior to birth comes from glucose taken from the mother's blood. The newborn's body stores enough glucose in the form of muscle and liver glycogen within hours of birth, providing all the energy the baby needs. Because the liver is still not developed enough at birth to carry out gluconeogenesis, the plasma glucose concentration can drop to as low as 30 to 40 mg/dl, or less than half of the normal level. Until two or three days later, when the mother's milk is available, the baby uses the proteins and fats it has stored for metabolism. In the first two or three days of life, the baby's weight drops by five to ten percent, and sometimes by as much as twenty percent. Instead of bodily solids, fluids account for the majority of this weight loss. An infant requires certain vitamins and minerals in order to ensure healthy growth and development.

- **Calcium and Vitamin D:** A calcium supply must be provided during infancy due to the rapid ossification of bones at birth. However, in the absence of vitamin D, the GI tract has a poor ability to absorb calcium. As a result, infants with a vitamin D deficiency may develop severe rickets within a few weeks. Premature babies should be especially concerned about this since their GI tracts absorb calcium even less efficiently than those of term babies.
- **Iron:** The infant's liver usually has enough iron stored to keep forming blood cells for 4–6 months after birth if the mother consumes an adequate amount of iron through her diet. After the baby is three months old, severe anemia can result from the mother's diet lacking in iron.
- **Vitamin C (Ascorbic Acid):** Although it is not stored in considerable amounts in the fetal tissues, it is necessary for the healthy formation of bone and cartilage. Enough vitamin C is usually found in the mother's breast milk, unless she has a severe deficiency. It is noteworthy that cow's milk contains only 1/4 the vitamin C of human milk and is not advised during the newborn stage.

7.2.4.4. Immunity

The mother's antibodies diffuse into the fetus prior to birth through the placenta. A newborn's ability to produce antibodies on its own is negligible after birth, and by the end of the first month of life, the newborn's antibody levels have dropped to less than half of what they were at birth, which is associated with a decline in the newborn's immunity. But for about six months after birth, the baby is protected from the majority of infectious diseases by the antibodies inherited from the mother. This covers defense against diphtheria, polio, and measles. For this reason, immunization against these diseases is not required for newborns right away. However, infants should be immunized against hepatitis B as soon as they are born. Between 12 and 20 months is when the baby's immune system produces its antibodies. A combination vaccination against diphtheria, tetanus, and acellular pertussis (DTaP) is advised for children ages 2 to 6 years old as well as at 4, 6, and 15 months.

7.3. Respiratory Distress in the Newborn

Up to 7% of all term newborns experience respiratory distress, and even mild prematurity is increasingly associated with respiratory distress. Well-researched preventive and therapeutic interventions can lessen the burden of disease when used for some of the most prevalent underlying causes. Short- and long-term complications, such as chronic lung disease, respiratory failure, and even death, can result from failing to promptly identify symptoms and treat the underlying cause of the newborn's respiratory distress. A newborn is most frequently admitted to the neonatal intensive care unit due to respiratory distress. In the neonatal intensive care unit, respiratory morbidity affects 15% of term babies and 29% of late preterm babies admitted; the percentage rises for babies born before 34 weeks of pregnancy. Neonatal respiratory disease is more likely to occur in babies who have certain risk factors. Prematurity, caesarian section delivery, gestational diabetes, meconium-stained amniotic fluid (MSAF), maternal chorioamnionitis, and abnormalities in the lungs or oligohydramnios observed on prenatal ultrasound are some of these factors. But it's not always possible to determine which newborns will exhibit symptoms prior to birth. Respiratory distress, no matter what the cause, can progress to respiratory failure and cardiopulmonary arrest if it is not identified and treated promptly. Thus, it is essential for any medical professional attending to neonates to be able to quickly identify respiratory distress symptoms, distinguish between different etiologies, and start treatment plans in order to avoid serious complications or even death.

7.3.1. Definition, Signs, Symptoms

Tachypnea, nasal flaring, chest retractions, or grunting are examples of signs of increased work of breathing that indicate respiratory distress in a newborn. A newborn breathes between 30 and 60 times per minute on average. If the breathing rate is more than 60 breaths per minute, you have tachypnea. In a wide range of respiratory, cardiovascular, metabolic, or systemic diseases, tachypnea is a common but nonspecific finding. It is a compensatory mechanism for hypercarbia, hypoxemia, or acidosis (both metabolic and respiratory). Tachypnea can be brought on by pulmonary illness, particularly in newborns. The lungs' elasticity naturally causes them to contract. Functional residual capacity (FRC), which keeps the alveoli from collapsing at the end of expiration, is triggered by the chest wall's outward recoil. Due to its greater pliability, the newborn lung's chest wall—which is mainly made of cartilage—predisposes it to pulmonary atelectasis and lower FRC. The ability of the alveoli to fill with air at a specific pressure is known as pulmonary compliance, and it is defined as a given change in volume (ΔVolume) for every given change in pressure (ΔPressure). Tidal volume decreases in cases where lung compliance is compromised, as in the case of transient tachypnea of the newborn (TTN), respiratory distress syndrome (RDS), pneumonia, or pulmonary edema. The respiratory rate needs to rise in order to attain adequate minute ventilation. Tachypnea gets worse with hypoxemia. As such, neonates with the condition exhibit noticeable tachypnea. Tachypnea is a nonspecific symptom; therefore, additional clinical findings help to rule out respiratory disorders as the cause.

Mismatched pulmonary mechanics resulting in decreased lung compliance (ΔVolume/ΔPressure), increased airway resistance (ΔPressure/Volumetric Flow), or both can cause increased work of breathing. There is an increase in airway resistance when there is an airflow obstruction. The equation $R = V(8l\eta/\pi r(4))$, where R is resistance, V is flow, l is length, η is viscosity, and r is radius, illustrates the critical importance of airway radius. The resistance multiplies sixteen times when the airway radius is cut half. As a compensatory symptom, nasal flaring widens the upper airway and lessens breathing resistance and effort. When airway resistance is high or lung compliance is low, retractions take place, which are demonstrated by the activation of accessory muscles in the neck, rib cage, sternum, or abdomen (Garbar & Newton, 2023). The type of noise auscultated may help localize airway obstruction, and noisy breathing may indicate increased airway resistance (Table 7.1). A sonorous snore that is audible over the extrathoracic airways and signifies nasopharyngeal blockage is called a stertor. A stridor is a high-pitched, monophonic breath sound that suggests a blockage in the subglottic, glottis, or larynx. While wheezing is usually polyphonic, it can also be high pitched. It is indicative of tracheobronchial blockage and occurs during expiration. In an effort to preserve FRC and avoid alveolar atelectasis, the glottis abruptly closes during expiration, producing the expiratory sound known as grunting. Achieving and maintaining physiologic FRC is crucial in the treatment of respiratory disorders with poor compliance, like RDS or TTN, because lung compliance deteriorates at very low or very high FRC. Conversely, a lower airway obstruction with air trapping is exemplified by meconium aspiration syndrome (MAS). These newborns' lung compliance is negatively impacted by their frequent high lung volumes. Whichever the cause, it's critical to identify the symptoms and take prompt action. Respiratory failure results if the newborn's breathing cannot be supported by the additional effort required to meet its needs. This malfunction could show up as respiratory acidosis or reduced oxygenation (cyanosis). Respiratory arrest is becoming imminent if action is not taken quickly.

Table 7.1. Noisy Breathing Characteristics in Term Infants

Type	Definition	Causes
Stertor	Sonorous snoring sound, mid-pitched, monophonic, may transmit throughout airways, heard loudest with stethoscope near mouth and nose	Nasopharyngeal obstruction—nasal or airway secretions, congestion, choanal stenosis, enlarged or redundant upper airway tissue or tongue
Stridor	Musical, monophonic, audible breath sound. Typically high-pitched. Types: Inspiratory (above the vocal cords), biphasic (at the glottis or subglottis), or expiratory (lower trachea)	Laryngeal obstruction—laryngomalacia, vocal cord paralysis, subglottic stenosis, vascular ring, papillomatosis, foreign body
Wheezing	High-pitched, whistling sound, typically expiratory, polyphonic, loudest in chest	Lower airway obstruction—MAS, bronchiolitis, pneumonia
Grunting	Low- or mid-pitched, expiratory sound caused by sudden closure of the glottis during expiration in an attempt to maintain FRC	Compensatory symptom for poor pulmonary compliance—TTN, RDS, pneumonia, atelectasis, congenital lung malformation or hypoplasia, pleural effusion, pneumothorax

FRC=functional residual capacity; MAS=meconium aspiration syndrome; RDS=respiratory distress syndrome; TTN=transient tachypnea of the newborn.

Source: https://www.ncbi.nlm.nih.gov/pmc/articles/PMC4533247/.

7.3.2. Pathogenesis

There are various reasons why a newborn may experience respiratory distress, often involving multiple systems. Issues with the lungs can stem from abnormalities during the development of the lungs or the transition to life outside the womb. There are 5 stages of normal lung development, and respiratory problems can arise from malformations that occur before or after birth. Conditions like tracheoesophageal fistula, bronchopulmonary sequestration, and bronchogenic cysts are examples of early developmental abnormalities. Later in gestation, issues like congenital cystic adenomatoid malformation or pulmonary hypoplasia can occur. Common respiratory diseases in newborns, such as transient tachypnea of the newborn, respiratory distress syndrome, neonatal pneumonia, meconium aspiration syndrome, and persistent pulmonary hypertension of the newborn, result from complications during the transition from prenatal to postnatal life. Even though mature alveoli are present at 36 weeks gestation, further development and maturation of the lungs continue after birth. The lungs are not fully developed until ages 2 to 5 years. As a result, developmental lung diseases like bronchopulmonary dysplasia can occur postnatally, particularly in premature infants who experience issues with lung development due to factors like mechanical ventilation and exposure to oxygen. Bronchopulmonary dysplasia affects a significant portion of premature infants, with up to 32% of them and 50% of very low-birth-weight infants experiencing the condition (Table 7.2).

Table 7.2. Developmental Stages of Lung Development and Respiratory Disease Pathogenesis

Developmental Stage	Embryonic	Pseudoglandular	Canalicular	Terminal Sac	Alveolar
Gestation	0–6 weeks	7–16 weeks	17–24 weeks	25–36 weeks	>37 weeks
Structural morphogenesis	Trachea, bronchi	Bronchioles, terminal bronchioles, lung circulation	Respiratory bronchioles, primitive alveoli	Alveolar ducts, thin-walled alveolar sacs, increasing functional type 2 cells[a]	Definitive alveoli and mature type 2 cells[a]
Disease manifestation	Tracheoesophageal fistula, pulmonary sequestration	Bronchogenic cyst, congenital diaphragmatic hernia, congenital cystic adenomatoid malformation	Pulmonary hypoplasia, RDS, BPD, alveolar capillary dysplasia	RDS, BPD	TTN, MAS, neonatal pneumonia, PPHN

BPD=bronchopulmonary dysplasia; MAS=meconium aspiration syndrome; PPHN=persistent pulmonary hypertension of the newborn; RDS=respiratory distress syndrome; TTN=transient tachypnea of the newborn;

[a]Type 2 pneumocytes are surfactant-producing cells

Source: https://www.ncbi.nlm.nih.gov/pmc/articles/PMC4533247/.

7.3.3. Differential Diagnosis

Newborn respiratory distress can have a variety of underlying causes, not all of which are related to the lungs (Table 7.3). As a result, it's critical to use a thorough history, physical examination, radiographic, and laboratory results to establish a more precise diagnosis and properly adjust management following initial resuscitation and stabilization. Finding risk factors linked to common causes of neonatal respiratory distress may be aided by a comprehensive medical history (Table 7.4). In order to rule out nonpulmonary causes of respiratory distress in a newborn, a thorough physical examination should go beyond the lungs.

Table 7.3. Differential Diagnosis of Respiratory Distress in the Newborn

Airway
Nasal obstruction, choanal atresia, micrognathia, Pierre Robin sequence, macroglossia, congenital high airway obstruction syndrome, including laryngeal or tracheal atresia, subglottic stenosis, laryngeal cyst or laryngeal web, vocal cord paralysis, subglottic stenosis, airway hemangiomas or papillomas, laryngomalacia, tracheobronchomalacia, tracheoesophageal fistula vascular rings, and external compression from a neck mass
Pulmonary
RDS,[a] TTN,[a] MAS,[a] neonatal pneumonia,[a] pneumothorax,[a] PPHN,[a] pleural effusion (congenital chylothorax), pulmonary hemorrhage, bronchopulmonary sequestration, bronchogenic cyst, congenital cystic adenomatoid malformation or congenital pulmonary airway malformation, pulmonary hypoplasia, congenital lobar emphysema, pulmonary alveolar proteinosis, alveolar capillary dysplasia, congenital pulmonary lymphangiectasis, and surfactant protein deficiency
Cardiovascular
Cyanotic and select acyanotic congenital heart defects,[a] neonatal cardiomyopathy, pericardial effusion or cardiac tamponade, fetal arrhythmia with compromised cardiac function, and high-output cardiac failure
Thoracic
Pneumomediastinum, chest wall deformities, mass, skeletal dysplasia, and diaphragmatic hernia or paralysis
Neuromuscular
Central nervous system injury (birth trauma or hemorrhage),[a] hypoxic-ischemic encephalopathy,[a] cerebral malformations, chromosomal abnormalities, medication (neonatal or maternal sedation, antidepressants, or magnesium), congenital TORCH infections, meningitis, seizure disorder, obstructed hydrocephalus, arthrogryposis, congenital myotonic dystrophy, neonatal myasthenia gravis, spinal muscular atrophy, congenital myopathies, and spinal cord injury
Other
Sepsis,[a] hypoglycemia,[a] metabolic acidosis,[a] hypothermia or hyperthermia, hydrops fetalis, inborn error of metabolism, hypermagnesemia, hyponatremia or hypernatremia, severe hemolytic disease, anemia, and polycythemia

BPD=bronchopulmonary dysplasia; MAS=meconium aspiration syndrome; PPHN=persistent pulmonary hypertension of the newborn; RDS=respiratory distress syndrome; TTN=transient tachypnea of the newborn.

[a]Relatively common causes of respiratory distress in the newborn.

Source: https://www.ncbi.nlm.nih.gov/pmc/articles/PMC4533247/.

These nonpulmonary causes include airway obstruction, abnormalities of the chest wall, cardiovascular disease, and neuromuscular disease. Diaphragmatic paralysis, congenital pulmonary malformations, and intrathoracic space-occupying lesions that can impair lung expansion, such as pneumothorax, mediastinal mass, and congenital diaphragmatic hernia, can all be identified by radiographic findings. Severe tachypnea without increased respiratory effort should initiate further testing in the lab to rule out sepsis or metabolic acidosis. Given that hypoglycemia, hypomagnesemia, and hematologic abnormalities can lead to decreased oxygen transport to peripheral tissues or a lowered ventilatory drive, laboratory evaluations should be taken into account in conjunction with clinical findings. Due to hypotonia, a decreased respiratory drive, or even apnea, hypermagnesemia can exacerbate respiratory distress and impair a newborn's ability to respond to resuscitation.

Table 7.4. Perinatal History Associated with Common Respiratory Diseases in the Newborn Infant

Respiratory Disease	Risk Factors
TTN	Caesarian section, precipitous delivery, late preterm or early term, maternal sedation or medication, fetal distress, gestational diabetes
Neonatal pneumonia	Maternal group B streptococcus carrier, chorioamnionitis, maternal fever, PROM, prematurity, perinatal depression
RDS	Prematurity, gestational diabetes, male infant, multiple gestation
MAS	MSAF, post term gestation, fetal distress or perinatal depression, African American ethnicity
Pulmonary hypoplasia	Oligohydramnios, renal dysplasia or agenesis, urinary outlet obstruction, premature PROM, diaphragmatic hernia, neuromuscular disorder (loss of fetal respirations/bell-shaped chest)

MAS=meconium aspiration syndrome; MSAF=meconium-stained amniotic fluid; PROM=prolonged rupture of membranes; RDS=respiratory distress syndrome; TTN=transient tachypnea of the newborn.

Source: https://www.ncbi.nlm.nih.gov/pmc/articles/PMC4533247/.

Distinguishing cardiovascular disease from pulmonary causes of respiratory distress may pose a challenge (Table 7.5). The majority of congenital heart defects (Budts et al., 2003) manifest as respiratory distress due to cardiac failure, tachypnea, or cyanosis. As the ductus arteriosus closes, congenital heart defects typically manifest hours or days after birth rather than right away, so timing may be a crucial indicator for differentiation. This differentiation is made easier by Table 7.5.

Table 7.5. Differentiation of Cyanotic Heart Disease from Pulmonary Disease among Infants in Respiratory Distress

Variable	Cyanotic Heart Disease	Pulmonary Disease
History	Previous sibling with congenital heart disease	Maternal fever
	Diagnosis of congenital heart disease by prenatal ultrasonography	MSAF
		Preterm delivery

Physical Examination	Cyanosis	Cyanosis
	Gallop rhythm or murmur	Severe retractions
	Single second heart sound	Split second heart sound
	Large liver	Temperature instability
	Mild respiratory distress	
Chest Radiograph	Increased heart size	Normal heart size
	Decreased pulmonary vascularity (except in transposition of the great vessels or total anomalous pulmonary venous return)	Abnormal pulmonary parenchyma, such as total whiteout or patches of consolidation in pneumonia, fluid in the fissures in TTN or ground glass appearance in RDS
Arterial Blood Gas	Normal or decreased $PaCO_2$	Increased $PaCO_2$
	Decreased PaO_2	Decreased PaO_2
Hyperoxia Test	PaO_2 <150 mm Hg	PaO_2 >150 mm Hg (except in severe PPHN)
Echocardiography	Abnormal heart or vessels	Normal heart and vessels

MSAF=meconium-stained amniotic fluid; PPHN=persistent pulmonary hypertension of the newborn; RDS=respiratory distress syndrome; TTN=transient tachypnea of the newborn.

Source: https://www.ncbi.nlm.nih.gov/pmc/articles/PMC4533247/.

Any infant exhibiting respiratory distress and cyanosis should be evaluated for pulmonary hypertension. Failure to switch from in utero to postnatal pulmonary circulation following delivery causes this condition. The persistence of elevated pulmonary vascular resistance leads to cyanosis due to compromised pulmonary blood flow and blood shunting from right to left across the ductus arteriosus and foramen ovale. Shunting exacerbates metabolic acidemia and systemic hypoxemia, which both lead to persistently elevated pulmonary vascular resistance. PPHN can result from respiratory diseases, specifically congenital diaphragmatic hernia, MAS, or RDS, either as a primary or secondary cause. It can be challenging to distinguish PPHN from cyanotic heart disease when there is no concurrent pulmonary disease. The hyperoxia test, which involves ventilation with 100% oxygen, can be used to differentiate between the two conditions. The PaO_2 will rise to above 100 mm Hg in some newborns with PPHN, but it won't rise above 45 mm Hg in babies with cyanotic heart defects who have circulatory mixing.

7.3.4. Common Case Scenarios

To assist in determining the most frequent causes of respiratory distress in newborns, four case scenarios are highlighted. Each disorder's pathophysiology, risk factors, prevention, and management techniques are then covered.

7.3.4.1. Case 1

A 32-kilogram baby girl is delivered via cesarean section at 38 weeks gestation without going through a labor trial. At one minute and five minutes, respectively, her Apgar scores are 9 and 9.

Within an hour of birth, she experiences nasal flaring, tachypnea, and subcostal retractions. At 97.9°F (36.06°C), the temperature is recorded.

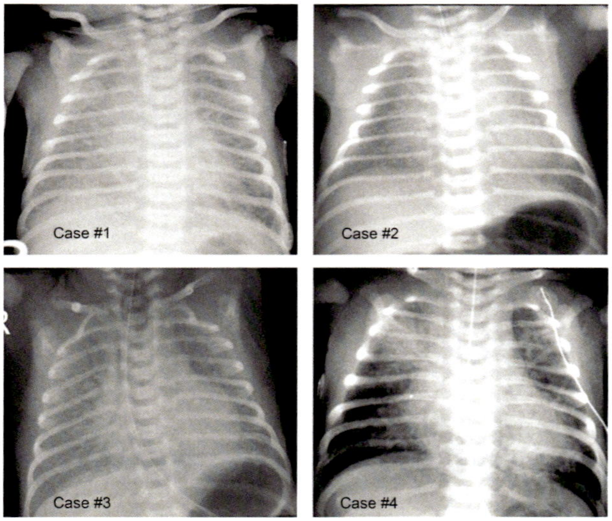

Figure 7.1. *Case 1: Transient tachypnea of the newborn is characterized by streaky, pulmonary interstitial markings and fluid in the fissure apparent on chest radiograph. Case 2: Neonatal pneumonia with bilateral opacities, air bronchograms, and pleural effusions is apparent. Case 3: Respiratory distress syndrome is characterized by diffuse, bilateral, ground glass fields with air bronchograms secondary to diffuse atelectasis. Case 4: Meconium aspiration syndrome causes a chemical pneumonitis, partial airway obstruction, and a localized surfactant inactivation that leads to areas of hyperinflation mixed with diffuse, patchy infiltrates radiographically.*

Source: https://www.ncbi.nlm.nih.gov/pmc/articles/PMC4533247/bin/pedsinreview.20140029f1.jpg.

The respiratory rate is 74 breaths per minute, and the pulse rate is 165 beats per minute. Her physical examination results are normal, except for an increased effort of breathing. Figure 7.1 displays the chest radiograph. For 36 hours, she needs to receive extra oxygen through a nasal cannula at a fraction of inspired oxygen (FiO_2) of 0.3. From room air, she weans herself off. She is breathing at a rate of 35 breaths per minute and is not experiencing any difficulty breathing.

7.3.4.1.1. Transient Tachypnea of the Newborn

Infants born full term or late preterm may exhibit early respiratory distress due to retained fetal lung fluid syndrome, or TTN. Because of poor fetal lung fluid clearance, TTN frequently results in respiratory distress in newborns. Air sacs and airspaces in a fetus are normally filled with fluid. It is necessary to remove this fluid from the alveolar airspaces in order for postnatal gas exchange to take place effectively. Fluid is removed from the lungs and fluid absorption takes place due to a reversal of the chloride and fluid-secreting channels in the lung epithelium late in gestation and just before birth. Retained fetal lung fluid is more likely in cases of preterm delivery because labor accelerates this process. Antenatal corticosteroids, uterine contractions that compress the fetal thorax, and the release of fetal adrenaline during labor—which improves lung fluid absorption—are factors that increase the clearance of lung fluid. Tachypnea and increased respiratory effort are typically seen in infants with TTN, and these symptoms last for 24 to 72 hours. On chest radiographs, fluid in the interstitium, fluid in the interlobar fissure, and occasionally pleural effusions are responsible for the excess diffuse parenchymal infiltrates (Figure 7.1). The administration offers assistance. For the purpose of preserving alveolar integrity and promoting fluid circulation, infants often need continuous positive airway pressure (CPAP) and additional oxygen. A slight respiratory acidosis and hypoxemia are frequently seen in blood gas analyzes. It is typically not necessary to use mechanical ventilation during the self-limited course of TTN. Avoiding elective cesarean sections in infants under 39 weeks gestation before labor begins is one way to take preventive action. This is due to the fact that fetal distress, premature delivery, sedation of the mother, diabetes in the mother, and delivery before 39 weeks of gestation are the most frequent risk factors for TTN. The risks associated with premature birth (37–38 weeks gestation) are widely known, but the effects of early-term delivery are less well understood. Early-term babies are more likely to need mechanical ventilation, respiratory support, and neonatal services; cesarean delivery is common in this population, which raises the risk even more. Furthermore, respiratory morbidity in infants is reduced by a single course of antenatal glucocorticoids (two doses of betamethasone) administered at least 48 hours prior to an elective term cesarean delivery. We encourage pediatricians to be aware of the increased risk of respiratory morbidity in late preterm and early-term newborns, and we recommend that elective deliveries be carefully considered before spontaneous onset of labor at less than 39 weeks' gestation, based on multiple cohort studies and expert opinion.

7.3.4.2. Case 2

After the membranes have ruptured for 22 hours, a 2.9 kg male baby is born vaginally at 39 weeks gestational age. At 1 and 5 minutes, the corresponding Apgar scores are 8 and 8. In the delivery room, he needs a FiO_2 of 0.4. He has both acrocyanosis and tachypnea. Bilaterally, coarse rales have been observed. There is a 98.6°F (37°C) temperature, a 144 beats per minute pulse, and a 65 breaths per minute respiratory rate. Even with CPAP, his tachypnea and grunting get worse, and over the course of the next six hours, he needs to be ventilated and put into an intubation due to increasing respiratory acidosis, increased work of breathing, and an increased need for oxygen. Figure 7.1 displays the chest radiograph.

7.3.4.2.1. Neonatal Pneumonia

A newborn's respiratory infections may be caused by bacteria, viruses, fungi, spirochetal infections, or protozoa. Pneumonia can strike infants nosocomially, transplacentally, through contaminated amniotic fluid, or through colonization at birth. The most prevalent type of neonatal pneumonia, perinatal pneumonia is contracted at birth. For term infants, the most common organism that causes illness is Group B streptococcus (GBS). When the causing organism is transferred transplacentally to the fetus, congenital pneumonia develops. The most prevalent pathogens include human immunodeficiency virus, varicella zoster, rubella, cytomegalovirus, adenovirus, enteroviruses, mumps, Toxoplasma gondii, Treponema pallidum, Mycobacterium tuberculosis, and Listeria monocytogenes. A newborn's increased risk of infection stems from their immature immune system as well as unique anatomical and physiological characteristics of their lungs. Pathogen removal from the respiratory system is impeded by underdeveloped respiratory cilia and a reduction in pulmonary macrophages. Additionally, newborns' cellular and humoral immune functions are compromised, and this is particularly evident in premature infants. Prematurity, maternal infection, and prolonged rupture of membranes (PROM) are risk factors for perinatal pneumonia. Infants have a greater need for oxygen and require more effort to breathe. Diffuse parenchymal infiltrates with air bronchograms or lobar consolidation are frequently seen on chest radiography. Furthermore possible are pleural effusions. Neonatal pneumonia, unlike infections in older infants and children, is a component of a generalized sepsis illness; therefore, for any infant exhibiting symptoms, obtaining cultures of blood and cerebrospinal fluid and starting broad-spectrum antibiotic therapy are advised.

The recommended initial treatment for a newborn with early-onset pneumonia or sepsis is a combination of penicillin and an aminoglycoside. Vancomycin therapy is necessary for infants who have spent more than four days in a neonatal intensive care unit due to the presence of methicillin-resistant Staphylococcus aureus and Staphylococcus epidermidis. The most common causes of infections in infants with pneumonia, whether in the nursery or at home, are respiratory viruses (like influenza, adenovirus, and respiratory syncytial virus), gram-positive bacteria (like streptococcal species and S aureus), and gram-negative enteric bacteria (like Klebsiella, Proteus, Pseudomonas aeruginosa, Serratia marcescens, and Escherichia coli). Pneumonia brought on by Chlamydia trachomatis in infants manifests later in the newborn period (4–12 weeks of age) as a staccato cough without fever or wheezing. It's also possible to have chlamydial conjunctivitis (5 to 14 days after birth). Diffuse bilateral infiltrates are seen on chest radiography, and eosinophilia is found on a complete blood cell count with a differential. In order to treat chlamydial pneumonia or conjunctivitis, systemic macrolide antibiotic therapy and ophthalmologic follow-up are necessary, even in cases where pneumonia is not present. Newborns with pneumonia need supportive care in addition to antibiotics, regardless of the causative organism. Many babies will need mechanical ventilation and CPAP in addition to extra oxygen. Vasopressors for cardiovascular support and intravenous nutrition are examples of additional supportive interventions. One frequent side effect of neonatal pneumonia is PPHN.

Based on compelling evidence, maternal GBS screening, intrapartum antibiotic prophylaxis, and appropriate postpartum follow-up of high-risk newborns are the main strategies for preventing neonatal pneumonia and its complications. It should be possible for anyone tending to newborns to identify at-risk babies and determine whether the proper intrapartum antibiotic prophylaxis has been given. They also need to be aware of which newborns need to be seen more closely, screened further, and given antibiotics right away. The American Academy of Pediatrics and the American College of Obstetrics and Gynecology have approved guidelines for the best practice management of at-risk infants, which were developed by the Centers for Disease Control and Prevention. Babies born to mothers who test positive for GBS (culture or polymerase chain reaction), those with a history of GBS bacteruria, those affected by GBS or with an unknown GBS status but delivered at a gestational age less than 37 weeks, those with a PROM of 18 hours or longer, and those with intrapartum fever (≥100.4°F [38°C]) are among those who need extra care. Intravenous penicillin (5 million units, followed by 2.5 million to 4.0 million units every 4 hours) is the recommended intrapartum antibiotic in these circumstances; cefazolin may be used for women who are penicillin-allergic and who are not at high risk of anaphylaxis. The injection should be given at least 4 hours prior to delivery. Clindamycin culture sensitivity testing should be done on women who are extremely penicillin-allergic, and clindamycin should be administered if the mother's strain is sensitive (which it is in 75% of cases). Vancomycin should only be given to women who have severe allergies and resistant strains. Promising GBS vaccines are in clinical trials and may be widely accepted by patients, but they are not yet prepared for general use. These treatments are in addition to intrapartum antibiotic prophylaxis.

After maternal GBS screening and intrapartum antibiotic prophylaxis were widely implemented, the incidence of early-onset GBS infection dropped from 1 in 8 cases per 1,000 live births to 0.3 cases per 1,000. GBS remains the most common cause of cases and deaths, though. The majority of affected term infants are born to mothers who had fever or PROM during labor but were not given antibiotics, and who may have had unknown GBS status. Some are born to mothers who were not given enough prophylactic care (using macrolide antibiotics or waiting less than four hours before giving birth). The burden of disease rises as a result of numerous missed opportunities for prevention. As a result, it is crucial to carefully manage any newborn who has any of the aforementioned risk factors after birth. Updated 2010 guidelines state that any infant exhibiting symptoms or signs of illness needs to have a complete diagnostic evaluation, which includes starting antibiotics and obtaining cultures of their spinal fluid and blood. It is advised to perform a limited evaluation (blood culture and complete blood cell count) and start antibiotic therapy for at least 48 hours if maternal chorioamnionitis is suspected but the infant shows no symptoms. A restricted assessment and 48 hours of observation are required for asymptomatic, at-risk infants who did not receive sufficient antibiotic prophylaxis; however, antibiotic initiation is not required unless a clinical suspicion develops. Infants who are at-risk and asymptomatic but have received sufficient intrapartum antibiotic prophylaxis ought to be monitored for a full 48 hours. Following these recommendations will reduce the number of cases of neonatal pneumonia and enable early diagnosis and treatment, which may avert fatalities or life-threatening consequences like PPHN.

7.3.4.3. Case 3

Due to preterm labor at 33 weeks gestation, a 1.5-kg male is delivered vaginally. At 1 and 5 minutes, the corresponding Apgar scores are 7 and 8. After delivery, the baby needs CPAP right away because they are cyanotic. He has nasal flaring, grunting, and subcostal retractions. Reduced air entry is detected throughout the lung fields by auscultation. The patient's temperature is 98.2°F (36.8°C), their pulse rate is 175 beats per minute, and their respiration rate is 70 breaths per minute. He needs a 0.4 FiO_2. Figure 7.1 displays his chest radiograph.

7.3.4.3.1. Respiratory Distress Syndrome

Respiratory diseases in premature infants are frequently caused by RDS, also referred to as hyaline membrane disease. Pregnant mothers with diabetes can also have babies with RDS. Alveolar surfactant deficiency leads to microatelectasis and low lung volumes by raising surface tension in alveoli, which is the cause of RDS. Diffuse fine granular infiltrates on radiographs are indicative of surfactant deficiency (Figure 7.1). The pathophysiology of RDS is largely dependent on pulmonary edema, which also aids in the formation of air bronchograms. The causes of excess lung fluid in premature infants are attributed to relative oliguria in the first two days after birth, epithelial injury in the airways, and decreased concentration of sodium-absorbing channels in the lung epithelium. By the fourth day following birth, infants usually show improvement in their diuresis.

RDS babies usually show symptoms in the first few hours of life, sometimes right after birth. In terms of clinical presentation, infant's exhibit marked respiratory distress accompanied by subcostal, intercostal, and/or suprasternal retractions, tachypnea, and nasal flaring. When an infant uses partial glottic closure to maintain an adequate FRC in the face of poorly compliant lungs, grunting is the result. There is a prolonged and increased residual volume that sustains the airway opening and an audible expiratory sound as the infant prolongs the expiratory phase against this partially closed glottis. Because of their cyanosis, infants with RDS need extra oxygen. In milder cases of RDS, the distending pressures of CPAP may be helpful;

however, in more severe cases, endotracheal intubation and the injection of an exogenous surfactant into the lungs are necessary. There aren't any established rules that specify when or if exogenous surfactant should be given. Certain establishments recommend giving prophylactic surfactant to premature infants born before 30 weeks of pregnancy within the first two hours of their lives. Some start with noninvasive ventilation (CPAP) and save the intubation and surfactant administration for babies who need more oxygen—between 35 and 45 percent—to keep their arterial pressure above 50 mm Hg. The administration of antenatal corticosteroids, the clinical presentation, radiographic findings, and the infant's oxygen requirements should all be taken into account when developing a management plan.

The diuresis phase mentioned earlier and the infant's start of producing endogenous surfactant are associated with the self-limiting nature of RDS, which usually improves by the age of 3 to 4 days. Prior to this, the use of mechanical ventilation is supportive and should be done so carefully to prevent lung damage from the ventilator. If surfactant treatment does not help an infant's condition, they should be examined for congenital heart disease, such as patent ductus arteriosus. The baby who receives surfactant treatment and improves at first, but then gets worse, needs to be checked for nosocomial pneumonia as well. As pneumonia and RDS can present clinically similarly and have similar findings on chest radiographs, it is appropriate to start antibiotic therapy as soon as the newborn is admitted. The incidence of RDS will decrease if premature births are avoided. Premature birth rates remain high, accounting for 11.5% of all births in 2012, despite widespread efforts to prevent them failing. Multiple randomized clinical trials strongly support the use of maternal antenatal corticosteroids to benefit infants who will deliver prematurely. In babies between the ages of 23 and 29 weeks gestation, two doses of betamethasone dramatically lower the risk of RDS, intraventricular hemorrhage, and mortality.

7.3.4.4. Case 4

Due to the baby's estimated large for gestational age status, a 4.4 kg female infant is delivered by cesarean section at 41 weeks gestational age. Thick meconium is present in the amniotic fluid. At birth, she is cyanotic, limp, and requires little effort to breathe. Apgar ratings are 2 and 7, respectively, at 1 and 5 minutes. Pulse rate is 177 beats per minute, respiratory rate is 80 breaths per minute, and temperature is 99°F (37.2°C). Physical examination findings include a barrel-shaped chest, subcostal and suprasternal retractions, nasal flaring, coarse rhonchi in bilateral lung fields, and a markedly increased work of breathing. The radiograph of her chest is displayed in Figure 7.1.

7.3.4.4.1. Meconium Aspiration Syndrome

Meconium passage before birth causes MSAF in the fetus. Meconium aspiration during pregnancy or in the first moments after birth is a risk for infants born through MSAF. A newborn diagnosed with MAS is any infant born with MSAF who experiences respiratory distress postpartum that cannot be attributed to any other cause. Meconium is made up of mucus, lanugo, bile, vernix, pancreatic enzymes, and desquamated epithelia. Since meconium can be found in the gastrointestinal tract as early as 16 weeks of pregnancy but does not appear in the lower descending colon until 34 weeks, MSAF is rarely observed in infants born before 37 weeks of pregnancy. Hypoxia or acidosis in the weakened fetus can cause a peristaltic wave and the anal sphincter to relax, which can lead to the passage of meconium in utero. Aspiration can happen while the fetus is still in the womb or right after birth when it gasps. Meconium poses a threat to newborn lungs as it moves through the airways. With a pH ranging from 7.1 to 7.2, it triggers inflammation and damage to the epithelial cells. The acidity of meconium leads to airway irritation and chemical pneumonitis, causing the release of cytokines. As meconium travels to the smaller airways, it causes partial blockages that result in air trapping and excessive air in the lungs. Initially, chest X-rays may show diffuse infiltrates throughout the lung tissue. Over time, the lungs may become overinflated with areas of collapsed lung tissue due to inactivation of surfactant by bile acids in meconium. This can present in X-rays similarly to respiratory distress syndrome with reduced lung volumes. While air leak syndromes can be present in various respiratory conditions in newborns, conditions like pneumomediastinum, pneumothorax, and persistent pulmonary hypertension are commonly seen in meconium aspiration syndrome (Figure 7.2).

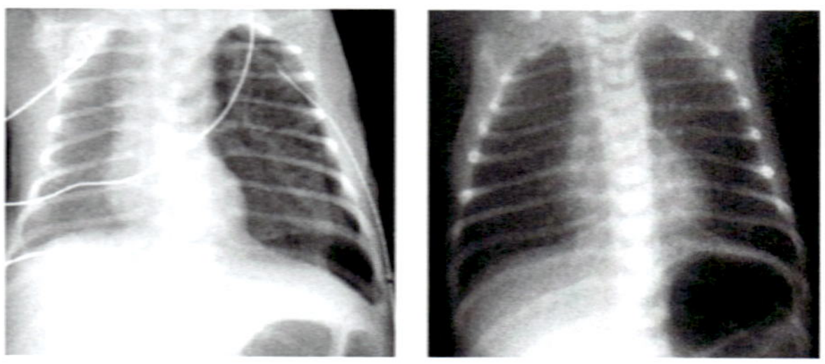

Figure 7.2. *Common complications of meconium aspiration syndrome include pneumothorax (left upper) and persistent pulmonary hypertension of the newborn (right upper) characterized by cyanosis with normal lung fields and decreased pulmonary vascular markings.*

Source: https://www.ncbi.nlm.nih.gov/pmc/articles/PMC4533247/bin/pedsinreview.20140029f2.jpg.

Strategies to support the infant are the focus of management. In severe cases, CPAP and mechanical ventilation may also be considered in addition to the need for additional oxygen. It is standard procedure to replace with exogenous surfactant, which lowers the risk of pneumothorax and the requirement for extracorporal membrane oxygenation (ECMO). Severe hypoxemia may occur as a result of MAS, which causes a ventilation-perfusion mismatch in which pulmonary blood vessels do not adequately supply ventilated alveolar units. This further raises the resistance of the pulmonary vascular system. Echocardiography reveals tricuspid regurgitation, right-to-left shunting at the patent ductus arteriosus, and flattening of the ventricular septal wall, all of which contribute to the confirmation of PPHN. Nitric oxide inhaled is a systemically inert selective pulmonary vasodilator. In severe cases of MAS, it is frequently used in conjunction with high-frequency ventilation to maintain appropriate ventilation and oxygenation and lessen the need for ECMO. Since gram-negative organisms grow in meconium, it is appropriate to start broad-spectrum antibiotic therapy. Following MAS, residual pulmonary compromise is typical. Reactive airway disease affects up to 50% of affected infants during the first six months of life, and children as old as eight years old can have persistent pulmonary insufficiency.

Preventive measures are important due to the significant morbidity associated with meconium aspiration syndrome (MAS). In the past, meconium-stained infants underwent oropharyngeal and nasopharyngeal suctioning, which was initially believed to be a successful preventive measure, following head delivery but prior to shoulder delivery. However, a sizable, multicenter randomized controlled trial conducted in 2004 discovered that neither the length of hospital stay nor the requirement for mechanical ventilation is reduced by this practice, nor does it prevent MAS. As a result, regular perineum suctioning is no longer recommended. Prior to the discovery in a sizable randomized controlled trial that intubating and suctioning vigorous infants born through MSAF increased the risk of complications, endotracheal suctioning was also a standard procedure for all meconium-stained newborns. Additional well-designed studies have confirmed this finding, leading to a change in practice guidelines in 2000. As long as the depressed infant exhibits low heart rate (less than 100 beats per minute), poor muscle tone, and no spontaneous respiratory effort, immediate endotracheal suctioning is still recommended. It is not advised to intubate and suction the restless, spontaneously breathing baby.

The MSAF is used in about 13% of live births worldwide. Notwithstanding a decline in cases over the previous ten years, 4–5% of cases will progress to MAS. Before, MAS was common in infants born after full term (births lasting more than 42 weeks). Induction of labor at 41 weeks gestation, however, appears to lower the risk of perinatal death and MAS without raising the risk of cesarean section, according to a recent meta-analysis. Consequently, a lot of obstetricians won't let a pregnancy progress past 41 weeks' gestation. Furthermore, innovations in fetal heart rate monitoring have made it possible to identify fetuses that are compromised, which has led to prompt obstetric intervention and the potential to prevent meconium aspiration in utero. There have been suggestions for a procedure to reduce the incidence of MAS, known as amnioinfusion, or transcervical infusion of saline into the amniotic cavity. Despite the fact that amnioinfusion helps fetuses in distress due to oligohydramnios, the best available data does not suggest a decreased risk of moderate to severe MAS or perinatal mortality (Drapkin et al., 2019).

A Closer Look

Sensory and Cognitive Development

Sensory and cognitive development in newborns is a dynamic process that begins at birth and progresses rapidly during the first few months of life. Sensory development lays the foundation for cognitive growth, enabling infants to interact with and learn from their environment. Each of the five senses—sight, hearing, smell, taste, and touch—plays a crucial role in this developmental phase.

At birth, a newborn's vision is quite limited. Infants can see only about 8 to 12 inches away, which is roughly the distance to a caregiver's face during feeding. This proximity allows newborns to focus on faces, which they find particularly engaging due to the high-contrast features. Over the first few months, their visual acuity improves, enabling them to track moving objects and recognize familiar faces. The ability to perceive depth and color also develops gradually, enhancing their interaction with the world.

Hearing is well-developed at birth, allowing newborns to recognize and respond to familiar sounds, such as their mother's voice, which provides comfort and security. This auditory recognition is crucial for early bonding and social interaction. Newborns are particularly attuned to high-pitched voices and will often quiet down when spoken to gently. They can also distinguish between different sounds, which lays the groundwork for language acquisition.

The senses of smell and taste are also highly developed in newborns. They can recognize their mother's scent, which is associated with feeding and comfort. This olfactory recognition helps in establishing early bonding. Newborns show a preference for sweet tastes, which is why they readily accept breast milk or formula. This preference is an evolutionary trait that encourages feeding and nutrition. Touch is perhaps the most developed sense at birth. Newborns respond positively to gentle handling and skin-to-skin contact, which is vital for emotional and physical comfort. Touch plays a critical role in early bonding, as well as in the development of motor skills and spatial awareness. Through touch, infants begin to explore their environment, learning about textures, shapes, and the physical properties of objects. Cognitive development in newborns is closely tied to these sensory experiences. Cognitive growth in this stage is marked by the development of basic concepts such as object permanence—the understanding that objects continue to exist even when they are out of sight. This concept typically begins to develop around the age of four to seven months. Initially, newborns rely on reflexive actions, but they gradually start to exhibit more purposeful behaviors as they learn from their sensory experiences.

Interaction with caregivers is crucial for cognitive development. Talking, singing, and reading to newborns, even though they do not yet understand the words, stimulates brain development and language acquisition. The repetition of sounds and words helps infants begin to recognize patterns, which is a fundamental aspect of cognitive growth. Moreover, social interactions help newborns develop emotional regulation and social awareness, laying the groundwork for future social skills.

Summary

- A newborn infant, often referred to as a neonate, is a child within the first 28 days of life, a critical period characterized by rapid physiological adjustments and developmental changes.
- Feeding is another critical aspect of newborn care. Breastfeeding is highly recommended due to the nutritional and immunological benefits of breast milk, which is tailored to the infant's needs and provides antibodies that help protect against infections.
- A newborn's shoulders and hips are wide, the abdomen protrudes slightly, and the arms and legs are relatively long with respect to the rest of the body.
- The way to measure a baby's length is to lay the baby down and stretch a measuring tape from the top of the head to the bottom of the heel.
- The umbilical cord of a newborn is bluish-white in color. After birth, the umbilical cord is normally cut, leaving a 1–2 inch stub.
- Infants cry as a form of basic instinctive communication. A crying infant may be trying to express a variety of feelings including hunger, discomfort, overstimulation, boredom, wanting something, or loneliness.
- Caregivers of an infant are advised to pick up on the infant's facial expressions and mirror them. Reproducing and empathizing with their facial expressions enables infants to experience effectiveness and to recognize their own actions more easily
- The behavior of a newborn infant is a fascinating and complex interplay of reflexes, sensory responses, and early developmental processes. Understanding these behaviors can help caregivers meet the infant's needs and promote healthy development.

References

1. Ansong-Assoku, B., Shah, S. D., Adnan, M., & Ankola, P. A. (2023). Neonatal jaundice. In *StatPearls*. StatPearls Publishing. Retrieved from: https://www.statpearls.com (accessed on 6 September 2024).
2. Araki, S., & Shirahata, A. (2020). Vitamin K deficiency bleeding in infancy. *Nutrients, 12*(3). https://doi.org/10.3390/nu12030814.
3. Asakura, H. (2004). Fetal and neonatal thermoregulation. *Journal of Nippon Medical School, 71*(6), 360–370. https://doi.org/10.1272/jnms.71.360.
4. Blue, G. M., Kirk, E. P., Sholler, G. F., Harvey, R. P., & Winlaw, D. S. (2012). Congenital heart disease: Current knowledge about causes and inheritance. *Medical Journal of Australia, 197*(3), 155–159. https://doi.org/10.5694/mja12.10126.
5. Budts, W., Gewillig, M., & Van de Werf, F. (2003). Left-to-right shunting in common congenital heart defects: Which patients are eligible for percutaneous interventions? *Acta Cardiologica, 58*(3), 199–205. https://doi.org/10.2143/AC.58.3.2005551.
6. Drapkin, Z., Franchek-Roa, K., Srinivas, G. L., Buchi, K. F., & Miescier, M. J. (2019). Is my baby normal? A review of seemingly worrisome but normal newborn signs, symptoms and behaviors. *American Journal of Emergency Medicine, 37*(6), 1153–1159. https://doi.org/10.1016/j.ajem.2019.01.025.

7. Dubay, K. S., & Zach, T. L. (2023). Newborn screening. In *StatPearls*. StatPearls Publishing. Retrieved from: https://www.statpearls.com (accessed on 6 September 2024).
8. Garbar, V., & Newton, B. W. (2023). Anatomy, abdomen and pelvis: Falciform ligament. In *StatPearls*. StatPearls Publishing. Retrieved from: https://www.statpearls.com (accessed on 6 September 2024).
9. Ginglen, J. G., & Doyle, M. Q. (2023). Immunization. In *StatPearls*. StatPearls Publishing. Retrieved from: https://www.statpearls.com (accessed on 6 September 2024).
10. Griese, M. (1999). Pulmonary surfactant in health and human lung diseases: State of the art. *European Respiratory Journal, 13*(6), 1455–1476. https://doi.org/10.1034/j.1399-3003.1999.13c26.x.
11. Hand, I., Noble, L., & Abrams, S. A. (2022). Vitamin K and the newborn infant. *Pediatrics, 149*(3). https://doi.org/10.1542/peds.2021-052915.
12. Hillman, N. H., Kallapur, S. G., & Jobe, A. H. (2012). Physiology of transition from intrauterine to extrauterine life. *Clinical Perinatology, 39*(4), 769–783. https://doi.org/10.1016/j.clp.2012.08.003.
13. Jain, L., & Eaton, D. C. (2006). Physiology of fetal lung fluid clearance and the effect of labor. *Seminars in Perinatology, 30*(1), 34–43. https://doi.org/10.1053/j.semperi.2006.01.005.
14. Kelly, D. H., Stellwagen, L. M., Kaitz, E., & Shannon, D. C. (1985). Apnea and periodic breathing in normal full-term infants during the first twelve months. *Pediatric Pulmonology, 1*(4), 215–219. https://doi.org/10.1002/ppul.1950010406.
15. Kondamudi, N. P., Krata, L., & Wilt, A. S. (2023). Infant apnea. In *StatPearls*. StatPearls Publishing. Retrieved from: https://www.statpearls.com (accessed on 6 September 2024).
16. LaFranchi, S. H., & Austin, J. (2007). How should we be treating children with congenital hypothyroidism? *Journal of Pediatric Endocrinology and Metabolism, 20*(5), 559–578. https://doi.org/10.1515/JPEM.2007.20.5.559.
17. Lidell, M. E. (2019). Brown adipose tissue in human infants. *Handbook of Experimental Pharmacology, 251*, 107–123. https://doi.org/10.1007/164_2018_223.
18. Ovalı, F. (2020). Molecular and mechanical mechanisms regulating ductus arteriosus closure in preterm infants. *Frontiers in Pediatrics, 8*, 516. https://doi.org/10.3389/fped.2020.00516.
19. Remien, K., & Majmundar, S. H. (2023). Physiology, fetal circulation. In *StatPearls*. StatPearls Publishing. Retrieved from: https://www.statpearls.com (accessed on 6 September 2024).
20. Sidhu, P. S., & Lui, F. (2023). Embryology, ductus venosus. In *StatPearls*. StatPearls Publishing. Retrieved from: https://www.statpearls.com (accessed on 6 September 2024).
21. Yadav, S., Lee, B., & Kamity, R. (2023). Neonatal respiratory distress syndrome. In *StatPearls*. StatPearls Publishing. Retrieved from: https://www.statpearls.com (accessed on 6 September 2024).

Chapter 8

ABNORMAL LABOR

Contents

Introduction

Dystocia, another name for abnormal labor, is the term used to describe any circumstance in which the natural course of labor is impeded, resulting in challenges during delivery. This can happen for a number of reasons, such as problems with the mother, the child, or the birthing environment. In order to ensure a safe delivery, abnormal labor frequently necessitates medical intervention and puts the mother and baby at risk. An insufficient number of uterine contractions is a common cause of abnormal labor. If these contractions are weak or erratic, labor may stall. These contractions are what force the baby through the birth canal. This may be the result of things like hormonal imbalances, tiredness in the mother, or overuse of painkillers that prevent contractions from progressing naturally. In these situations, medical interventions like oxytocin augmentation or assisted delivery methods like forceps or vacuum extraction might be required to make the birth easier.

One of the factors that can lead to abnormal labor is when the fetus is in a malposition or presentation. It is best for the baby to be head-down in the uterus, facing the mother's back. If the baby is in a breech position (feet or buttocks first) or laying sideways (transverse position), labor may become prolonged or blocked. In some cases, techniques like external cephalic version or a cesarean section may need to be performed to manually turn the baby and ensure a safe delivery.

Dystocia can also result from abnormalities in the mother's pelvis. Labor complications can arise from an obstruction in the baby's path through the birth canal, such as a narrow pelvis or an abnormal shape. In such circumstances, the mother and the unborn child may need to be carefully monitored and may require surgical intervention, such as a cesarean delivery. Atypical labor can also be more likely in women with health conditions like diabetes, hypertension, or obesity. These ailments may make it more difficult for the mother to endure labor or raise the possibility of problems like uterine rupture, fetal distress, or macrosomia (large baby).

Abnormal labor can also be caused by psychological factors, such as fear, anxiety, or traumatic experiences in the past. These factors can interfere with the normal progression of contractions and make it difficult for the mother to relax and cooperate during childbirth. Emotional support, assurance, and pain management methods like hypnobirthing or relaxation exercises can help reduce these problems and facilitate a more seamless labor experience. Numerous factors, such as insufficient contractions, fetal malposition, pelvic abnormalities, maternal health conditions, and psychological factors, can cause abnormal labor. It is crucial to identify dystocia as soon as possible and treat it appropriately to protect the mother and child during childbirth. Effective risk management and timely interventions by healthcare providers can help ensure a successful delivery outcome.

Orientation and Directional Terms

Terms	Definition	Illustration
Hormonal	A hormonal imbalance happens when you have too much or too little of one or more hormones — your body's chemical messengers.	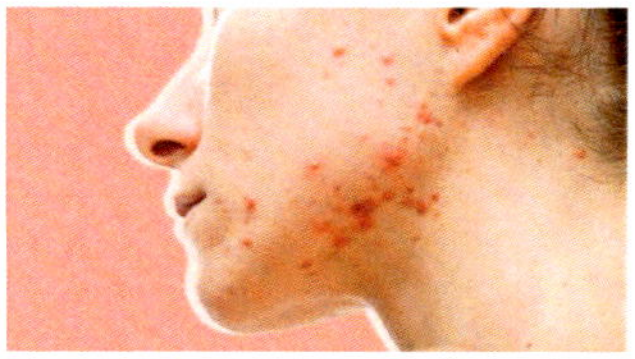
Macrosomia	Macrosomia is an obstetric condition associated with other potentially life-threatening complications to both the mother and the fetus.	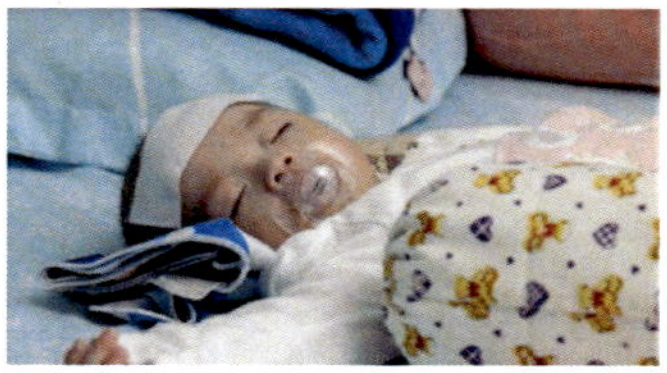
Hypnobirthing	Hypnobirthing is a method of pain management that can be used during labor and birth.	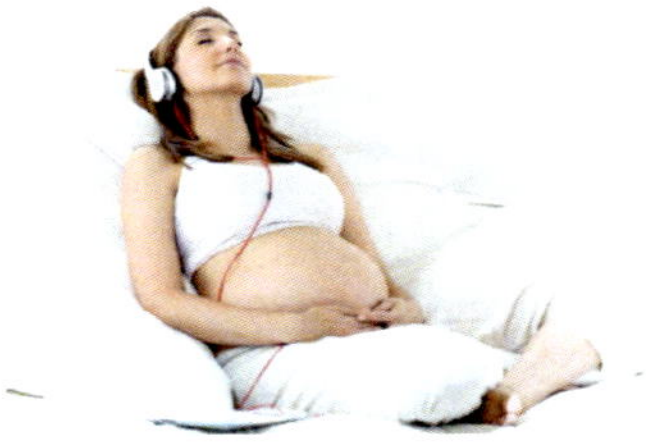
Malpresentation	Malpresentation is when your baby is not facing head-first down the birth canal as birth approaches.	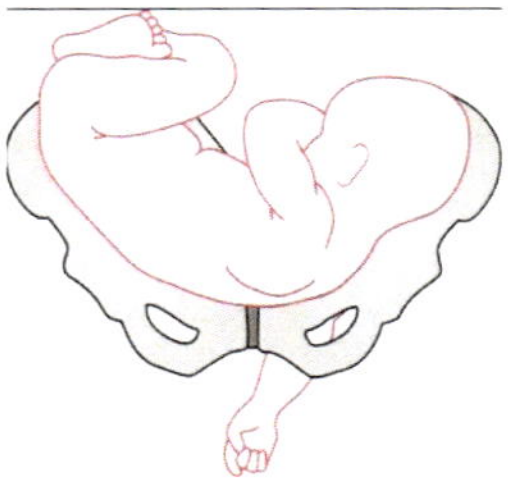
Dystocia	Dystocia is an abnormal or difficult childbirth or labor. Dystocia may arise due to incoordinate uterine activity, abnormal fetal lie or presentation, or absolute or relative cephalopelvic disproportion.	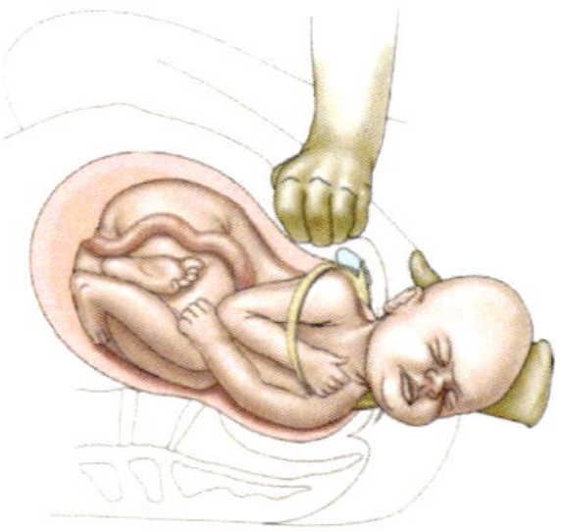

8.1. Basic Concept of Malpresentation

The term "malpresentation" during childbirth refers to the fetus's abnormal positioning inside the uterus, which can cause issues with labor and delivery. A baby should ideally make the vertex presentation, which is when it presents head-first with its chin tucked into its chest. When the baby is not in this ideal position, malpresentation happens, which raises the possibility of obstructed labor and birth-related injuries.

The transverse lie is another form of malpresentation in which the baby is not positioned vertically across the uterus, but rather horizontally. The baby cannot descend through the birth canal due to this presentation, so emergency medical attention is required. Transverse lies have the potential to cause uterine rupture, protracted labor, or fetal distress if they are not promptly corrected. To enable safe delivery, techniques like cesarean sections or external cephalic versions—in which the infant is manually turned onto the mother's abdomen so that it is head-down—might be necessary.

Less common malpresentations during childbirth include the face presentation, where the baby's face comes out first instead of the head, and shoulder presentation, where the baby is positioned sideways in the birth canal. These positions increase the risk of birth injuries like facial bruising or shoulder dystocia, a situation where the baby's shoulder gets stuck behind the mother's pubic bone during delivery, necessitating immediate medical attention to avoid complications.

Factors that can lead to malpresentation include abnormalities in the mother's pelvis, such as pelvic tumors or a contracted pelvis, as well as issues related to the amount of amniotic fluid or the position and size of the placenta. Fetal anomalies or genetic predispositions can also play a role in determining the likelihood of malpresentation.

Careful management of the challenges posed by malpresentation during childbirth is necessary to ensure a safe delivery for both the mother and the baby. Appropriate medical interventions, comprehensive fetal assessment, and prompt identification of malpresentation are essential for improving outcomes and lowering the risk of problems brought on by aberrant fetal positioning. It is imperative that expectant mothers and healthcare professionals work closely together to address any concerns and decide on the best delivery plan.

8.1.1. Dystocia

Dystocia is also a common problem in guinea pigs and the most common cause of perinatal mortality. Guinea pigs give birth to one to two large precocious pups per litter; in fact, female guinea pigs may gain up to 60% of their body weight during gestation. One common treatment for incoordinate uterine activity is oxytocin. But dystocia-complicated pregnancies frequently result in assisted deliveries, such as ventouses, forceps, or, more frequently, cesarean sections. Fetal death, respiratory depression, hypoxic ischemic encephalopathy, and brachial nerve damage are among the known risks associated with dystocia. Shoulder dystocia is a particular type of dystocia in which the infant's anterior shoulder either cannot pass below the pubic symphysis or requires substantial manipulation in order to do so. Another type of optician is a prolonged second stage of labor, in which the mother's cervix has not fully dilated and the fetus has not been delivered within three hours. Synonyms for challenging labor include abnormal labor, dysfunctional labor, difficult labor, and difficult childbirth.

A condition called labor dystocia, or obstructed labor, occurs when the baby is unable to emerge from the pelvis during childbirth. It's a dangerous illness that can cause issues for the mother as well as the unborn child. It is a reasonably common labor complication that affects approximately 10% of women worldwide. Dystocia is a condition where the normal progression of childbirth is hindered, resulting in difficulties during the delivery process. It is also referred to as difficult or prolonged labor. It can happen for a number of reasons pertaining to the mother, the child, or both, and frequently calls for medical attention to guarantee the mother's and the child's safety.

Ineffective contractions of the uterus are one of the main causes of dystocia. The uterus contracts rhythmically during labor in order to force the baby through the birth canal. On the other hand, labor may stall and become prolonged if these contractions are weak, irregular, or insufficient in strength. Ineffective contractions can be caused by a number of things, including maternal tiredness, dehydration, or the use of specific medications. To advance labor, medical procedures like oxytocin augmentation—which is giving synthetic oxytocin to induce stronger contractions—might be required.

Inappropriate fetal positioning is another frequent cause of dystocia. The baby should ideally be facing the mother's back and positioned head-down in the uterus. However, labor may become obstructed if the baby is positioned transversely, or sideways, or breech, with the feet or buttocks first. It might be necessary to perform a cesarean section or adjust the fetal position using methods like external cephalic version in order to facilitate delivery.

Dystocia may also be caused by the mother's abnormal pelvis. A baby may have difficulty passing through the birth canal due to a narrow pelvis or other abnormalities in the pelvic structure, which could cause complications during labor. Interventions like cesarean delivery might be required in these situations to guarantee a safe delivery for the mother and the child.

Maternal health issues like diabetes, hypertension, or obesity can also cause dystocia because they can impede the course of labor and raise the possibility of complications. Psychological elements like anxiety, fear, or traumatic past experiences can also obstruct labor's normal course and result in dystocia.

In order to effectively manage dystocia, it is usually necessary to closely monitor both the mother and the infant and to act quickly to address any potential complications. This could involve methods to induce contractions, adjustments to the fetal position, or surgical procedures like cesarean sections. For the purpose of promoting a safe delivery outcome, expectant mothers and healthcare providers must work closely together to ensure that the right interventions are implemented. A safe delivery for both the mother and the child is ensured by careful management of dystocia, a difficult condition that can result from a variety of factors. Timely identification of dystocia and suitable medical interventions are crucial for improving results and lowering the likelihood of complications related to challenging labor.

8.1.1.1. Causes

Labor dystocia can be caused by several factors, including:

- **Fetal Malpresentation**: This means that the baby is not in the optimal position for delivery, such as breech or face presentation.
- **Cephalopelvic Disproportion (CPD)**: This means that the baby's head is too large to fit through the mother's pelvis.
- **Uterine Inertia:** This is when the uterus does not contract strongly

enough to dilate the cervix and push the baby through the birth canal.

- **Cervical Dystocia**: This is when the cervix does not dilate properly.

Other factors include multiple gestation (twins or triplets), maternal obesity, and gestational diabetes.

8.1.1.2. Symptoms

The main symptom of labor dystocia is a prolonged or difficult labor. Other symptoms may include:

- Slow or no dilation of the cervix
- Weak or infrequent uterine contractions
- Fetal distress (such as a decrease in heart rate)
- Painful contractions that do not produce progress

8.1.1.3. Complications

Labor dystocia can lead to many complications for both the mother and the baby, including:

- **Maternal Complications**: such as postpartum hemorrhage, infection, and uterine rupture.
- **Fetal Complications**: such as hypoxia (lack of oxygen), birth injury, and stillbirth.

8.1.1.4. Diagnosis

During labor, labor dystocia is typically identified through monitoring the mother's contractions, the baby's heart rate, and the dilation progress of the cervix. If the labor does not progress as expected, a healthcare provider may conduct a vaginal exam to determine the underlying cause of the dystocia.

8.1.1.5. Treatment

The treatment for labor dystocia will vary depending on the underlying cause. Sometimes, the healthcare provider can manually reposition the baby for a smoother delivery. If the baby is too big for the mother's pelvis, a cesarean section might be required.

8.1.2. Role of a Physiotherapist in Relation to Labor Dystocia

When it comes to labor dystocia, physiotherapists can be an invaluable part of the multidisciplinary healthcare team. They can help women manage pain and accelerate the course of labor, as well as offer them information and support before, during, and after labor.

Here are some of the ways that physiotherapists can help with labor dystocia:

- **Education**: Physiotherapists can educate women about the different causes and signs of labor dystocia. They can also teach women about different positions and techniques that can help to manage pain and improve the progression of labor.
- **Pain Management:** Physiotherapists can use a variety of techniques to help manage pain during labor, such as massage, acupressure, and heat therapy. They can also teach women about relaxation techniques and breathing techniques that can help to reduce pain and anxiety.
- **Positioning:** Physiotherapists can help women to find positions that are comfortable and that help to promote the progression of labor. They can also teach women about different positions that can be used to manage pain and avoid complications.
- **Movement:** Physiotherapists can help women to move around during labor, which can help to improve the progression of labor and reduce the risk of complications. They can also teach women about different exercises

that can be used to manage pain and improve their overall well-being.

- **Postpartum Care**: Physiotherapists can also provide postpartum care to women who have experienced labor dystocia. They can help women to manage pain, improve their mobility, and recover from any injuries that may have occurred during labor.

8.1.3. Cephalo Pelvic Disproportion

When a mother's pelvis is not proportionately large for the size of her baby's head, it is known as cephalopelvic disproportion (CPD), which can make it difficult or impossible for the baby to pass through the birth canal during labor. This imbalance raises the possibility of problems for the mother and the unborn child by causing protracted or obstructed labor.

During childbirth, the baby must pass through the pelvis, which is a bony structure. It is made up of multiple bones joined together by joints and ligaments to form a strong yet flexible structure. Women's pelvises can differ in size and shape; while most can allow a baby's head to pass through during labor, some may have pelvises that are too small or malformed to allow for a safe vaginal delivery.

CPD can result from various factors, including:

1. **Maternal Pelvis Abnormalities**: Structural abnormalities in the pelvis, such as a contracted or android (heart-shaped) pelvis, can restrict the passage of the baby's head. This can be due to genetic factors, pelvic injuries, or developmental anomalies.
2. **Fetal Macrosomia**: When the baby is larger than average (macrosomic), particularly in relation to the size of the mother's pelvis, it can increase the risk of CPD. Factors contributing to macrosomia include maternal diabetes, excessive maternal weight gain, or genetics.
3. **Malpresentation**: If the baby is not in the optimal position for delivery, such as being in a breech or transverse position, it can exacerbate the challenge of CPD by presenting a larger fetal part to pass through the pelvis.
4. **Previous Pelvic Surgery**: Surgical procedures involving the pelvis, such as pelvic fractures or previous cesarean sections, can alter pelvic dimensions and increase the likelihood of CPD in subsequent pregnancies.

A variety of clinical evaluations, including pelvic exams and ultrasound measurements of the baby's size and position, are commonly used to diagnose CPD. The degree of the disproportion, the stage of labor, and the general health of the mother are some of the variables that affect how CPD is managed. In certain instances, a cesarean delivery may be advised in order to reduce the possibility of complications from vaginal delivery, such as protracted labor, fetal distress, or birth injuries. Despite being relatively uncommon, CPD is nevertheless a major concern in obstetrics because it can result in serious complications during childbirth. To guarantee the best possible outcomes for the mother and the unborn child, CPD must be identified and managed with the help of early detection, appropriate prenatal care, and close monitoring during labor.

8.1.4. Cardiotocograph Findings

A cardiotocograph (CTG) is a monitoring tool used to measure uterine contractions and the fetal heart rate (FHR) during pregnancy and labor. It offers important details regarding the baby's health and the status of labor. In order to guarantee a safe delivery for both the mother and the child, the results of a cardiotocograph interpretation are essential for informing clinical decisions and interventions.

The key findings from a cardiotocograph include:

1. Fetal Heart Rate (FHR) Patterns:

- **Baseline Fetal Heart Rate:** This is the average heart rate of the fetus over a 10-minute period. A normal baseline FHR typically ranges between 110 and 160 beats per minute (bpm). Deviations from this range may indicate fetal distress or other underlying issues.
- **Variability:** Variability refers to the fluctuations in the fetal heart rate around the baseline. It is an important indicator of fetal well-being, with moderate variability considered reassuring. Absent or decreased variability may suggest fetal compromise.
- **Accelerations:** Accelerations are transient increases in the fetal heart rate, typically associated with fetal movement or sympathetic nervous system activity. They are a reassuring sign of fetal well-being.
- **Decelerations:** Decelerations are temporary decreases in the fetal heart rate. They can be classified as early, late, or variable depending on their relationship to uterine contractions. Late or variable decelerations may indicate fetal hypoxia and require further evaluation.

2. Uterine Contractions:

- **Frequency:** This refers to the number of contractions occurring within a specified time frame, usually measured in minutes.
- **Duration:** Duration indicates how long each contraction lasts, typically measured in seconds.
- **Strength:** The strength of uterine contractions can be assessed subjectively by palpation or objectively using intrauterine pressure catheters. Strong, regular contractions are necessary for effective labor progression.

Clinical judgment and consideration of several variables, such as gestational age, maternal and fetal conditions, and labor stage, are necessary when interpreting the results of a cardiotocograph. Unusual FHR patterns or contractions may indicate the need for additional testing, which may include fetal ultrasound, fetal scalp blood collection, or emergency procedures like cesarean delivery. All things considered, cardiotocography is essential for tracking fetal health and directing obstetric care choices throughout pregnancy and labor. To interpret cardiotocograph results and ensure the best possible outcomes for mother and child, close collaboration between healthcare providers and expectant mothers is necessary.

8.1.5. Categorization of Cardiotocography – Category

A pregnancy monitoring technique called cardiotocography (CTG) is used to measure the fetal heart rate and the force of the uterine contractions. Healthcare practitioners can detect possible fetal distress and make prompt clinical decisions with the aid of the CTG categorization. Based on recommendations from groups such as the American College of Obstetricians and Gynecologists (ACOG), the National Institute for Health and Care Excellence (NICE), and the International Federation of Gynecology and Obstetrics (FIGO), the categories can be broadly categorized.

- **FIGO Classification**
1. **Normal (Reassuring)**
   - **Baseline Fetal Heart Rate (FHR)**: 110–160 bpm
   - **Variability**: 5–25 bpm
   - **Accelerations**: Present (≥15 bpm for ≥15 seconds)
   - **Decelerations**: None or early decelerations
2. **Suspicious (Non-Reassuring)**
   - **Baseline FHR**: 100–109 bpm or 161–180 bpm
   - **Variability**: <5 bpm for 30–50 minutes, >25 bpm for 15–25 minutes
   - **Accelerations**: None over 40 minutes
   - **Decelerations**: Variable decelerations without concerning features, occasional late decelerations
3. **Pathological (Abnormal)**
   - **Baseline FHR**: <100 bpm or >180 bpm
   - **Variability**: Sinusoidal pattern, <5 bpm for >50 minutes, >25 bpm for >25 minutes
   - **Accelerations**: Absence of accelerations after stimulation
   - **Decelerations**: Repeated late decelerations, prolonged deceleration (>3 minutes)

- **NICE Classification**
1. **Normal**
   - **Baseline FHR**: 110–160 bpm
   - **Variability**: 5–25 bpm
   - **Accelerations**: Present (≥15 bpm for ≥15 seconds)
   - **Decelerations**: None or occasional variable decelerations with no concerning features
2. **Suspicious**
   - **Baseline FHR**: 100–109 bpm or 161–180 bpm
   - **Variability**: <5 bpm for 30–50 minutes, >25 bpm for 15–25 minutes
   - **Accelerations**: None for 40 minutes
   - **Decelerations**: Variable decelerations with concerning characteristics for less than 90 minutes
3. **Pathological**
   - **Baseline FHR**: <100 bpm or >180 bpm
   - **Variability**: Sinusoidal pattern, <5 bpm for more than 90 minutes
   - **Accelerations**: Absent
   - **Decelerations**: Late decelerations for more than 30 minutes, prolonged deceleration for more than 3 minutes, severe variable decelerations

- **ACOG Classification**
1. **Category I (Normal)**
   - **Baseline FHR**: 110–160 bpm
   - **Variability**: Moderate

- o **Accelerations**: Present or absent
- o **Decelerations**: No late or variable decelerations, early decelerations may be present

2. **Category II (Indeterminate)**
   - o **Baseline FHR**: Bradycardia not accompanied by absent variability, tachycardia
   - o **Variability**: Minimal, absent (without decelerations), or marked
   - o **Accelerations**: Absent after fetal stimulation
   - o **Decelerations**: Prolonged, variable with slow return to baseline, late decelerations with moderate variability
3. **Category III (Abnormal)**
   - o **Baseline FHR**: Absent variability with any of the following: recurrent late decelerations, recurrent variable decelerations, bradycardia
   - o **Variability**: Sinusoidal pattern

8.2. Reasons for Studying Abnormal Labor

Researching abnormal labor is essential for improving clinical outcomes, improving maternal and fetal health, and streamlining medical procedures. The management and avoidance of potential labor complications is the main justification. Comprehending anomalous labor enables medical professionals to promptly identify and manage conditions like protracted labor, ruptured uterus, and hemorrhage after delivery. Prompt interventions have the potential to greatly lower the likelihood of severe morbidity and mortality among mothers. Early detection of labor abnormalities is critical in order to protect the fetus from long-term neurological damage or even death due to fetal distress, hypoxia, and acidosis. Better neonatal outcomes, such as increased Apgar scores and fewer admissions to neonatal intensive care units (NICU), are ensured by improved identification and management of abnormal labor.

Moreover, evidence-based clinical decision-making is supported by the study of abnormal labor. In order to provide consistent and efficient care, healthcare professionals can create standardized guidelines and protocols by identifying patterns and risk factors linked to labor abnormalities. Additionally, by using this knowledge in risk assessment, care plans can be customized to meet the individual needs of each patient. For example, anticipating and managing potential issues more effectively can be aided by recognizing risk factors such as maternal obesity, advanced maternal age, or a history of obstetric complications. In terms of education, researching abnormal labor is essential for preparing medical professionals. To provide safe and effective care, obstetricians, midwives, and nurses need to be well-versed in the warning signs, symptoms, and techniques of abnormal labor. Their readiness is increased through simulation training based on actual cases of abnormal labor, which improves their capacity to act quickly and wisely in emergency situations. This part of education is essential for developing teamwork and communication in labor and delivery units in addition to individual competency.

From the standpoint of the healthcare system, managing costs and allocating resources requires an understanding of abnormal labor. Costs associated with healthcare can be considerably decreased by effectively managing labor, which also shortens hospital stays, minimizes the need for emergency interventions, and lowers the likelihood of long-term complications. Furthermore, more efficient resource allocation guarantees that healthcare providers have the tools necessary to address labor issues in a timely and efficient manner. This includes proper staffing and the availability of equipment.

Studying abnormal labor patterns not only leads to new treatments and technologies but also promotes innovation in the field. By investigating the causes and management of labor complications, researchers can pinpoint areas where current practices fall short and strive for improved solutions. This research fosters the creation of more advanced and minimally invasive techniques for labor management, ultimately resulting in better patient care.

It is impossible to ignore the psychosocial effects of researching abnormal labor. Better mental health outcomes can result from mothers experiencing less stress and anxiety during childbirth when labor complications are effectively managed. Furthermore, making sure the delivery process is safe and healthy has a positive effect on the family's overall wellbeing.

The study of abnormal labor has significant implications worldwide. Complications from abnormal labor are major factors in maternal and infant mortality rates in many regions. It is essential to prioritize research and education in this area to enhance global health outcomes and address healthcare disparities for pregnant women and their babies. By identifying and managing the risks linked to abnormal labor, we can make strides in lowering maternal and infant mortality rates on a global scale and securing a healthier future for both mothers and children.

8.2.1. Abnormal Labor: Diagnosis and Management

8.2.1.1. Passage—the Obstetric Pelvis

The shape of the mother's pelvis influences the positions and attitudes the fetus adopts throughout labor. The inlet, midpelvis, and outlet make up the "true" pelvis. At the pubic symphysis, the anterior wall measures about 5 cm, while the posterior wall measures about 10 cm.

- **Pelvic Inlet:** The iliopectineal lines, which run anteriorly along the pectineal eminence and pubic crest to the symphysis, bounded the pelvic inlet laterally. The sacrum at the level of the iliopectineal lines makes up the posterior boundary. The shortest path between the sacral promontory and the pubic symphysis is known as the anteroposterior diameter (obstetric conjugate). If the greatest transverse diameter is less than 12 cm or the obstetric conjugate is less than 10 cm, the inlet is typically regarded as contracted. The incidence of dystocia is significantly higher when both diameters are contracted than when just one diameter is.
- **Midpelvis:** The sacrum at the level of S3 or S4 borders the midpelvis posteriorly, and the posterior aspect of the pubis and symphysis bounded it anteriorly. The pelvic sidewalls and ischial spines form the lateral boundary. The ischial spine distance, which typically measures 10 cm or more, is the smallest diameter of the pelvis. The midpelvis has an average anteroposterior diameter of at least 11.5 cm, extending from

the inferior aspect of the pubic symphysis to the sacral hollow at the level of the ischial spines. When the interspinous diameter is less than 10 cm, midpelvic contraction should be suspected. It is considered that the midpelvis is definitely contracted when the diameter is less than 9 cm. Compared to inlet contraction, midpelvic contraction is more frequent.

- **Pelvic Outlet:** Two triangle regions that do not lie in the same plane but have a common base make up the pelvic outlet. The pubic arch forms the anterior triangle. The sacral sciatic ligaments and ischial tuberosities form the sides of the posterior triangle, with the sacrum serving as its apex. The anteroposterior diameter typically measures about 11.5 cm, extending from the inferior edge of the pubic symphysis to the tip of the sacrum. The transverse diameter, or the space between the ischial tuberosities' inner edges, is roughly 10 cm. Finding outlet contraction in the absence of midplane contraction is uncommon.
- **Contracted Pelvis:** The pelvis of the gynecoid is the most ideal for a normal delivery out of the four types of pelves: android, anthropoid, platypelloid, and gynecoid. The bony pelvis may also be impacted by additional anomalies. If kyphosis affects the lumbar region, it may be linked to a pelvis that resembles a funnel, which causes labor to stop late. Because scoliosis affects the lower back, it can result in an irregular inlet that obstructs labor. When unilateral lameness occurs, the pelvis is typically not contracted. Although the pelvis is short and wide in people with bilateral lameness, most women can give birth vaginally. The pelvis may be asymmetrical in poliomyelitis patients, who are now very rare, but most can give birth vaginally. Cesarean delivery is typically the norm in dwarfism due to a noticeable fetopelvic disproportion. Women who have previously experienced a pelvic fracture, particularly a bilateral pubic rami fracture, are more likely to have cesarean sections. Imaging pelvimetry may be useful to further assess the pelvis in the aforementioned uncommon pelvic abnormalities.
- **Soft Tissue Dystocia:** Dystocia can sometimes be caused by abnormalities in the soft tissues of the pelvis. The most frequent pelvic masses linked to dystocia are uterine myomas. They could cause the fetus to be malpresented or obstruct the birth canal. Ovarian tumors, bladder distention, a pelvic kidney, excess adipose tissue, uterine malposition, and cervical stenosis or neoplasm are among the other potential causes of upper genital tract dystocia. The following conditions can result in lower genital tract dystocia: vaginal septum, large condylomata, hematomas, neoplasms, Bartholin's or Gartner's duct cysts, partial vaginal or vulvar atresia, severe edema or inflammation.
- **Pelvimetry:** A clinician may

become aware of the potential risk of pelvic dystocia by performing a clinical estimation of the pelvis' adequacy. A 2.5-fold increase in primary cesarean sections is linked to a clinically small pelvis. The real diameters of the pelvis have a greater bearing on the labor's outcome than the pelvis's form and composition. Clinical measures of pelvic diameters include the diagonal conjugate (distance from the sacral promontory to the inferior edge of the pubic symphysis), prominence of the ischial spines, convergence of the pelvic sidewalls, angle of the subpubic arch, and sacral curvature. In general, suspicion of a contracted pelvis is increased with the conditions listed in Table 8.1.

Table 8.1. Clinical Indices that Increase the Suspicion of Potential for Disproportion During Labor

Pelvic sidewalls are convergent
Ischial spines are prominent
Diagonal conjugate is <11.5 cm
Subpubic arch angle is <90 degrees
Sacrum is flat
No descent of vertex with Valsalva or fundal pressure (Müller-Hillis maneuver)

Source: Drennan, K, Blackwell, S, et al., Glob. libr. women's med., (ISSN: 1756–2228) 2008; DOI 10.3843/GLOWM.10132.

8.2.1.2. Passenger—the Fetus

Important aspects of labor include the fetus's size, position, and presentation. The fetal position and presentation can be affected by the size, shape, and abundance of soft tissue in the pelvis. While babies that are macrosomic are more likely to experience dystocia, most abnormal labor cases involve fetuses that weigh less than 4,000 g.

Among term fetuses, the biparietal diameter (BPD), the smallest transverse dimension of the fetal skull, averages between 9.5–9.8 cm. The suboccipitobregmatic diameter, which also averages about 9.5 cm, is the shortest anteroposterior dimension. Pelvic contracture to a minor degree can be overcome by the fetal head molding. Major suture lines allow the skull bones to overlap, which can reduce the BPD by 0.5 cm without endangering the fetus. Severe molding can cause intracranial hemorrhage and tentorial tears.

Fetal scalp necrosis or skull fractures can result from prolonged, intense pressure exerted on the fetus inside the birth canal. A rectovaginal, vesicocervical, or vesicovaginal fistula may form in the mother. Fetopelvic disproportion can also result from cord prolapse, prolonged labor associated with a higher risk of infections in both the mother and the fetus, uterine rupture, postpartum hemorrhage, abnormal presentation or position, and trauma to the mother and the newborn.

8.2.1.3. Malposition and Malpresentation

Dystocia may be the cause of, or a result of, fetal malpresentation. The possibility of pelvic dystocia should be brought to the clinician's attention by nonvertex presentations. A light pinch may be used to induce a fetal hand next to the head to withdraw in compound presentations. Even more uncommon is a fetal foot next to the head, though if the pelvis is large enough, vaginal delivery might still be feasible. Transverse lie deliveries necessitate cesarean delivery, with the exception of extremely preterm cases. The average term fetus presents with a partially extended head and an occipitomental diameter of 13 points

5 cm in a brow presentation. Nuchal masses, small or large fetuses, and pelvic contraction are linked to brow presentations. Of them, two thirds automatically change to an occipital or facial presentation. Conversion by hand or with forceps is no longer recommended. If the brow presentation continues, cesarean delivery is advised, with the exception of small fetuses.

A face presentation involves a fully extended fetal head. There are roughly 1:600 deliveries per year. Brow presentations and anencephaly are associated factors. A cesarean delivery is required if the mentum (chin) remains posteriorly, as the fetal neck is unable to hyperextend any further to accommodate the pelvic curve. When mentum anterior presentations are present, vaginal delivery is an option. It is no longer recommended to convert face presentations using forceps or a manual method.

About 25% of early labors and 10–15% of active labors have the fetal occiput present posteriorly. This position is predisposed by the pelvis of the anthropoid type. A prolonged second stage, ineffective contractions, a persistent anterior cervical lip, and an accentuated backache in the mother are clinical indicators of an occiput posterior position. When occiput posterior position is uncertain based only on clinical examination, ultrasound is a valuable tool for confirmation. Regional anesthesia and insufficient voluntary effort can prevent spontaneous rotation to the occiput anterior from occurring. The baby can deliver naturally from the occiput posterior position if the posterior triangle of the pelvic outlet has enough room, but an episiotomy might be required. Rotating manually or with forceps are additional choices. The best forceps are Kielland forceps because they don't have a pelvic curve. The vertex can be rotated using the Scanzoni maneuver with traditional forceps. In modern clinical practice, forceps rotations are infrequent and call for specific training and knowledge. A persistent occiput posterior position is linked to a higher risk of vaginal deliveries via surgery and cesarean sections; spontaneous vaginal deliveries occur in approximately 25% of nulliparous women and 57% of multiparous women. Adverse neonatal outcomes such as a 5-minute Apgar score of less than 7, neonatal acidemia, birth trauma, admission to the intensive care nursery, and prolonged hospitalization of the neonate have also been linked to persistent occiput posterior position. Lower rates of cesarean sections can be achieved by manually rotating an occiput posterior fetus to an occiput anterior position. Multiparity is the main element linked to manual rotation attempts' success. Occipital posterior position raises the risk of severe perineal lacerations both with and without operative delivery attempts, which is another reason to try manual rotation from the posterior position.

Because of internal rotation, the occiput transverse position is typically ephemeral. Due to their small anteroposterior diameters, platypelloid and android pelvises might not be able to rotate normally. A cesarean delivery is required if it is thought that the transverse arrest is caused by a contracted pelvis. Should the pelvis be deemed sufficient, an attempt at a forceps rotation could be made. In cases of transverse arrest, such as uterine inertia and compromised pelvic floor muscles, oxytocin may be helpful. Asynclitism may occur if the pelvis has a noticeable sacral promontory; in this case, the sagittal suture is not oriented by the vertex in the midplane of descent. Small amounts of pelvic inlet contraction may be overcome by asynclitism of the fetal head. When asynclitism is anterior, the sagittal suture is closer to the sacrum, and the result is better than when it is posterior, when the sagittal suture is closer to the pubic symphysis. A deep transverse arrest occurs if the asynclitism is unable to overcome the contracted anteroposterior diameter.

8.2.1.4. Fetal Anomalies

The majority of anomalies that can cause disproportion are identified prior to the onset of labor thanks to the widespread use of ultrasound. One common developmental anomaly that results in dystocia is hydrocephalus. There is evidence linking a biparietal diameter of more than 120 mm to a genuine cephalopelvic disproportion. Cerebrospinal fluid may be extracted to enable a vaginal delivery if the fetus is in a fatal condition; this is an uncommon practice in contemporary obstetrics. Premature closure of the cranial sutures, or craniosynostosis, can result in distortion but is not usually associated with dystocia. Poorly prognosed encephaloceles are typically fragile and can burst during delivery. Conjoined twins that have the potential to live must be delivered via cesarean section. Hydrops fetalis, posterior urethral valves, Wilms's tumor, polycystic kidneys, ovarian and hepatic tumors, and ascites are among the abdominal masses that can result in dystocia. In order to facilitate vaginal delivery during labor, ascitic fluid and other cystic masses can be percutaneously drained. But ascitic fluid can reabsorb quickly. Although the best obstetric care for individuals with meningomyeloceles, omphaloceles, and gastroschisis is debatable, these conditions typically do not prevent labor. An undetected sacrococcygeal teratoma may be the cause of an abrupt incapacity to deliver the fetus outside of the abdomen. To provide more space for the mass to deliver in such circumstances, it might be possible to flex and deliver the legs. Another option is to perform a cesarean delivery in place of resuscitation and infant stabilization on the perineum.

8.2.1.5. Fetal Macrosomia

The literature does not define fetal macrosomia consistently. The definition that is most frequently used is birth weight greater than 4,000 g. The prevalence of babies born weighing more than 4,000 grams has been rising. Fetuses weighing over 4,000 g typically make up approximately 10% of all deliveries, while fetuses weighing 4,500 g or more typically make up 1%. Infants with macrosomia experience a three-fold rise in morbidity. They are more susceptible to brachial plexus injury, placenta previa, traumatic midforceps, asphyxia, shoulder dystocia, and fetopelvic disproportion. The head has less potential for molding because it is larger than average and more calcified. The fetal trunk's size may also play a role in dystocia and mechanical issues during delivery. Shoulder dystocia and arrest and protraction disorders are examples of labor abnormalities.

8.2.1.6. Estimation of Fetal Weight

Accurately estimating fetal weight (EFW) is a challenging task. A precise EFW would be beneficial for making important clinical decisions regarding the management of macrosomic fetuses, such as preventing shoulder dystocia, using oxytocin in abnormal labor, and utilizing midforceps. Clinical EFW is typically determined through abdominal palpation and fundal height measurements. Research shows that clinical EFW tends to estimate closer to the average birth weight, which can be problematic for extreme birth weights. Errors in estimating fetal weight in preterm and macrosomic fetuses can lead to critical obstetric interventions. Despite experience, accuracy in estimating fetal weight does not improve significantly, and there is substantial variability among examiners. Using clinically estimated fetal weight in individual cases is challenging, but it can be valuable in selecting cases for further ultrasound evaluation.

Fetal weight estimation by ultrasonography has significantly outperformed and replaced clinical estimation. Numerous researchers have released formulas for estimating fetal weight via sonography. Hadlock et al., published a formula that combines abdominal circumference and femur length that is likely the most widely used. Since then, a great deal of research has been done utilizing a variety of complex formulas, but the accuracy of sonographic EFW has not significantly improved. Ultrasound-derived birth weight predictions have a tendency to overestimate low-birth-weight infants and underestimate macrosomic infants, which is comparable to the tendency observed in the clinical EFW. To identify the macrosomic fetus, numerous mathematical models have been tested using various fetal measurements. Because different fetal parameters, statistics, populations, and definitions of macrosomia are used in the studies, comparisons become challenging. Ultrasonographic EFW has a variability of ± 15% even with technological advancements, and it can be as much as ± 20% when EFW exceeds 4000 g. Other clinical factors should be taken into consideration when using ultrasonographic EFW.

8.2.2. Power—Uterine Contractility

Uncertainty surrounds the causes of purely dysfunctional dystocia, a condition in which uterine contractility is insufficient to produce dilation and descent. Abdominal palpation requires a pressure greater than 10 mmHg above resting pressure in order to detect uterine contractions. An external electronic monitoring device is a tocodynamometer that is placed over the fundus on the abdomen. It can give information about the frequency and approximate duration of contractions, but not about their tone or intensity. One way to monitor internal pressure is by inserting a disposable pressure transducer into the amniotic cavity after membrane rupture, or by transcervically inserting an open-ended plastic cannula that is filled with fluid and connected to a pressure transducer. Estimates of the length, frequency, and intensity of contractions as well as the resting uterine tone can be obtained through internal intrauterine pressure monitoring. The uterus is not a closed fluid system when the membranes are ruptured, and the patient's position also affects intrauterine pressure, which is why the term "estimates" is used.

About every 3–5 minutes, contractions in early labor happen, and they have a pressure of 20–30 mmHg higher than resting tone. Typically, contractions in active labor occur every 2–4 minutes and have pressures between 30 and 50 mmHg above resting tone. The pressures may increase to 100–150 mmHg when pushing. In the early stages of labor, the resting pressure is 5 to 10 mmHg; later, it is 12 to 14 mmHg. The length of contractions increases from 30 to 60 seconds in early labor to 60–90 seconds in later labor, along with an increase in frequency and tone. It has been determined that contractions must occur at least more frequently than once every five minutes and develop pressure greater than 25 mmHg to qualify as minimal effective uterine contractility.

The most accurate method of obtaining information about the strength and intensity of uterine activity is through direct monitoring using an intrauterine pressure catheter. A stiff catheter guide that is inserted only slightly beyond the fetal presenting portion is a feature of the majority of commercially available systems. After inserting the pressure catheter into the uterus, the catheter guide is taken out. A mark on the catheter, which should be at the level of the introitus following insertion, can be used to determine the proper depth of insertion. The area of the fetus that is presenting should be posterior to the catheter. Anterior insertion may be attempted if the presenting part is well engaged in the pelvis, making posterior insertion unlikely. It is not recommended to insert laterally because lateral perforation can cause uterine artery compromise and all of its related problems, such as broad-ligament hematoma. Catheters currently on the market connect to the fetal monitor using a reusable cable that is specific to the manufacturer. The majority of systems include a lumen in the catheter to enable simultaneous monitoring of intrauterine pressure and amnioinfusion. The setup and calibration procedures are simple.

Numerous researchers have created objective uterine contractility measures, but none have been widely used in clinical settings. The Montevideo unit is the most basic way to estimate uterine work. The peak intensity above resting pressure multiplied by the quantity of contractions within a 10-minute period yields the Montevideo unit. A wide range of uterine work, including 95–395 Montevideo units, is involved in normal labor. The average length of each contraction over a 10-minute period multiplied by the Montevideo unit yields the Alexandria unit.

Two distinct forms of aberrant contraction patterns have been linked to functional dystocia. A hypertonic pattern is characterized by higher resting pressures, more frequent contractions, poorer coordination, and a delayed return to baseline uterine tone. Fetal malpresentation and uterine overdistention are associated with a higher frequency of this pattern. Although it is generally not advised, oxytocin has occasionally been demonstrated to transform this pattern into productive labor. The condition known as hypotonic uterine dysfunction is more prevalent and often reacts to oxytocin. The contractions occur at the same time but may be weak, infrequent, or both. It is assumed that contractions were never normally established in cases of primary dysfunction. It is hypothesized that in cases of secondary dysfunction, contractions were once strong but grew weaker as labor went on, usually after 4 cm of dilation.

8.2.3. Provider/Patient

Although absolute fetopelvic disproportion is rare, cesarean delivery is frequently performed for that indication. In order to diagnose dystocia, it is thought that the physician factor is important. A patient's attitude, the time of day, anesthesia support, the medicolegal environment, and the doctor's own education and experience can all have an impact. The nature and length of labor may also be influenced by the patient's anxiety level and pain threshold.

During labor, medications may change the contractility of the uterus. Labor inhibition has been achieved through the use of magnesium sulfate, calcium channel blockers, β-mimetics, and anti-prostaglandins. Ethanol directly depresses smooth muscle and prevents the release of oxytocin. Caffeine and theophylline may cause labors to last longer. Barbiturates have dose-related effects. Phenobarbital has minimal effect, while pentobarbital and thiopental in anesthetic doses may stop labor. The lower uterine segment is relaxed and contraction frequency is reduced by atropine and scopolamine. Tranquilizers work in different ways; high dosages typically cause labor to be delayed. Cocaine has been "marketed" as a medication that shortens labor. While there is growing evidence linking cocaine abuse to a higher risk of preterm birth, the length of labor is not considerably shortened by cocaine abuse. There is evidence that patients with dysfunctional labor may safely require fewer cesarean sections when propranolol is administered in small doses in addition to oxytocin for augmentation. The mechanism is believed to be related to propranolol's production of β-blockade.

For ten to thirty minutes, contractility may temporarily decrease as a result of epidural anesthesia. If anesthesia is administered during the latent phase, or if there is fetopelvic disproportion or malposition, this effect is significantly stronger. It may be more difficult for voluntary muscles to correct malposition. Intervention is not advised unless the second stage of labor lasts longer than three hours in a nulliparous woman or two hours in a parous woman under a regional anesthetic due to the association between epidural anesthesia and a prolonged second stage of labor. There have been reports of an increase in instrumental deliveries and malpresentations when epidural anesthesia is used. When comparing patients receiving epidural anesthesia to controls in 1989, Thorp and colleagues found that the incidence of cesarean sections for dystocia and the frequency of oxytocin augmentation were significantly higher. The use of oxytocin, gestational age, cervical dilation, and birth weight were not found to be significant confounding factors in the increased rate of cesarean delivery for dystocia. There hasn't been any evidence of an increase in cesarean deliveries from other randomized trials examining the administration of epidural anesthesia at different times of day.

The latent phase of labor is especially susceptible to the effects of drugs. While the latent phase is far more sensitive than active labor, heavy sedation may slow the dilation process and increase the risk of protraction and dilation arrest. Inhalation agents exhibit a diverse range of dose-dependent effects. Contractions are not affected by nitrous oxide, but they are strongly inhibited by halothane and other halogenated substances. Subjecting 50 μg of nitroglycerin intravenously causes uterine relaxation that happens quickly and deeply. In order to enable internal podalic version of a second twin, delivery of an entrapped breech head, or manual placenta removal, halothane and nitroglycerin can be used to relax the uterus. However, there is a chance that using these medications will result in postpartum hemorrhage. The onset of spontaneous labor is closely correlated with the cervical score. Myometrial oxytocin sensitivity may be reflected in the condition of the cervix. Encouraging cervical ripening may soften the cervix and make the myometrium more sensitive. Numerous substances have been studied and discovered to cause cervical ripening with differing degrees of success. These substances include relaxin and estradiol gels, Foley catheters, Laminaria tents, and prostaglandin E_2 and $F_{2\alpha}$ through different pathways. Other more recent induction agents may induce and stimulate labor as well as cervical ripening. One such agent is misoprostol, an analog of prostaglandin E_1.

8.2.3.1. Obesity

Obesity is predicted to become a major cause of labor dystocia due to rising obesity rates in the developed world and the United States. There is strong evidence that dystocia is predisposed to obesity. It has been demonstrated that being overweight prior to pregnancy increases the risk of cesarean delivery in nulliparous women giving birth to singletons at term, especially in extremely obese women. According to more research, there is a significant increase in the risk of primary cesarean section for women whose BMI rises from the normal range to the obese range between their first two pregnancies (i.e., when they fail to lose the weight gained from the first pregnancy before getting pregnant again). The OR for women who went from being normal weight to being obese was 1.96 (95% confidence interval [CI]: 1.71–2.26–26–26). For women who went from being underweight to being obese, the magnitude of the increased risk was even higher. Crucially, women who lost weight and went from being obese to normal weight also had a 1 in 51 chance of needing a cesarean section.

8.2.3.2. Advancing Maternal Age

Given the aging of the parturient population, it is critical to recognize that older women are more likely to undergo cesarean sections. Although the exact mechanism causing this elevated risk is unknown, older women seem to have longer labors and greater rates of primary cesarean sections, both elective and non-elective (i.e., indications (breech and myomectomy).

We might soon be living in the era of customized labor curves, following the age of customized medicine. It's interesting and useful to know that labor curves can differ by ethnic group, with African Americans typically having a shorter duration of the second stage than other groups, as we continue to learn that older and obese women have different and longer labors.

8.2.3.3. Oxytocin

An octapeptide called oxytocin is produced in the hypothalamus and then sent to the posterior pituitary gland's axonal terminals. Regarding maternal plasma oxytocin concentrations during pregnancy and spontaneous labor, there is a great deal of variation in reports. During a typical labor, oxytocin is released in pulses at intervals of three to five minutes in addition to a tonic baseline release. Fetal transfer of oxytocin to the maternal side may be a significant physiological source of this release. The majority of researchers note that plasma oxytocin levels increase gradually during gestation and peak in the second stage of labor. The onset of uterine contractions appears to be facilitated by human myometrial oxytocin receptors, which reach their peak during early spontaneous labor. Most likely, the main factor influencing the uterine response to either endogenous or exogenous oxytocin is receptor concentration.

When used properly, oxytocin is a powerful uterotonic agent that can be both safe and effective. Friedman recommended using oxytocin in cases where there is no suspicion of cephalopelvic disproportion in conjunction with a secondary arrest of labor or failure of descent. For prolonged active phase disorders or prolonged latent phase disorders, many doctors also prescribe oxytocin. There is some evidence that using oxytocin to shorten labor duration improves outcomes for both the mother and the fetus. Because a diagnosis of cephalopelvic disproportion may be made sooner, this better outcome appears to hold true even in cases where it is clinically suspected. Augmentation of labor may be indicated generally when there is dysfunctional labor and vaginal delivery is judged possible by the enhancement of uterine contractions.

According to in vivo research, it takes 40–60 minutes from the start of the infusion to reach a steady-state concentration of oxytocin in plasma (and the maximal response). Oxytocin has a half-life of roughly ten to fifteen minutes in vivo. Research on the kinetics of first-order saturation in plasma oxytocin levels during continuous intravenous infusion reveals a progressive, linear, stepwise increase with each increase in the infusion rate. The infusion rate of oxytocin should begin low (0.5–2 mU/min), according to pharmacologic data, and increase arithmetically by 1–2 mU/min every 40–60 minutes. However, this rate of increase is inefficient in a significant number of patients due to individual differences in clearance rates and sensitivities resulting in varied response ranges. Clinically, in 31% of patients who needed more than 4 mU/min, this variation caused an intolerable delay in reaching an effective maintenance dose of oxytocin. The rate of infusion should be checked for hyperstimulation every 30 minutes. Term nulliparas and multiparas with dysfunctional labor were used to test this proposal. The frequency of stopping or reducing the oxytocin infusion due to hyperstimulation or fetal distress increased twofold when the oxytocin infusion rate was increased at intervals shorter than thirty minutes. It was also discovered that the most significant factor leading to a higher maximum dose of oxytocin and a real delivery delay of an average of three hours was a brief (less than thirty minutes) rate increase interval. The sensitivity of the preterm uterus to oxytocin is lower compared to the term uterus, often necessitating larger doses. Research by Theobald and colleagues found that at 32 weeks' gestation, a 2 mU/min infusion induced mild contractions, while just before, during, or after spontaneous labor, the uterus responded to 0.5 mU/min regardless of gestational age. Typically, an infusion rate of 2–8 mU/min is sufficient for successful labor induction at term. Lower doses of 5 mU/min or less have shown to improve delivery outcomes without causing hyperstimulation. It is rare for doses higher than 20 mU/min to be needed at term. Additionally, higher doses required for effective contractions are associated with lower success rates. In a study on oxytocin augmentation of labor, Seitchik and Castillo found that the majority of multiparas and nulliparas required less than 4 mU/min when starting with an initial dose of 1 mU/min and increasing by 1 mU/min every 30 minutes until a dilation rate of 1 cm/h was achieved.

Increased intrauterine resting pressure and contraction strength, velocity, and frequency are among the myometrium's oxytocic effects. Once maximal efficiency is achieved, additional oxytocin increases may lead to excessive frequency of contractions and an increase in baseline tone, which will reduce the effectiveness of the contractions and cause fetal distress. In cases where cervical dilation is insufficient but the contraction pattern appears adequate (one every 3–5 minutes), clinical experience suggests that reducing the oxytocin dosage may sometimes increase efficacy. The quantification of uterine activity is far from ideal in detecting hypocontractile labor, identifying excessive stimulation, or directing oxytocin therapy. However, the uterine contractile pattern may offer an initial assessment of response. Additional criteria for titrating oxytocin are also advised, as uterine activity varies greatly within and between individuals during normal labor. Among nulliparas who were laboring spontaneously, the initial cervical dilation rate was at least 1 cm/h, and 93% of them delivered their babies vaginally. In contrast, if the cervical dilation rate was less than 1 cm/h, 67% of patients needed forceps, vacuum delivery, or a cesarean section.

Advocates of "active management of labor" base their oxytocin dosage on the cervical dilation rate of 1 cm/h in nulliparas. According to O'Driscoll and colleagues, early routine amniotomy and oxytocin infusions, starting at 6 mU/min and increasing every 15 minutes to 40 mU/min, were included in the active management of labor for dilation rates less than 1 cm/h, as long as there was no fetal distress. Just 1 percent of the 3106 nulliparas had dystocia diagnosed during a cesarean section. A 1 cm/h rate of dilation may be a helpful guide to determine the most effective dose of oxytocin in induction or augmentation in nulliparous women, despite some asserting that this policy for oxytocin use might result in too many patients receiving oxytocin. While shorter labor times were the outcome of this active management approach in the US, the rate of cesarean sections did not decline.

Fetal heart rate response offers an additional, and possibly more suitable, basis for titrating oxytocin than does uterine contractility, particularly in the nulliparous patient. It has been demonstrated that placental venous outflow stops during contractions, but good relaxation and adequate exchange occur afterwards. Arterial inflow may cease entirely at pressures between 30 and 70 mmHg. The fetus keeps drawing oxygen from the intervillous blood, but eventually it might turn to anaerobic metabolism in order to wait for the contraction to end and for oxygen to be restored. The frequency, intensity, duration, and resting pressure of contractions all have an indirect impact on uterine blood flow. Fetal reserve varies greatly, but even in healthy fetuses, high uterine tone and frequent contractions can cause acidosis, distress, and even fetal death. More contractions are required if the power and frequency of contractions must be kept low to protect a fetus with "decreased reserve," but the patient may still be able to deliver the baby vaginally with cautious oxytocin dose titration.

If there is excessive uterine activity or fetal distress during oxytocin induction or augmentation, it might not be a pathologic condition necessitating an emergency cesarean delivery. A patient may experience less severe but more frequent contractions when they are in the supine position. Additionally, there may be a higher chance of fetal hypoxemia and less cervical dilation advancement in this position. For hyperstimulation and fetal distress, positioning the patient in a left lateral position might be the only necessary corrective action. Starting oxygen and reducing or stopping the oxytocin infusion are examples of additional actions. Rather than stopping the oxytocin dose, reducing it could rectify the abnormal pattern and avoid an unnecessary delivery delay. We advise cutting the previous rate in half or less when starting the oxytocin again.

Once labor has been established, the oxytocin dosage might be reduced. The risk of postpartum uterine atony may be reduced if oxytocin is administered continuously during labor and delivery. The uterine activity and fetal heart rate should be monitored prior to and during the induction or augmentation of oxytocin. In the current medicolegal environment, this monitoring is essential and could help determine the optimal oxytocin dosage. It's also advised to accurately record the oxytocin rate, the frequency and duration of contractions, and the tones of the fetal heart (Drennan et al., 2008).

8.3. Dystocia—Functional Definition of Labor Abnormality

In the preceding sections, the limitations of pelvimetry, EFW, and uterine contractility to predict dystocia were discussed. For clinical purposes, other means must be employed to identify dystocia.

8.3.1. Labor Graph

Caldeyro-Barcia and Friedman were pioneers in assessing labor based on functional rather than anatomic/physiologic features. They determined that the essential features of labor are cervical dilation and fetal descent as a function of time. They outlined normal labor progress and identified specific abnormal patterns, linking them to causative factors and recommending tailored management strategies (Table 8.2).

Table 8.2. Diagnostic Criteria for Abnormal Labor Patterns

Labor Pattern	Nulliparous	Parous
Protraction disorders	–	–
Dilation	<1.2 cm/h	<1.5 cm/h
Descent	<1.2 cm/h	<1.5 cm/h
Arrest disorders	–	–

Dilation	>2 h	>2 h
Descent	>1 h	>1 h

Source: Drennan, K, Blackwell, S, et al., Glob. libr. women's med., (ISSN: 1756–2228) 2008; DOI 10.3843/GLOWM.10132.

Friedman developed the "graphico/statistical" method of labor analysis in the 1950s; the doctor was advised to plot the fetal presenting part's station and the uterine cervix's dilation against time (Figure 8.1). displays an idealized labor. Depending on the method used for station, dilation can extend from 0 to 10 cm, while station can extend from −3 to +3 finger breadths or −5 to +5 cm. For stations, we advise using the −5 to +5 cm system. The diagnosis of arrest and protraction disorders is greatly aided by a graphical representation of labor (Figure 8.2). The attending doctor or nurse should note the time, dilation, and station on the labor graph at the time of each examination. It is not beneficial to construct the graph after the labor has been finished.

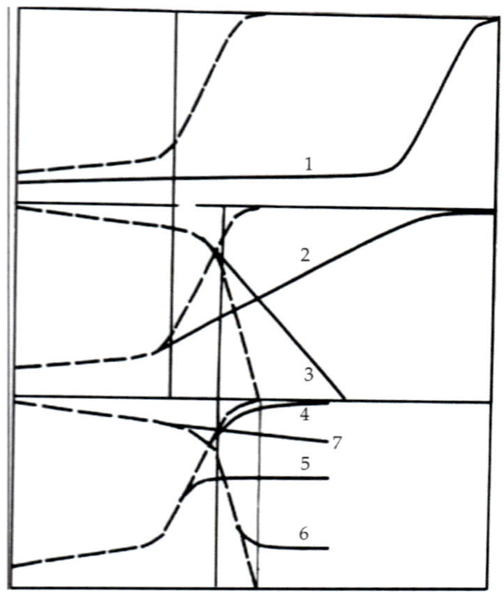

Figure 8.1. *An idealized labor pattern. The normal patterns of cervical dilation (solid line) and descent (broken line) as they are traced against elapsed time in labor. The distinctive phases of the first stage are shown. The active phase comprises the interval from the onset of the acceleration phase to the beginning of the second stage.*

Source: Drennan, K, Blackwell, S, et al., Glob. libr. women's med., (ISSN: 1756–2228) 2008; DOI 10.3843/GLOWM.10132.

The time at which regular uterine contractions begin is known as the "onset of labor," and it is represented by the number 0 on the labor graph. The patient's estimation of the start of labor (latent phase) is used since she is usually at home when contractions start. Cervical dilation typically occurs at 2 cm for both nulliparas and multiparas at the onset of labor, though it can occasionally be closed due to premature rupture of the membranes. Nonetheless, some multiparas may start labor with cervical dilations as small as 4–5 cm. Compared to multiparas, the station of the fetal presenting part in nulliparas usually occurs lower in the pelvis. While it is commonly stated that a nullipara should have an engaged fetal head when labor begins, this is often not the case. When labor begins, the presenting portion should typically be −1 in the nullipara as opposed to −1 to −2, or even marginally higher, in the multipara.

It becomes unclear how long it should be between exams once the patient has been admitted while in labor. This is a contentious topic. According to some experts, doing vaginal exams frequently raises the possibility of postpartum endometritis. Using multivariate analyzes, other authorities have proposed that the issue is not so much repeated examination as it is prolonged labor, which in turn results in more examinations. In the latent phase, we advise exams every two hours; in the active phase, we advise exams every hour. When combined with proper documentation of the examinations, this general approach helps guarantee that developing labor abnormalities are neither overlooked nor disregarded. Thousands of deliveries using this method have not resulted in any evidence of an elevated risk for infection.

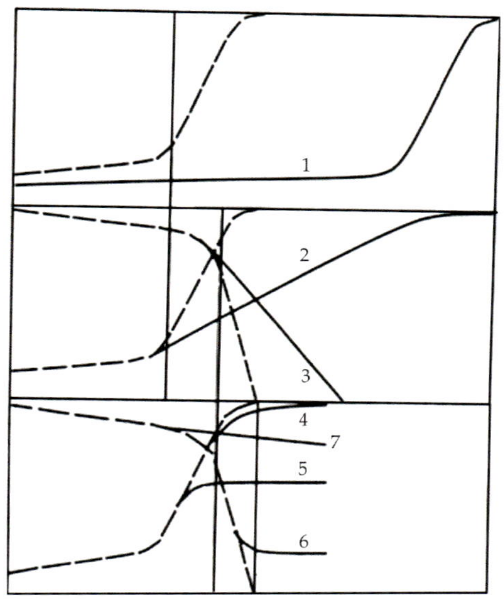

Figure 8.2. *Graphic representation of disorders of the functional divisions of labor. Cervical dilation and fetal station as the ordinate and time as the abscissa. At the top, the normal dilation curve is compared with the preparatory division abnormality of prolonged latent phase.*

Note: (1). The middle group presents the protraction disorders of the dilational division—protracted active-phase dilation (2) and protracted descent (3). At the bottom are the pathologic states of the pelvic division, including prolonged deceleration phase (4), secondary arrest of dilation (5), arrest of descent (6); and failure of descent (7). The broken portions of the curves represent mean normal patterns; the unbroken portions represent abnormal patterns.

Source: Drennan, K, Blackwell, S, et al., Glob. libr. women's med., (ISSN: 1756–2228) 2008; DOI 10.3843/GLOWM.10132.

Despite service policy, in our experience, clinicians frequently refuse to create labor graphs while the labor is progressing. In reaction to this resistance, a method has been created that permits a comparable decision-making procedure without requiring the creation of a labor graph. The only things required of the clinician are to ascertain whether labor is latent or active and to retain a few basic numerical guidelines. The patient should be classified as being in the latent phase if the cervix is less than 4 cm and the dilation is greater than l cm/h in the nullipara and 1.5 cm/h in the multipara. In the latent phase, the average dilation slope is less than 0.6 cm/h. If the cervix dilates at a rate of at least 1 cm/hr in the nullipara and 1+5 cm/h in the multipara, or if the cervical dilation is greater than 5 cm, the patient is in the active phase. Although they are not all-inclusive, the two definitions for latent and active phases are mutually exclusive. Intermediate lengthenings (i.e., from 4 to 5 cm) and slopes provide an imprecise image of the labor phase. These patients frequently move from the latent to the active phase (i.e., they are in the stage of acceleration.

The phase of maximum slope, during which there is rapid cervical dilation, comes after the acceleration phase. Ultimately, the deceleration phase is defined as a dilation of 9–10 cm (full dilation). The fetal presenting portion may not descend until 9 cm of dilation has been reached, at which point it should be actively proceeding (i.e., in terms of descent, the deceleration phase is an acceleration phase). Complete dilation marks the start of the second stage of labor.

According to traditional definitions, there are six dysfunctional labor patterns: (1) prolonged latent phase; (2) protracted active phase dilation; (3) secondary arrest of dilation; (4) prolonged deceleration phase; (5) protracted descent; and (6) arrest of descent (refer to Figure 8. 2). Certain authorities would supplement this list with the additional diagnoses of failure to descend as an anomaly distinct from arrest of descent and prolonged acceleration phase. Precipitous labor, which is typically defined as labor lasting less than three hours, is occasionally added to the list as well. However, there are only two ways that labor can be abnormal from a functional standpoint: either dilation and descent can be prolonged or arrested.

8.3.2. First Stage of Labor

8.3.2.1. Prolonged Latent Phase

Regular contractions that dilate and efface the cervix signal the start of the latent phase, which concludes with the onset of active labor. Latent phase duration depends on a number of variables. The latent phase and cervical dilation at the beginning of labor are typically inversely correlated. Likewise, the shorter the latent phase, the lower in the pelvis the fetal presenting part is at the beginning of labor. It's important to keep in mind that sedation has the potential to cause prolonged latent phase. After the effects of sedation wear off, labor typically resumes in these patients.

Prolonged latent phase is typically diagnosed after 21 hours in nulliparous women and 14 hours in multiparous women, based on standard criteria. This condition is not very common, occurring in only 3–4% of labors. Patients usually find these long intervals unacceptable, leading to maternal exhaustion. One approach is to carefully evaluate the patient as they approach 12 hours in the latent phase. If there has been progress in cervical effacement and dilation or fetal descent, oxytocin augmentation can be considered. Starting at a low dose of 1–2 mU/min and increasing by 1–2 mU/min every 30 minutes is recommended. In most cases, an oxytocin infusion of 16 mU/min or less successfully brings the patient into active labor. Prolonged latent phase has been found to be relatively harmless in epidemiological studies, but it is associated with a 2.5-fold increase in the risk of primary cesarean section. Despite this, the fetus generally tolerates prolonged latent phase well, with no significant increase in morbidity or mortality.

8.3.3. Active Phase

8.3.3.1. Protracted Active Phase Dilation

When the dilation rate is less than 1 cm/h, protracted active phase dilation should be diagnosed in nulliparas. The lower bound of normal for the multipara is 1 point 5 cm/h. A limit of 1.2 cm/h for nulliparas could be applied based on Friedman's original definition; however, in our experience, this limit might be unduly sensitive and more difficult to remember than the 1 cm/h limit.

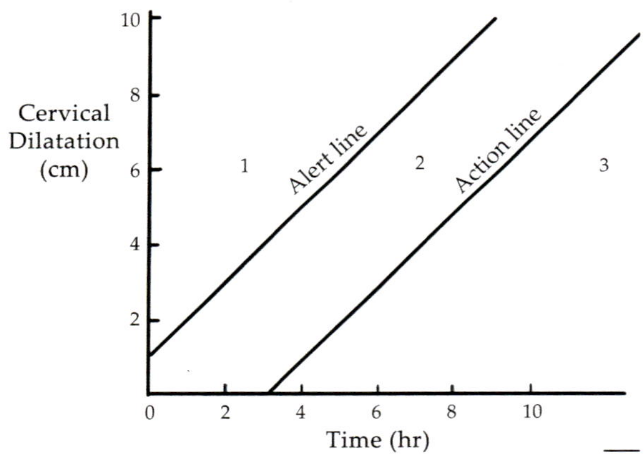

Figure 8.3. *Cervicograph for evaluating the active phase of labor.*

Note: Zone 1 represents normal labor (>1 cm/h). Zone 2 indicates the possibility of dysfunctional labor. Zone 3 indicates a need for intervention.

Source: Drennan, K, Blackwell, S, et al., Glob. libr. women's med., (ISSN: 1756–2228) 2008; DOI 10.3843/GLOWM.10132.

Furthermore, Philpott and Castle, who suggested a different and straightforward method of graphing labor progress, have validated the 1 cm/hr limit (Figure 8.3). When a patient is actually in the latent phase of labor, a common mistake is to diagnose them with a protracted active phase. Rouse et al., reported that the fifth percentile rate for nulliparas and parous women may be lower (0.5 cm/h) due to changes in the increased use of epidural anesthesia and its "slowing effect." The fact that Friedman reported on patients with "normal labor," which did not require oxytocin, while Rouse described patients with "abnormal labor," which required augmentation, could also be the cause of the lower rate of dilation (Figure 8.3). An often occurring pattern of dysfunctional labor is prolonged active phase dilatation. It appears to be linked to a mild disproportion of the cephalopelvis. Many cases of prolonged active phase dilation may have previously been referred to as primary uterine inertia or hypertonic uterine inertia, indicating some sort of uterine dysfunction, according to clinical experience with intrauterine pressure catheters. An iatrogenic factor could also be involved in this labor anomaly; lying down could reduce uterine contractility and consequently slow cervical dilation. Furthermore, even though analgesia is generally ineffective during active labor, the use of opioids has been linked in certain instances to precipitating slow dilation during the active phase. An increased risk of this labor abnormality is also linked to early epidural anesthesia, especially if the station of the presenting part is greater than −1.

Prolonged active phase dilation should be regarded as a significant risk factor for subsequent labor dysfunction. Nulliparas and multiparas may have an 8- to 25-fold increased risk of protracted descent, prolonged deceleration phase, and subsequent arrest of dilation or descent. As a general clinical guideline, when active labor starts later than usual, complications should be expected. There is little information available regarding the use of oxytocin to treat prolonged dilation, despite the fact that it occurs rather frequently.

However, there is strong evidence that the "active management of labor" is a safe and effective strategy. 552 nulliparas with singleton pregnancies who had established labor and amniotomy were compared with 533 previously delivered patients of a similar nature in a 1988 study conducted by Akoury and colleagues. Amniotomy and oxytocin augmentation, up to 40 mU/min for dilation rates less than 1 cm/h, were administered to the study group. The actively managed group experienced an almost threefold decrease in the frequency of labor lasting longer than 12 hours, from 20% to 7 percent, according to the results of this historically controlled study. The rate of cesarean births dropped from 13% to 4.3 percent, or one-third of the previous rate. The percentage of forceps operations was reduced from 29% to 19%. There was no rise in perinatal morbidity or mortality in the study group linked to these variations in surgical delivery rates.

Even though the exact cause of protraction is unknown, fetal monitoring, lateral positioning, cautious oxytocin use, and early detection of abnormal labor progress during the active phase are all reasonable strategies. The best course of action is unclear, much like the causative factors for prolonged active phase dilation. Taking into account the possibility that slight disproportion and malposition (i.e., for example, occiput posterior and occiput transverse), this can present challenges for both the doctor and the patient. A prudent course of action would be to stay away from needless anesthesia and sedation.

8.3.3.2. Secondary Arrest of Dilation

When cervical dilation has not changed for at least two hours, secondary arrest of dilation is diagnosed. This time criterion, which applies to both nulliparas and multiparas, is based in part on the degree of confidence with which digital examination can detect cervical dilation. Secondary arrest is more common with larger than smaller fetuses and with term versus preterm labors; it occurs in 5–10% of labors in most series. This anomaly happens less frequently than prolonged active-phase dilatation but more frequently than prolonged latent phase. Due to its correlation with a higher risk of cesarean delivery and an increased risk of fetal morbidity and mortality, it has been acknowledged as the most severe of the dilation abnormalities.

The correlation between fetopelvic disproportion and secondary arrest is widely acknowledged. It has been recommended that the diagnosis not be made until the cervix is dilated more than 4 cm, labor is active, and there has been no cervical change for at least 2 hours with 200 Montevideo units or more every 10 minutes. There is statistical evidence linking the development of secondary arrest to the occurrence of persistent malposition (i.e., both the persistent occiput transverse and posterior. However, it's unclear if the arrest disorder causes or results from the associated malposition.

Prolonged active phase dilation complicating nulliparous labors carries an eight-fold increased risk of secondary arrest of dilation compared to a five-fold increase in multiparous labors. This increase raises the possibility that "uterine inertia" is the cause. Neither mechanically nor electrophysiologically, however, has this situation been thoroughly examined. When compared to the information currently available regarding the cause, numerous studies have produced clearly defined findings regarding the best course of action for treating secondary arrest of dilation. The traditional indication for a "trial of labor" is a secondary arrest of dilation; this includes the diagnosis of failure to progress and the augmentation of labor with oxytocin in patients who have an arrest but no evidence of disproportion.

Following a secondary arrest of dilation, Friedman reported a primary section rate of about 40%. He hypothesized that this rate might be decreased with the right management, and later research has supported this finding. Sokol and colleagues found that 255 primary cesarean sections and 2362 vaginal deliveries resulted in a primary cesarean section rate of 25.5% following a secondary arrest of dilation. This rate was an increase of 2 to the power of 6. Bottoms and colleagues examined 4573 spontaneous, vertex, and singleton labors. In this study, 593 labors (11 percent) experienced arrest disorders. Amniotomy, oxytocin, and ambulation were all part of the "conservative" medical protocol used to treat patients with arrest disorders. It was discovered that half of the arrests ended on their own and that the other half needed to be stimulated with oxytocin. In total, 83% of the women either gave birth naturally or with minimal forceps. The rate of midforceps was raised fivefold to about 4 percent. Additionally, the rate of cesarean sections was raised fivefold to roughly 13 percent. There was no rise in low Apgar scores at 5 minutes (1.5 percent) or perinatal mortality in this series. When comparing cases treated conservatively to those delivered via cesarean section, neonatal morbidity was comparable. It was determined that oxytocin augmentation combined with conservative management could result in improved maternal and infant outcomes and a higher, albeit still low, rate of cesarean deliveries.

Cervical examinations should be performed on patients at least every two hours while they are in active labor in order to expeditiously diagnose secondary arrest. To identify early arrest, examinations that occur closer to every hour might be necessary. In cases of disorders related to secondary arrest, electronic monitoring for assessment of uterine contractions and fetal heart rate is necessary. The goal of oxytocin augmentation is to mimic normal uterine contractility during the active phase. Infusion rate is increased every 30 minutes, starting at 1–2 mU/min. Maternal and fetal status needs to be regularly observed. Little cervical dilation may occur during the first hour of augmentation; however, in certain cases, cervical dilation resumes quickly, usually resulting in a spontaneous vaginal delivery without further incident. Nonetheless, fetal descent typically occurs during the first hour, with cervical dilation starting up again after that. More than 90% of patients undergoing oxytocin labor augmentation attain a value of more than 200 Montevideo units, with 40% achieving a value of more than 300. It was previously proposed that a patient needed to exhibit a uterine contraction pattern with more than 200 Montevideo units for at least two hours in order to be diagnosed with labor arrest in active labor. If oxytocin is continued, about 60% of women who undergo labor arrest for two hours and have more than 200 Montevideo units ultimately give birth vaginally. Research suggests that extending this time to four hours can safely and effectively lower the number of patients experiencing active labor arrest.

The fetus may be assessed biochemically if there is evidence of fetal distress, but cesarean delivery is frequently required. A cesarean section may be necessary if labor does not proceed normally two to three hours after the oxytocin augmentation starts. Nonetheless, cesarean deliveries are not very common. When oxytocin is administered after waiting for up to four hours of sufficiently strong contractions, the chances of a vaginal birth increase. According to his research, a vaginal delivery was eventually accomplished by more than 60% of patients who had an arrest of active phase lasting longer than two hours. Though there was a higher risk of shoulder dystocia in his research, no brachial plexus palsies were observed. At least three out of every four patients with this complication may have a successful vaginal delivery, according to the clinician. It appears that a secondary arrest does not warrant an immediate cesarean delivery. Medical management that is conservative can yield positive results.

8.3.3.3. Prolonged Deceleration Phase

Following the phase of maximum slope, the deceleration phase is the third stage of active labor. The deceleration phase in both nulliparous and multiparous labor starts at 9 cm. Although active descent often starts earlier in active labor, it should start by the start of the deceleration phase. Engagement that doesn't happen before the deceleration phase starts (i.e., 9 cm) in nulliparas and abnormally high by the end of the deceleration phase in multiparas. In nulliparous labor, a prolonged deceleration phase diagnosis takes at least three hours, while in multiparous labor, it takes one hour. The clinician's attention should be directed more toward descent than toward dilation at this point in labor because descent should be active by this point in a normal labor and because the intervals required for the diagnosis of descent abnormalities are shorter than those required for the diagnosis of prolonged deceleration phase.

In cases where there is no dilation of 9 cm and engagement, there is a higher chance of a second-stage abnormality. Descent disorders are strongly correlated with a prolonged deceleration phase. Generally speaking, secondary arrest appears to be most closely associated with prolonged deceleration phase as a labor anomaly. It is frequently necessary to carefully augment labor with oxytocin, following the previously mentioned protocol. A prolonged deceleration phase only happens in 1–3% of labors, which is relatively uncommon. Based on clinical experience, it appears that these cases are often linked to pelvic abnormalities that can be commonly detected through clinical pelvimetry, such as persistent occiput transverse or posterior. Patients with this anomaly may experience significant molding of the fetal skull along with cervical edema. In this case, fetal heart rate decelerations happen more frequently, which increases the temptation to insert forceps through an almost but not quite dilated cervix. Refusing this impulse is necessary because there is a significant risk of severe trauma to both the mother and the fetus (Drennan et al., 2008).

8.3.4. Second Stage of Labor

When the cervix fully dilates, the second stage of labor begins. The unintervened second stage of labor is expected to last, on average, one hour for nulliparas and fifteen minutes for multiparas. There have been suggestions for "clinical limits" for second-stage durations, which indicate when the clinician should start to worry and foresee delivery issues. This clinical limit is two hours for nulliparas and one hour for multiparas; however, the clinician should become concerned if the second stage lasts longer than forty-five minutes. These deadlines are not meant to imply that delivery must occur by these dates. A maximum of two hours of the second stage was thought to be safe for the fetus by many clinicians prior to the availability of electronic fetal monitoring. This belief was supported by epidemiologic data showing that when the second stage lasted at least 2.5 hours, there was an increase in fetal morbidity and mortality in nulliparas.

8.3.4.1. Protracted Descent

When descent is occurring at less than l cm/h in nulliparous labor or less than 2 cm/h in multiparous labor, it is recommended to diagnose prolonged descent. It is true that estimating the station of the fetal presenting part is more challenging than accurately estimating dilation, but for the nullipara, this diagnosis can be made in one hour, and for the multipara, in 0–5 hours. Since treatment may require significant intervention, a careful balance between overdiagnosis and failing to diagnose prolonged descent as soon as possible should be sought. Absolute fetopelvic disproportion is uncommon; malposition and relatively mild degrees of fetopelvic disproportion are common causes of protracted descent. Epidural anesthesia is frequently used in conjunction with slow descent.

A protracted descent needs to be managed with skill and attention. It usually precedes other abnormal labor patterns, which could be signs of uterine dysfunction, significant disproportion, or both. It's debatable whether trying oxytocin stimulation makes sense in these situations. Each case must be addressed individually in the response. It is reasonable to propose that a cesarean delivery might be the best course of action if protracted descent occurs in a labor that has already been complicated by prior dysfunctional labor patterns in the presence of oxytocin augmentation.

Coach effectively and give more time if the patient also receives an epidural anesthetic or voluntary pushing seems insufficient. While it may be debatable, many medical professionals reduce or stop the epidural anesthetic to improve the parturient's pushing ability. Some medical professionals think that the patient benefits from gravity and can push more effectively when they are upright. On these points, however, there is inconsistency in the literature and clinical experience.

Electronic fetal monitoring is one appropriate management strategy for prolonged descent, which has been linked to a worsened infant outcome. When a patient is transferred from the labor and delivery room, fetal monitoring is often stopped. Making a paper tracing in the delivery room for documentation is crucial since the period immediately before delivery is the one when fetal monitoring most closely correlates with neonatal status. It is probably reasonable to augment with oxytocin if a labor that has otherwise been normal experiences a prolonged descent. The likelihood of an atraumatic vaginal delivery is significantly decreased in the nullipara if complete cervical dilation has not been accomplished and there is a persistent anterior cervical lip that becomes edematous. It is occasionally possible to achieve full dilation and a significant descent in the multipara by supporting the anterior lip and having the patient bear down. This latter strategy appears to be especially successful if labor has progressed normally prior and there has been a positive response to oxytocin stimulation.

Prolonged posterior occiput persistence is often linked to prolonged descent. In the past, forceps rotation was frequently used to treat occiput posterior. Nonetheless, manual rotation and direct occiput posterior delivery are suitable and possibly less traumatic methods. About half of cases complicated by protracted descent result in a normal spontaneous vaginal delivery and low forceps procedures.

8.3.4.2. Arrest of Descent

When descent has completely stopped for at least one hour in the nullipara and zero to five hours in the multipara, the diagnosis of arrest of descent should be made. Prolonged descent often precedes it and shares the same causative factors. Experience indicates that, like secondary arrest of dilation, arrest of descent is extremely sensitive to oxytocin augmentation when it is not preceded by other dysfunctional labor patterns. Spontaneous vaginal birth is often linked to low-dose intravenous oxytocin. Electronic monitoring is appropriate in cases of augmentation for other labor abnormalities.

The situation is similar to prolonged descent when arrest of descent is preceded by other dysfunctional labor patterns. The best course of action is probably to proceed with a cesarean section if the patient is already receiving oxytocin augmentation or if full dilation has not been achieved. Vaginal birth is possible occasionally, but in these cases, extreme caution must be used when trying midforceps delivery or vacuum extraction. It is important to carefully assess the maternal outlet prior to attempting an operative vaginal delivery, especially with regard to the angle of the pubic arch and the separation between the ischial tuberosities. It's also important to consider the potential for shoulder dystocia and macrosomia. It is not uncommon for the vertex to be below +1 cm but for the descent to have stopped. Cervical and lower uterine lacerations are common after a cesarean section involving the delivery of a fetal head with such a deep engagement. In such cases, the option of an operative vaginal delivery still merits consideration.

8.3.5. Third Stage of Labor

Manual removal of the placenta has complicated most studies on the third stage of labor. Dombrowski and colleagues employed life-table analysis in a 45,852 gravidas study to account for the confounding effects of manual placenta removal. This analysis showed that the apparent duration of the third stage of labor was reduced when the placentas were manually removed, particularly in cases of preterm deliveries (Table 8.3). The third stage of labor complications, such as retained placenta (undelivered for more than 30 minutes), manual removal, and hemorrhage (estimated blood loss greater than 500 mL), were significantly more likely to occur in cases of premature delivery.

Table 8.3. Life-Table Analysis with Censoring of Manual Placenta Removal: Predicted Third-Stage Duration in Minutes and Predicted Incidence of Retained Placenta

	Percentiles			**Undelivered at 30 Minutes**	
Gestational age (wk)	10th	50th	90th	%	N
20	2	19	180	42.5	17
21	4	25	180	47.1	32
22	3	19	180	37.7	34
23	3	17	240	40.7	44
24	4	16	80	32.2	38
25	3	11	60	24.7	23
26	3	8	40	11.5	12
27	3	6	19	6.8	6
28	3	8	25	7.4	9
29	3	6	24	8.2	12
30	3	6	21	5.9	13
31	3	6	17	3.8	10
32	3	6	19	6.4	26
33	3	6	20	6.2	36
34	3	6	17	3.5	28

35	3	6	16	3.7	42
36	3	6	17	3.8	72
37	3	6	15	3.2	112
38	3	6	14	2.4	142
39	3	6	14	2.1	183
40	3	6	14	2.1	280
41	3	6	14	2.1	115
42	3	6	14	1.6	35
43	3	5	15	1.3	4

Source: Drennan, K, Blackwell, S, et al., Glob. libr. women's med., (ISSN: 1756–2228) 2008; DOI 10.3843/GLOWM.10132.

The way the third stage of labor is managed (i.e., It's debatable whether placentas should be handled expectantly or manually removed. According to life-table analysis, only 2.2% of term placentas would remain undelivered at 30 minutes, while 90% spontaneously deliver by 15 minutes (i.e., a "placenta retained." In term gestations, a 30-minute threshold would lead to a low intervention rate. Several factors influence how third-stage labor is managed today, such as the belief that term placentas should be delivered within 30 minutes and the worry that a prolonged third stage could result in hemorrhage. Anxiety among doctors and patients is a factor, but the desire to minimize maternal bleeding and transfusion needs is the most significant one. The use of preventive oxytocin, controlled cord traction, fundal massage, and early cord clamping to aid in placenta delivery has reduced the incidence of bleeding.

Regardless of gestational age, the frequency of bleeding peaks 40 minutes before delivery. This peak could be the result of manually removing the placenta from patients who were experiencing active uterine bleeding, though in certain circumstances, manual removal may actually result in more blood loss. It would be challenging to defend the routine manual removal of the placenta before 10 minutes for any gestational age based on these data. We think the possibility of more maternal trauma and bleeding must be taken into consideration when deciding whether to remove the placenta manually. The best time for intervention can only be established by a prospective clinical trial; it is unknown whether manual placental removal can reduce the risk of bleeding or the amount of blood lost (Althous et al., 2006; Drennan et al., 2008).

A Closer Look

Macrosomia

A fetus that is abnormally large—typically defined as weighing more than 8 pounds, 13 ounces (4,000 grams) at birth—is said to have macrosomia. Numerous health risks are associated with this condition for both the mother and the child. Shoulder dystocia, in which the baby's shoulders become stuck during delivery and may result in fractures or nerve damage, is more common in babies with macrosomia. Additionally, low blood sugar, respiratory problems, and a higher chance of obesity and diabetes in later life are all associated with macrosomic infants.

Macrosomic babies can have complications during delivery, including prolonged labor, a higher risk of cesarean delivery, and severe perineal tears. Maternal obesity, diabetes, excessive weight gain during pregnancy, and a history of prior macrosomic births are among the factors that lead to macrosomia. A major contributing factor is gestational diabetes, which frequently results in elevated blood sugar levels that may encourage uncontrollably rapid fetal growth. The prevention of macrosomia-related complications depends heavily on early detection and treatment. Essential preventive measures include controlling blood sugar levels, eating a healthy diet, and getting regular prenatal care. To reduce the risks involved with vaginal delivery of a large baby, doctors may in some cases advise an early delivery or cesarean section.

Summary

- Abnormal labor, also known as dystocia, refers to any situation during childbirth where the progression of labor is hindered, leading to difficulties in the delivery process.
- Malpresentation during childbirth refers to the abnormal positioning of the fetus within the uterus, which can lead to complications during labor and delivery.
- Cephalopelvic disproportion (CPD) refers to a condition where the size or shape of the mother's pelvis is not adequately proportionate to the size of the baby's head, making it difficult or impossible for the baby to pass through the birth canal during labor.
- A cardiotocograph (CTG) is a monitoring device used during pregnancy and labor to assess the fetal heart rate (FHR) and uterine contractions.
- Studying abnormal labor is crucial for advancing maternal and fetal health, improving clinical outcomes, and refining healthcare practices.
- The causes of purely dysfunctional dystocia, in which uterine contractility is inadequate in effecting dilation and descent, are not well understood.
- Absolute fetopelvic disproportion is uncommon, but the performance of cesarean delivery for that indication is common. It is assumed that the physician factor is significant in the diagnosis of dystocia.

References

1. Althous, J. E., et al. (2006). Cephalopelvic disproportion is associated with an altered uterine contraction shape in the active phase of labor. *American Journal of Obstetrics and Gynecology, 195*(3), 739–742. https://doi.org/10.1016/j.ajog.2006.05.034.
2. Bergholt, T., et al. (2007). Maternal body mass index in the first trimester and risk of cesarean delivery in nulliparous women in spontaneous labor. *American Journal of Obstetrics and Gynecology, 197*(2), 163.e1–163.e5. https://doi.org/10.1016/j.ajog.2007.02.042.
3. Cheng, Y. W., Shaffer, B. L., & Caughey, A. B. (2006). The association between persistent occiput posterior position and neonatal outcomes. *Obstetrics & Gynecology, 107*(4), 837–844. https://doi.org/10.1097/01.AOG.0000207363.14262.73.
4. Dietz, P. M., et al. (2005). Population-based assessment of the risk of primary cesarean delivery due to excess prepregnancy weight among nulliparous women delivering term infants. *Maternal and Child Health Journal, 9*(3), 237–244. https://doi.org/10.1007/s10995-005-0052-1.
5. Ecker, J. L., et al. (2001). Increased risk of cesarean delivery with advancing maternal age: Indications and associated factors in nulliparous women. *American Journal of Obstetrics and Gynecology, 185*(4), 883–887. https://doi.org/10.1067/mob.2001.118722.
6. Getahun, D., et al. (2007). Changes in prepregnancy body mass index between pregnancies and risk of primary cesarean delivery. *American Journal of Obstetrics and Gynecology, 197*(4), 376.e1–376.e7. https://doi.org/10.1016/j.ajog.2007.08.020.
7. Greenberg, M. B., et al. (2006). Are there ethnic differences in the length of labor? *American Journal of Obstetrics and Gynecology*. Retrieved from: https://doi.org/10.1016/j.ajog.2006.04.001.

8. Greenberg, M. B., et al. (2007). Does length of labor vary by maternal age? *American Journal of Obstetrics and Gynecology, 197*(2), 428.e1–428.e7. https://doi.org/10.1016/j.ajog.2007.04.031.

9. Ohel, G., et al. (2006). Early versus late initiation of epidural analgesia in labor: Does it increase the risk of cesarean section? A randomized trial. *American Journal of Obstetrics and Gynecology, 194*(2), 600–605. https://doi.org/10.1016/j.ajog.2005.08.007.

10. Ponkey, S. E., et al. (2003). Persistent fetal occiput posterior position: Obstetric outcomes. *Obstetrics & Gynecology, 101*(5), 915–920. https://doi.org/10.1016/S0029-7844(03)00240-5.

11. Rouse, D. J., Owen, J., Savage, K. G., & Hauth, J. C. (2001). Active phase labor arrest: Revisiting the 2-hour minimum. *Obstetrics & Gynecology, 98*(4), 550. https://doi.org/10.1016/S0029-7844(01)01464-7.

12. Shaffer, B. L., et al. (2006). Manual rotation of the fetal occiput: Predictors of success and delivery. *American Journal of Obstetrics and Gynecology, 194*(6), e7–e9. https://doi.org/10.1016/j.ajog.2006.01.016.

13. Wong, C. A., et al. (2005). The risk of cesarean delivery with neuraxial analgesia given early versus late in labor. *New England Journal of Medicine, 352*(7), 655–665. https://doi.org/10.1056/NEJMoa042330.

14. Wu, J. M., et al. (2005). Occiput posterior fetal head position increases the risk of anal sphincter injury in vacuum-assisted deliveries. *American Journal of Obstetrics and Gynecology, 193*(2), 525–529. https://doi.org/10.1016/j.ajog.2005.04.031.

Chapter

GYNECOLOGICAL DIAGNOSIS

9

Contents

Introduction

Gynecological diagnosis encompasses a wide range of procedures and evaluations aimed at identifying conditions affecting the female reproductive system. This field is crucial as it deals with disorders that can have significant implications for a woman's overall health, fertility, and quality of life. A thorough gynecological diagnosis typically begins with a comprehensive patient history, where the clinician gathers detailed information about the patient's menstrual cycle, sexual history, and any symptoms such as pain, abnormal bleeding, or discharge. This initial step is fundamental as it guides the clinician towards potential diagnoses and informs the subsequent choice of diagnostic tests.

Physical examination is another cornerstone of gynecological diagnosis. During this examination, the clinician assesses the external genitalia, vagina, cervix, uterus, and ovaries. Techniques such as palpation, speculum examination, and bimanual examination allow the healthcare provider to identify abnormalities such as masses, lesions, or tenderness that may indicate underlying conditions. These examinations can help detect a variety of issues, from infections and benign growths like fibroids to more serious conditions such as cancers of the reproductive organs.

In addition to these standard diagnostic methods, genetic and molecular testing are increasingly becoming integral to gynecological diagnosis. These advanced tests can identify specific genetic mutations associated with hereditary conditions like BRCA-related breast and ovarian cancers, guiding both preventative and therapeutic measures. By integrating these various diagnostic approaches, healthcare providers can offer personalized and effective care, improving outcomes and ensuring that women receive the most appropriate treatments for their specific conditions.

Overall, gynecological diagnosis is a multi-faceted and dynamic field, continuously evolving with advances in medical science. It requires a careful and systematic approach to ensure that conditions are accurately identified and managed, thereby enhancing women's health and well-being.

Orientation and Directional Terms

Term	Definition	Illustration
Cervical Biopsy	A cervical biopsy is performed to evaluate abnormal cervical tissue found during a Pap test or colposcopy.	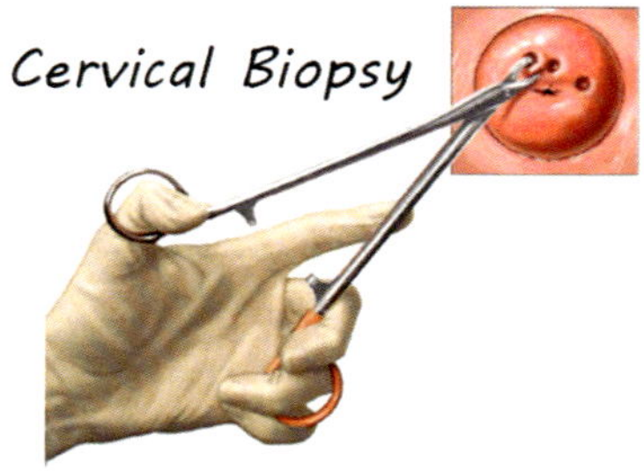
Polycystic Ovary Syndrome (PCOS)	Polycystic ovary syndrome (PCOS) is a condition in which the ovaries produce an abnormal amount of androgens, male sex hormones that are usually present in women in small amounts.	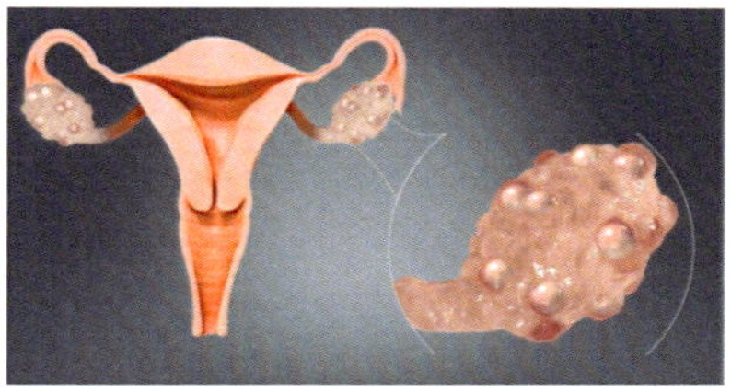
Hormone Replacement Therapy (HRT)	Hormone replacement therapy, or HRT, is a treatment that helps people with symptoms of menopause. Healthcare providers also call it hormone therapy (HT), especially when you receive treatment after age 50. Most often, hormone replacement therapy (HRT) is the term providers use when you receive the treatment at a younger age, especially before age 40.	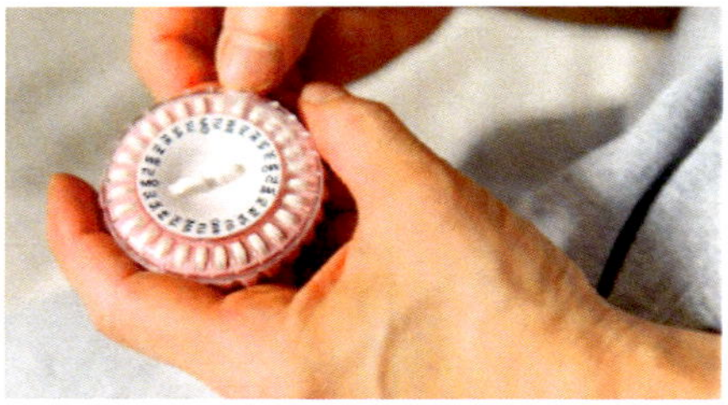
Breast Cancer	Breast cancer is a disease in which abnormal breast cells grow out of control and form tumors. If left unchecked, the tumors can spread throughout the body and become fatal.	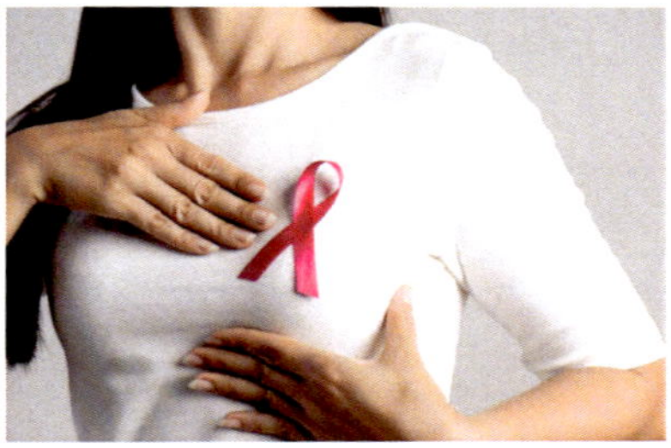
Abdominal Muscles	Abdominal muscles are the muscles forming the abdominal walls, the abdomen being the portion of the trunk connecting the thorax and pelvis. An abdominal wall is formed of skin, fascia, and muscle and encases the abdominal cavity and viscera.	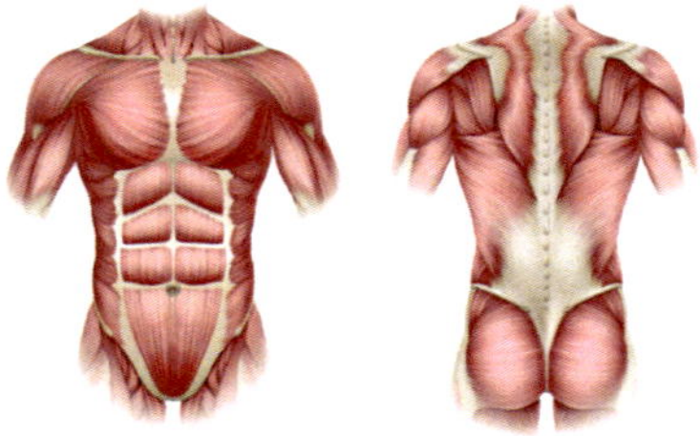

9.1. History

A gynecological history is a critical component of a woman's medical record, providing vital information about her reproductive health. This history encompasses multiple facets, including personal and family history, menstrual and obstetric history, sexual health, lifestyle factors, and more. Collecting a detailed and accurate gynecologic history enables healthcare providers to understand the patient's health status comprehensively, leading to better clinical decisions and personalized care (Nustaum & Hamilton, 2002).

9.1.1. Personal Information

Basic Identifiers

- **Name**: Full legal name of the patient.
- **Age**: Current age and date of birth.
- **Contact Information**: Address, phone number, and email.
- **Occupation**: Job title, work environment, and any occupational hazards.
- **Marital Status**: Single, married, divorced, widowed, or in a domestic partnership.
- **Sexual Orientation**: Heterosexual, homosexual, bisexual, or other.

Lifestyle

- **Diet**: Typical dietary habits, including vegetarian or vegan preferences, and any dietary restrictions or allergies.
- **Exercise**: Frequency, type, and duration of physical activities.
- **Stress Levels**: Sources of stress, coping mechanisms, and overall mental health.
- **Sleep Patterns**: Average hours of sleep per night, quality of sleep, and any sleep disorders.

9.1.2. Menstrual History

- **Menarche**
  - o **Age at Menarche**: Age when the patient had her first menstrual period.
- **Menstrual Cycle Characteristics**
  - o **Regularity**: Whether menstrual cycles are regular or irregular.
  - o **Cycle Length**: Number of days from the start of one period to the start of the next.
  - o **Duration of Flow**: Number of days bleeding lasts.
  - o **Volume of Flow**: Light, moderate, or heavy bleeding; number of pads or tampons used per day.
  - o **Pain During Menstruation (Dysmenorrhea)**: Presence and severity of menstrual cramps, and the impact on daily activities.
- **Menstrual Irregularities**
  - o **Amenorrhea**: Absence of menstruation for more than three months.
  - o **Oligomenorrhea**: Infrequent menstrual periods (cycles longer than 35 days).
  - o **Polymenorrhea**: Frequent menstrual periods (cycles shorter than 21 days).
  - o **Menorrhagia**: Excessive menstrual bleeding.
  - o **Metrorrhagia**: Bleeding between periods.

9.1.3. Obstetric History

- **Gravida and Para**
  - o **Gravida (G)**: Total number of pregnancies, including current pregnancy.
  - o **Para (P)**: Outcomes of those pregnancies, broken down into:
    - ▪ **Full-Term Births (T)**: Number

of deliveries at 37 weeks or later.

- **Preterm Births (P)**: Number of deliveries before 37 weeks.
- **Abortions (A)**: Number of spontaneous (miscarriages) and elective abortions.
- **Living Children (L)**: Number of living children.

- **Pregnancy Complications**
  - **Gestational Diabetes**: Occurrence and management during pregnancy.
  - **Preeclampsia**: High blood pressure and signs of damage to another organ system, often the kidneys.
  - **Eclampsia**: Severe preeclampsia that leads to seizures.
  - **Preterm Labor**: Labor that begins before 37 weeks of pregnancy.
  - **Placental Issues**: Placenta previa, placental abruption.
  - **Infections**: Any infections during pregnancy (e.g., urinary tract infections, sexually transmitted infections).
  - **Delivery Complications**: Difficult labor, need for cesarean section, postpartum hemorrhage.

9.1.4. Gynecologic History

- **Previous Gynecologic Conditions**
  - **Infections**: History of bacterial vaginosis, yeast infections, pelvic inflammatory disease (PID).
  - **Surgeries**: History of gynecologic surgeries such as hysterectomy, myomectomy, laparoscopy for endometriosis.
  - **Other Conditions**: Endometriosis, polycystic ovary syndrome (PCOS), fibroids, ovarian cysts.
- **Pap Smear History**
  - **Last Pap Smear**: Date of the last test and results.
  - **Abnormal Results**: History of abnormal Pap smears and follow-up procedures like colposcopy or biopsy.
- **Contraceptive Use**
  - **Current Method**: Type of contraception currently used (e.g., oral contraceptives, IUD, implants).
  - **Past Methods**: History of contraceptive use, reasons for discontinuation, and any complications or side effects experienced.
- **Sexually Transmitted Infections (STIs)**
  - **History of STIs**: Type, treatment received, and any complications.
  - **Screening**: Frequency of STI screenings and results.
- **Menopausal Status**
  - **Age at Menopause**: Age when menstrual periods ceased permanently.
  - **Symptoms**: Hot flashes, night sweats, vaginal dryness, mood changes.
  - **Hormone Replacement Therapy (HRT)**: Use of HRT, type, dosage, and duration.

9.1.5. Sexual History

- **Sexual Activity**
  - **First Intercourse**: Age at first sexual intercourse.
  - **Number of Partners**: Total number of lifetime sexual partners.
  - **Current Sexual Activity**: Frequency and nature of sexual activity.
- **Sexual Function**
  - **Libido**: Level of sexual desire.
  - **Arousal**: Ability to become sexually aroused.

- **Orgasm**: Ability to achieve orgasm and any difficulties.
- **Dyspareunia**: Pain during intercourse, its location, intensity, and frequency.

9.1.6. Medical History

- **Chronic Conditions**
  - **Systemic Diseases**: Presence of conditions like diabetes, hypertension, thyroid disorders, autoimmune diseases.
  - **Psychiatric Conditions**: History of mental health issues such as depression, anxiety, bipolar disorder.
- **Surgeries and Hospitalizations**
  - **Major Surgeries**: Dates, reasons, and outcomes of significant surgeries, particularly those affecting the reproductive system.
  - **Hospitalizations**: Reasons for past hospital admissions.
- **Medications**
  - **Current Medications**: Prescription and over-the-counter medications, herbal supplements, and vitamins.
  - **Past Medications**: Any significant past medications that have impacted gynecologic health.
- **Allergies**
  - **Drug Allergies**: Specific medications and types of allergic reactions.
  - **Other Allergies**: Latex, foods, environmental allergens (Marrazzo & Stine, 2004).

9.1.7. Family History

- **Genetic Conditions**
  - **Cancers**: Family history of gynecologic cancers (e.g., breast, ovarian, endometrial).
  - **Other Hereditary Conditions**: Conditions like endometriosis or PCOS in family members.
- **Reproductive Health**
  - **Mother and Siblings**: Menstrual and reproductive health of mother and siblings, any significant issues.

9.1.8. Lifestyle and Social History

- **Substance Use**
  - **Tobacco**: Type, amount, and duration of use.
  - **Alcohol**: Type, frequency, and amount of consumption.
  - **Recreational Drugs**: Type, frequency, and amount of use.
- **Diet and Exercise**
  - **Dietary Habits**: Daily intake, food preferences, and any recent changes in diet.
  - **Exercise Routine**: Type of exercise, frequency, and duration.
- **Mental Health and Stress**
  - **Mental Health History**: Previous diagnoses, treatments, and current mental health status.
  - **Stressors**: Major life stressors, sources of support, and coping mechanisms.

9.2. Physical Examination

If the physical examination takes place in an environment that the patient finds visually pleasing, it will be most beneficial. Sufficient drapes and gowns help shield against embarrassment. Frequently, a PA leads the patient to the changing room, where she receives detailed instructions on what to remove and how to put on her gown. The PA may then help drape the patient.

A doctor may ask a female assistant to stay in the examination room to help out when needed, but whether or not she stays only as a chaperone depends on local custom as well as the doctor's and patient's preferences. Although it is not legally required, both male and female doctors must exercise caution, particularly when performing pelvic and breast exams. Unless the doctor determines that the patient's request to have her partner, family member, or friend present will interfere with the examination or the taking of an accurate history, the request should be honored. Especially during the pelvic examination, when the patient may not be able to make direct eye contact with the doctor, it is highly advised that the doctor explain the actions and steps that will be taken.

9.2.1. General Examination

If the patient's gynecologist serves as their primary care physician, a yearly or as needed general physical examination should be conducted. Obviously, a thorough examination yields more information, shows the doctor's thoroughness, and builds rapport with the patient (Bayrak & Saadat, 2005).

9.2.1.1. General Evaluation

9.2.1.1.1. Vital Signs

The patient should be weighed and have her blood pressure taken as part of every examination, regardless of whether it is for a specific issue, a routine yearly examination, or a follow-up visit for a previously diagnosed issue. It is important to measure postmenopausal patients' height in order to record any height loss caused by osteoporosis and vertebral fractures. It should be decided if the urine needs to be sent for a urinalysis, culture, or pregnancy test before the patient empties her bladder for the examination. The visual assessment of any skin lesions and symmetry of movement should be part of the examination of the chest. Purposeful lung auscultation and percussion are crucial in ruling out primary pulmonary issues like pneumonia and asthma. Auscultation is used to check for arrhythmias and significant murmurs, and percussion is used to measure the size of the heart.

9.2.2. Breast Examination

As part of the physical examination, a routine breast examination should be performed. In the US, one in eight women will develop breast cancer at some point in their lives. As one of the most reliable ways to screen for breast disease is for a patient to be well-prepared, doctors who treat women should teach their patients how to do self-examinations. The physical examination offers a convenient opportunity to determine the frequency and technique of self-examination of the breast. Additionally, it's a great opportunity to instruct the patient in breast self-examination techniques. The patient should be instructed to carefully palpate each quadrant of the breast after examining herself in the mirror to check for skin changes or dimpling. When taking a shower or bath, the majority of women like to do this with soapy hands. Postmenopausal women should self-examine on the same day each month. The examination should be repeated at the same time each month, preferably one week after the start of the menses, when the breasts are least nodular.

The individual woman and her family history determine the frequency of mammography or the earlier use of mammography. Patients should get screened for breast cancer at an earlier age if there is a positive family history of the disease, especially if their mother, aunt, or sister had premenopausal breast cancer. Generally speaking, a mammogram should be taken every 1–2 years starting in the 40s and every year after that. These days, ultrasonography can accurately distinguish between solid and cystic lesions; it is a complementary method that does not replace mammography. The early detection of breast cancer should benefit from the complementary use of mammography, ultrasonography, breast self-examination, and physician examination. Patients with BRCA1/2 mutations or those with a strong family history of breast cancer should only have annual breast magnetic resonance imaging (MRI) exams. That being said, this test is not a replacement for the other methods for early breast cancer detection; rather, it is an addition to them.

Figure 9.1 displays an accurate breast examination technique. If anomalies are found, unless the gynecologist is skilled in doing breast biopsies, a decision should be made regarding the necessity of mammography (or other imaging techniques) or a direct referral to a breast surgeon. Skin lesions should be closely monitored, especially eczematous lesions around the nipple. If these lesions cannot be resolved with over-the-counter remedies, a biopsy should be performed. A nipple or areola eczematous lesion could be Paget's carcinoma.

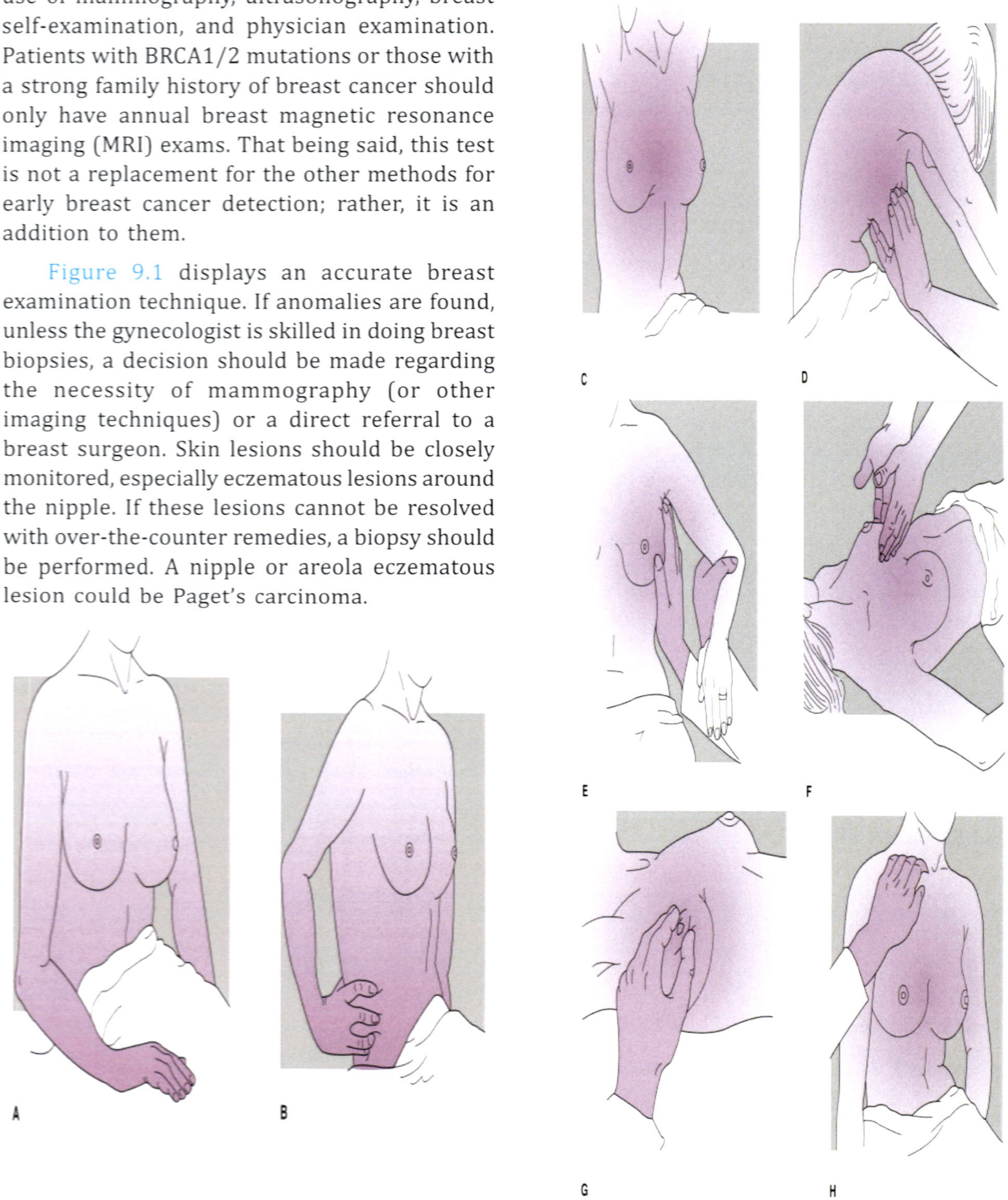

Figure 9.1. *Breast examination by the physician.*

Note: A: Patient is sitting, arms at sides. Perform visual inspection in good light, looking for lumps or for dimpling or wrinkling of skin. B: Patient is sitting, hands pressing on hips so that pectoralis muscles are tensed. Repeat visual inspection. C: Patient is sitting, arms above head. Repeat visual inspection of breasts and perform visual inspection of axillae. D: Patient is sitting and leaning forward, hands on examiner's shoulders, the stirrups, or her own knees. Perform bimanual palpation, paying particular attention to the base of the glandular portion of the breast. E: Patient is sitting, arms extended 60–90 degrees. Palpate axillae. F: Patient is supine, arms relaxed at sides. Perform bimanual palpation of each portion of breast (usually each quadrant, but smaller sections for unusually large breasts). Repeat examinations C, E, and F with patient supine, arms above head. G: Patient is supine, arms relaxed at sides. Palpate under the areola and nipple with the thumb and forefinger to detect a mass or test for expression of fluid from the nipple. H: Patient is either sitting or supine. Palpate supraclavicular areas.

Source: Charles Kawada & Drorith Hochner-Celnikier; Gynecologic History, Examination, & Diagnostic Procedures; ISBN: 978–0-07–163969–9.

9.2.3. Abdominal Examination

The patient should be fully supine and at ease; to help the abdominal muscles relax, the knees may be supported and slightly flexed. An examination should reveal any irregularities in color or contour. Inspection should come first, but auscultation should come before palpation because the latter may alter the nature of intestinal activity. When the entire abdomen is palpated, tenderness, masses, and voluntary guarding should all be felt. Palpate gently at first, then firmly as directed. The examiner should ask the patient to point with one finger the location of her greatest pain or tenderness if she reports having abdominal pain or if she exhibits unexpected tenderness. The purpose of suprapubic palpation is to find enlargements of the uterus, ovaries, or bladder. Deep palpation should only be performed on a painful area last; otherwise, the entire abdomen can be voluntarily guarded. The doctor should thoroughly examine the abdomen as a last step to look for any abnormalities in the kidneys, intestines, liver, gallbladder, or spleen. When an abnormality of the abdominal muscle reflexes is demonstrated, it can sometimes aid in the diagnosis. An abdominal percussion should be used to detect ascites, tumors, or enlargement of the organs.

9.2.4. Pelvic Examination

Many women are afraid of the pelvic examination, so it needs to be done in a way that calms her fears. It can be particularly unsettling for a patient to have their first pelvic examination, so it's critical for the doctor to try to calm anxiety and encourage cooperation. A satisfactory gynecologic examination is typically not a problem by the time the history has been taken and a painless, embarrassing general examination has been completed, according to the compassionate doctor. Cozy surroundings, a nurse or chaperone in attendance if necessary, warm instruments, and a slow, gentle approach with ongoing explanation and comfort are all beneficial in ensuring patient relaxation and cooperation. This is particularly valid for women who have never had a pelvic exam before. A narrow speculum and a one-finger examination are frequently required in these patients. When vaginal examination is not feasible, the only option is to palpate the pelvic structures through rectal examination. When a patient is unable to relax their abdominal muscles sufficiently, an ultrasound examination can occasionally be useful in determining whether the pelvic organs are normal in size and configuration. The patient can be given anesthesia if a more thorough pelvic examination is required (Bazot, Darai, and Hourani, 2004).

9.2.4.1. External Genitalia

Examining the pubic hair for abnormalities such as infected hair follicles, pubic lice nits, and pattern (masculine or feminine) is recommended. Vera, mons pubis, and perineal skin should all be checked for signs of discoloration or dermatitis. You can reveal the glans clitoridis by carefully pulling back the surrounding skin folds. The clitoris, which is located at the ventral confluence of the two labia, should measure no more than 2.5 cm, the majority of which should be subcutaneous. Although the major and minor labia are typically the same size on both sides, a slight variation in size is acceptable. Subcutaneous nodules or small protuberances could be tumors or sebaceous cysts. In this region, external condylomata are frequently observed. The urethra, which is located directly below the clitoris, should have no protuberances and the same color as the surrounding tissue (Figure 9.2).

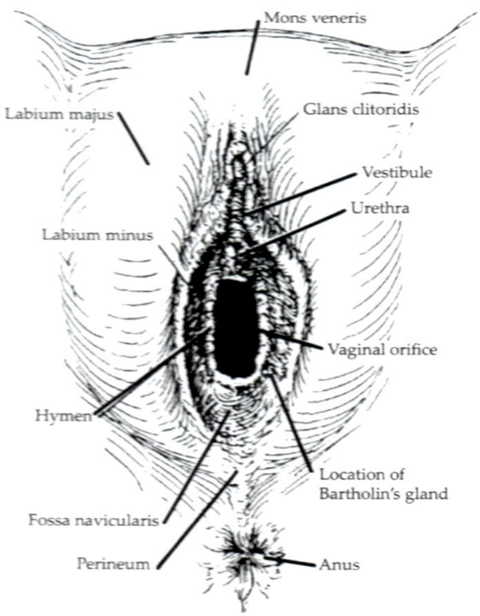

Figure 9.2. *Normal external genitalia in a mature woman.*

Source: Pernoll ML. Benson & Pernoll's Handbook of Obstetrics and Gynecology. 10th ed. New York, NY: McGraw-Hill; 2001.

Vestibular (Bartholin's) glands are normally neither felt nor seen, so their enlargement may be a sign of a problem with this gland system. Palpating the vestibular gland area with the thumb outside and the index finger inside the vagina will allow you to feel for any enlargement or tenderness (Figure 9.3). A vaginal or vulvar infection may cause redness in the perineal skin. Scars could be an indication of surgery or obstetric cuts. At this point, the anus should be examined for hemorrhoids, fissures, irritation, or perianal infections (e.g., such as herpesvirus lesions or condylomata).

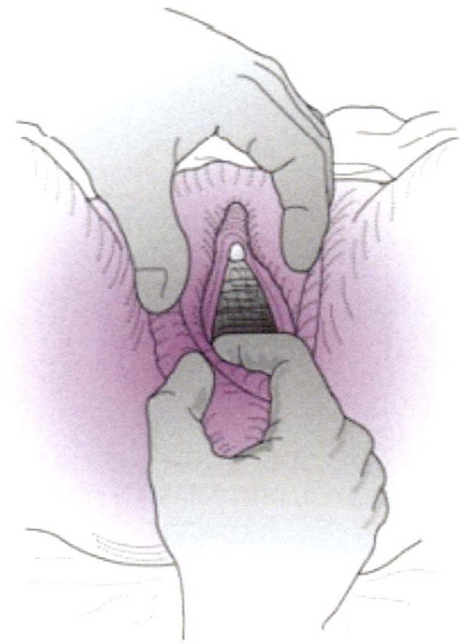

Figure 9.3. *Palpation of vestibular glands.*

Source: Charles Kawada & Drorith Hochner-Celnikier; Gynecologic History, Examination, & Diagnostic Procedures; ISBN: 978-0-07-163969-9.

9.2.4.2. Hymen

There are various ways in which an unruptured hymen can appear, but only a fully imperforate, cribriform, or septate hymen is pathologic. The hymen can appear in a variety of ways following rupture (Figure 9.4). The hymen may almost disappear after multiple childbirths.

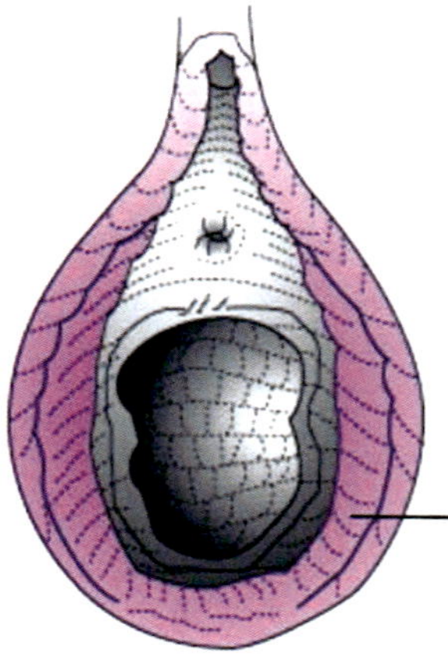

Figure 9.4. *Ruptured hymen (parous introitus).*

Source: Charles Kawada & Drorith Hochner-Celnikier; Gynecologic History, Examination, & Diagnostic Procedures; ISBN: 978-0-07-163969-9.

9.2.4.3. Perineal Support

The doctor separate the labia with two fingers and instructs the patient to "bear down" in order to assess the presence of pelvic relaxation. This will show uterine prolapse, cystocele, rectocele, or urethrocele; however, in certain cases, an upright posture might be required to show significant prolapse.

9.2.4.4. Urethra

An infection, urethral caruncle, or carcinoma may be indicated by redness of the urethra. The paraurethral glands empty into the urethra just inside the meatus, and they are located beneath the urethra. The urethra may be "stripped"—that is, pressure applied by the examining finger as it moves from the proximal to the distal urethra—to express discharge from the urethra or paraurethral glands after the labia have been sufficiently spread for improved vision.

9.2.5. Vaginal Examination

Prior to any further testing, the vagina should be examined with a speculum to check for anomalies and to get a Pap smear. A speculum that has been lightly moistened with warm water but not lubricated is gently inserted into the vagina to provide a clear view of the cervix and fornixes. Examining the cervix for discharge, color, erosion, and other lesions is important. Any discharge can then be obtained for a Pap smear and tested for microbiology, virology, or microscopy. The vaginal wall is examined once more closely as the speculum is removed following the preparation of the Pap smear (Figure 9.5).

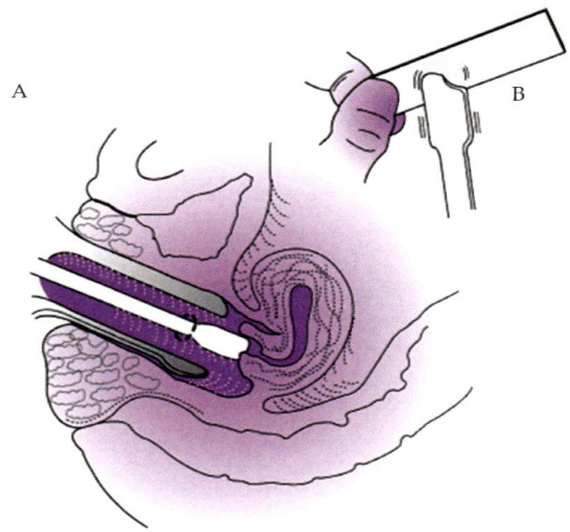

Materials Needed

One cervical spatula, cut tongue depressor, cotton swab, or small brush made especially for obtaining endocervical cells.
One glass slide (one end frosted). Identify by writing the patient's name on the frosted end with a lead pencil.
One speculum (without lubricant).
One bottle of fixative (75% ethyl alcohol) or spray-on fixative, eg, Aqua-Net or Cyto-Spray.

Figure 9.5. *Preparation of a Papanicolaou (Pap) smear.*

Source: Pernoll ML. Benson & Pernoll's Handbook of Obstetrics and Gynecology. 10th ed. New York, NY: McGraw-Hill; 2001.)

Note: A: Obtain cervical scraping from complete squamocolumnar junction by rotating 360 degrees around the external OS. B: Place the material 1 in from the end of the slide and smear along the slide to obtain a thin preparation. Place a saline-soaked cotton swab or small endocervical brush into the endocervical canal and rotate 360 degrees. Place this specimen onto the same slide and quickly fix with fixative.

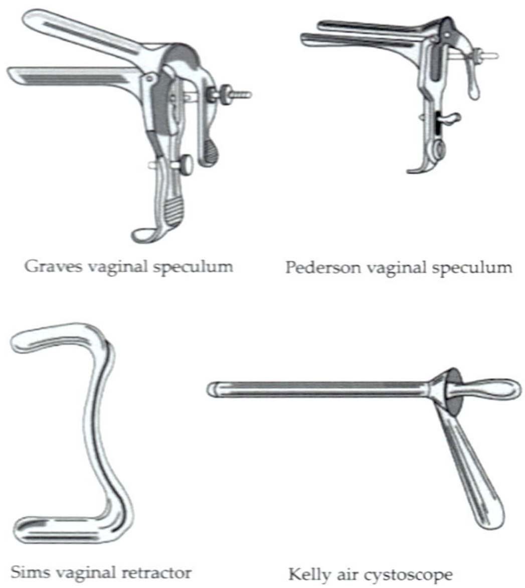

Figure 9.6. *Specula.*

Source: Pernoll ML. Benson & Pernoll's Handbook of Obstetrics and Gynecology. 10th ed. New York, NY: McGraw-Hill; 2001.).

Although the doctor's preference will determine which type of speculum is used, the Pederson speculum is the most effective tool for sexually active patients, though a wider Graves speculum might be required to provide sufficient visualization (Figure 9.6). It is best to use the narrow-bladed Pederson speculum for patients who have a small introitus. An extra-large Graves speculum is available when exposure beyond that of the usual course is required. A large otoscope, a Kelly air cystoscope, or a Huffman or nasal speculum are all very useful tools for visualizing a child's vagina.

9.2.6. Bimanual Examination

Between the two fingers of the hand in the vagina and the flat of the other hand, which is positioned on the lower abdominal wall, the uterus and adnexal structures should be indicated (Figure 9.7). Position, size, shape, mobility, consistency, and tenderness of the pelvic structures can all be determined with gentle palpation and manipulation of the structures—with the exception of obese or uncooperative patients and those whose abdominal muscles are tense due to discomfort or fear. One can feel tenderness through direct palpation, as well as through movement or stretching of the pelvic structures.

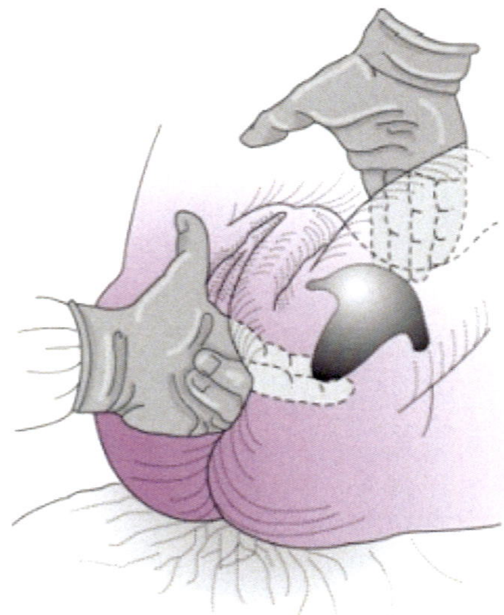

Figure 9.7. *Bimanual pelvic examination.*

Source: Charles Kawada & Drorith Hochner-Celnikier; Gynecologic History, Examination, & Diagnostic Procedures; ISBN: 978–0-07–163969–9.

9.2.6.1. Cervix

The cervix is a hard structure that is sometimes compared to the consistency of the nose tip. Its normal shape is round, with a diameter of about 3.4 cm. Figure 9.8 depicts the cervix in various appearances. The outer orbit is circular and almost completely closed. Women who are multiparous could have a lacerations on their os. One or more Nabothian cysts may be the cause of an irregularity in form or nodularity.

Extremely firm cervical tissue could be the result of a tumor or even cancer. Since the cervix and uterine body are normally fairly mobile, a 2–4 cm movement in any direction can be made without causing undue discomfort. (It is helpful to inform a patient during an examination that although she may feel her uterus moving, this procedure usually doesn't hurt. Limited cervix or corpus mobility frequently follows neoplasia, surgery, or inflammation.

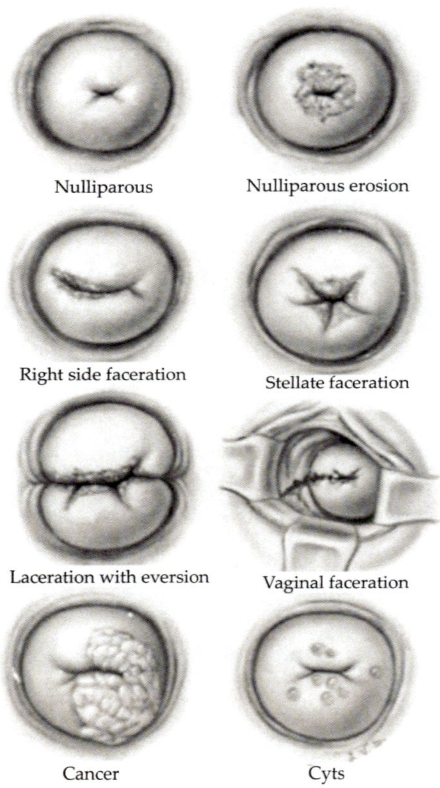

Figure 9.8. *Uterine cervix: normal and pathologic appearance.*

Source: Charles Kawada & Drorith Hochner-Celnikier; Gynecologic History, Examination, & Diagnostic Procedures; ISBN: 978-0-07-163969-9.

9.2.6.2. Corpus of the Uterus

The uterine corpus weighs between 70 and 90 g and is about half the size of the patient's fist. Its outline is regular, and it moves moderately and is not sensitive to pressure. The uterus is anteverted in the majority of women and retroverted in about one-third of them. Generally speaking, a retroverted uterus is not pathologic. The "tipped" uterus in some endometriosis or salpingitis cases may be the consequence of adhesions brought on by the illness. Typically, the uterus is described in terms of its consistency, size, shape, location, and mobility.

9.2.6.3. Adnexa

Many overweight women are unable to palpate their adnexal structures, which include their ovaries and fallopian tubes, because the average tube measures only 7 mm in diameter and the ovary no larger than 3 cm. But the ovaries and, in some cases, the oviducts are almost always palpable in extremely thin women. In postmenopausal women, adnexal structures are typically not palpable. Any adnexal structure that exhibits unusual tenderness or enlargement warrants additional diagnostic testing; any woman who has an adnexal mass should have it looked into.

9.2.7. Rectovaginal Examination

It is always recommended to perform a rectovaginal examination following the bimanual pelvic examination, particularly if the patient is over 40. The examining hand's middle finger, which has been well-lubricated, should be gently inserted into the rectum to feel for any irregularities, masses, or tenderness. The index finger can then be inserted into the vagina until the depth of the vagina is reached after the examining finger has been inserted a brief distance (Figure 9.9). Examining certain areas of the posterior part of the pelvis with a rectovaginal examination is far simpler than doing so with a vaginal examination alone. The uterosacral ligaments are stretched when the index finger raises the cervix toward the anterior abdominal wall. This procedure is usually painless; however, if it hurts, particularly if there are sensitive nodules along the uterosacral ligaments that can be felt with the finger in the rectum, endometriosis may be present.

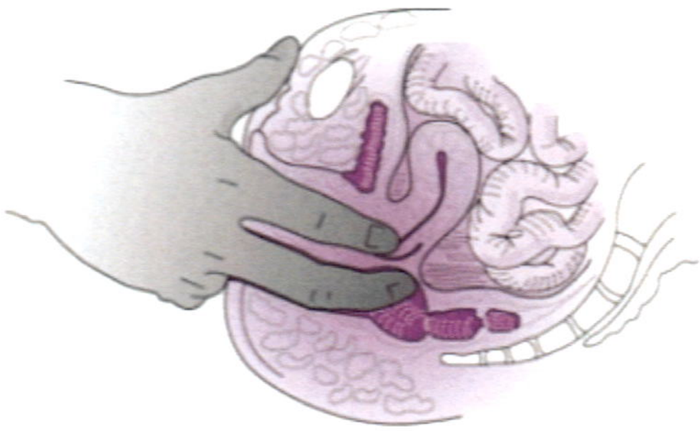

Figure 9.9. *Rectovaginal examination.*

Source: Charles Kawada & Drorith Hochner-Celnikier; Gynecologic History, Examination, & Diagnostic Procedures; ISBN: 978-0-07-163969-9.

9.2.8. Rectal Examination

The rectal examination includes a visual inspection of the perianal skin, digital palpation of the rectum, and evaluation of the perineum's neuromuscular function (Henry, Parks, and Swash, 1982).

9.2.8.1. Technique

The choice of method to use for the rectal examination depends on the examiner's experience and the clinical situation. When the patient is in the lithotomy position, they should be lying supine with their legs pulled in toward their trunk and their knees left loose. This may provide a more thorough examination of the anterior rectum and is the standard position for examining the pelvic organs in women. For examinations where the patient is too sick or unable to assume other positions, the lateral decubitus, also known as Sim's position, is the best option. With their right knee and hip slightly bent, the patient is positioned on their left side, their buttocks close to the edge of the examination table or by their bed. Proper examination of the perineum and rectum is best performed in the proctologic (knee-chest or prone jackknife) position. The easier access to the anorectum in this position allows the patient to undergo additional studies with ease, including sigmoidoscopy and anoscopy. Both inspection and palpation are used in the rectal examination, regardless of the position taken. Examiners first check the buttocks for fistulous tracts, skin tags from hemorrhoids, excoriations, blood, and rectal prolapse with gloved hands. In order to confirm that there is no rectal prolapse and that the perineum—the space between the thighs that runs from the coccyx to the pubis—is properly descended, the patient is then asked to bear down. Approximately 2.5 cm above the ischial tuberosities is where the perineum is located in healthy individuals. The perineum will descend to a level approximately 1.5 cm above the ischial tuberosities when straining at stool, or about 1 and a half centimeter. In order to assess an early abscess or fistual formation associated with inflammatory bowel disease, the examiner then applies firm pressure to the ischial tuberosities. To obtain additional evidence of an abscess or fistula, the patient is asked to bear down again while maintaining pressure on the perineum.

The evaluation of neuromuscular integrity is the next step in the rectal examination process. Initially, the gloved finger is used to scratch the buttocks on both sides in order to trigger the superficial anal reflex, which is a function of L_1 and L_2. A generous amount of water-soluble gel is then used to lubricate the area before the gloved index finger is carefully inserted into the rectum. Examiners should assess anterior contraction of the puborectalis muscle and external anal sphincter while the patient consciously resists defecation (similar to stopping midstream during urination). After the patient has calmed down, the examiner notes that the internal anal sphincter has relaxed by pushing the puborectalis muscle posteriorly. The internal anal sphincter relaxes and the puborectalis muscle moves posteriorly when the patient finally bears down once more, ejecting the examining finger. This technique frequently makes it possible to palpate a woman's cervix and gauge how tender the organ is.

Using digital palpation, the final step of the rectal examination evaluates anatomic integrity. Once more, the rectum is gently probed with the gloved finger, and in two stages, the entire circumference is methodically palpated. The first stage covers the region 1 to 2 cm (the length of the fingerpad) beyond the external sphincter, and the second stage covers the remaining 7 to 8 cm of the rectum that is within the examining finger's reach. With a focus on the posterior rectal shelf, particular attention should be paid to any masses, tenderness, hemorrhoids, fissures, ulcers, and stool color and consistency. Men's prostates should be observed for their size, consistency, and presence of nodules. The rectovesicular pouch's area should also be evaluated. It is recommended to palpate the Douglas rectouterine pouch in women to check for lumps or soreness. Examining the lower abdomen and genitourinary structures is often made easier with a bimanual examination (rectoabdominal or rectovaginal).

9.2.8.2. Basic Science

Starting approximately 12 centimeters from the anal verge, the rectum is formed at the end of the sigmoid colon (Figure 9.10). During defecation, two muscle bundles called the internal and external anal sphincters are involved. The colon's circular smooth muscle enlarges to form the internal anal sphincter, which contracts automatically. The puborectalis muscle voluntarily controls the striated muscle bands that make up the external anal sphincter. The internal and external anal sphincters are controlled by the internal pudendal nerve (S_3–S_4), while the hypogastric nerves innervate the rectum. These nerves are the same ones that innervate the bladder. As a result of the shared innervation, dysuria is frequently reported in relation to disorders of the rectal area.

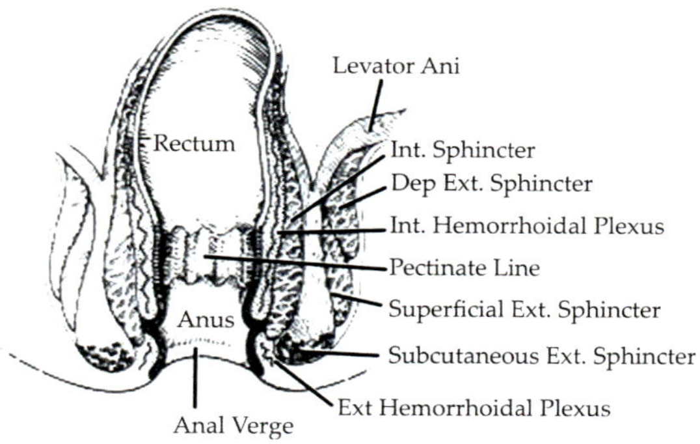

Figure 9.10. *Anatomy of the anus.*

Source: Lieberman DA. (1984). Common anorectal disorders. Ann Intern Med., 101, 838.

The pectinate line, located about 3 to 4 cm from the skin and marking the merger of the anus and rectum, is a significant anatomical and clinical landmark. It acts as a boundary for the nerve supply as well as for lymphatic and venous drainage. The veins drain into the portal and caval systems, the lymph drains to the superior rectal and iliac nodes, and sympathetic nerves are present but not producing pain above the pectinate line. Below the pectinate line, lymph drains into the inguinal nodes, somatic nerves provide innervation (pain is present), and veins empty into the caval system alone.

The purpose of the rectum is to enable voluntary defecation. The sigmoid colon's stool is propelled into the rectum by peristalsis. The internal anal sphincter relaxes involuntarily in response to increased intraluminal pressure, causing the external anal sphincter to reflexively contract, preventing incontinence and alerting the user to impending defecation. The feces are then expelled when the external anal sphincter voluntarily relaxes. Larger fecal bulk may aid in the evacuative process, according to studies, which supports the recommendation that patients eat diets rich in bulk and fiber (Porter & Liechty, 1976).

9.2.9. Clinical Significance

Many otherwise perplexing clinical situations are resolved when a rectal examination is performed, as Major hinted as early as 1937. It is true that the rectal examination is necessary and should not be skipped; the history and physical examination are insufficient without it. Any individual experiencing stomach issues (e.g., diarrhea, constipation, nausea, vomiting, or bleeding) must have a rectal examination in order to determine the best course of action for additional diagnostic and therapeutic procedures. The American Cancer Society suggests yearly rectal examination and testing for occult blood in the stool for all individuals over 40 as a screening procedure for both colorectal and prostate carcinoma, though there is disagreement regarding the exact age and frequency of testing.

Examining the buttocks can reveal symptoms of a variety of conditions, such as syphilis or herpes simplex superficial ulcers, fistulous tracts, skin tags from hemorrhoids, fissures in patients with inflammatory bowel disease, and rectal prolapse. In addition, generalized conditions like vitiligo and psoriasis, as well as infectious diseases like candidiasis and syphilitic dermatitis, can impact the perianal skin.

In many cases, assessing neuromuscular function is required because palpating the external anal sphincter alone is insufficient to diagnose dysfunction and is a poor indicator of strength. Because the anal canal cannot hold a typical volume of stool or because the urge to urinate is not strongly felt, patients with fecal incontinence frequently complain of diarrhea. These people frequently report traumatic childbirth experiences or surgically repaired hemorrhoids, which led to subsequent disruption of the innervation or musculature of the sphincter. Examining the perineum reveals that it descends much more than is typical, frequently below the ischial tuberosity plane. Furthermore, neuropathies, multiple sclerosis, primary or metastatic spinal cord tumors, and other serious systemic diseases may present with fecal incontinence as their initial symptom.

Palpation of the rectum can reveal fistulae or fissures not visible on inspection, as well as ulcers from syphilis, herpes, or inflammatory bowel disease. Because the rectum is the site of 22% of colorectal cancers and may also harbor metastatic disease, careful palpation of the rectum is necessary to detect the presence of masses. Not all masses are neoplastic; some could be abscesses. The mass's fluctuating consistency and the fever point to an abscess.

During a rectal examination, one of the more useful indicators is tenderness. The location and intensity of the tenderness may offer further or compelling evidence of conditions like ovarian cysts, pelvic inflammatory disease, prostatitis, ectopic pregnancy, tubo-ovarian abscesses, and inflammatory bowel disease. Although rectal tenderness has been hailed as a crucial diagnostic indicator in cases of suspected appendicitis, the overwhelming body of research indicates that this finding is not very helpful.

It cannot be overstated how important it is to record the color, consistency, and presence of frank or occult blood in the stool. Rectal examination may reveal that diarrhea in elderly patients—with or without a history of chronic constipation—is the result of fecal impaction. Degraded blood (melena), iron, licorice, bismuth, rhubarb, or overindulging in chocolate cookies are the causes of black stools. Red-colored stools can be caused by hematochezia, a rapid bleeding condition that typically occurs distal to the ligament of Treitz; on the other hand, patients receiving rifampin therapy for tuberculosis may report red- or orange-colored stools. Tan stools and dark urine are two of the earliest signs of hepatobiliary disease. Seldom does a patient with carcinoma of the Vater's ampulla complain of having silver stools.

For a variety of reasons, busy practitioners frequently neglect the rectal examination. There are claims that the procedure is not esthetically pleasing, takes too long, and hurts the patient. Nonetheless, a rectum examination can often lead a doctor to the right diagnosis in many cases. Consequently, there might be no need for costly and pointless laboratory and/or radiologic evaluation. A careful, meticulous, and industrious doctor will consider the rectal examination an essential component of a full assessment of the patient. Relevant is a quote from an unidentified source that states that most diagnoses can be made with just a pound of thoroughness, an ounce of knowledge, and an ounce of intelligence.

9.3. Laboratory Tests

9.3.1. Tests for Vaginal Infection

A sample of vaginal discharge should be examined if abnormal vaginal discharge is evident. Applying a sterile cotton-tipped applicator to the suspected area and then moving the suspect material to a suitable culture medium is how a culture is obtained. Most laboratories provide a prepackaged kit that enables the doctor to place the cotton-tipped applicator into a sterile container, which is then sent to the laboratory, because performing this procedure in the doctor's office is inconvenient. The pH of the vaginal discharge can also be measured. Fungal infections are typically associated with an acidic pH of 4–5, while bacterial vaginosis and Trichomonas infections are suggested by an alkaline pH of 5–7. A vaginal infection can frequently be mistaken for an endocervical infection. It is recommended to take a swab from the endocervix in order to test for chlamydia and gonorrhea.

a. **Saline (Plain Slide):** On a slide, the doctor combines one drop of vaginal discharge with one drop of normal saline that has been warmed to about body temperature in order to show Trichomonas vaginalis organisms. There should be a coverslip on the slide. When examining the smear while it's still warm, actively moving trichomonads are typically visible. The mycelia of the fungus Candida albicans, which resemble segmented and branching filaments, can also be found on the saline slide. By searching for "clue cells," or epithelial cells that have short coccobacilli type bacteria covering them from edge to edge, the slide can be helpful in the detection of bacterial vaginosis.

b. **Potassium:** Hydroxide: On a sterile slide, one drop of vaginal discharge is combined with one drop of an aqueous 10% potassium hydroxide solution, and a coverslip is placed on top. Potassium hydroxide helps to visualize the mycelia of a fungus that causes vaginal infections by dissolving epithelial cells and debris. You can put the slide up to your nose to find out if the discharge smells "fishy." Bacterial vaginosis, a common vaginal infection linked to a mixed anaerobic bacterial flora, is strongly suggested by this odor. Additionally, using just the saline smear, mycelia that may have been obscured by debris can be seen when this coverslip-equipped slide is magnified under a microscope.

c. **Bacterial Infection:** A patient may

have a bacterial infection, particularly if there is an ischemic lesion, as happens after radiation therapy for cervical carcinoma, or if they may have gonorrhea, bacterial vaginosis, or a Chlamydia trachomatis infection. Samples from the cervix, urethra, or vaginal lesion can be cultured, smeared, stained, and analyzed under a microscope.

9.3.2. Fern Test for Ovulation

The fern test can identify whether ovulation is occurring, whether it is not, and when it occurs.

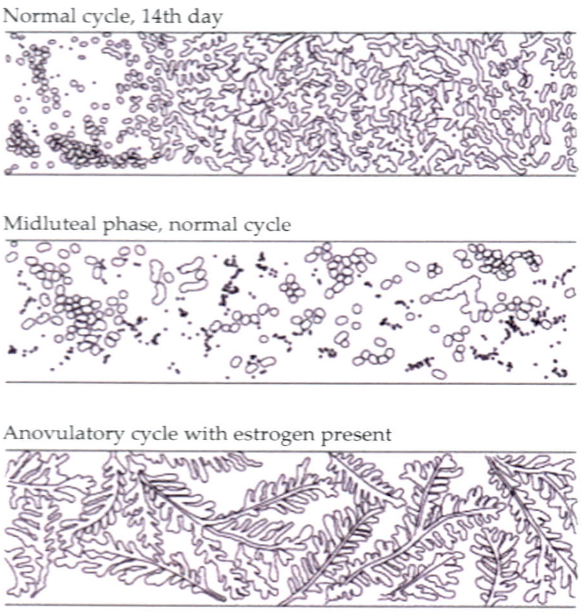

Figure 9.11. *Patterns formed when cervical mucus is smeared on a slide, permitted to dry, and examined under a microscope. Progesterone makes the mucus thick and cellular. In the smear from a patient who failed to ovulate (bottom), there is no progesterone to inhibit the estrogen-induced fern pattern.*

Source: Ganong WF. Review of Medical Physiology. 20th ed. New York, NY: McGraw-Hill; 2003.

Under a microscope, cervical mucus may or may not take on a frond-like pattern after being spread out on a clean, dry slide and allowed to dry in the air (occasionally, it can be seen grossly). A non-frondlike pattern can be interpreted as evidence that ovulation has occurred, as the fern frond pattern indicates an estrogenic effect on the mucus without the influence of progesterone (Figure 9.11).

9.3.3. Schiller Test for Neoplasia

The Schiller test may be carried out when cancer or precancerous changes of the cervix or vaginal mucosa are suspected, even though colposcopy is a more accurate method. The cervix's glycogen-rich epithelial cells are marked and interacting when Lugol's (strong iodine) solution is applied to the suspicious area. Because of scar tissue, neoplasia and precursors, and columnar epithelium, any area of the epithelium that rejects the dye is aberrant. If there is even a remote possibility of cancer, samples taken from this region should be biopsied.

9.3.4. Biopsy

A biopsy involves removing a small piece of tissue from the body for microscopic examination and testing.

a. **Vulva and Vagina:** A 1–2% aqueous solution of a typical local anesthetic solution can be injected around a small, suspicious area for vulva or vaginal biopsies, and a sample can be taken using a sharp scalpel or skin punch. Usually, applying pressure or using Monsel's solution can stop bleeding, but occasionally suturing is required.

b. **Cervix:** The preferred method for diagnosing cervical lesions—which may be suspected upon visualization or may become necessary following an abnormal Pap smear—is a colposcopically directed biopsy.

The entire columnar-squamous "transformation zone" (TZ) at the intersection of the exocervix and endocervix should be visible on a colposcopy. Furthermore, it might be wise to use a curettage to obtain an endocervix sample. Particular tools have been developed for endocervical curettage and cervical biopsies (Figure 9.12). Since the cervix is less sensitive to cutting techniques than the vagina, the patient may experience little to no discomfort when one or more tiny biopsy samples are taken from the cervix. Usually, bleeding is kept to a minimum and managed with Monsel's solution or light pressure for a few minutes. In the event that colposcopy is not available, a "4-quadrant" biopsy sample of the squamocolumnar junction can be obtained at the 12, 3, 6, and 9 o'clock positions. The area that needs to be biopsied can frequently be found more quickly by the doctor using a Schiller test.

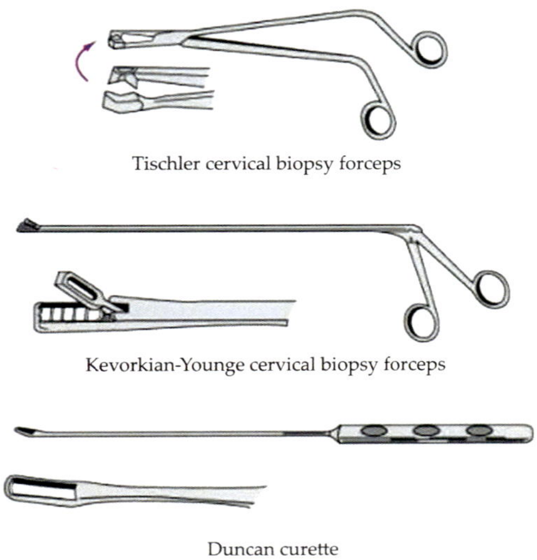

Figure 9.12. *Biopsy instruments.*

Source: Charles Kawada & Drorith Hochner-Celnikier; Gynecologic History, Examination, & Diagnostic Procedures; ISBN: 978-0-07-163969-9.

c. **Endometrium:** An endometrial biopsy can be used to screen for uterine corpus carcinoma as well as to diagnose ovarian dysfunction (such as infertility) or irregular uterine bleeding. Flexible disposable cannulas like the Pipelle, which have supplanted the majority of previously used metal curettes, can be used to perform endometrial biopsies (Figure 9.13). Since endometrial biopsies are almost as accurate as formal dilatation and curettage (DandC), the need for them has actually decreased significantly. The patient should be informed that the procedure will cause cramps and should take an ibuprofen or other pain medication an hour before the procedure.

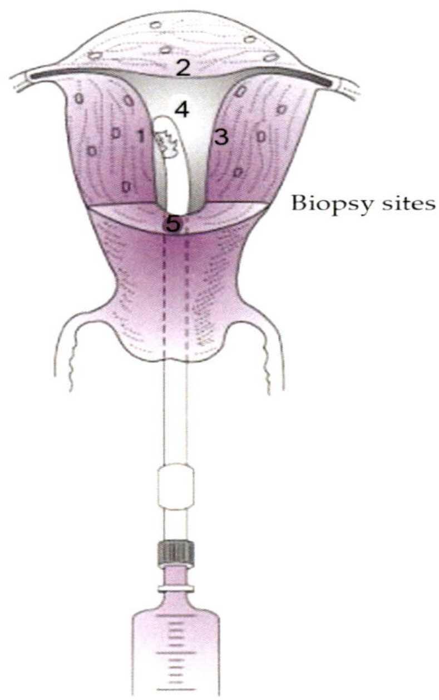

Figure 9.13. *Sites of endometrial biopsy.*

Source: Pernoll ML. Benson & Pernoll's Handbook of Obstetrics and Gynecology. 10th ed. New York, NY: McGraw-Hill; 2001.

9.4. Diagnostic Laboratory Procedures

A complete blood count (including differential white cell count), glucose screening, lipid profile, thyroid function tests, and other routine procedures are not covered here but should be taken into consideration during routine primary care visits. Based on risk factors and presenting complaints, the doctor should determine how frequently these tests are conducted.

9.4.1. Urinalysis

Patients who exhibit symptoms should have a urinalysis, which should include microscopic and gross examinations. Crystals or bacteria may be seen under a microscope, but the presence of bacteria has no significance if the specimen is not obtained in a way that prevents vaginal discharge.

9.4.2. Urine Culture

Research has indicated that a considerable proportion of women (roughly 3% of non-pregnant and 7% of pregnant) experience urinary tract infections without any symptoms. Urinary tract infection diagnosis and treatment are guided by culture and antibiotic sensitivity testing.

The "clean-catch" method is often a reliable way to obtain urine specimens for culture: the patient is instructed to carefully wash their urethral meatus with soap and water, to urinate briefly to remove any debris from their urethra, and then to collect a portion of their urine that is "midstream." Urine must not trickle over the labia, but some patients may find this challenging to achieve.

A sterile catheterization by a doctor or nurse is a more dependable way to collect pee for culture. Catheterization requires caution, though, to reduce the possibility of infection.

9.4.2.1. Other Cultures

a. **Urethral:** Urethral cultures are indicated if an STD is suspected.

b. **Vaginal:** A culture is typically not required to diagnose vaginal infections because the doctor can usually make the diagnosis based on microscopic examination or visual inspection, such as in the case of curd-like vaginal material that reveals mycelia (candidiasis). Nonetheless, in dubious situations, a culture ought to be acquired. When vaginal candidiasis is resistant to standard treatment, it is advisable to identify the type of yeast and determine its specific sensitivity to different antimycotic medications. This will help eradicate the problematic infection.

c. **Cervical:** As in the case of the urethra, the usual indication for a culture of cervical discharge is the suspected presence of an STD.

9.4.2.2. Specific Tests

a. **Herpes Simplex Virus (HSV):** Herpes genitalis (types 1 and 2), also known as herpesvirus hominis (HSV), is a common vulvar lesion. The cytopathologist can make the diagnosis based on the typical cellular changes they observe. Other, more reliable, and frequently employed techniques for detecting HSV infection include culturing the virus and identifying it with the polymerase chain reaction (PCR) method.

b. **Human Papillomavirus:** Genital warts and intraepithelial lesions in the vagina and cervical regions are linked to human papillomavirus (HPV) infection. Precancerous or cancerous lesions are present in some of these lesions. Epithelial alterations that are benign or more aggressive are associated with different HPV subtypes. The distinct fingerprints derived from the PCR products can be used to distinguish between the various subtypes.

c. **Chlamydia & Gonorrheal Infections:** There are two most common sexually transmitted infections, chlamydia being the most common. They are more common in women who do not use barrier methods of contraception and in those who have several sexual partners. With a sensitivity of more than 90%, nucleic acid amplification testing is the most widely utilized diagnostic technique.

d. **Human Immunodeficiency Virus:** AIDS, or acquired immunodeficiency syndrome, is currently one of the most challenging conditions that clinicians of all stripes must deal with. Given that young heterosexually active females without any other risk factors are experiencing the highest increase in HIV incidence, it is imperative that HIV screening be done on the general population. For diagnosis, a precise blood test is available. The doctor has to explain to the patient how accurate the blood test is at detecting HIV before taking any blood. The patient needs to be informed that false-positive tests are rare and that there is a "window" in which a test could be falsely negative before antibodies develop. Currently, the patient has to sign a written consent form before their blood can be drawn.

9.4.3. Papanicolaou Smear of Cervix

A crucial component of the gynecologic examination is the Pap smear. Recently, the requirement for this test's frequency was changed. Based on epidemiologic statistics, the US Preventive Services Task Force suggests that a Pap test every two or three years is sufficient for a typical woman who has had three normal Pap smears. The majority of cervical cancers are observed to grow slowly, which provides support for this recommendation. Annual Pap smear screenings are advised by the American College of Obstetricians and Gynecologists starting three years after the initiation of sexual activity and no later than age 21. After three consecutive negative Pap smears, the frequency of screening for women aged 30–64 years may be lowered to every 2–3 years. Patients who are at risk should continue to undergo annual screenings. These patients include women who have had multiple sexual partners, a history of STDs, genital condylomata, or abnormal Pap smears; women on immune suppression therapy; women living with HIV; and women exposed to diethylstilbestrol (DES) in utero. Cervical cytology testing should be performed on HIV-positive women every six months following diagnosis, and then yearly following two consecutive normal test results. These recommendations for cervical cytology screening remain unchanged based on HPV vaccination status. If a patient is 65 to 70 years old, has had three or more consecutive normal test results, no abnormal test results in the previous ten years, has no history of cervical cancer, has not previously been exposed to DES in utero, is HIV negative, is not immunodepressed, and has no other risk factors for new STD acquisition, the doctor may consider stopping cervical cytology at that age. If cervical cytology has been discontinued, the doctor should review risk factors every year to determine whether resuming screening is necessary.

The cytologist may suspect additional local conditions in addition to premalignant and malignant changes. Mucosal alterations can be observed in cases of viral infections, including condylomata acuminata, HPV, and HSV. A Pap smear can identify infections caused by Trichomonas and actinomycosis. The Pap test is just a screening procedure. Additional diagnostic procedures like a colposcopy, endocervical curettage, cervical biopsy or conization, endometrial biopsy, or D&C are indicated by positive test results. In about 95% of cases, a properly collected Pap smear can reliably result in the diagnosis of cervical carcinoma. Although it only detects less than 50% of cases, the Pap smear is useful in identifying endometrial abnormalities such as polyps, hyperplasia, and cancers.

The patient should not be menstruating and should not have had a period for at least 24 hours before the examination. After lubricating the vagina with only water, the speculum is inserted into the vagina. After the cervix is exposed, a specially made plastic or wooden spatula is applied, and it is rotated 360 degrees to slightly abrade the surface and collect cells from the cervical os's squamocolumnar area. Subsequently, a tiny brush or cotton-tipped applicator is placed inside the endocervix and turned 360 degrees. Depending on the examiner's preference, these two specimens can be combined or placed separately on the slide. Preservative is applied right away to avoid air drying, which could cause the interpretation to become compromised. Together with an identification sheet that includes relevant findings and history, the slide is sent to the lab. In order to eliminate the variability caused by the clinician preparing the slide, another technique called ThinPrep automates the Pap smear slide preparation process. By using this technique, the sample is sent to the lab in a liquid-based medium. Furthermore, fewer smears with atypical squamous cells–undetermined significance (ASCUS) are required after using the ThinPrep technique, which reduces the need for colposcopic examinations. For these reasons, the traditional Pap smear has been superseded by the ThinPrep technique in many regions of the nation. It's unclear, though, whether the liquid-based approach has any sensitivity or specificity advantages over the traditional approach.

Testing for high-risk HPV is possible using the liquid-based medium; the most prevalent subtypes are 16, 18, 31, 33, and 35. The American Society for Colposcopy and Cervical Pathology has suggested testing for high-risk HPV as a means of classifying and assessing patients with ASCUS Pap smear results. Similar to those who have a negative Pap smear, these people can have a follow-up Pap smear in a year if the ASCUS Pap smear reveals no high-risk HPV. Individuals with a high-risk HPV subtype would be evaluated colposcopically.

To reduce the number of false-positive and false-negative Pap smear results, alternatives to the conventional Pap smear are being investigated. Research suggests that computerized Pap smear screening can reduce the risk of overlooking important pathologies. A number of computerized screening techniques have been developed to assist the human eye in identifying anomalies, but no system has gained widespread acceptance as of yet.

9.4.4. Colposcopy

A binocular microscope called a colposcope is used to directly view the cervix (Figure 9.14). Although there are instruments with magnifications as high as 60 ×, the most widely used one in clinical settings has a 13.5 × magnification, which effectively fills in the gaps between what the unaided eye and a microscope can see. A camera is a feature of certain colposcopes that allows for the single or sequential photography of pathologic conditions.

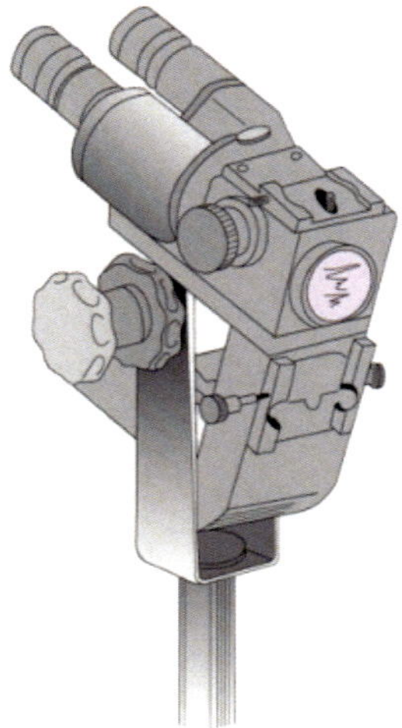

Figure 9.14. *Zeiss colposcope.*

Source: Charles Kawada & Drorith Hochner-Celnikier; Gynecologic History, Examination, & Diagnostic Procedures; ISBN: 978-0-07-163969-9.

Colposcopy is an additional and crucial tool for diagnosing cervix abnormalities; it does not take the place of other techniques in this regard. DES-exposed daughters, who may have dysplasia of the vagina or cervix, and patients with abnormal Pap smears are the two most significant patient groups that can benefit from its use.

The areas most suitable for biopsy can be chosen because a doctor can see areas of cellular dysplasia and vascular or tissue abnormalities that are not visible in other light. Additional chemical agents and stains are also used to enhance visualization. The use of blind cervical biopsies, which have a poor success rate, has decreased thanks to the colposcope. Furthermore, there is no longer as much need for a cone biopsy, a procedure that has a high rate of morbidity. Because of this, a skilled doctor can identify focal cervical lesions, take directed biopsies at the best locations, and determine the best course of treatment primarily based on what is visible through the colposcope.

9.4.5. Hysteroscopy

With hysteroscopy, a gynecologist can use a fiberoptic device called a hysteroscope to examine the uterine cavity. Furthermore, the hysteroscope can be used to execute surgical procedures like polypectomy, myomectomy, septectomy, and resection of intrauterine adhesions. The uterine cavity is inflated using a solution (typically saline, but other solutions like glycine or dextran can be used) or by carbon dioxide insufflation in order to examine the interior of the uterus with a hysteroscope. While general anesthesia, paracervical block, or intravenous sedation are frequently sufficient for operative hysteroscopies, diagnostic hysteroscopies are typically performed without any kind of sedation.

Evaluation for abnormal uterine bleeding, uterine synechiae and septa resection, polyp and intrauterine device (IUD) removal, submucous myoma resection, and endometrial ablation are among the applications of hysteroscopic procedures. Since the majority of these therapeutic techniques involve substantial manipulation, either regional or general anesthesia is necessary.

Only doctors who have received the necessary training should perform hysteroscopy. After inserting the instrument tip slightly past the internal cervical, it should be slowly advanced with sufficient distention under direct vision. Hysteroscopy frequently works in tandem with other surgical techniques like curettage and laparoscopy.

Bleeding, excessive mucus secretion, cervical stenosis, and insufficient uterine cavity distention can all lead to hysteroscopy failure. Bleeding, infection, and perforation are the most frequent side effects. Uterine perforation typically happens at the fundus. Surgery may not be necessary unless there is internal bleeding or damage to a viscus. Although bleeding usually stops, in certain situations fulguration may be necessary after attempts to remove polyps or myomas. Seldom observed parametritis or salpingitis typically requires antibiotic therapy. Although intravascular extravasation of gas or fluid from hysteroscopy has been linked to serious outcomes like cerebral edema, air embolism, hyponatremia, and even death, it frequently does not reach a clinically significant level.

9.4.6. Culdocentesis

A diagnostic procedure that can be carried out in a hospital treatment room or an office involves passing a needle into the cul-de-sac (culdocentesis) to extract fluid from the Douglas pouch (Figure 9.15). The fluid obtained can reveal the type of intraperitoneal lesion (e.g., pus with acute salpingitis, bloody with ruptured ectopic pregnancy, or ascitic fluid with malignant cells in cancer). Nowadays, culdocentesis is seldom done because advancements in ultrasonography technology allow for a more thorough assessment of pelvic pathology (Wright et al., 2004).

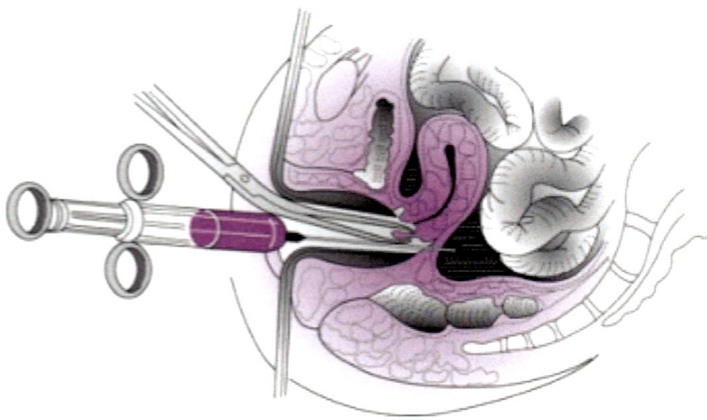

Figure 9.15. *Culdocentesis.*

Source: Charles Kawada & Drorith Hochner-Celnikier; Gynecologic History, Examination, & Diagnostic Procedures; ISBN: 978-0-07-163969-9.

A Closer Look

Radiographic Diagnostic Procedures

Radiographic diagnostic procedures are essential tools in medical imaging that help healthcare professionals diagnose and monitor various conditions. These procedures use X-rays to create images of the internal structures of the body, providing valuable insights that are not visible through external examination. One of the most common radiographic procedures is the standard X-ray, which is often used to detect fractures, infections, and abnormalities in bones and joints. This technique is also employed in the examination of the chest to identify conditions such as pneumonia, lung tumors, and heart problems.

Another significant radiographic procedure is computed tomography (CT) scanning. CT scans combine X-ray images taken from different angles to produce cross-sectional views of the body. This advanced imaging technique allows for a more detailed examination of soft tissues, blood vessels, and organs, making it indispensable in diagnosing diseases such as cancer, cardiovascular diseases, and internal injuries. The high-resolution images generated by CT scans enable doctors to detect small abnormalities that might be missed with standard X-rays.

Fluoroscopy is another vital radiographic diagnostic procedure, which provides real-time moving images of the internal structures of the body. During fluoroscopy, a continuous X-ray beam is passed through the body, and the images are displayed on a monitor. This technique is particularly useful in guiding procedures such as catheter insertions, joint injections, and barium studies of the gastrointestinal tract. Fluoroscopy enhances the precision and safety of these procedures by allowing the physician to see the exact placement of instruments within the body.

Mammography is a specialized radiographic technique used primarily for the early detection and diagnosis of breast cancer. This procedure involves compressing the breast tissue to obtain clear X-ray images, which can reveal tumors, cysts, and calcifications. Regular mammograms are recommended for women, especially those over the age of 40, as they can detect breast cancer at an early, more treatable stage.

Lastly, angiography is a radiographic procedure used to visualize the inside of blood vessels and organs of the body, particularly the arteries, veins, and heart chambers. During this procedure, a contrast dye is injected into the bloodstream, making the blood vessels visible on the X-ray images. Angiography is crucial in diagnosing and managing conditions such as aneurysms, blockages, and other vascular diseases. By providing detailed images of the blood vessels, angiography helps in planning surgical interventions and other treatments.

Summary

- To adequately evaluate the gynecologic patient, it is important to establish a rapport during the history taking. The patient needs to tell her story to an interested listener who does not allow body language or facial expressions to imply disinterest or boredom. One should avoid cutting off the patient's story, because doing so may obscure important clues or other problems that may have contributed to the reasons for the visit.
- The physical examination is most useful if it is conducted in an environment that is esthetically pleasing to the patient. Adequate gowning and draping assist in preventing embarrassment. Often a physician's assistant escorts the patient to the dressing area and gives explicit instructions about what to take off and how to put on her gown and then may assist in draping the patient.
- Breast examination should be a routine part of the physical examination. Breast cancer will occur in 1 in 8 women in the United States during her lifetime. Physicians who treat women should educate patients on the technique of self-examination because the well-prepared patient is one of the most accurate screening methods for breast disease.
- The pelvic examination is a procedure feared by many women, so it must be conducted in such a way as to allay her anxieties. A patient's first pelvic examination may be especially disturbing, so it is important for the physician to attempt to allay fear and to inspire confidence and cooperation.
- The cervix is a firm structure traditionally described as having the consistency of the tip of the nose. Normally it is round and approximately 3–4 cm in diameter.
- Two muscle bundles, known as the internal and external anal sphincters, participate in defecation. The internal anal sphincter is an enlargement of the circular smooth muscle of the colon and functions involuntarily.
- Tenderness is one of the more helpful signs on rectal examination. The location and degree of tenderness may provide additional or convincing evidence of such disorders as prostatitis, pelvic inflammatory disease, tubo-ovarian abscesses, ovarian cysts, ectopic pregnancy, and inflammatory bowel disease.
- One drop of an aqueous 10% potassium hydroxide solution is mixed with 1 drop of vaginal discharge on a clean slide and a coverslip is applied. The potassium hydroxide dissolves epithelial cells and debris and facilitates visualization of the mycelia of a fungus causing vaginal infection.
- An endometrial biopsy can be helpful in the diagnosis of ovarian dysfunction (eg, infertility) or irregular uterine bleeding and as a test for carcinoma of the uterine corpus.
- Reliable specimens of urine for culture often can be obtained by the "clean-catch" method: The patient is instructed to cleanse the urethral meatus carefully with soap and water, to urinate for a few seconds to dispose of urethral contaminants, and then to catch a "midstream" portion of the urine. It is essential that the urine not dribble over the labia, but this may be difficult for some patients to accomplish.
- Acquired immunodeficiency syndrome (AIDS) has become one of the most difficult issues confronting all kinds of clinicians. The need to screen for HIV in the general population has become more pressing given that the largest increase in incidence is seen in young heterosexually active females with no other risk factors.

References

1. American Cancer Society. (2003). American Cancer Society guidelines for breast cancer screening: Update 2003. *CA: A Cancer Journal for Clinicians, 53*(3), 141–169. https://doi.org/10.3322/canjclin.53.3.141.
2. American College of Obstetricians and Gynecologists. (2003). Cervical cytology screening. *Obstetrics & Gynecology, 102*(2), 417. https://doi.org/10.1016/S0029-7844(03)00663-3.
3. Bayrak, A., Saadat, P., Mor, E., Chong, L., Paulson, J. P., & Sokol, R. Z. (2005). Pituitary imaging is indicated for the evaluation of hyperprolactinemia. *Fertility and Sterility, 84*(1), 181–185. https://doi.org/10.1016/j.fertnstert.2005.01.092.
4. Bazot, M., Darai, E., Hourani, R., Thomassin, I., Cortez, A., Uzan, S., & Buy, J. N. (2004). Deep pelvic endometriosis: MR imaging for diagnosis and prediction of extension of disease. *Radiology, 232*(2), 379–389. https://doi.org/10.1148/radiol.2322030601.
5. Henry, M. M., Parks, A. G., & Swash, M. (1982). The pelvic floor musculature in the descending perineum syndrome. *British Journal of Surgery, 69*(8), 470–472. https://doi.org/10.1002/bjs.1800690808.
6. Lieberman, D. A. (1984). Common anorectal disorders. *Annals of Internal Medicine, 101*(6), 837–846. https://doi.org/10.7326/0003-4819-101-6-837.
7. Marrazzo, J. M., & Stine, K. (2004). Reproductive health history of lesbians: Implications for care. *American Journal of Obstetrics and Gynecology, 190*(5), 1298–1304. https://doi.org/10.1016/j.ajog.2004.01.007.
8. Nustaum, M. R., & Hamilton, C. D. (2002). The proactive sexual health history. *American Family Physician, 66*(9), 1705–1712. https://www.aafp.org/afp/2002/1101/p1705.html (accessed on 6 September 2024).
9. Porter, S. D., & Liechty, R. D. (1976). The anorectum. In R. D. Liechty & R. D. Soper (Eds.), *Synopsis of Surgery* (pp. 385–396). C. V. Mosby.
10. Schrock, T. R. (1983). Examination of the anorectum, rigid sigmoidoscopy and flexible fibroptic sigmoidoscopy. In M. H. Sleisenger & J. S. Fordtran (Eds.), *Gastrointestinal Disease* (pp. 1276–1280). W. B. Saunders.
11. Vassilakos, P., Schwartz, D., de Marval, F., et al. (2000). Biopsy-based comparison of liquid-based, thin-layer preparations to conventional Pap smear. *Journal of Reproductive Medicine, 45*(1), 11–16. https://pubmed.ncbi.nlm.nih.gov/10664916/ (accessed on 6 September 2024).
12. Wright, T., Massad, L. S., Dunton, C. J., et al. (2004). Interim guidelines for the use of human papillomavirus DNA testing as an adjunct to cervical cytology screening. *Obstetrics & Gynecology, 103*(3), 304–309. https://doi.org/10.1097/01.AOG.0000117104.45568.59.

Chapter

PEDIATRIC AND ADOLESCENT GYNECOLOGY

10

Contents

Introduction

Pediatric and adolescent gynecology is a specialized field of medicine that addresses the unique gynecological needs of children and adolescents. This discipline encompasses a broad range of issues, from congenital anomalies and menstrual disorders to the management of puberty and reproductive health. The focus is on providing age-appropriate care that considers the physiological, psychological, and developmental stages of young patients.

Children and adolescents face distinct gynecological challenges that differ significantly from those of adults. Congenital anomalies, such as Müllerian duct anomalies, can present early in life and require careful diagnosis and management. Conditions like labial adhesions, vulvovaginitis, and ovarian cysts are also common in this age group and necessitate specific approaches to treatment that minimize discomfort and psychological impact.

Menstrual disorders, including amenorrhea (absence of menstruation), dysmenorrhea (painful menstruation), and abnormal uterine bleeding, are frequent concerns among adolescents. These issues can significantly impact the quality of life and require thorough evaluation to rule out underlying conditions such as polycystic ovary syndrome (PCOS), coagulation disorders, or thyroid dysfunction. Hormonal therapies, lifestyle modifications, and, in some cases, surgical interventions are part of the treatment spectrum.

Puberty, a critical phase in an adolescent's life, involves a series of complex physiological changes. Delayed or precocious puberty can lead to significant physical and emotional distress. Early identification and appropriate intervention are crucial in managing these conditions to ensure normal development and psychosocial well-being.

Reproductive health education forms a cornerstone of pediatric and adolescent gynecology. Providing comprehensive, age-appropriate information about sexual health, contraception, and sexually transmitted infections (STIs) is vital for fostering informed and healthy decision-making among young individuals. Sensitive and confidential communication is essential to build trust and encourage open discussions about gynecological and sexual health issues.

Pediatric and adolescent gynecology is dedicated to addressing the specific gynecological and reproductive health needs of young patients. By combining medical expertise with a compassionate, developmentally appropriate approach, healthcare providers can effectively support the well-being and healthy development of children and adolescents.

Orientation and Directional Terms

Term	Definition	Illustration
Vaginoscopy	Vaginoscopy is performed to see lesions, investigate potential sexual abuse, remove foreign bodies, perform rectovaginal examinations, and drain cysts.	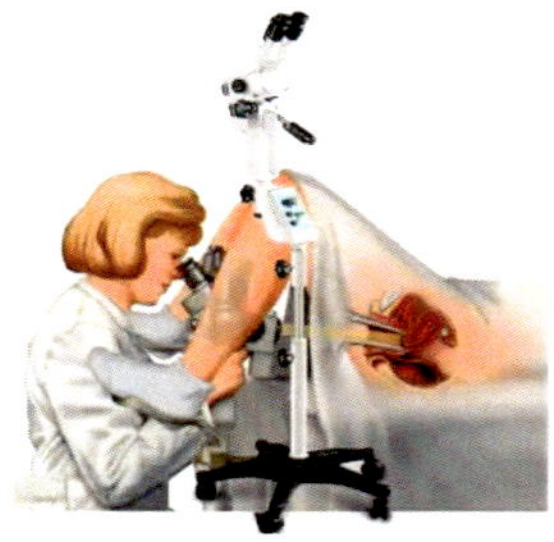
Precocious puberty	Precocious puberty is when children's bodies start to change into adult bodies too early.	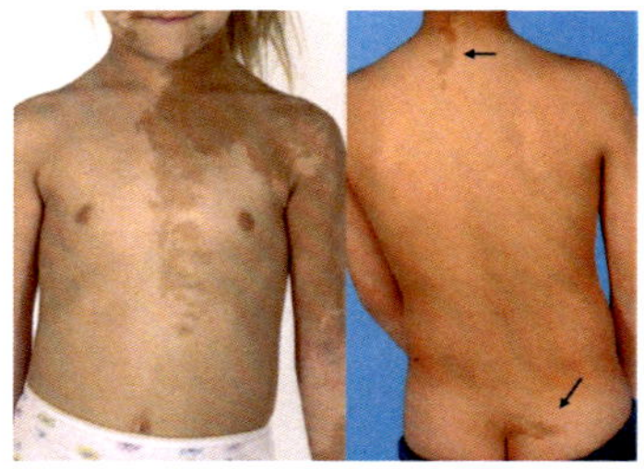
Vulvovaginitis	Vulvovaginitis is an inflammation of both the vulva and the vagina.	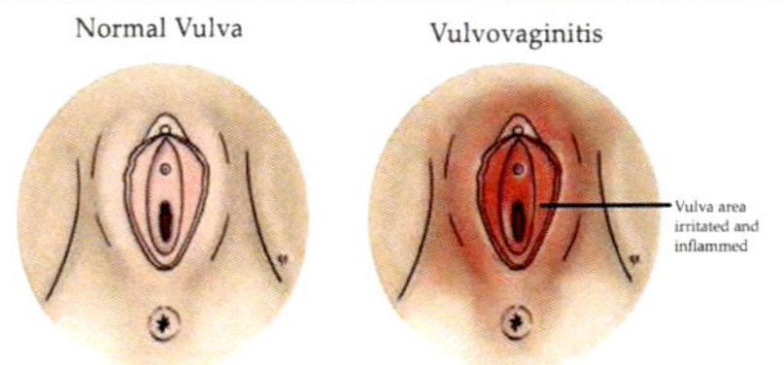
Labia minora	The labia minora are the smaller inner folds of skin on the outside of the vulva, or female genitals.	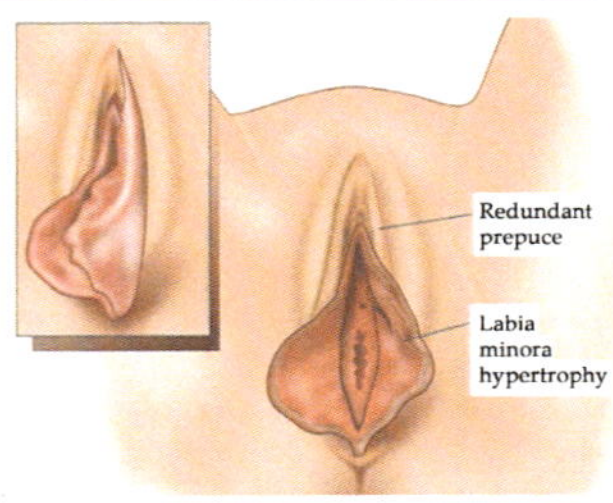
Mons pubis	The mons pubis is a triangular area of fatty tissue and hair-bearing skin that covers the pubic bone and symphysis pubis in both sexes.	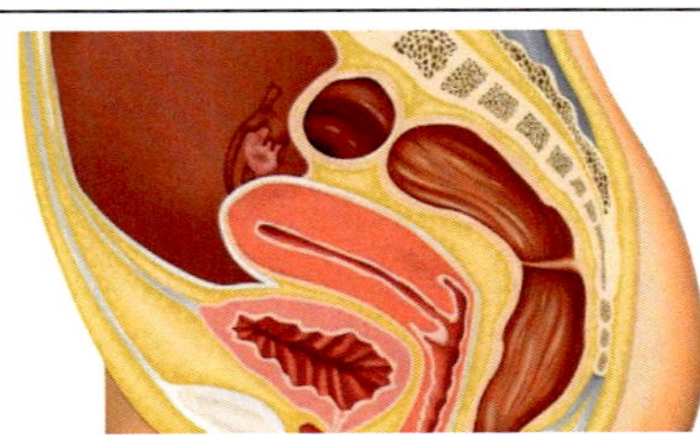

10.1. The Pediatric Gynecological Examination

Gynecologic care includes the subspecialty of pediatric and adolescent gynecology as a crucial component. It is typically the first gynecologic encounter a female will ever have. In an attempt to set the standard for all gynecologic care in the future, it is imperative that this be a positive experience. This chapter covers the history, physical examination procedure, and fundamentals of common gynecologic issues found in pediatric patients. One cannot stress the significance of a thorough examination enough. The physician needs to continue to be aware of the physical issue at hand as well as its psychological implications. An understanding of the psychological effects the patient and parents experience, for example, is essential to the evaluation process when dealing with precocious puberty. It is crucial that the obstetrician/gynecologist diagnoses and treats the condition appropriately because it may turn out to be potentially fatal, such as in the case of congenital adrenal hyperplasia.

10.1.1. General Principles

The patient should be actively involved in the process as long as it is age-appropriate, and it is crucial to get the history from the parent or parents. Building rapport and communication is the main strategy; it is crucial for the patient to gain confidence in the healthcare professional. Prioritizing education over the examination procedure will pay off in a way that will improve patient compliance and the overall evaluation of the issue at hand. The idea of "show and tell" is frequently beneficial in obtaining a sufficient evaluation. The office staff's identity (i.e., A successful evaluation is facilitated by the medical assistant or nurse who spends time with the patient and parent prior to the physical examination. Knowledge of the equipment that will be utilized during the examination process (e.g., cotton swab, or otoscope) could ease the patient's discomfort. The equipment's nonthreatening nature should be emphasized. Frequently, a simple vulvovaginal examination suffices. It is important to reassure the patient and parent that the evaluation will end if it becomes uncomfortable or painful.

With rare exceptions, most patients can undergo evaluation without sedation, though it may occasionally be necessary to ensure a thorough assessment. Parents and patients should be informed that it is often not necessary to perform an "internal" exam. Pediatric conscious sedation, however, may be used if the child needs a certain level of sedation and trained personnel are on hand, or in conjunction with anesthesia for an examination. The choice to have an examination without the parent present should be presented to the pediatric patient as they get closer to puberty. An assistant's actual physical presence (i.e., nurse, or medical assistant) needs to be highlighted.

10.1.2. Positioning and Initial Assessment

The general assessment ought to be conducted in the same manner as a physical examination, meaning that the skin should be examined and any lesions or disfigurements should be noted. It is not appropriate to restrain the child while they are being examined. Once more, a cooperative attitude (i.e., "Show and tell") is frequently beneficial in starting the examination procedure. The best course of action is to give the child a sense of control over the examination and to promise not to cause them any discomfort.

10.1.3. Breast Examination

During the neonatal period, breast examination often shows signs of maternal estrogen influence, such as palpable breast tissue and milky discharge. This discharge typically disappears within a few days after birth. It is advisable not to massage the breast tissue as it may increase the risk of abscess formation, particularly with staphylococcal organisms.

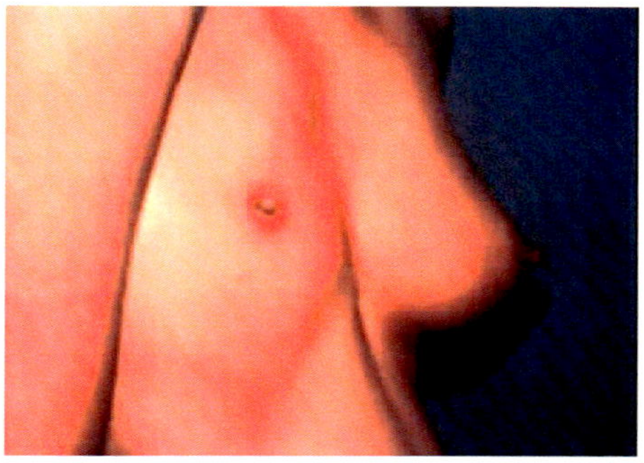

Figure 10.1. *Breast asymmetry in a 16-year-old girl.*

Source: Syed-Ansari, T, Murray, P, et al., Glob. libr. women's med., (ISSN: 1756–2228) 2008; DOI 10.3843/GLOWM.10010.

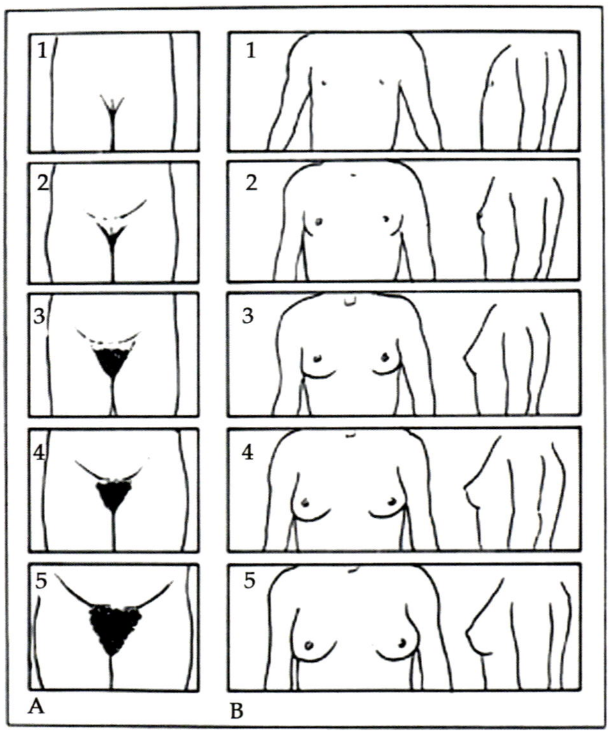

Figure 10.2. *Female tanner staging.*

Source: Syed-Ansari, T, Murray, P, et al., Glob. libr. women's med., (ISSN: 1756–2228) 2008; DOI 10.3843/GLOWM.10010.

For white girls, thelarche typically starts at age nine, whereas it starts a little earlier for African American girls. The onset age is 9 +/- 8 years old on average. (Kaplowitz, 2006) It is not unusual for breast development to be asymmetrical, particularly in the early phases of breast formation. Breast tanner staging is advised (Figures 10.1 and 10.2).

10.1.4. Abdominal Examination

Examining the abdomen for skin lesions is the first step in the evaluation process. Palpation for masses comes after the evaluation of bowel sounds. Since the prepubertal child's ovaries are situated at the pelvic brim, an intra-abdominal mass is the typical presentation of an adnexal enlargement. Ultrasonography is a helpful addition to the examination process to detect abnormalities of the reproductive tract (Muram, 1987).

10.1.5. Pelvic Examination

The supine position with the buttocks on the end of the gynecologic examination table is the best position for achieving a clear view of the external genitalia. The legs are positioned like "frog legs." If the child is not cooperating, the parent may sit in a chair and hold the child, or the child may be placed on the parent's lap. Should additional visualization be required, the patient can assume a knee-chest position and be instructed to expel their stomach by pushing it out while holding their breath. Valsalva). In both positions, the Valsalva maneuver may help with visualization. Visualizing the entire vaginal canal, including cervix identification, is often possible. To further involve the patient in the examination process, a hand-held mirror can be used. To examine the introitus and the lower third of the vagina, the clinician should gently grasp the labia in the "frog-leg" position and move them laterally and downward. This portion of the examination is frequently made easier with the use of an otoscope or a colposcope. It is recommended to stage pubic hair using tanner; any discharge, edema, erythema, or congenital anomalies should be noted. Furthermore, physical signs such as cuts, scrapes, bruises, or scars may suggest sexual abuse even in the absence of the primary complaint from the parent or guardian (Christensen et al., 1971) (Figure 10.3).

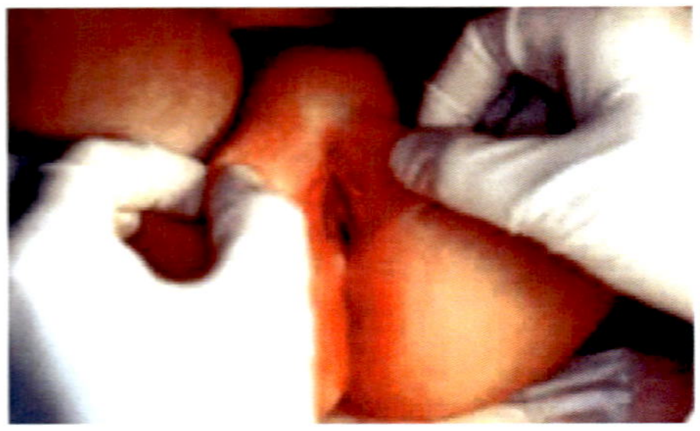

Figure 10.3. *Normal female external genital examination.*

Source: Syed-Ansari, T, Murray, P, et al., Glob. libr. women's med., (ISSN: 1756–2228) 2008; DOI 10.3843/GLOWM.10010.

It is not recommended to manipulate the labia forcefully, and any pain or discomfort should cause the evaluation method to be reevaluated. It matters what the hymenal diameter, configuration, and symmetry are. It is important to record the clitoris' dimensions and shape as well as any urethral anomalies. In order to rule out the presence of a foreign body, trauma, neoplasm, or other congenital anomaly, an external light source such as a vaginoscope, hysteroscope, or otoscope is particularly helpful. The most frequent past complaints reported by the parent or guardian are recurrent vaginal discharge and bleeding, but a clinician needs to be prepared to consider a wide range of possibilities. In order to evaluate vaginal discharge, a wet preparation is helpful.

In most cases, a speculum is not required when evaluating a pediatric patient. Body-temperature saline irrigation of the vaginal region frequently lavages out foreign bodies if one is suspected of having one. The most frequent foreign object is rolled toilet paper, which is easily removed with water (Leung et al., 1993) (Figure 10.4).

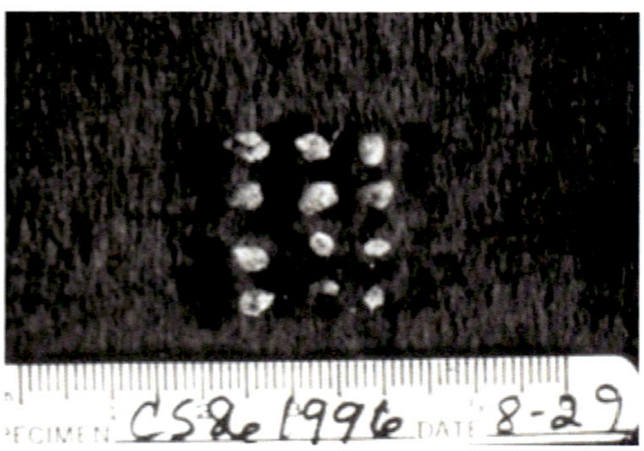

Figure 10.4. *Rolling toilet paper—the most common foreign body in pediatric vagina.*

Source: Syed-Ansari, T, Murray, P, et al., Glob. libr. women's med., (ISSN: 1756–2228) 2008; DOI 10.3843/GLOWM.10010.

In certain situations, a rectal examination should be considered, particularly if a pelvic-abdominal mass is suspected (Table 10.1).

Table 10.1. Tips for Getting Through the Pediatric Gyn Exam

Obtain the patient's cooperation; this is necessary for teachable moments and adequate examinations.
• Give her as much control as possible.
• Give a realistic description of what to expect in regards to what will happen and when during the exam.
• Describe what she might feel and talk with her about it.
• Explain who will be in the room.
• Define the information that is to be obtained.
Special aspects of the prepubertal female's examination
• Inform the child that the genital examination is sanctioned.
• Involve the child by giving them a hand-held mirror and magnification device.
• Be open to different types of positioning for the exam. Consider the child with the feet in the stirrups, with the feet on the examiner's lap, or sitting on the parent's lap, with the child's legs dropped over the parent's thighs.
• Attempt both the supine and knee-chest positions.
• Be knowledgeable about the various visualization methods to see the vestibule.
• There is only a limited need to use instruments.
Special aspects of the peripubertal genital examination
• Understand the impact of estrogen.
• Choose the proper speculum width after the introitus is evaluated.

Source: Syed-Ansari, T, Murray, P, et al., Glob. libr. women's med., (ISSN: 1756–2228) 2008; DOI 10.3843/GLOWM.10010This.

10.1.6. First Pelvic Examination

Many experts in the field have addressed the question of when a virginal adolescent should have her first pelvic examination. Present guidelines suggest a Pap smear and pelvic exam be performed on a virgin patient three years after coitarche, or at age 21. However, regardless of coitarche, routine evaluations for sexually transmitted infections (STIs) should be performed on any young woman who is sexually active. Urine, vaginal, or cervical specimens are available for STI testing. The clinician will determine whether visualization of the external genitalia, vagina, or cervix is necessary in a patient who is sexually active if a Pap smear is not recommended. Remember that even if a patient is not "sexually active," they may have experienced sexual abuse as a youngster. If the event happened three years or longer ago, a Pap smear might be recommended for these patients. The therapist may be able to discuss sexuality, preventive health issues, and build rapport with teenage patients in a non-threatening way during counseling sessions.

10.2. Normal Genital Anatomy

10.2.1. Newborn Infant

The effects of maternal hormones acquired transplacentally are primarily responsible for the typical appearance of the female genitalia in newborns. The labia minora have thickened and the labia majora are full. The hymenal folds seem superfluous and thick. The vaginal mucosa has an acidic pH and is pink and moist. In most cases, physiological leukorrhea is evident. Parents may become anxious and concerned when their child experiences vaginal bleeding due to the natural decrease in maternal estrogen during the first week of life. It should be clarified that this is a typical process brought on by the effects of maternal hormones and that it usually goes away in 7–9 days. In addition, breast tissue development and, in certain situations, nipple discharge in the newborn are brought on by the mother's estrogen circulation. The baby might therefore be more vulnerable to infection and inflammation of the breasts. The labia majora become less full, the labia minora and hymen become flatter and thinner, and the amount of breast tissue decreases as the levels of maternal hormones drop (Christensen et al., 1971) (Figure 10.5).

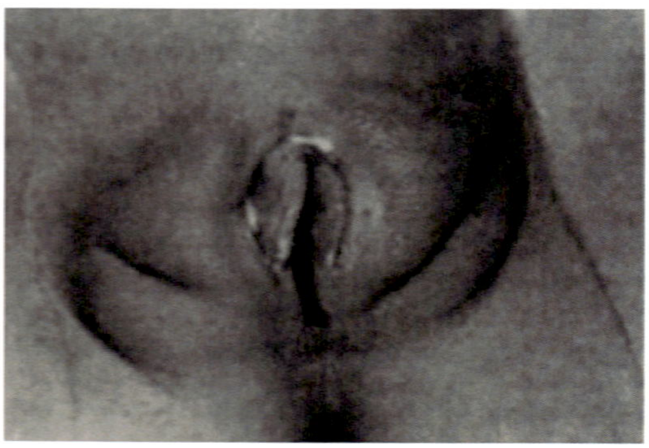

Figure 10.5. *Normal newborn female external genitalia.*

Source: Syed-Ansari, T, Murray, P, et al., Glob. libr. women's med., (ISSN: 1756-2228) 2008; DOI 10.3843/GLOWM.10010.

10.2.2. Prepubertal Girls

The labia get smaller as the baby gets older. Because of this, the vaginal vestibule is less shielded from germs and outside allergens, particularly when the child is sitting or squatting. The mucosa of the vagina becomes relatively atrophic and thin. The pH of the vagina is either neutral or alkaline, and there are less secretions. The hymen becomes smooth-edged, thin, and translucent by the time the child is 18 to 24 months old. At this point, the vaginal orifice's typical variations in shape are visible. (Leung A. K., and others. 1993) The hymen, for instance, could have an annular, crescentic, or fimbriated appearance. Furthermore, there is a higher chance of tearing due to trauma because the perineum, perivaginal tissues, and pelvic supporting structures become relatively rigid and inelastic. Furthermore, the ovaries are situated above the pelvic brim prior to the onset of puberty. Thus, rather than pelvic complaints, abdominal pain is more typical presentation of ovarian disorders in young children (Figures 10.6 and 10.7).

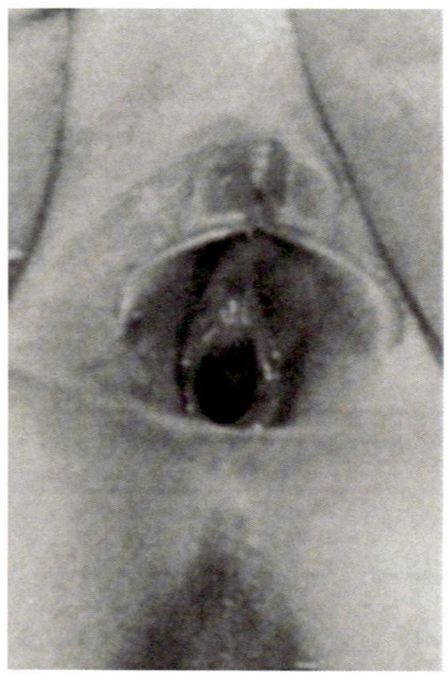

Figure 10.6. *Normal prepubertal female external genitalia.*

Source: Syed-Ansari, T, Murray, P, et al., Glob. libr. women's med., (ISSN: 1756-2228) 2008; DOI 10.3843/GLOWM.10010.

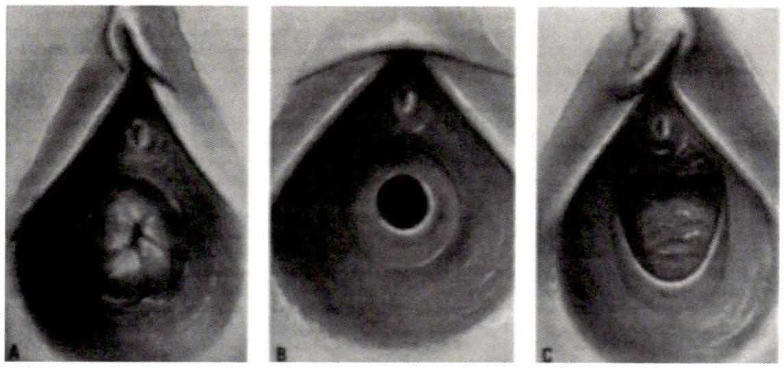

Figure 10.7. *A. Fimbriated hymen, normal variant. B. Circumferential hymen, normal variant. C. Posterior rim hymen, normal variant. (Pokorny SF: Configuration of the prepubertal hymen. Am J Obstet Gynecol 157:950, 1987).*

Source: Syed-Ansari, T, Murray, P, et al., Glob. libr. women's med., (ISSN: 1756-2228) 2008; DOI 10.3843/GLOWM.10010.

10.2.3. Peripubertal Girls

Ovarian estrogen is mostly responsible for the development of secondary sex traits during puberty. Hair grows in the midline of the abdomen and the mons pubis becomes full. Both the labia majora and minora get thicker, softer, and rounder as they age. The urethra becomes more noticeable, and the clitoris slightly enlarges. Along with its central opening enlarging, the hymen thickens. Additionally, the vaginal mucosa softens and thickens. The mucosa becomes moist as vaginal secretions rise. In addition, the pH levels drop and it starts to appear pink. The ovaries shift into the pelvis and the perineal and pelvic tissues become more elastic. Physiologic leukorrhea, a white discharge containing mature epithelial cells, is stimulated by rising estrogen levels in the months before menarche and frequently causes concern for patients and their parents. Reassure them that this is a typical stage of development and does not indicate an infection (Figure 10.8).

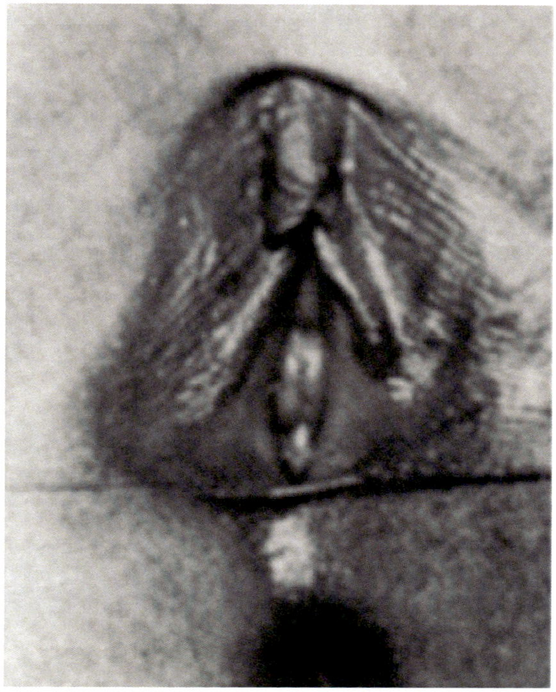

Figure 10.8. *Normal female peripubertal genitalia.*

Source: Syed-Ansari, T, Murray, P, et al., Glob. libr. women's med., (ISSN: 1756-2228) 2008; DOI 10.3843/GLOWM.10010.

Body odor and facial acne appear as androgen levels rise. Breast development is the first outward manifestation of puberty, which is followed by the onset of pubic hair, a maximum rate of linear growth, and menarche.

10.3. Labial Agglutination

It has been reported that 1 in 4 infants develop labial adhesions. (Christensen et al., 1971) Additional writers (Leung et al., 1993) have discovered that infants and early children were the most common age group to experience labial fusion, with a peak incidence of 3.3% in children between the ages of 13 and 23 months. The hypoestrogenic state seems to have a role in the etiology. Another possible factor is inflammation. The posterior aspect of the labia is typically involved in incomplete fusion, resulting in the labia minora becoming adherent. In severe situations, the only exposed region might be a tiny hole directly beneath the clitoris. Minor friction injuries that deplete the delicate hypoestrogenic surface of the labia can exacerbate trauma. Adherence happens when the epithelium regenerates. Due to the increased estrogen levels, the condition is rare in newborns and people who have reached puberty. When a hypoestrogenic state reappears in a postmenopausal patient, it may be seen once more (Table 10.2).

Table 10.2. Age Range of Children with Labial Adhesion

Reference	Age Range	Peak Incidence
Capraro and Greenberg,[5](1972)	2 months–14 years	24 months
Leung et al. (1993)	3–48 months	13–27 months
Nag (1972)	3–90 months	24–60 months
Aribarg (1975)	2–24 months	Not quoted
Khanam et al. (1977)	3–48 months	12–24 months
Jenkinson and Mackinnon (1984)	10–22 months	Not quoted
Berkowitz et al. (1987)	–	Sexually abused children 2.9–3%
Muram (1988)	3–36 months	Not quoted

Source: Syed-Ansari, T, Murray, P, et al., Glob. libr. women's med., (ISSN: 1756–2228) 2008; DOI 10.3843/GLOWM.10010This.

A thin, lucent vertical line can be seen inside the labia's central region upon physical examination. Since labial adhesions have been linked to urinary tract infections, it is important to inquire about any symptoms and signs related to the urinary tract. *Lichen sclerosus*, child sexual abuse, and less common causes like childhood cicatricial pemphigoid are included in the differential diagnosis.

During a physical examination, the labia should be gently tractioned; however, this procedure should be carried out in a way that causes the child no trauma. Any discomfort should cause you to stop trying to separate your labia (Figure 10.9).

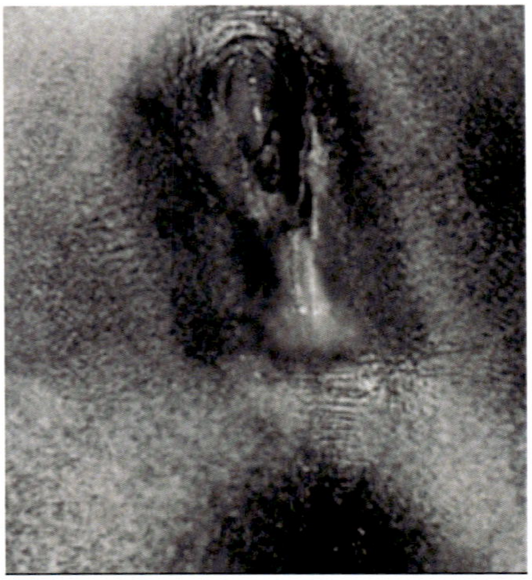

Figure 10.9. *Labial agglutination.*

Source: Syed-Ansari, T, Murray, P, et al., Glob. libr. women's med., (ISSN: 1756–2228) 2008; DOI 10.3843/GLOWM.10010.

Reassure the parent that once puberty hits, this will be a self-limiting issue. Labial adhesions frequently recur after separation up until that point. For two to four weeks, a fingertip application of estrogen cream should be made over the adhesions once or twice a day, provided there is no urinary tract-related issue. Possible side effects include temporary hyperpigmentation of the vulvar area and, in rare cases, systemic absorption of estrogen leading to precocity. Maintaining good perineal hygiene is crucial, and secondary infection should be avoided at all costs. Applying a preparation like AandDTM or zinc oxide ointment every night is beneficial once separation has taken place. Applying the ointment to the adhesion area can be done gently using an applicator with a cotton tip (Droegemueller et al., 1987).

88 to 90% of patients receive topical estrogen therapy successfully. Between 20 and 100% of patients experience recurrence. Labial adhesions have been referred to by many medical professionals as "physiologic fusion," which suggests that observation alone is a suitable form of treatment. In one series of ten patients, ages 13 to 22 months, all of the patients experienced spontaneous resolution in less than 18 months, requiring only reassurance as treatment. Biopsies are seldom, if ever, necessary. A pelvic mass with a distended bladder is typically identified in cases of acute urinary retention; ultrasound is frequently useful in making this diagnosis. Urinary decompression and catheterization are necessary in this emergency. The urethral meatus may need to be identified by examination while under anesthesia, and the meatus may need to be distinguished by sharp dissection. In order to accelerate healing and stop the adhesion and urine retention from returning, a 7–10 day course of estrogen cream application is administered to the vulvar area following surgery. Separation may be achievable in an office setting with specific patients if other clinicians recommend applying Xylocaine gel to the line of fusion using a cotton-tipped applicator. Reevaluating patients who don't improve after applying topical agents is a good idea. According to a recent retrospective study, betamethasone 0.05% cream seemed to be a secure and successful treatment option as well (Myers et al., 2006).

10.4. Vulvovaginitis

10.4.1. Pathophysiology and Clinical Presentation

Inflammation of the labia majora, minora, clitoris, and introitus is referred to as vulvitis, whereas vaginal mucosa inflammation is known as vaginitis. The primary care physician frequently diagnoses pediatric vulvovaginitis, which affects the vulvar and vaginal tissues. If initial treatment is ineffective, the physician will frequently refer the patient to a specialist. It is crucial to comprehend the pathophysiology, be aware of the different etiologies in relation to the clinical manifestation, and develop a methodical approach for vulvovaginitis evaluation.

An increased risk of vulvovaginitis occurs in prepubertal girls due to behavioral and anatomical factors. First, the vaginal vestibule and vulva are less shielded from outside irritants when squatting or sitting due to the lack of pubic hair and labial fat pads. Second, the vulva and vaginal mucosa have thinner, more delicate skin, making it more susceptible to irritation from chemicals, the environment, and allergies. Third, the vaginal cavity is warm and moist, with a neutral pH range of 6 to 7, and it contains unestrogenized epithelium that is devoid of glycogen and lactobacilli. Each of these elements promotes the growth of bacteria. Finally, a lack of proper hand washing and perineal cleaning practices among prepubertal children can result in autoinoculation with fecal bacteria or, less frequently, with organisms linked to respiratory or urinary tract infections.

The most common symptoms of pediatric vulvovaginitis are vaginal itching and excoriation, malodorous vaginal discharge, widespread vulvar, vaginal, or perianal discomfort, pain, or dysuria. In addition, parents might mention stains, smells, or colors on their child's underwear. When determining the etiology and guiding treatment, the history is crucial. The beginning, timing, and duration of symptoms, past home treatments, medications (including prescription and over-the-counter oral and topical therapies), and previous laboratory testing or evaluation procedures should all be questioned of the parents. It is important to evaluate the potential for sexual abuse in addition to thoroughly reviewing the behavioral, psychological, and developmental histories. It is important to assess the child's past medical or surgical history for allergies, dermatoses, and other skin infections. It's important to evaluate any allergies, contact sensitivities, and family histories of chronic illness. Investigations should be conducted into any lotions, powders, fabric softeners, hair products, and washcloth usage that may have leaked into the bathwater.

A thorough physical examination should be performed on the child to record the pubertal stage and look for signs of chronic illness or other abnormalities of the skin. The perineum and vulva can be checked for erythema, discharge, odor, and edema while the patient is in the knee-chest or frog-leg position. An otoscope or colposcope can help the examiner by giving magnification and focused light. When vaginal discharge occurs, it can range from heavily dried secretions to very little.

Examining the vaginal discharge is frequently beneficial, but getting a specimen from a child can be difficult. When saline is injected into the vagina, it can be "recollected" because it builds up in the vestibule and lower vagina. Alternatively, and more frequently, the discharge can be directly collected using a thin, dry or saline-moistened bacteriostatic swab; however, extreme caution must be taken to avoid touching the delicate hymenal tissue. Asking the child to carry out a Valsalva technique (e.g., cough) could facilitate this process. Because of the initial burning sensation, topical anesthetics should be used carefully as this could agitate the child and prevent further examination. EMLA cream is an exception to this rule. It is usually applied painlessly, but in the case of older cooperative children, it needs to be applied 30 to 60 minutes before the evaluation, specimen collection, or even biopsy. Following collection, the sample needs to be analyzed using cultures, potassium hydroxide (KOH), saline wet mount inspection, Gram stain, and vaginal pH.

The causes of pediatric vulvovaginitis are most easily divided into noninfectious (or nonspecific) and infectious (or specific) groups based on the history, physical examination, and laboratory evaluation; the latter group is further divided into nonsexually and sexually transmitted infections (Slupik, 1991) (Table 10.3).

Table 10.3. Prepubertal Vulvovaginitis

Noninfectious
• Chemical irritants (e.g., bubble baths, perfumes, soaps, and hair products in the bathwater)
• Allergic contact
• Poor hygiene
• Poor perineal aeration
• Foreign body
• Urologic anatomic abnormalities
Infectious
Nonsexually Transmitted
• Bacteria: group A beta-hemolytic streptococcus, *Haemophilus influenzae*, *Staphylococcus aureus*, *Streptococcus pneumoniae*, *Streptococcus viridans*, *Shigella sonnei*, methicillin-resistant *Staphylococcus aureus*
• Viral: adenovirus, varicella zoster, echovirus, non-sexually acquired human immunodeficiency virus
• Fungal: *Candida albicans*
• Helminths: *Enterobius vermicularis*
Sexually Transmitted
• *Neisseria gonorrhoeae*, *Chlamydia trachomatis*, *Trichomonas*, *Mycoplasma hominis*, *Ureaplasma urealyticum*, herpesvirus (1 and 2), human papillomavirus, human immunodeficiency virus, molluscum contagiosum, *Treponema pallidum*

Source: Syed-Ansari, T, Murray, P, et al., Glob. libr. women's med. (ISSN: 1756–2228) 2008; DOI 10.3843/GLOWM.10010This.

10.4.2. Noninfectious Vulvovaginitis

Poor perineal hygiene is one of the most common causes of noninfectious vulvovaginitis, also known as nonspecific vulvovaginitis. Upon examination, patients typically present with mild, nonspecific vulvar inflammation, soiled underwear, and possibly bits of toilet paper or stool on the perineal tissue. The main stays of treatment are supportive care and education about good hygiene. It is recommended by the clinician that the child be given ample opportunities to urinate, that she wipes with soft, white, unscented toilet paper from front to back, and that she regularly washes her hands, particularly after using the restroom. Undergarments ought to be made entirely of cotton, fitted loosely, and carefully cleaned or rinsed with a mild, hypoallergenic detergent that is unscented and doesn't contain fabric softener. When used to gently wash the perineal area, mild hypoallergenic cleansers free of dyes and perfumes leave the skin feeling more moisturized than when using ordinary soap. Cleaning products should never be applied with a washcloth since it can irritate already sensitive areas or spread pathogens. The perineal area should be patted dry with a towel or allowed to air dry after bathing, but not rubbed.

Most patients can be treated symptomatically with frequent sitz baths containing colloidal oatmeal or baking soda, or with wet compresses of Burrow's solution for acute nonspecific vulvovaginitis of any cause. A course of 1–2 weeks of estrogen cream can be used to promote healing of excoriation, or a 1% hydrocortisone cream can be applied once or twice a day for up to 2 weeks to relieve itching in extremely severe cases where other etiologies have been ruled out.

Prolonged or excessive exposure to moisture combined with inadequate perineal tissue aeration is another common cause of vulvovaginitis. This type of vulvovaginitis is predisposed to by obesity, wearing tight or synthetic undergarments, and being exposed to wet underwear for extended periods of time (e.g., swimwear, enuresis, etc.). Physical examination results could range from mild excoriation to nonspecific inflammation, all of which could be signs of secondary bacterial infections—most often from Staphylococcus aureus. It is important to review sitz baths as well as appropriate methods for cleaning and drying the perineum. Patients may find it more comfortable to sleep without underwear if they wear loose-fitting cotton underwear.

Table 10.4. Bloody Genital Discharge

Infectious vulvovaginitis: group A beta-hemolytic streptococcus, *Haemophilus influenzae*, *Shigella sonnei*, *Shigella flexneri*
• Foreign body
• Sexual abuse
• Trauma
• Urethral prolapse
• Exogenous hormone exposure
• *Lichen sclerosus*
• Tumor

Source: Syed-Ansari, T, Murray, P, et al., Glob. libr. women's med. (ISSN: 1756-2228) 2008; DOI 10.3843/GLOWM.10010This.

The most common symptom of allergic vulvovaginitis or contact dermatitis is pruritus. Typically, topical creams, lotions, scented soaps, toilet paper, and poison ivy are considered acute or chronic offending agents. The vulva may get fissures or cracks after prolonged exposure, and eventually it will take on a lichenified appearance. When an allergic reaction occurs, vaginal fluid may contain eosinophils. A similar clinical picture is produced by chemical irritants found in fabric softeners, bubble baths, laundry detergents, and soaps. The course of treatment includes sitz baths, eradication of the offending agent, education on hygiene, and a short course of 1% hydrocortisone cream, which can last up to two weeks (Slupik, 1991).

In prepubescent children, vaginal foreign bodies may also manifest as nonspecific vulvovaginitis. Blood-stained discharge that is persistent, foul-smelling, and prolific are possible symptoms (Table 10.4).

Antibiotics may offer brief respite from superinfection, but this is often followed by a return of symptoms. Therefore, a vaginoscopy to rule out a foreign body may be necessary if symptoms are persistent and need for repeated medication trials in addition to the aforementioned history. Even though firm foreign objects might be palpable during a rectal examination, a child might resist the process. In addition, irrigation is typically required to loosen and remove all debris because foreign bodies can be multiple or fragmented. Additionally, objects may become embedded in and covered by granulation tissue, which increases the risk of erosion or puncture into the tissue of the bowel or bladder. Therefore, a full evaluation for the presence of a vaginal foreign object may require an examination while the child is sedated. As is always the case, there should be a high degree of suspicion for sexual abuse when vulvovaginitis is diagnosed, but this is especially true when foreign bodies are involved. Curative action occurs when the offending agent—most frequently toilet paper—is removed. Certain individuals may discover that utilizing larger objects (e.g., using disposable wipes) to keep themselves clean helps stop recurrences.

Rare causes of vulvovaginitis include anatomic abnormalities like fistulas, urethral prolapse, and ectopic ureter. An ectopic ureter opens somewhere else, usually along the urethra, as opposed to the bladder's trigone. In addition, it may open into the vagina or near the vaginal vestibule, where a second meatal opening is visible around the urethral meatus. It has a strong correlation with other congenital defects like dilatation and multiple systems. Patients usually have a history of urine leakage and a persistently damp lower leg. These kids can accumulate urine in their bladders and go about their regular lives because their contralateral ureters are functioning normally. These patients may not receive a diagnosis until adulthood, even though the diagnosis can be made during pregnancy because they are susceptible to being misdiagnosed as having stress incontinence or primary enuresis. The diagnosis is confirmed by a voiding cystourethrogram; associated müllerian structural anomalies can be identified by ultrasound; and functioning can be detected by renal scan. For this condition, surgery is required for correction.

Due to the continuous presence of urine, patients with vesicovaginal fistulas typically present with nonspecific vulvovaginitis and excoriation on physical examination, as well as a history of a constantly wet perineum. Fecund vaginal discharge is indicative of a rectovaginal fistula. Blood stains on underwear are typically seen in patients with urethral prolapse. Additional indications consist of open vaginal bleeding accompanied by dysuria or vulvar pain. This issue is frequently brought on by actions that raise intra-abdominal pressure (e.g., sobbing, coughing, and straining during bowel motions). An everted, red, circular mass at the external urethral meatus is usually visible upon examination. African-American children under the age of ten are most likely to experience it. The combination of episodes of elevated intra-abdominal pressure and weak attachments of the various layers of urethral muscle is hypothesized to put young children at increased risk (Lowe et al., 1986). Urethral prolapse can be treated medically with sitz baths or by applying estrogen cream twice or three times a day for two to four weeks. When it doesn't go away or keeps coming back, surgical excision is taken into consideration (Figure 10.10).

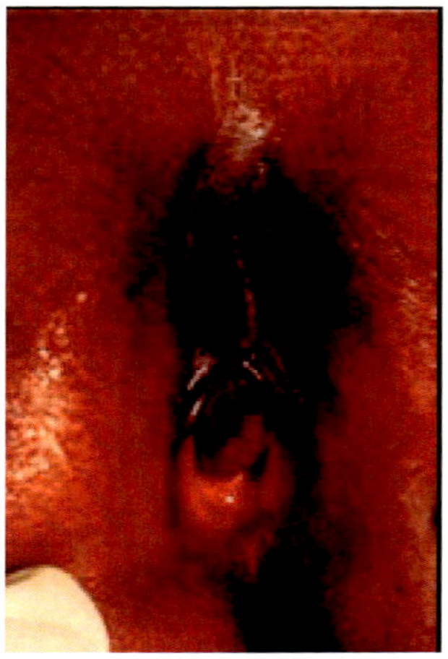

Figure 10.10. *Urethral prolapse with periurethral adhesions.*

Source: Syed-Ansari, T, Murray, P, et al., Glob. libr. women's med., (ISSN: 1756-2228) 2008; DOI 10.3843/GLOWM.10010.

10.4.3. Infectious Vulvovaginitis, Nonsexually Transmitted

When it comes to infectious versus non-infectious causes of vulvovaginitis, vaginal discharge is a more common finding. It is preferable to diagnose infections based on culture rather than treating cases based on observation in order to provide a conclusive diagnosis and prescribe the right antibiotics. Furthermore, if specific organisms are recovered, it might lead to a sexual abuse evaluation that wouldn't have happened otherwise. Information regarding the typical vaginal flora in a prepubescent child is scarce. Enteric bacteria, lactobacilli, Staphylococcus epidermidis, and other Bacteroides species have all been cultured from prepubertal asymptomatic "control" subjects. When these organisms are discovered in the cultures of patients whose symptoms do not improve with supportive care, antibiotic treatment may be necessary, despite the fact that this is a poorly researched topic.

The unprotected, unestrogenized prepubertal vaginal tissues support the growth of respiratory, gastrointestinal, or urinary pathogens that are often autoinoculated by young children with poor hygiene practices. Haemophilus influenzae, Streptococcus pneumoniae, and group A beta-hemolytic streptococci (GAS) are a few examples of bacterial respiratory pathogens that can induce vulvovaginitis along with a purulent vaginal discharge, either alone or in conjunction with other symptoms. Particularly GAS can present dramatically, with severe vulvovaginal erythema, edema, and discharge; it may or may not be linked to a positive throat culture and concomitant scarlet fever. Additionally, it is linked to desquamation, which may occur a few weeks later. The diagnosis can be verified with perineum bacterial cultures. For ten days, amoxicillin 40 mg/kg, divided three times a day, can be used to treat gas vulvovaginitis. Methicillin-resistant Staphylococcus aureus (MRSA) is a pathogen that is becoming more and more prevalent in communities, so the likelihood of this organism causing an infection should be taken into consideration when selecting an antibiotic. When thinking about empiric therapy, a family history of MRSA infection may be relevant. Clindamycin usually has an effect on MRSA. Bacterial sensitivities and culture results should guide the antibiotic selection process.

In the vaginal region, viral pathogens typically manifest as ulcerative lesions. Adenovirus, varicella, echovirus, Epstein-Barr virus, and herpesvirus 1 and 2 are among the harmful viral pathogens. A conclusive diagnosis requires a viral culture. While waiting for culture results, a direct florescent antibody evaluation of a swab of the lesion may provide an instantaneous indication as to whether or not HSV is present. While cultures are being obtained, presumptive acyclovir treatment should be taken into consideration. Acute or chronic vaginal discharge that is bloody, purulent, and odorous, along with vulvovaginal erythema, can be caused by gastrointestinal pathogens like Shigella. It can occasionally be linked to diarrhea in the patient or relatives. Sensitivities should be determined in order to administer systemic antibiotics appropriately, as a culture of the vaginal discharge serves a diagnostic purpose (Smith, 1986) (Figure 10.11).

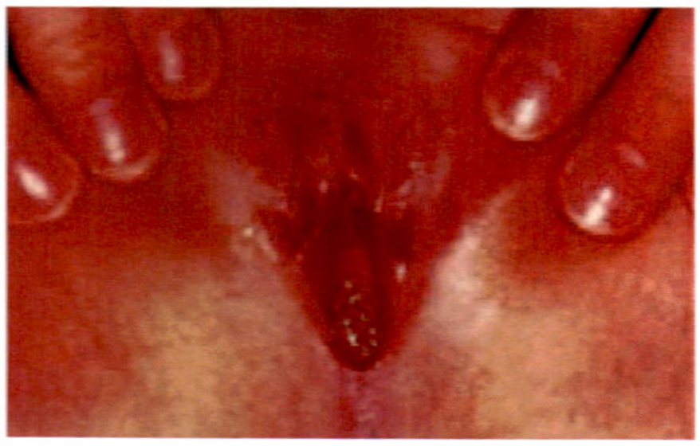

Figure 10.11. *Ulcerative lesions on vaginal mucosa.*

Source: Syed-Ansari, T, Murray, P, et al., Glob. libr. women's med., (ISSN: 1756–2228) 2008; DOI 10.3843/GLOWM.10010.

While perianal itching is typically the result of an intestinal infestation with *Enterobius vermicularis* (pinworms), vulvovaginitis has also been documented. The pinworms may crawl into the vagina (or be transferred by scratching) due to their close proximity, bringing eggs and attached enteric organisms with them. Upon physical examination, vaginal discharge, generalized inflammation, and scratch-related excoriation may be observed. The best time to observe pinworm ova and/or adults is during the night, when the worms emerge to feed, and this can be done with a saline wet mount or by using Scotch tape testing. These methods confirm the diagnosis. Mebendazole is used to treat the patients; in order to prevent reinfection, the entire family receives empirical care.

Although quite common after puberty, candidal vulvovaginitis is incredibly uncommon in healthy prepubertal children and is frequently over diagnosed and overtreated. Predisposing factors include immunodeficiency syndromes, diabetes mellitus, inflammatory skin conditions like seborrheic dermatitis, poor perineal aeration, and recent antibiotic use. The most frequent complaints are pruritus and dysuria; other common complaints include diffuse vulvar erythema, thick, cheesy vaginal discharge, scratch-induced excoriation, and white plaques on the mucosa of the vagina. Candidal rashes are characterized by "satellite lesions" and erythematous prominence in the creases, particularly in diaper-wearing individuals. A saline wet mount and KOH preparation can reveal budding yeast and pseudohyphae in a patient with a candidal infection, who will also have a low vaginal pH. Topical or oral antifungal medications, such as fluconazole, are used as a form of treatment; the affected area should be kept as dry as possible. Chronic candidal infections should raise suspicions of diabetes, HIV, or other immunodeficiency syndromes, particularly in prepubescent children.

10.4.4. Infectious Vulvovaginitis, Sexually Transmitted

If organisms linked to sexual transmission are discovered in prepubescent girls, they should be evaluated for potential sexual abuse. Professionals ought to maintain a high degree of suspicion at all times and ask routine history questions that address sexual abuse. They should also be aware of the mandatory reporting laws in their area, conduct a comprehensive physical examination, and compile a detailed psychosocial history. Referrals to community-based child abuse specialists should be made upon the discovery of sexual abuse in order to guarantee appropriate and comprehensive care, particularly since the office guidelines may not always be followed when gathering evidence. Acute injuries and infections need to be treated right away, and they may need to be referred to an emergency room. Before beginning treatment, cultures for chlamydia and gonorrhea should always be obtained.

In this age group, the absence of estrogenized epithelium may prevent STDs from growing upward into the pelvis. The "lower tract" symptoms of pruritus, dysuria, vaginal discharge, and odor are thus commonly present. External lesions, vaginal discharge, and vulvovaginitis are the physical findings. Neisseria gonorrhoeae infections in the genitalia are practically pathognomonic for sexual abuse. It is typically accompanied by inguinal lymphadenopathy, vulvar erythema, edema, and excoriation in addition to a purulent, thick yellow discharge. A cervical or vaginal culture or nucleic acid amplification testing (NAAT) of a cervical, vaginal, or urine specimen are used to confirm the diagnosis. For patients allergic to penicillins, the patient is treated with ceftriaxone, cefixime, or azithromycin. A prepubertal child may also contract chlamydia trachomatis from infected atrophic vaginal squamous cells, which can result in a vaginal discharge and a similar vulvovaginitis with pruritus. The existence of *C. trachomatis* is a sign of sexual abuse as well. It can also be acquired during pregnancy; it has been demonstrated that children born to chlamydia carriers can carry the infection asymptomatically for up to 18 months. Cervical or vaginal culture or NAAT of a cervical, vaginal, or urine specimen will confirm the diagnosis, just like in the case of gonorrhea. Treatment for the patient should involve either doxycycline or azithromycin.

Diagnosing Trichomonas vaginalis can be accomplished through culture or, for ease of use, by looking at the organisms using a saline wet mount. When potassium hydroxide is added to the vaginal discharge sample, there is a fishy smell (positive "whiff"). It is given metronidazole as a treatment. One should be suspicious of sexual abuse.

Although bacterial vaginosis has been documented in "control" subjects, it is often linked to sexual abuse. The presence of a higher-than-normal vaginal pH, a positive "whiff" (when KOH is added to a specimen), and "clue cells"—vaginal epithelial cells covered in bacteria that can be seen with a saline wet mount—are the diagnostic criteria. Metronidazole is the treatment of choice.

Herpes simplex virus (HSV) typically causes inguinal lymphadenopathy along with systemic symptoms, vesicular lesions, and ulcerative vulvovaginitis. Genital lesions can be caused by either serotype, and both should raise the possibility of child abuse for the clinician. Acyclovir is a treatment option for HSV.

Condyloma acuminata, or painless, soft, moist, granular, and friable lesions, are primarily found in the perianal area and vaginal vestibule and are caused by the human papilloma virus (HPV). It is possible for the lesions to secondary infect and cause pruritus, pain, and discharge. Cryotherapy, repeated TCA applications, podophyllin, or imiquimod cream are the available forms of therapy. Immunization against high-risk HPV strains linked to both genital warts and cervical dysplasia may be made available to older children (age 11 and up).

Molluscum contagiosum are 2.5–5 mm in diameter, waxy, centrally umbilicated lesions. Curettage or imiquimod cream are possible forms of treatment.

The development of condyloma Lata on the vulva and anus, as well as a rash over the perineum and inner thighs, are typical symptoms of secondary syphilis, which is the cause of vulvovaginitis from syphilis. Cerebrospinal fluid and serologic testing establish the course of treatment and validate the diagnosis.

10.5. Noninfectious Dermatologic Conditions

10.5.1. Lichen sclerosus

All parts of the body are affected by *Lichen sclerosus* in people of all ages and genders. Although the exact cause is unknown, autoimmune diseases are thought to be linked to it. *Lichen sclerosus* is currently associated with certain HLA types; a significant and well-known familial incidence is present. Borrelia burgdorferi has also received attention, but more clarification is required. Although it is more common in the hypoestrogenic prepubertal state, it is primarily observed in women who have gone through menopause. It manifests as white sores. The average age of onset in children is five years old. It begins as tiny, pink-white papules that converge to form plaques with prominent, follicular keratinous plugs and a wrinkled, atrophic "cigarette paper" surface. It's normal to have an hourglass or figure-of-eight shape. The biopsy sample frequently shows an edematous, hyalinized area in the dermis with red cells and an underlying band of inflammatory cells. The dermatopathology is reflected in the clinical appearance of ivory-colored, flat-topped polygonal papules that aggregate into plaques. The Koebner effect is widely known, and purpuric speckling and frank ecchymosis are frequent (Ridley et al., 1994) (Figure 10.12).

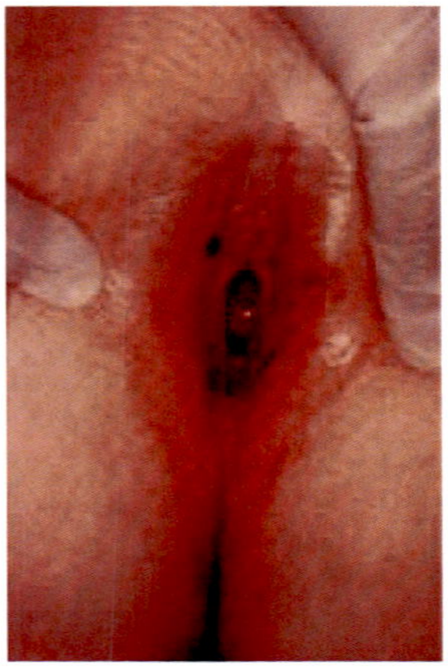

(A)

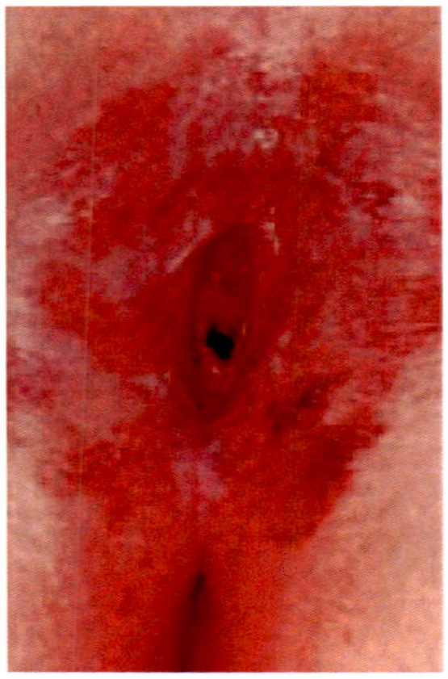

(B)

Figure 10.12. *A. Lichen sclerosus, mild atrophy with thin, pale skin. B. Lichen sclerosus, severe with hemorrhage and mild scarring.*

Source: Syed-Ansari, T, Murray, P, et al., Glob. libr. women's med., (ISSN: 1756–2228) 2008; DOI 10.3843/GLOWM.10010.

The most common complaint is pruritus and vulvar irritation, which can lead to a cycle of itching and scratching. In severe cases, the vulvar architecture may be destroyed, resulting in scarring, labial agglutination, and kraurosis.

Perineal cleanliness and trauma reduction are two aspects of management (i.e., scraping the affected region). The use of a strong topical corticosteroid, such as clobetasol propionate 0.05%, applied to the affected area once a day for about two weeks, has been recommended, depending on the symptomatology. In addition, betamethasone dipropionate 0.05% was administered three times a day for three weeks, and then twice a day until the vulva's appearance returned to normal. It might take one to six months of therapy for this. The corticosteroid preparation may be lowered to 1% to 2% hydrocortisone cream or ointment applied daily to the affected area as needed when symptoms improve. A vulvar biopsy is advised if the diagnosis is unclear. Exams after puberty should be conducted twice a year, although opinions vary. A slight but possible long-term risk of cancer exists.

It has been discussed how sexual abuse is related to *Lichen sclerosus*. The question is whether false allegations of abuse could serve as a "trigger" for the development of *Lichen sclerosus*, potentially through the Koebner phenomenon. Gynecologists may see patients with both *Lichen sclerosus* and sexual abuse; the two conditions are not necessarily mutually exclusive.

Lichen simplex is a condition where the skin thickens in response to scratching, becoming lichenified due to repeated irritation. It may also involve elements of psoriasis, eczema, or *Lichen sclerosus*. Clinically, the lesions appear pale with increased skin margin markings. Histologically, the skin shows hyperkeratosis and acanthosis with dermal inflammation. Treatment typically involves applying topical corticosteroids (1% to 2% hydrocortisone) and antihistamines until the underlying causes are addressed. Breaking the itch/scratch cycle is crucial for managing this condition.

10.5.2. Lichen Planus

Lichen planus has been reported in pediatric patients, despite its uncommon manifestation as vulvar involvement in premenarchal children in general. Angular, violaceous flap papules that are demarcated are used to classify lichen planus. A remarkable linear distribution is produced by Koebner's phenomenon along scratch-traumatized sites. The inner thighs, forearms, and wrist flexor surfaces are the most frequently affected areas. Less noticeable vulvar lesions can have varying degrees of excoriation, maceration, or verrucous thickening, similar to leukoplakia. There may be a lacy pattern of tiny white papules on the buccal mucosa. An biopsy confirms the diagnosis. Most treatment plans, which mainly involve topical and intralesional corticosteroid administration along with antihistamines, have limited success rates due to exacerbations and recurrences. Long-term hypertropic vulvar lichen planus is a risk factor for squamous cell carcinoma. It is advised to carefully follow up with a biopsy when necessary.

10.5.3. Psoriasis

One of the contributing factors to psoriasis, a papulosquamous skin disease, is an increased turnover of epidermal cells accompanied by excessive cell proliferation. It affects 1% to 3% of the population overall, with 2% of cases beginning before the age of two. Up to one-third of patients have a family member who has the illness, proving that it can be inherited. Although the precise etiology of psoriasis remains unclear, the alterations observed are believed to arise from a T-cell lymphocyte immune response that incites the production of cytokines and other mediators to induce inflammation.

The genital area may be the only part of the body affected by psoriasis. However, comparable lesions are usually found in other symmetrically characteristic locations on the body, such as the scalp, anogenital area, lumbosacral area, and extensor surfaces of the extremities. Well-defined erythematous papules or plaques with adherent gray or silvery scales are the outward manifestation of psoriatic lesions. Up to 5–7% of patients have arthritis as an associated finding, which can manifest up to 2 years after the start of skin findings. If the vagina is sufficiently moist, vaginal psoriasis may not appear scaly, but it typically manifests as scaly, well-defined patches. When scales are removed, capillaries high in the papillary dermis burst, resulting in the Auspitz sign—a distinctive pattern of punctate bleeding points. The Koebner phenomenon, an aberrant skin reaction in which a localized injury or trauma results in an extension of the lesion, is another feature of psoriatic lesions.

The first step in treatment is to inform the parents about the potential emotional impact of the disease and its course, which includes remissions and exacerbations with variable onset and duration. Topical treatment is the cornerstone of therapy. Emollients help to retain moisture, and tar preparations work as anti-inflammatory agents to reduce the growth of new skin cells. Even at low potencies, topical corticosteroids can yield remarkable outcomes. Topical corticosteroids should be used with caution, though, as there is a higher risk of side effects, particularly in the genital area. In cases of severe exacerbations, higher potencies should be saved and quickly tapered down to a lower dose. Treatment should also be restricted to two-week courses spaced at least two weeks apart. Patients with complex and widespread involvement should be referred to a dermatologist.

10.5.4. Seborrheic Dermatitis

The hallmarks of seborrheic dermatitis are erythematous, scaly, crusting, or greasy-looking eruptions that mostly affect the scalp, face, neck, axillae, and intertriginous areas—areas with high concentrations of sebaceous glands. The effects of maternal hormones acquired transplacentally can cause infantile seborrheic dermatitis as early as the second week of life. It goes away on its own and can last for up to 12 months. With the exception of the groin region, where severe itching can result in secondary bacterial infections, pruritus is not a common feature of seborrheic dermatitis. This disorder is distinguished from atopic dermatitis and psoriasis by its early onset, greasy, scale-like appearance, preference for the scalp and intertriginous areas, and general lack of pruritus.

Treatments for seborrhea include lubricants, antifungal medications, and preparations containing selenium sulfide to soften the scales. If the diagnosis is unclear or the case is refractory, a dermatologist referral might be required.

10.5.5. Atopic Dermatitis

Atopic dermatitis, which affects 10–15% of children, is one of the most prevalent skin conditions in newborns and young children. It is a chronic illness that frequently coexists with asthma and allergies. There is evidence that the primary immunologic abnormality is altered T-cell immune function, even though the precise pathophysiology is unknown. Atopic dermatitis patients also have structurally abnormal skin, which compromises the skin's defenses against outside irritants.

Based on the patient's age, atopic dermatitis can be divided into three basic forms. The erythema, papules, vesicles, and severe pruritus on the face, trunk, or extremities are the hallmarks of the infantile form, which appears between the ages of two and six months. Because the diaper area is moist, atopic dermatitis in this age group typically spares that area. Atopic dermatitis in childhood typically affects the wrists, ankles, antecubital and popliteal fossas, and manifests during the prepubertal years.

Usually more parched, the lesions have the potential to lichenify over time. Additionally, "wet" lesions in patients may be erythematous, edematous, oozing, or weepy. Pruritus and an increased risk of secondary bacterial (mostly GAS) or fungal infections are common when the vulva is involved.

The first step in treating an allergy is to control potential triggers, such as foods or environmental allergens. Dry areas should be regularly moistened and rehydrated with lubricants. Skin that is extremely irritated can also be soothed with wet compresses containing Burrow's solution. Patients should be advised to keep their child's fingernails neat and short in order to lower the risk of a secondary infection. Antihistamines that are systemic in nature may be useful in managing extreme pruritus. The cornerstone for treating atopic dermatitis has been topical corticosteroids; however, due to potential long-term side effects, including immune suppression, telangiectasias, striae, skin atrophy, and pigment changes, these medications should not be used in the genital area. The length, strength, and location of use all affect these negative effects, particularly in intertriginous areas. A dermatologist referral can be required for cases that are severe or resistant to treatment.

10.6. Obstructive Vaginal Disorders

There are two types of vaginal obstructive disorders: longitudinal and transverse fusion issues. Septate vagina, in relation to longitudinal fusion issues, is a condition in which the vagina is duplicated and asymptomatic. The septum may occasionally need to be removed if dyspareunia brought on by vaginal narrowing is experienced.

A transverse septum in the vagina can lead to a blockage in the outflow tract. This can cause severe pain during menstruation in adolescents, as well as swelling in the vagina, which may be a sign of hematocolpos.

Transverse fusion disorders are more prevalent, with imperforate hymen being the most common. Labial adhesions are one differential for an imperforate hymen. Microperforate and imperforate hymens are the most frequent issues seen in pediatric patients. The newborn exhibiting the Valsalva maneuver (crying) and bulging at the introitus is known to have an imperforate hymen. The hymenal membrane's mucocolpos distention is linked to the obstruction (Figure 10.13).

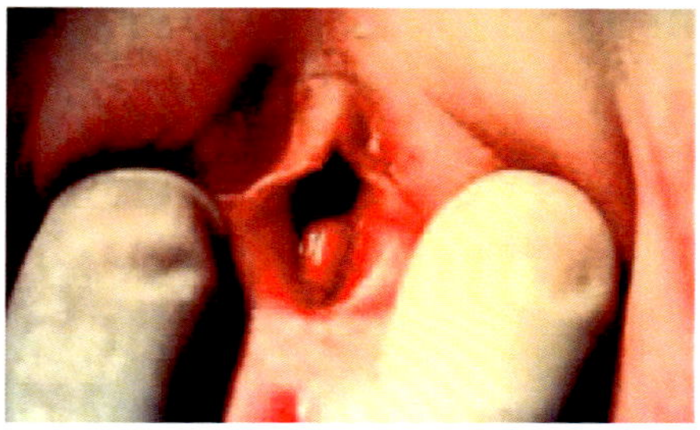

Figure 10.13. *Imperforate hymen in prepubertal girl.*

Source: Syed-Ansari, T, Murray, P, et al., Glob. libr. women's med., (ISSN: 1756–2228) 2008; DOI 10.3843/GLOWM.10010

When a girl ages 9 or older experiences periodic pelvic and/or abdominal pain and has normal secondary sexual development, imperforate hymen should be taken into consideration. Hematocolpos, hematometra, hematosalpinx, and frequently related endometriosis as a result of retrograde menstruation are manifestations of endometrial fluid accumulation. Examining the vulvar reveals a taut, protruding, blue membrane at the introitus. The menstrual fluid is reflected in the blue discoloration. A stellate incision is made into the membrane and any redundant segments are removed following the diagnosis. There is no need for further surgery, and endometriosis, hematocolpos, and hematometra stop when the obstruction is removed.

Although it is appropriate to correct an imperforate hymen in a prepubertal patient, it is usually avoided in the first six months of life due to increased anesthesia risks. Some authors recommend delaying surgery until the premenarchal stage, partly due to the possibility that estrogenization will speed up the healing process.

The intersection of the middle and upper thirds of the vagina can result in the transverse vaginal septum. The septum can be detected using sonography or magnetic resonance imaging. Before undergoing surgery to repair the vaginal septum, an intravenous pyelogram or other renal ultrasonographic evaluation should be done to rule out renal abnormalities, such as pelvic kidney. Any accompanying obstruction is relieved by surgically removing the septum.

One in 80,000 females have a transverse vaginal septum, which is indicative of a vertical fusion disorder. To relieve the obstruction in the tract's outflow, surgical resection is recommended. It is advised to reanastomose the upper and lower vaginal mucosa. If this is not possible, safe excision and resection can be accomplished by using a transfundal uterine sound that is inserted through the cervix and along the vaginal septum. Primary reanastomosis may be facilitated by Z-plasty procedures or mucosal undermining and mobilization. By using a hollow mold, the so-created space is kept patent until the patient starts engaging in sexual activity.

10.7. Ambiguous Genitalia

In a neonate, ambiguous genitalia is a real emergency that could be fatal. It is crucial to evaluate in the right way. Since adrenal hyperplasia can be fatal, it needs to be ruled out. If vomiting and diarrhea are not treated, adrenal failure can quickly lead to dehydration, shock, and even death.

A parent finds it upsetting when they are unable to respond to the question, "Is it a boy or a girl?" in the delivery room. Parents may put pressure on the doctor to designate a gender in the delivery room, but it's better to wait than to be forced to change the sex assignment later, leaving parents uncertain about which sex they should raise their child for the rest of their lives. A tactful approach is essential. It is preferable to refer to the infant's sexual development as "incomplete" rather than using derogatory terms like "hermaphrodite." The phrase "disorders of sex development" is suggested by the American Academy of Pediatrics in a recent consensus statement on the treatment of intersex disorders. Multidisciplinary methods work best.

The history is the first place to look for a cause, particularly in relation to any drugs taken during pregnancy that might have masculinizing effects. Pregnancy-related seizure disorders have been linked to drugs like P-450 inhibitors, testosterone, and some 19-nortestosterone derivatives. Examining the systems may reveal endogenous maternal androgen excess indicators, like hirsutism or acne, which indicate a virilizing ovarian tumor. In cases of virilizing adrenal hyperplasia, an autosomal recessive gene, a family history of a previously affected fetus or a previous neonatal death may be revealed (Lee et al., 1997) (Table 10.5).

It is appropriate to evaluate the genital system step-by-step. The genital tubercle's entire length and width are measured. Depending on the situation, one can determine if the phallus symbolizes the penis or the clitoris. In contrast to a penis, which has a midline ventral frenulum, a clitoris has two folds that extend laterally to the labia minora. The urethral meatus can be found in a variety of places, including the urogenital sinus, the perineal area, and mild hypopadias.

Table 10.5. Ambiguous Genitalia in Neonates

Partially Virilized 46, XX: Female Pseudohermaphrodite	
1.	Congenital adrenal hyperplasia
•	21-Hydroxylase deficiency
•	11-β-Hydroxylase deficiency
•	3-β-Hydroxysteroid dehydrogenase deficiency
2.	Maternal drug intake
•	Testosterone
•	Ethisterone
•	Norethindrone
•	Oral contraceptives
•	Danocrine
3.	Maternal ovarian tumor
•	Luteoma of pregnancy
•	Sertoli Leydig cell tumor
•	Leydig cell tumor
4.	Maternal adrenal tumor
Incompletely Virilized 46, XY: Male Pseudohermaphrodite	
1.	Müllerian duct inhibitory factor defect
2.	Impaired androgenization
•	Testicular feminization
•	5-α-Reductase deficiency
3.	Testosterone biosynthesis defects
•	20,22-Desmolase deficiency
•	3-β-Hydroxysteroid dehydrogenase deficiency
•	17-α-Hydroxylase deficiency
•	17,20-Desmolase deficiency
•	17-Hydroxysteroid dehydrogenase deficiency

Source: Syed-Ansari, T, Murray, P, et al., Glob. libr. women's med.,(ISSN: 1756–2228) 2008; DOI 10.3843/GLOWM.10010This.

Gonadal protuberances are felt in the labioscrotal folds and inguinal canals. A normal ovary herniates infrequently, but these ovaries do not migrate into the labioscrotal folds; instead, they appear just outside the inguinal ring. Until proven otherwise, palpable masses in the lower inguinal or scrotal regions are almost always testicles; their absence warrants a provisional diagnosis of virilizing adrenal hyperplasia. A 46,XY baby with undescended intra-abdominal testes is not completely ruled out by this anatomy, but true bilateral cryptorchidism is extremely uncommon and is not typically linked to ambiguous genitalia. There are multiple methods to define the degree of the Müllerian system presence. A rectal examination may reveal a uterus, especially in the newborn stage when the effects of recent maternal estrogen administration may have caused some hypertrophy. Ultrasonography or urogenital sonography can provide additional confirmation.

A newborn's blood should be drawn as soon as possible for diagnostic evaluation in order to obtain samples for karyotype, electrolytes, 17-hydroxyprogesterone, androstenedione, and dehydroepiandrosterone sulfate (DHEAS). When diagnosing an ovarian or adrenal neoplasm, maternal blood levels of DHEAS and testosterone may also be useful; if these levels are elevated, ultrasonography is necessary. 21-hydroxylase is the most commonly deficient enzyme in congenital adrenal hyperplasia. Virilization of a 46, XX infant is frequently linked to it, similar to 11-β-hydroxylase deficiency. Serum 17-hydroxyprogesterone levels will rise significantly in both cases. Naturally, regardless of the steroid pattern, evidence of adrenal failure in a hyperkalemic, hyponatremic infant confirms the diagnosis of adrenal hyperplasia. Since metabolic disturbances may not manifest for seven to ten days, electrolytes should be constantly watched during this time (Table 10.6).

Table 10.6. Laboratory Workup: Ambiguous Genitalia in Neonates

Maternal
• Serum testosterone
• Serum DHEAS (dihydroepiandrosterone sulfate)
• Pelvic/abdominal ultrasonography
Newborn
• Karyotype
• Serum electrolytes
• Serum 17-hydroxyprogesterone
• Serum androstenedione
• Serum DHEAS (dihydroepiandrosterone sulfate)

Source: Syed-Ansari, T, Murray, P, et al., Glob. libr. women's med.,(ISSN: 1756–2228) 2008; DOI 10.3843/GLOWM.10010This.

A team consisting of a pediatrician, reproductive endocrinologist, geneticist, surgeon, and psychologist is best suited to oversee in-depth counseling with the parents. Determining the sex of rearing involves a great deal of anxiety, and if gender assignment is later changed, the patient and family may suffer irreversible trauma. Regardless of gonadal sex, the adequacy of the phallus may limit reconstructive surgical procedures, so this could affect the ultimate decision. The parents' acceptance and support play a major role in the affected child's successful psychological development and adjustment. It is crucial that parents receive education and continuous support throughout their diagnosis and course of treatment.

10.8. Precocious Puberty

The onset of puberty in girls before the age of eight is known as precocious puberty. Puberty, however, appears to be beginning as much as one year earlier in white girls and two years earlier in African-American girls, according to recent data. Girls who show signs of puberty before the age of eight should be investigated until more prospective studies using similar evaluative methods are conducted. Breast or pubic hair development, along with an accelerated rate of linear growth or early bone maturation, are indicators of precocious puberty. It's possible that these kids don't develop in the typical pubertal sequence. They can be categorized as having contrasexual precocity, in which the predominance of male androgen effects predominates, or isosexual precocity, in which there is progression of normal female development.

The early development of isolated breast tissue without other puberty-related symptoms is known as premature thelarche. It may be mistaken for the initial indication of early puberty. The early development of body odor, axillary hair, and isolated pubic hair without the presence of other pubertal symptoms is known as premature adrenarche. Usually, there is no correlation between these two conditions and a higher rate of linear growth.

There are two primary etiologic categories for precocious puberty: those that are GnRH-independent and those that are GnRH-dependent. An early activation of the hypothalamic-pituitary-gonadal axis, which regulates puberty, is referred to as GnRH-dependent precocious puberty, also known as central or true precocious puberty. Girls are far more likely to experience premature puberty, which is typically idiopathic. However, early puberty must not be caused by life-threatening conditions. Pathology involving the central nervous system (CNS) is the most frequent cause of nonidiopathic precocity. CNS processes include trauma, encephalitis, meningitis, hydrocephalus, neurofibromatosis, and CNS tumors, most commonly hypothalamic hamartomas and rickets-related abnormal skull development can result in precocious puberty that is GnRH-dependent. Several neurologic disorders, like spina bifida, are frequently linked to early puberty. Additional causes include severe, chronic hypothyroidism, ectopic gonadotropin production, and most frequently, hCG-producing chorioepitheliomas and dysgerminomas of the ovary or liver (Doron et al., 1999) (Table 10.7).

Table 10.7. Precocious Puberty Classification

GnRH-dependent, central, or true precocious puberty
1. Idiopathic
2. Central nervous system lesions
• —Cranial trauma
• —Encephalitis, meningitis
• —Rickets
• —Tumors: hypothalamic hamartomas, craniopharyngioma, optic glioma, suprasellar teratoma, astrocytoma
• —Hydrocephalus
• —Neurofibromatosis type I
3. Gonadotropin-producing tumors
• —Ovary, liver, mediastinum
4. Prolonged untreated primary hypothyroidism
5. GnRH-independent processes
GnRH-independent, peripheral or pseudoprecocious puberty
1. Ovarian cyst
2. Ovarian tumor: granulosa cell, theca cell, gonadoblastoma, teratoma, chorioepithelioma, lipid cell tumor
3. Feminizing adrenal tumor
4. Congenital adrenal hyperplasia
5. Drug ingestion: synthetic estrogens, oral contraceptives, anabolic steroids
6. McCune–Albright syndrome

Source: Syed-Ansari, T, Murray, P, et al., Glob. libr. women's med.,(ISSN: 1756–2228) 2008; DOI 10.3843/GLOWM.10010This.

Sex steroids are secreted independently of pituitary gonadotropin in GnRH-independent precocious puberty, also referred to as peripheral or pseudoprecocious puberty. The majority of these cases are caused by ovarian tumors that secrete estrogen, most often granulosa cells, which are frequently palpable during an abdominal examination. On an abdominal examination, large ovarian luteal or follicular cysts that secrete estrogen are typically palpable in patients who have reached early puberty. Congenital adrenal hyperplasia and feminizing adrenal tumors are two other etiologies.

Genetic syndromes like McCune-Albright (polyostotic fibrous dysplasia), which is characterized by multiple cystic bone lesions, café-au-lait spots, and sexual precocity, are also linked to GnRH-independent precocity. Fractal abnormalities may appear later in life in this syndrome, with premature menarche possibly the first indication of pubertal development.

The hypothalamic-pituitary-gonadal axis can be secondary activated by almost all causes of GnRH-independent precocious puberty, leading to additional GnRH-dependent effects.

The diagnostic evaluation starts with a thorough medical history that includes information on growth rate, acne, body odor, vaginal discharge or bleeding, pubertal progression rate, and family history of medical issues, including early unexplained deaths (which may have been caused by salt-losing congenital adrenal hyperplasia). A thorough physical examination should be performed, which should include an assessment of the Tanner stage, growth progression and percentiles, as well as examinations of the abdomen, skin, nervous system, and external genitalia. The scope of the evaluation is determined by the clinical situation, which should always begin with a radiographic assessment to ascertain bone age.

Table 10.8. Precocious Puberty: Diagnostic Evaluation

Physical examination

- Growth velocity and percentiles
- Tanner staging
- Abdominal, neurologic, genital, and skin examination
- Palpation of thyroid
- Evidence of androgen excess (hirsutism, clitoromegaly)

Radiologic

- X-ray for bone age
- Brain MRI
- Abdominal or pelvic CT or ultrasound

Serologic

- Follicle-stimulating hormone
- Luteinizing hormone
- Human chorionic gonadotropin
- Thyroid-stimulating hormone
- Free T_4
- Dehydroepiandrosterone sulfate
- Testosterone
- Estradiol
- Progesterone
- 17-hydroxyprogesterone
- Prolactin

Testing

- Gonadotropin releasing hormone stimulation test
- ACTH stimulation test

Source: Syed-Ansari, T, Murray, P, et al., Glob. libr. women's med.,(ISSN: 1756–2228) 2008; DOI 10.3843/GLOWM.10010This.

Additional tests that could be helpful include follicle-stimulating hormone, luteinizing hormone, hCG, thyroid function tests, prolactin, DHEAS, testosterone, estradiol, progesterone, and 17-hydroxyprogesterone, as well as brain magnetic resonance imaging and abdominal/pelvic computed tomography or ultrasound. It is advised to consult an endocrinologist for assistance in planning, assessing, and interpreting tests. A GnRH stimulation test measures the levels of serum luteinizing hormone, administers 100 micrograms of GnRH subcutaneously, and then measures the levels of serum luteinizing hormone again 40 minutes later. This test determines the activity of the hypothalamic-pituitary-gonadal axis. Serum luteinizing hormone levels in patients with GnRH-dependent processes will be higher than the pubertal range. An ACTH stimulation test is required to confirm the diagnosis of congenital adrenal hyperplasia, which is suggested by elevated levels of 17-OH progesterone and adrenal androgens (Speroff et al., 1989) (Table 10.8).

The management of precocious puberty aims to minimize final adult height, postpone the development of secondary sexual development and bone maturation, rule out life-threatening etiologies, and screen for potential emotional and psychosocial effects of early puberty. The cornerstone of treatment for precocious puberty is GnRH agonists; if a particular etiology is found, treatment should be customized to manage that process first. Excision, radiation, chemotherapy, and careful waiting may be recommended for CNS tumors. GnRH agonists can regulate pubertal effects in some CNS tumors, such as hypothalamic hamartomas. Surgical exploration and removal are typically necessary for any suspicion of an abdominal neoplasm or ovarian cysts that may be large enough to undergo torsion or rupture. The majority of individuals experiencing idiopathic true precocious puberty end up being shorter than five feet as adults due to the early epiphyseal closure caused by estrogen. The most common medication used to postpone this process is a GnRH agonist, which has been demonstrated to dramatically slow down the rate of growth and postpone the development of secondary sexual traits. Serum estradiol levels, which should remain in prepubertal ranges (less than 10 pg/mL), or a negative GnRH stimulation test can be used to track the efficacy of exogenous GnRH administration.

Treatment should continue until the patient reaches the appropriate pubertal versus chronologic age or until the epiphyses close. Impaired fertility or an early menopause are not linked to idiopathic precocious puberty. The patient may experience emotional effects from looking different from her peers or from feeling socially, intellectually, and sexually expected because the chronologic age does not match the pubertal age. It is important to discuss these issues as well as the potential need for contraception (Lee, Houk, Ahmed, 2006).

A Closer Look

Speculum Exam

A speculum exam is a gynecological procedure used to visualize the vaginal walls and cervix, crucial for routine health checks and for diagnosing various conditions. During the exam, a speculum, a hinged instrument typically made of metal or plastic, is gently inserted into the vagina. The device is then opened to spread the vaginal walls, allowing the healthcare provider a clear view of the cervix and upper vaginal canal. This procedure is fundamental in conducting Pap smears, screening for cervical cancer, and collecting samples for testing sexually transmitted infections (STIs) and other vaginal infections.

The speculum exam begins with the patient lying on an examination table, usually in a lithotomy position with feet in stirrups to provide better access to the pelvic area. After explaining the procedure to the patient and obtaining informed consent, the healthcare provider warms the speculum to enhance comfort. Lubrication may be applied to ease the insertion. Once the speculum is in place, it is gently opened, and a light source is used to illuminate the vaginal canal and cervix.

During the exam, the provider may perform a Pap smear by using a small brush or spatula to collect cells from the cervix's surface. These cells are then sent to a laboratory to check for abnormalities that could indicate cervical dysplasia or cancer. Additionally, swabs may be taken from the vaginal walls to test for infections like bacterial vaginosis, yeast infections, or STIs such as chlamydia and gonorrhea.

The speculum exam, while generally quick and simple, can cause discomfort or anxiety for some patients. Healthcare providers strive to minimize discomfort by using appropriate-sized specula, applying sufficient lubrication, and maintaining clear communication throughout the procedure. Empathy and a gentle approach are essential to ensure a positive experience.

In summary, the speculum exam is a pivotal procedure in gynecological practice, essential for preventive health care, early detection of cervical cancer, and diagnosis of infections. It enables thorough assessment and sample collection from the cervix and vagina, playing a critical role in women's reproductive health management.

Summary

- Pediatric and adolescent gynecology is a specialized field of medicine that addresses the unique gynecological needs of children and adolescents.
- The breast examination in the neonate frequently reveals evidence of maternal estrogen effect in that palpable breast tissue is noted.
- The ideal positioning for good visualization of the external genitalia is in the supine position with the buttocks on the end of the gynecologic examination table.
- The typical appearance of the newborn female genitalia is primarily due to the effects of maternal hormones acquired transplacentally. The labia majora are full and the labia minora thickened.
- As the infant matures, the labia decreases in size. This leaves the vaginal vestibule less protected from bacteria and external irritants, especially when the child is in the sitting or squatting position.
- Vulvitis is defined as inflammation of the labia majora, labia minora, clitoris, and introitus; vaginitis is inflammation of the vaginal mucosa.
- One of the most common causes of noninfectious vulvovaginitis, usually referred to as nonspecific vulvovaginitis, is poor perineal hygiene.
- Vaginal discharge is a more prominent finding associated with infectious causes of vulvovaginitis than with noninfectious causes.
- The lack of estrogenized epithelium in this age group may inhibit sexually transmitted organisms from extending upward into the pelvis.
- *Lichen sclerosus* is a condition that affects all areas of the body in both sexes and in all ages. Its etiology is unknown, but it is believed to be associated with autoimmune disease.
- Psoriasis is a papulosquamous skin disease caused in part by a marked increase in epidermal cell turnover, with excessive cell proliferation.
- A transverse septum can create an outflow tract obstruction in the vagina. This presents in the adolescent with severe dysmenorrhea; in addition, there may be vaginal "swelling" indicative of hematocolpos.

References

1. American Academy of Pediatrics, & Pickering, L. D. (2007). *2007 Red book: Report of the Committee on Infectious Diseases* (25th ed.). American Academy of Pediatrics.
2. Aribarg, A. (1975). Topical oestrogen therapy for labial adhesions in children. *British Journal of Obstetrics and Gynaecology, 82*(5), 424. https://doi.org/10.1111/j.1471-0528.1975.tb01367.x.
3. Bartley, D., Morgan, L., & Rimsza, M. (1987). Gardnerella vaginalis in prepubertal girls. *American Journal of Diseases of Children, 141*(10), 1014. https://doi.org/10.1001/archpedi.1987.04460010078018.
4. Berkowitz, C., Elvik, S., & Logan, M. (1987). Labial fusion in prepubescent girls: A marker for sexual abuse? *American Journal of Obstetrics and Gynecology, 156*(1), 16. https://doi.org/10.1016/0002-9378(87)90048-8.

5. Bogaerts, J., Lepage, P., De Clercq, A., et al. (1992). Shigella and gonococcal vulvovaginitis in prepubertal central African girls. *Pediatric Infectious Disease Journal, 11*(10), 890. https://doi.org/10.1097/00006454-199210000-00013.

6. Brown, J. (1989). Hair shampooing technique and pediatric vulvovaginitis. *Pediatrics, 83*(1), 146. https://pediatrics.aappublications.org/content/83/1/146 (accessed on 6 September 2024).

7. Burden, A. (1999). Management of psoriasis in childhood. *Clinical and Experimental Dermatology, 24*(5), 341. https://doi.org/10.1046/j.1365-2230.1999.00527.x.

8. Capraro, V. J., & Greenberg, H. (1972). Adhesions of labia minora: A study of 50 patients. *Obstetrics & Gynecology, 39*(1), 65. https://doi.org/10.1097/00006250-197201000-00016.

9. Christensen, E., & Oster, J. (1971). Adhesions of labia minora (synechia vulvae) in childhood. *Acta Paediatrica Scandinavica, 60*(6), 709. https://doi.org/10.1111/j.1651-2227.1971.tb07192.x.

10. Clark, J., & Muller, S. (1967). *Lichen sclerosus* et atrophicus in children. *Archives of Dermatology, 95*(5), 476. https://doi.org/10.1001/archderm.1967.01600200032003.

11. Conn, P., & Crowley, W. (1994). Gonadotropin-releasing hormone and its analogs. *Annual Review of Medicine, 45*, 391–405. https://doi.org/10.1146/annurev.me.45.020194.002135.

12. Cox, R. (1997). Haemophilus influenzae: An underrated cause of vulvovaginitis in young girls. *Journal of Clinical Pathology, 50*(9), 765–766. https://doi.org/10.1136/jcp.50.9.765.

13. Cronje, H., Niemand, I., Bam, R., & Woodruff, J. (1998). Granulosa and theca cell tumors in children: A report of 17 cases and literature review. *Obstetrical and Gynecological Survey, 53*(4), 240–245. https://doi.org/10.1097/00006254-199804000-00004.

14. Dhar, V., Roker, K., Adhami, Z., & McKenzie, S. (1993). Streptococcal vulvovaginitis in girls. *Pediatric Dermatology, 10*(5), 366–369. https://doi.org/10.1111/j.1525-1470.1993.tb00185.x.

15. Doron, C., Shohat, M., Metzker, A., & Dickerman, Z. (1999). Growth, puberty, and endocrine functions in patients with sporadic or familial neurofibromatosis type 1: A longitudinal study. *Pediatrics, 103*(5), 1257–1263. https://doi.org/10.1542/peds.103.5.1257.

16. Droegemueller, W., Herbst, A., & Mishell, D. (1987). *Comprehensive Gynecology* (1st ed.). C.V. Mosby.

17. Edmonds, D. K. (1994). Sexual developmental anomalies and vary construction: Upper and lower tracts. In J. Sanfilippo, D. Muram, P. Lee, & J. Dewhurst (Eds.), *Pediatric Adolescent Gynecology* (pp. 555–572). W.B. Saunders.

18. Emans, S., & Goldstein, D. (1980). The gynecologic examination of the prepubertal child with vulvovaginitis: Use of the knee-chest position. *Pediatrics, 65*(5), 758–762. https://pediatrics.aappublications.org/content/65/5/758 (accessed on 6 September 2024).

19. Farber, E., & Jacobs, A. (1977). Infantile psoriasis. *American Journal of Diseases of Children, 131*(11), 1266. https://doi.org/10.1001/archpedi.1977.02120110038007.

20. Fischer, G., & Rogers, M. (1997). Treatment of childhood vulvar lichen sclerosis with potent topical corticosteroids. *Pediatric Dermatology, 14*(3), 235–239. https://doi.org/10.1111/j.1525-1470.1997.tb00989.x.

21. Fleischer, A. (1999). Treatment of atopic dermatitis: Role of tacrolimus ointment as a topical noncorticosteroidal therapy. *Journal of Allergy and Clinical Immunology, 104*(5), S126. https://doi.org/10.1016/S0091-6749(99)70076-5.

22. Friedrich, E. (1983). *Vulvar Disease* (2nd ed.). W.B. Saunders.

23. Gardner, J. (1992). Comparison of the vaginal flora in sexually abused and nonabused girls. *Journal of Pediatrics, 120*(6), 872–876. https://doi.org/10.1016/S0022-3476(05)80412-4.

24. Gregory, G. (1989). *Pediatric Anesthesia* (2nd ed., p. 15). Churchill Livingstone.

25. Hurwitz, S. (1993). *Clinical Pediatric Dermatology* (2nd ed.). W.B. Saunders.

26. Jaquiery, A., Stylianopolis, A., Hogg, G., & Grover, S. (1999). Vulvovaginitis: Clinical features, aetiology, and microbiology of the genital tract. *Archives of Disease in Childhood, 81*(1), 64–68. https://doi.org/10.1136/adc.81.1.64.

27. Jenkinson, S. D., & Mackinnon, A. E. (1984). Spontaneous separation of fused labia minora in prepubertal girls. *British Medical Journal, 289*(6445), 160. https://doi.org/10.1136/bmj.289.6445.160.

28. Jones, K. (1997). *Smith's Recognizable Patterns of Human Malformation* (p. 510). W.B. Saunders.

29. Kaplowitz, P. (2006). Pubertal development in girls: Secular trends. *Current Opinion in Obstetrics and Gynecology, 18*(5), 487–491. https://doi.org/10.1097/01.gco.0000243381.64475.5d.

30. Kaplowitz, P., & Oberfield, S. E. (1999). Reexamination of the age limit for defining when puberty is precocious in girls in the United States: Implications for evaluation and treatment. *Pediatrics, 104*(4), 936–941. https://doi.org/10.1542/peds.104.4.936.

31. Katz, H. (1995). Topical corticosteroids. *Dermatologic Clinics, 13*(4), 805–811. https://doi.org/10.1016/S0733-8635(21)00123-5.

32. Khanam, W., Chogtu, B., Mir, Z., & Shawl, F. (1977). Adhesion of the labia minora: A study of 75 cases. *Australian and New Zealand Journal of Obstetrics and Gynecology, 17*(3), 176–179. https://doi.org/10.1111/j.1479-828X.1977.tb01560.x.

33. Klein, P., & Clark, R. (1999). An evidence-based review of the efficacy of antihistamines in relieving pruritus in atopic dermatitis. *Archives of Dermatology, 135*(12), 1522–1526. https://doi.org/10.1001/archderm.135.12.1522.

34. Lee, M., & Donahoe, P. K. (1997). *The Infant with Ambiguous Genitalia* (6th ed.). C.V. Mosby.

35. Lee, P. A., Houk, C. P., Ahmed, S. F., & Hughes, I. A.; International Consensus Conference on Intersex organized by the Lawson Wilkins Pediatric Endocrine Society and the European Society for Paediatric Endocrinology. (2006). Consensus statement on management of intersex disorders. *Pediatrics, 118*(2), e488–e500. https://doi.org/10.1542/peds.2006-0738.

36. Leung, A. K., Robson, W. L., & Tay-Uyboco, J. (1993). The incidence of labial fusion in children. *Journal of Paediatric and Child Health, 29*(3), 235–236. https://doi.org/10.1111/j.1440-1754.1993.tb00114.x.

37. Linden, K., & Weinstein, G. (1999). Psoriasis: Current perspectives with an emphasis on treatment. *American Journal of Medicine, 107*(6), 595–605. https://doi.org/10.1016/S0002-9343(99)00225-6.

38. Lippe, B. (1979). Ambiguous genitalia and pseudohermaphroditism. *Pediatric Clinics of North America, 26*(1), 91–103. https://doi.org/10.1016/S0031-3955(16)34080-1.

39. Lorenz, B., Kaufman, R. H., & Kutzner, S. K. (1998). *Lichen sclerosus*. Therapy with clobetasol propionate. *Journal of Reproductive Medicine, 43*(9), 790–794. https://pubmed.ncbi.nlm.nih.gov/9757010/ (accessed on 6 September 2024).

40. Lowe, F., Hill, G., Jeffs, R., & Brandler, C. (1986). Urethral prolapse in children: Insights into etiology and management. *Journal of Urology, 135*(1), 100–103. https://doi.org/10.1016/S0022-5347(17)45061-7.

41. Merke, D., & Cutler, G. B. (1996). Evaluation and management of precocious puberty. *Archives of Disease in Childhood, 75*(4), 269–273. https://doi.org/10.1136/adc.75.4.269.

42. Meyrick Thomas, R., Ridley, C., McGibbon, D., & Black, M. M. (1998). *Lichen sclerosus* et atrophicus and autoimmunity: A study of 350 women. *British Journal of Dermatology, 118*(1), 41–46. https://doi.org/10.1111/j.1365-2133.1998.tb01507.x.

43. Mogielnicki, N., Schwartzman, J., & Elliot, J. (2000). Perineal group A streptococcal disease in a pediatric practice. *Pediatrics, 106*(2), 276–278. https://doi.org/10.1542/peds.106.2.276.

44. Moraes, P. (1998). Allergic vulvovaginitis induced by house dust mites: A case report. *Journal of Allergy and Clinical Immunology, 101*(5), 557–558. https://doi.org/10.1016/S0091-6749(98)70125-5.

45. Mroueh, S. M., & Muram, D. (1999). Common problems in pediatric gynecology, new developments. *Current Opinion in Obstetrics and Gynecology, 11*(5), 463–468. https://doi.org/10.1097/00001703-199910000-00006.

46. Muram, D. (1987). Pediatric and adolescent gynecology. In M. L. Pernoll & R. C. Benson (Eds.), *Current Gynecologic and Obstetric Diagnosis and Treatment* (pp. 563–585). Appleton & Lange.

47. Muram, D. (1988). Labial adhesions in sexually abused children. *Journal of the American Medical Association, 259*(2), 252–254. https://doi.org/10.1001/jama.259.2.252.

48. Muram, D. (1999). Treatment of labial adhesions in prepubertal girls. *Adolescent Pediatric Gynecology, 12*(2), 67–70. https://doi.org/10.1016/S1054-139X(99)00019-3.

49. Murray, P. J., Davis, H. W., & Hamp, M. (2007). *Pediatric and adolescent gynecology*. In *Atlas of Pediatric Physical Diagnosis* (5th ed., pp. 525–561). Mosby-Wolfe.

50. Myers, J. B., Sorensen, C. M., Wisner, B. P., et al. (2006). Betamethasone cream for the treatment of prepubertal labial adhesions. *Journal of Pediatric and Adolescent Gynecology, 19*(6), 407–411. https://doi.org/10.1016/j.jpag.2006.08.008.

51. Nag, R. N. (1972). Labial adhesion in children. *Indian Journal of Pediatrics, 39*(188), 33–36. https://doi.org/10.1007/BF02759728.

52. Orss, S., Sanchez, J., & Taboas, J. (1990). Spirochetal forms in the dermal lesions of morphea and *Lichen sclerosus* et atrophicus. *American Journal of Dermatopathology, 12*(5), 357–362. https://doi.org/10.1097/00000372-199010000-00003.

53. Paradise, J., Campos, J., Friedman, H., & Frishmuth, G. (1982). Vulvovaginitis in premenarchal girls: Clinical features and diagnostic evaluation. *Pediatrics, 70*(2), 193–198. https://doi.org/10.1542/peds.70.2.193.

54. Paul, J., Wojnarowska, F., Winsey, S., Marren, P., & Welsh, K. (2000). *Lichen sclerosus* premenarche: Autoimmunity and immunogenetics. *British Journal of Dermatology, 142*(3), 481–485. https://doi.org/10.1046/j.1365-2133.2000.03427.x.

55. Pokorny, S. P. (1987). Configuration of the prepubertal hymen. *American Journal of Obstetrics and Gynecology, 157*(4), 950–955. https://doi.org/10.1016/S0002-9378(87)80128-8.

56. Powell, J. (2006). Paediatric vulval disorders. *Journal of Obstetrics and Gynecology, 26*(7), 596–602. https://doi.org/10.1080/01443610600967970.

57. Purcell, K., Spence, L., Simpson, P., et al. (1990). HLA antigens in *Lichen sclerosus* at atrophicus. *Archives of Dermatology, 126*(8), 1043–1046. https://doi.org/10.1001/archderm.126.8.1043.

58. Rau, F. J., & Muram, D. (2001). Vulvovaginitis. In J. Sanfilippo (Ed.), *Pediatric and Adolescent Gynecology* (2nd ed., pp. 199–215). W.B. Saunders.

59. Redmond, C., Cowell, C., & Krafchick, B. (1988). Genital *Lichen sclerosus* in prepubertal girls. *Adolescent Pediatric Gynecology, 1*(3), 177–179. https://doi.org/10.1016/S1054-139X(88)80017-4.

60. Reindollar, R., Tho, S., & McDonough, P. (1987). Abnormalities of sexual differentiation: Evaluation and management. *Clinical Obstetrics and Gynecology, 30*(4), 697–717. https://doi.org/10.1097/00003081-198712000-00006.

61. Ridley, C. J. (1994). Vulvar disorders. In J. Sanfilippo, D. Muram, P. Lee, & J. Dewhurst (Eds.), *Pediatric and Adolescent Gynecology* (pp. 217–231). W.B. Saunders.

62. Ridley, C. M. (1987). *Lichen sclerosus* et atrophicus. *British Medical Journal, 295*(6603), 1295. https://doi.org/10.1136/bmj.295.6603.1295.

63. Rock, J. (1984). Surgical correction of uterovaginal anomalies. In J. J. Sciarra (Ed.), *Gynecology and obstetrics* (Vol. 1, pp. 123–134). Harper & Row.

64. Rock, J., & Azziz, R. (1987). Genital anomalies in childhood. *Clinical Obstetrics and Gynecology, 30*(4), 682–696. https://doi.org/10.1097/00003081-198712000-00005

65. Schachter, J., Grossman, M., Sweet, R., et al. (1986). Prospective study of perinatal transmission of *Chlamydia trachomatis*. *Journal of the American Medical Association, 255*(24), 3374–3377. https://doi.org/10.1001/jama.1986.03370240034012.

66. Singleton, A. (1980). Vaginal discharge in children and adolescents: Evolution and management: A review. *Clinical Pediatrics, 19*(12), 799–804. https://doi.org/10.1177/000992288001901207.

67. Slupik, R. (1991). Pediatric gynecology. In J. Sciarra (Ed.), *Gynecology and Obstetrics* (pp. 1–19). Lippincott Williams & Wilkins.

68. Smith, R., McNamara, J., & Ladd, M. (1986). Shigella and child abuse. *Pediatrics, 78*(5), 953–955. https://doi.org/10.1542/peds.78.5.953.

69. Sobel, J. D. (1997). Current concepts: Vaginitis. *New England Journal of Medicine, 337*(26), 1896–1903. https://doi.org/10.1056/NEJM199712253372606.

70. Speroff, L., Glass, R. H., & Kase, N. G. (1989). *Clinical Gynecologic Endocrinology & Infertility* (5th ed.). Williams & Wilkins.

71. Starr, N. (1997). Pediatric gynecology urologic problems. *Clinical Obstetrics and Gynecology, 40*(1), 181–192. https://doi.org/10.1097/00003081-199703000-00015.

72. Stovall, T., & Muram, D. (1988). Urinary retention secondary to labial adhesions. *Adolescent Pediatric Gynecology, 1*(2), 203–205. https://doi.org/10.1016/S1054-139X(88)80026-5.

73. Stylianopoulos, J., Hogg, G., & Grover, S. (1999). Vulvovaginitis: Clinical features, etiology, and microbiology of the genital tract. *Archives of Disease in Childhood, 81*(1), 64–67. https://doi.org/10.1136/adc.81.1.64.

74. Todd, P., Halpern, S., Kirby, J., & Pembroke, A. (1994). *Lichen sclerosus* and the Koebner phenomenon. *Clinical and Experimental Dermatology, 19*(4), 262–263. https://doi.org/10.1111/j.1365-2230.1994.tb01562.x.

75. Williams, T., Callen, J., & Owen, L. (1986). Vulvar disorders in the prepubertal female. *Pediatric Annals, 15*(8), 588–596. https://doi.org/10.3928/0090-4481-19860801-04.

INDEX

C

D

G

H

I

R

FSC
www.fsc.org
MIX
Papier | Fördert gute Waldnutzung
FSC® C083411

Kolibri 360 GmbH
Ferdinand-Jühlke-Straße 7
99095 Erfurt, Deutschland
produktsicherheit@kolibri360.de

LIST OF FIGURES

1.0 INTRODUCTION

On 7th February 1984, the Secretary of State for Transport announced that a study would be instituted into how a second crossing of the Severn Estuary might be provided in the general corridor of the existing bridge. The announcement continued "This is not a decision to build a second crossing. Before such a decision were taken, the Government would need to take full account of the outcome of the Study, forecast traffic requirements at the time, as well as of progress of the work on the existing crossing. But the completion of the work will ensure that there is no unnecessary delay in providing a second crossing as soon as it is needed."

The Second Severn Crossing Group was appointed by the Department of Transport on 16th August 1984 to undertake this study.

The brief for the Study requires three forms of crossing to be examined, viz: bridge, driven tunnel and immersed tunnel. For each type of crossing, the optimum location, capacity and timing of the construction are to be recommended in relation to the highway strategy of the region.

Of all the estuaries of the British Isles the Severn has probably the most difficult conditions for the construction of a major highway crossing. The difficulties occur below ground, in the waterway and as a result of frequent high winds. Consequently, all forms of crossing would have to surmount major obstacles and the following summary indicates the formidable challenge presented by the combined difficulties:

i) Ancient hard rocks at depth are contorted and occasionally faulted while overlying strata are appreciably softer and weakened by weathering. All the rocks are heavily-jointed and water-bearing. Limestones in the older strata contain fissures which can widen to cavernous proportions

ii) The physical form of the bed of the estuary is complex, with abrupt variations in bathymetry reflecting differences in rock properties and the distribution of sediment in a high energy tidal regime. The direction of turbulent, high velocity currents varies with location and time over the exceptionally large tidal range of 12 metres

iii) The wide expanse of the estuary is very exposed. The width varies from under 2 kilometres near the existing bridge from Beachley to Aust to 3 kilometres south of Beachley. It increases to 4 kilometres further south before narrowing to 3.5 kilometres at the English Stones. The total length of the Beachley to Aust crossing, combined with a crossing of the Wye and a high level viaduct across Beachley is nearly 3 kilometres, which approaches the width of the estuary at the English Stones

iv) The estuary has many important uses such as navigation and the disposal of land drainage and industrial effluents. The natural environment of the estuary margins is important and sensitive to change. There are also public amenity considerations. All these interests are the responsibility of a number of authorities and national organisations.

The object of the second crossing is to provide the most appropriate means of conveying traffic as part of the national highway network. Selection of locations and types of crossing to meet this requirement has necessitated complex investigations which have been affected by the following considerations:

i) The highways network includes the M4 and the M5, offering the possibility of linking a new crossing to either or both on the east bank and to the M4 on the west bank

ii) Traffic flow analyses including the complex Bristol road network with its links to the national motorways and consideration of the M4 and A40 routes in Wales

iii) Possible variations of the class of road required for the crossing and highway links ranging from single two-lane carriageways, with one-way or two-way operation, to dual carriageway motorways

iv) The possibility of phased construction of the schemes and the potential for increased capacity

v) Regional planning proposals and the safeguarding of the environment.

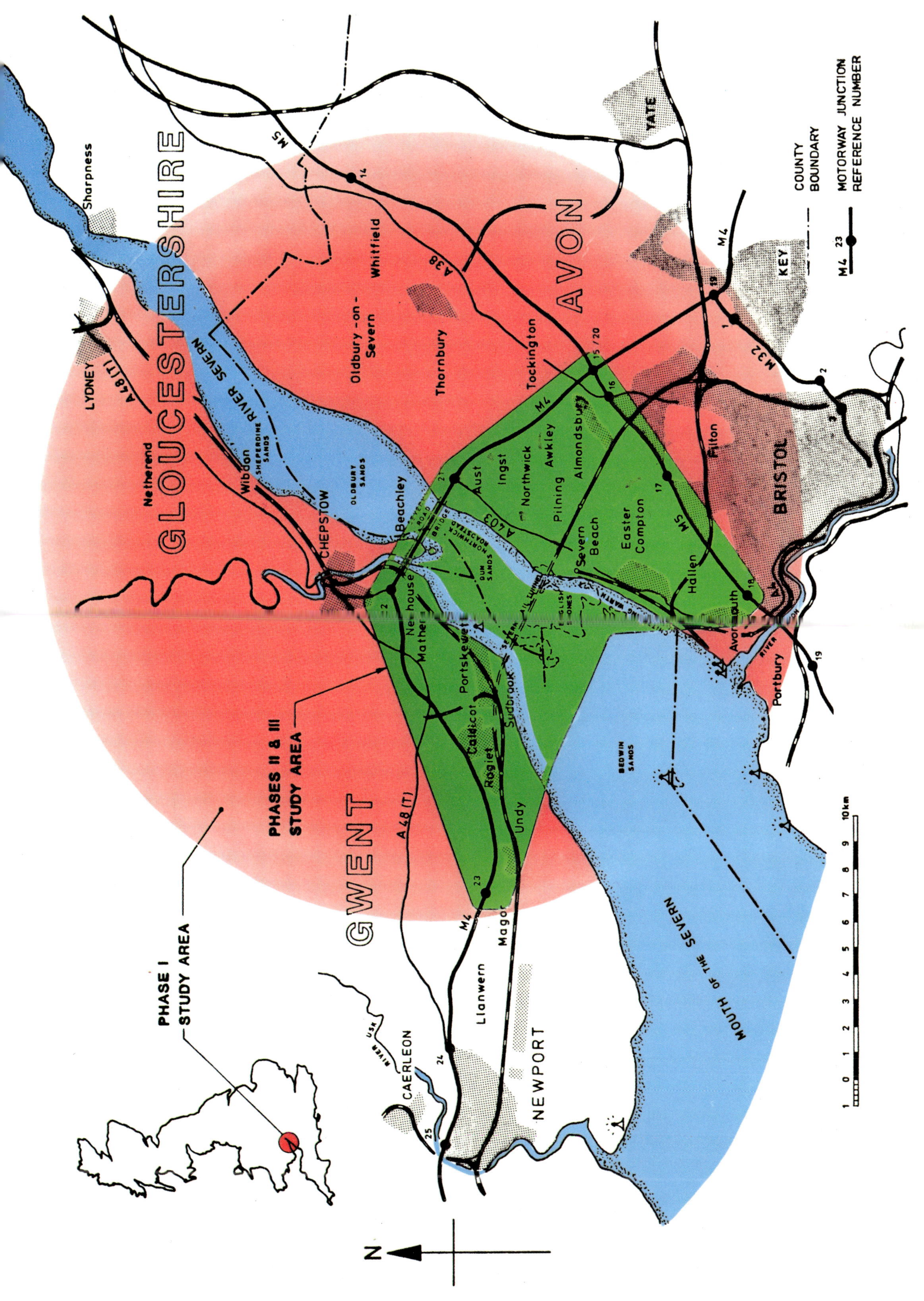
GLOUCESTERSHIRE
AVON
GWENT
BRISTOL
NEWPORT
CHEPSTOW
LYDNEY
CAERLEON
YATE
Sharpness
Netherend
Wibdon
Oldbury-on-Severn
Whitfield
Thornbury
Tockington
Beachley
Aust
Ingst
Northwick
Awkley
Pilning
Almondsbury
Severn Beach
Easter Compton
Hallen
Filton
Avonmouth
Portbury
Newhouse
Mathern
Portskewett
Sudbrook
Caldicot
Rogiet
Undy
Magor
Llanwern
RIVER SEVERN
SHEPERDINE SANDS
OLDBURY SANDS
DUN SANDS
BEDWIN SANDS
MOUTH OF THE SEVERN
RIVER USK
SEVERN ROAD BRIDGE
NORTHWICK ROADSTEAD
A48(T)
A38
A403
M4
M5
M32
PHASE I STUDY AREA
PHASES II & III STUDY AREA
KEY
COUNTY BOUNDARY
MOTORWAY JUNCTION REFERENCE NUMBER
M4 23
10km
N

Study Area **1**

2.0 CHARACTERISTICS OF THE SEVERN ESTUARY FROM ENGLISH STONES TO BEACHLEY

The banks of the estuary in the Study Area, shown in Figure 1, are generally a flat expanse of geologically recent sediment which overlies the bed rock to a depth of about 10 metres. The surface level is near to that of the highest tides and the area is protected from flooding by low earth embankments. A few kilometres inshore the ground on both banks rises appreciably, generally as the outcrop of the underlying rock. Nearer the shore line there are also occasional small outcrops of rock projecting above the plane of sedimentation.

Extensive banks of recent sediment also occur in the waterway where they are largely exposed at low tide. Areas of the pre-existing rock topography, denuded of the later cover of sediment are similarly exposed in the inter-tidal zone, forming the extensive English Stones and several smaller ledges. A deep ravine-like channel known as The Shoots has been eroded through the rocks of the estuary bed and forms an abrupt edge to the English Stones in the downstream half of the Study Area. Upstream of The Shoots the bed topography is less severe and channels such as Northwick Roadstead are relatively wide and shallow and they are generally flanked by banks of sediment.

The bedrock of the region is entirely sedimentary. Geologically ancient Carboniferous strata, composed of hard, dense rocks have been folded and faulted and subsequently overlain by relatively soft Triassic rocks. The latter have not been significantly affected by folding or faulting and they remain essentially flat-bedded.

The visible outcrops in the Study Area are almost entirely Triassic. Apart from a small outcrop exposed at low tide below Severn Road Bridge, the underlying Carboniferous strata are only encountered in the two existing tunnels below the estuary. The C.E.G.B. cable tunnel near the Severn Road Bridge penetrated dolomitic limestones from near the base of the Carboniferous Series while the rail tunnel 5 kilometres downstream passed through Coal Measures from near the top of the series. Between the tunnels the Carboniferous geology beneath the estuary is conjectural.

Seismic activity of low intensity occurs in the region to a sufficient degree to necessitate its consideration in the design of cross-estuary structures.

The most noticeable characteristic of the estuary is the behaviour of the tide, the average range at Springs of 12.3 metres being among the largest in the world. The resulting tidal flow includes streams with velocities of 4 metres/second (8 knots), with abrupt changes of direction at the turn of the tide. The flow pattern is dominated by the barrier presented by the English Stones and the confinement of a high proportion of the total discharge of the waterway to The Shoots channel and its vicinity. Constriction of the flow, with attendant high velocities, also takes place below the Severn Road Bridge. The high degree of turbulence of the estuary within the Study Area promotes a thorough mixing of the freshwater of the Rivers Severn and Wye with the seawater of the Bristol Channel.

Extreme tide levels can arise as a result of surges in the Irish Sea and Bristol Channel and a 1 in 1000 years event could involve an increase in water height of 3 metres above the mean tide level. Such an event would cause extensive inundation of the low-lying land on both sides of the estuary. The observed wave pattern in the estuary suggests that storm waves in the Study Area could reach a height in excess of 2.5 metres, with a probability of this occurring once in 100 years.

There are approximately 1400 ship movements per year through the Study Area length of estuary. Vessel size is generally from 650 to 1500 d.w.t., although there is occasional passage of a 6,500 d.w.t. vessel. The navigation channel follows the difficult and hazardous passage through The Shoots, upstream of which navigation is affected by shifting sand banks.

Navigation can be affected by the weather. Gales may blow from any direction for up to 15 per cent of the time through the winter months. Fog which reduces visibility to less than 100 metres can persist for 3 or 4 days and there is an average occurrence of 15 to 20 days of such fog per year.

The inter-tidal mud flats and adjacent saltings provide an important source of nutrients which support a very large biomass. The area is of international importance as a feeding ground for wild fowl and waders and much of the estuary above low water mark is designated a Site of Special Scientific Interest.

3.0 THE STUDY

The programme of work over the two year study period was undertaken in three phases. Phase I was an initial investigation leading to the recommendation of a limited range of bridge, driven tunnel and immersed tunnel options. Phase II was devoted to detailed study of those options and Phase III completed the investigation of the leading options, including the final evaluation and appraisal.

A description of the initial studies and a preliminary appraisal of the crossing options is given in the Phase I Report, published in January 1985.

3.1 Phase I - Initial Studies

The first phase of the Study included preliminary investigations, the collection of available data and consultation with County Councils, relevant statutory authorities and other organisations. In particular, discussions were held with Gwent County Council, Avon County Council and, the South Wales Standing Conference on regional policy issues.

The preliminary engineering studies and assessments involved the collation of such available data on geotechnical, topographical, hydrographical, planning, environmental and navigational matters as were considered sufficient for the initial investigation of possible crossing options. A number of crossing corridors, appropriate to each crossing type, were identified within the Study Area, together with some suitable crossing locations outside those limits.

An analysis of the various options for crossing and highway corridors, based on engineering feasibility, economic and non-economic cost and benefit, enabled a reduction to be made in the number of schemes which were finally recommended for further evaluation during the second phase of the Study. The options that were proposed for further consideration were:

i) Crossings between the existing Severn Road Bridge and Dun Sands, which would all have west and east links to the M4, namely

- a long span bridge adjacent to the existing Severn Road Bridge
- a combination of long span bridge south of the confluence of the Rivers Severn and Wye with a medium-length span across Northwick Roadstead
- a driven tunnel to the south of the Severn Road Bridge
- an immersed tunnel across the Dun Sands

ii) Crossings in the area of the English Stones, which would link to the M4 west of Caldicot on the Welsh Bank and to the M4 west of Almondsbury and/or the M5 north of Avonmouth on the English bank, namely

- a bridge across the English Stones with a medium-length navigation span
- a driven tunnel to the south of the existing British Rail tunnel

iii) Crossings south of the English Stones and north of Avonmouth, which would link to the M4 west of Caldicot and the M5 north of Avonmouth, namely

- a bridge with a medium-length navigation span
- a driven tunnel
- an immersed tunnel.

3.2 Phase II - Detailed Studies

The Department of Transport agreed with the options identified in the Phase I Report for further consideration, but they decided that those crossings in the area of the estuary between the English Stones and Avonmouth, which had been shown to be of high capital cost, would not be considered further. Thus, in the 6 kilometres of estuary between the existing bridge and the downstream limit of the English Stones, crossings by both bridge and tunnel were the subject of detailed study in Phase II. Included in those crossings was one by immersed tunnel over the southern edge of the English Stones, which was shown by hydraulic and geophysical investigations to be a favourable location for that form of construction.

The background data for the studies were extended in Phase II by a number of investigations involving site measurements or model testing, as follows:

- investigations of the estuary using seismic reflection techniques to establish the bed profile and significant geological boundaries
- a computational tidal model of the estuary within the Study Area to establish the existing hydraulic behaviour and to assess the effects of new construction on the hydraulic regime of the estuary. Measurements were also made in the estuary for calibration purposes
- wind tunnel tests of models of specific bridge superstructures to assess the aerodynamic response of the bridges. Wind shielding devices were included on some of the model decks and comparative tests on the effectiveness of these devices were also made.

During Phase II, engineering, traffic and other studies were carried out in sufficient depth to support a level of scheme development that enabled valid comparisons to be made within each crossing type, and the number of crossing options to be reduced to a logical minimum at the end of the phase. An analysis and evaluation of the proposed crossings and highway links - based on engineering feasibility, traffic operation and management, planning, environmental aspects, economic and non-economic costs and benefits - resulted in the identification of the following schemes for further study and appraisal in Phase III:

- a bridge crossing from Newhouse to Aust
- a bridge crossing at the English Stones
- a driven tunnel from Mathern beneath Northwick Roadstead
- an immersed tunnel from Mathern beneath Northwick Roadstead.

3.3 Phase III - Confirmatory Studies and Final Appraisal

In the final stage of the Study, attention was concentrated on the reduced number of crossing options indicated above, which made possible a fuller consideration of the highway links, operational characteristics, including one-way single carriageways and phasing of bridges and driven tunnels, as well as the completion of the engineering and traffic studies. Cost and sensitivity evaluations were made and the final evaluation, appraisal and financial assessment were undertaken.

The engineering appraisal of a restricted number of schemes was completed by confirmatory studies, which included further wind tunnel testing of wind shielding devices and a study of interference effects of an adjacent second crossing bridge on the existing bridge.

The engineering, traffic and financial implications of modified schemes for alternative connections and interchanges were reappraised, where such modifications were able to offer an increased net present value.

At the end of Phase III the final recommended proposals for each type of crossing have been sufficiently developed for valid comparisons to be made of crossing types and schemes.

4.0 BRIDGE AND TUNNEL CROSSINGS

The essential characteristics of those crossing schemes, including highway links, that have proved to be the best of the immersed tunnel and the driven tunnel proposals are summarised below. In the case of the bridge crossing, the characteristics are described of two schemes which have merited full consideration.

The engineering of what is potentially the longest and most difficult motorway crossing of an estuary in the UK, is summarised by presenting the essential characteristics of each crossing in terms of site conditions, construction, effects on existing features, and where relevant, phasing, services and operation.

4.1 Bridges

It has been determined that it would be possible to design with confidence bridge crossings which would be able to give a high level of performance, even under adverse conditions and which could be constructed using well-proven construction techniques. It would be feasible to design the bridges so that cable stays and suspension bridge hangers could be replaced while the crossing remains operational. The provision of wind shielding to protect traffic from strong cross winds should be feasible in all crossings, and phased provision of traffic capacity could be achieved by widening to provide additional carriageway breadth at a later date. The feasibility of adding even more width by twinning would need to be investigated by wind tunnel testing.

Crossing lengths, structural forms and site conditions would vary significantly from one crossing location to another, affecting the extent of site investigation, construction methods and programme. The effect of each crossing on existing features would also vary with location. These aspects are summarised below.

4.1.1 Newhouse to Aust Crossing - Adjacent to the Existing Bridge

The overall length of 3480 metres would include a 988 metres main span suspension bridge across the River Severn and a 240 metres main span cable stayed bridge across the River Wye. (See Fig 2). The crossing would be located approximately 250 metres south of the existing bridge and would match the attractive lines of the existing crossing.

Site Conditions

- This crossing would have 2000 metres of viaduct and 6 piers which would be exposed to a marine environment.

- Site investigation would be required at 6 foundations in water depths up to 13 metres at MHWS and at 26 foundations on land. However, conditions likely to be encountered during construction should be predictable from experience gained during the construction of the Severn Road Bridge.

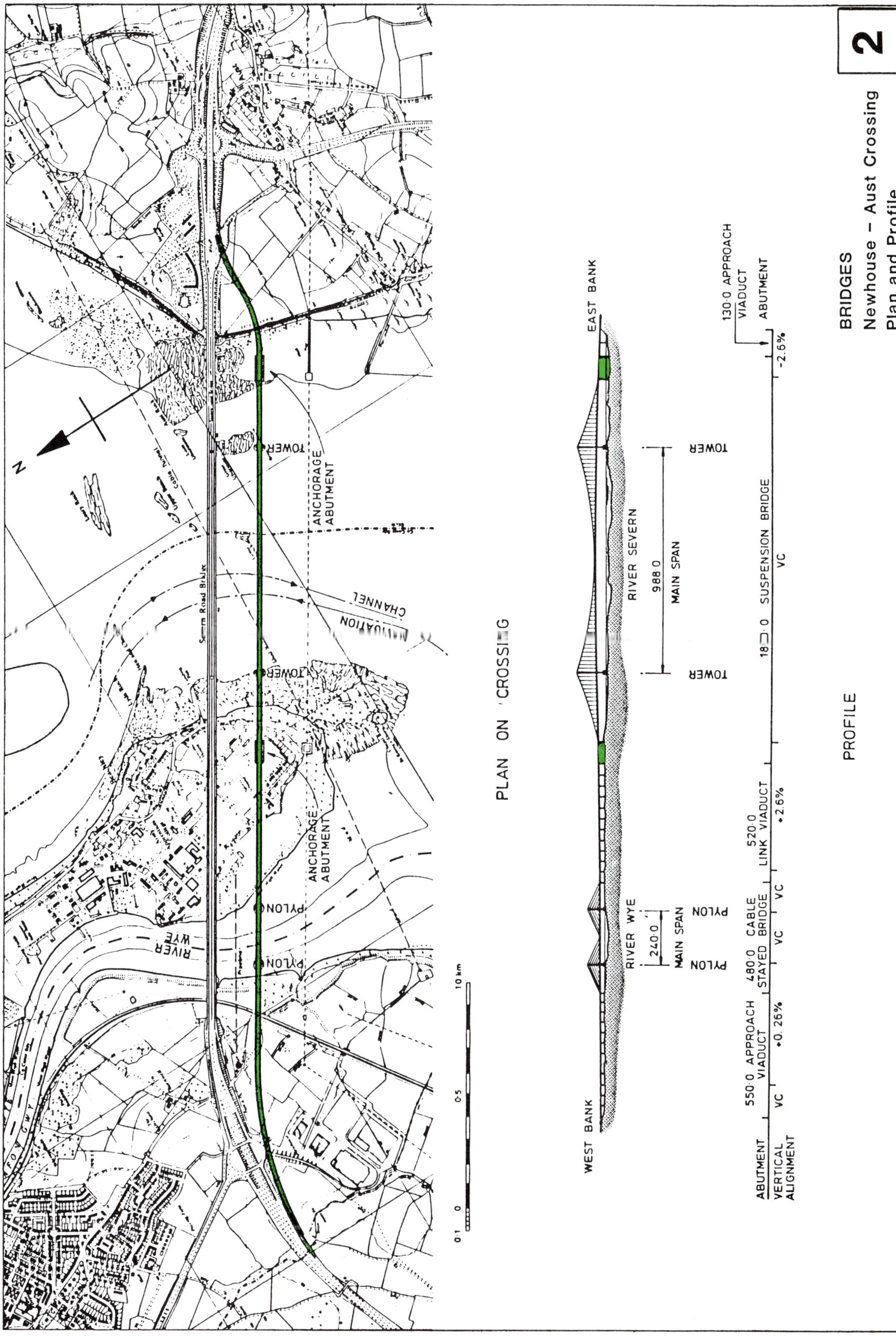

Newhouse – Aust Bridge Crossing
Plan and Profile

Construction

- The opportunity would exist for about 35 per cent of the construction work to be carried out in factory-like conditions, including slip forming of pylons, this part of the work being relatively unaffected by site conditions. Decks could be prefabricated to facilitate rapid erection.

- Foundation construction would be within cofferdams and therefore little affected by wind and tide conditions, but high level cable erection for the suspension bridge would be susceptible to wind and weather conditions which would need to be allowed for in the management and programming of the works.

- Construction would take approximately 54 months, with the installation of cables and erection of the superstructure for the suspension bridge being the key activities.

Effects on Existing Features

- The possibility of detrimental aerodynamic interference with the Severn Road Bridge is discussed further in Section 7.2.3.

4.1.2 English Stones Crossing

The overall length of 4900 metres would comprise a 456 metres main span, cable stayed bridge across The Shoots and approach viaducts with varying span lengths up to 130 metres (see Fig 3). The crossing would form an interesting new feature in the estuary remote from the Severn Road Bridge, with the long approach viaducts sweeping up from the banks to the high level main span with its cable stay supports. Alternative arrangements would allow the eastern approaches to remain at low level for approximately 1400 metres before rising to meet the main span.

Site Conditions

- This crossing would have 4700 metres of viaduct, including the main span and 56 piers which would be exposed to a marine environment.

- Site investigation would be required at 56 foundations in water depths generally up to 13 metres at MHWS and 3 foundations on land. The bedrock in the estuary is exposed at low water over 75 per cent of the crossing length, which would allow the condition and profile of the rock to be determined by visual inspection during the investigation.

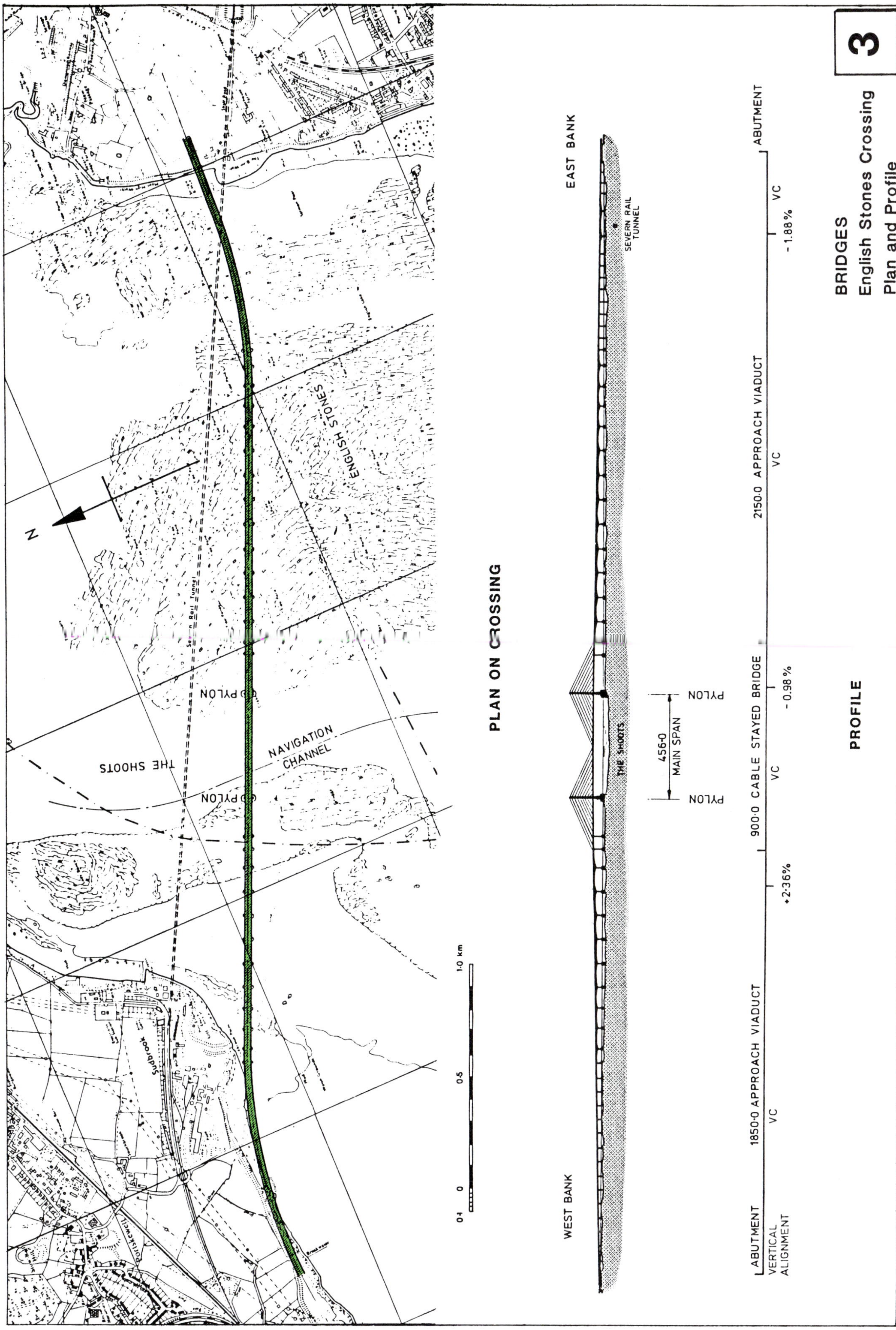

English Stones Bridge Crossing
Plan and Profile

Construction

- The opportunity would exist for about 50 per cent of the construction work to be carried out in factory-like conditions, including slip forming of pylons, and thus being relatively unaffected by site conditions. Decks could be prefabricted to facilitate rapid erection.

- Construction plant would need to be designed carefully for the floating out and positioning of a large number of foundation structures, taking account of variable wind, tide, estuarine currents and weather conditions.

- Construction would take approximately 38 months. Construction of the foundations, while being a major part, would benefit from the economy and flexibility of plant appropriate to the repetitious nature of the works.

Effects on Existing Features

- Piers adjacent to the rail tunnel could be located sufficiently far away to not affect the tunnel adversely.

4.2 Driven Tunnels - Northwick Roadstead Crossing

The driven tunnel beneath Northwick Roadstead would be located a few hundred metres downstream of Severn Road Bridge, as shown in Figure 4. Tunnels of circular cross-section are envisaged and the single bore, 11 metres internal diameter, required for a single carriageway highway of two-lane motorway standard would necessitate an opening of 12 to 12.5 metres diameter. Twin tunnels of this diameter would be required for a dual two lane motorway.

Tunnels would be driven beneath the full width of the estuary and would be 4.4 kilometres long between portals. The horizontal alignment would be curvilinear due to the influence of physical constraints, but this would have no significant effect on construction or operation.

Site Conditions

- The site investigation for the adjoining CEGB cable tunnel and the subsequent tunnel construction provide a substantial level of understanding of the site geology. A site investigation covering the area of a proposed road tunnel would be a direct extension of the earlier area of information.

- Beachley Point is a very advantageous location for an intermediate shaft, for both construction and ventilation purposes.

- Postulated buried channels beneath the alluvial beds of the Severn and the Wye are constraints on the envisaged vertical alignment, which consequently might have to be changed as a result of the site investigation.

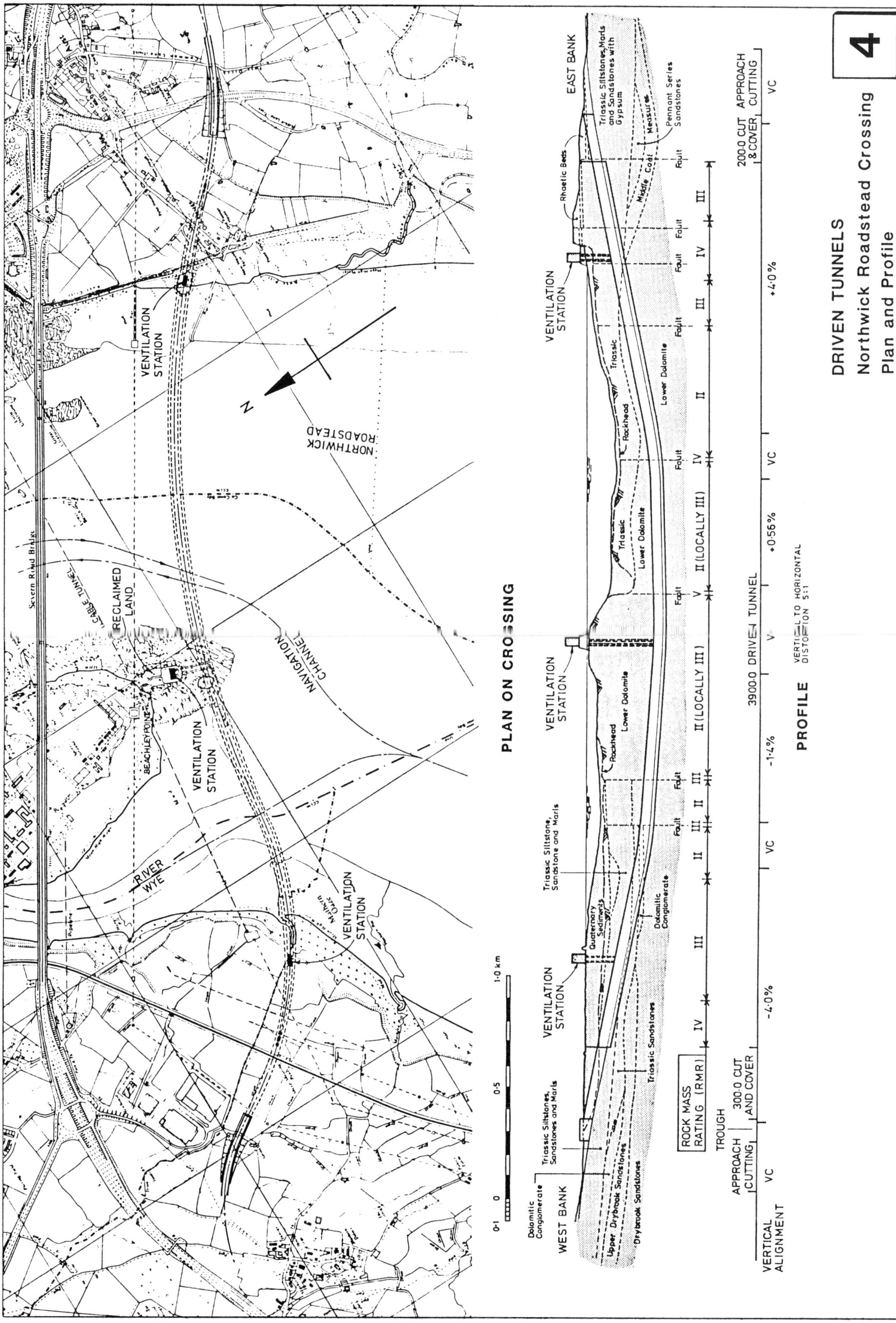

Northwick Roadstead Driven Tunnel Crossing
Plan and Profile

4

- The depth of Quaternary sediments at the western portal is an alignment consideration and the results of the site investigation might necessitate changed arrangements for the approaches.

- Beneath the western bank the tunnel would be within 150 metres of the cable tunnel and it would be necessary to avoid any possibility of damage to the structure or interference with the CEGB transmission.

Construction

- Traditional drill and blast tunnelling methods could be used. It would be possible to use a tunnel boring machine but the length of drive makes this questionable.

- The area of the western portal is overlain by 10 metres or more of soft Quaternary sediments which if actually deeper would necessitate more expensive construction or change of alignment. A shallower depth of sediment would simplify the approach works.

- Outcropping rock at the eastern portal would facilitate construction as it limits the need for cut-and-cover or soft ground tunnelling.

- Most of the tunnel beneath the estuary would probably be excavated in the Lower Dolomite, a thick bed of massive character with excellent tunnelling properties in which primary support would not be a major factor.

- At higher levels at both ends of the tunnel it would pass through Triassic strata which may require substantial primary support.

- Potential water ingress, including possible strong inflow from solution channels in the Lower Dolomite, would require pre-treatment by grout injection from a pilot tunnel.

- The presence of methane is not expected.

- Spoil from the shafts near to the two banks could be conveyed by road to the highway works.

- Part of the tunnel spoil from the Beachley shaft could be used for reclamation on the peninsula. The dolomitic limestone could be used for the in situ concrete lining of the tunnel. The remainder would probably be removed by barge to dumping grounds in the estuary downstream of Avonmouth.

- Construction would take approximately 60 months for a dual two-lane motorway scheme.

Effects on Existing Features

- The effect on the estuary would be slight except for small areas of reclamation which would be required for ventilation stations at Beachley and Aust.

- The area of the construction site at Beachley would be reinstated leaving the ventilation station as a permanent feature.

- There would be visual intrusion and noise from the three ventilation stations.

Phasing

- Phased construction would be straight-forward and would be effected by the later addition of a second tunnel. Construction would be in general little affected by the presence of the first tunnel, except for necessary control on the use of explosives. Where the ends of the tunnels converge, a separating wall would be formed from bored piles to protect the first tunnel during the second phase excavation.

- Cross-adits between the two tunnels would be provided by connecting to stub ends built in the first phase.

Services and Operation

- The 4.4 kilometre length of tunnel would impose high demands on operating and maintenance facilities.

  Emergency services would be faced with problems of access with single bore tunnels, particularly those carrying uni-directional traffic. The potential for incidents increases with the length of the tunnel.

- Beachley ventilation station, which is offset from the tunnel axis, would require long horizontal adits, resulting in high friction losses.

4.3 Immersed Tunnel - Northwick Roadstead Crossing

It is envisaged that an immersed tunnel crossing of the Severn Estuary could use adaptations of existing well-proven construction techniques.

This crossing would include a 3.1 kilometres long tunnel traversing the complete width of the estuary as shown in Fig 5. Either semi-transverse/transverse or reduced transverse ventilation systems would be employed, requiring the addition of ventilation ducts to the tunnel cross-section.

Site Conditions

- The sub-bed geology would be favourable for normal dredging techniques. The estimated depth of dredgeable material would generally be well in excess of that required for trench excavation, and the possibility of encountering hard rock is considered slight.

- The site would be sheltered from wave action by the presence of the English Stones downstream of the crossing.

- Weak foundation conditions for the immersed tunnel units might exist over part of the inter-tidal zone, requiring additional excavation followed by backfilling with suitable material.

Construction

- Construction facilities for the immersed tunnel units could be established on the bank of the estuary close to the tunnel alignment, with good access to the existing road and rail network.

- It is envisaged that the tunnel units, representing some 95 per cent of the crossing length, would be fabricated under factory-like conditions, offering the potential for a high degree of quality control and minimising delays due to adverse weather conditions.

- The fabrication of tunnel units in existing facilities remote from the crossing location could involve the towing of units through The Shoots as most of these facilities have been identified downstream of the English Stones.

- Suitable spoil grounds would be remote from the site and spoil disposal could involve passage through The Shoots.

- A large number of tunnel units, probably about 25, would have to be handled and joined within the estuary.

- A more detailed study of trench accretion would be required in order to evaluate the construction techniques for placing the tunnel units.

- The narrowness of the navigation channel over the line of the tunnel might impose some restriction on shipping movements during construction.

- Construction would take approximately 60 months for a dual two-lane motorway crossing.

Effects on Existing Features

- There would be little protrusion of the tunnel above the bed of the estuary, resulting in minimal change to the existing estuarine conditions and no effect on navigation.

- There would be minimal visual intrusion on the surroundings, even at low water.

- Aerodynamic studies would be required to assess the possible effects of noise and air pollution from the ventilation stations, particularly on the Avon bank, due to the proximity of existing habitation.

Phasing

- Minimal provision would be required in the first phase of construction to facilitate the construction of a second separate tunnel to provide additional traffic capacity.

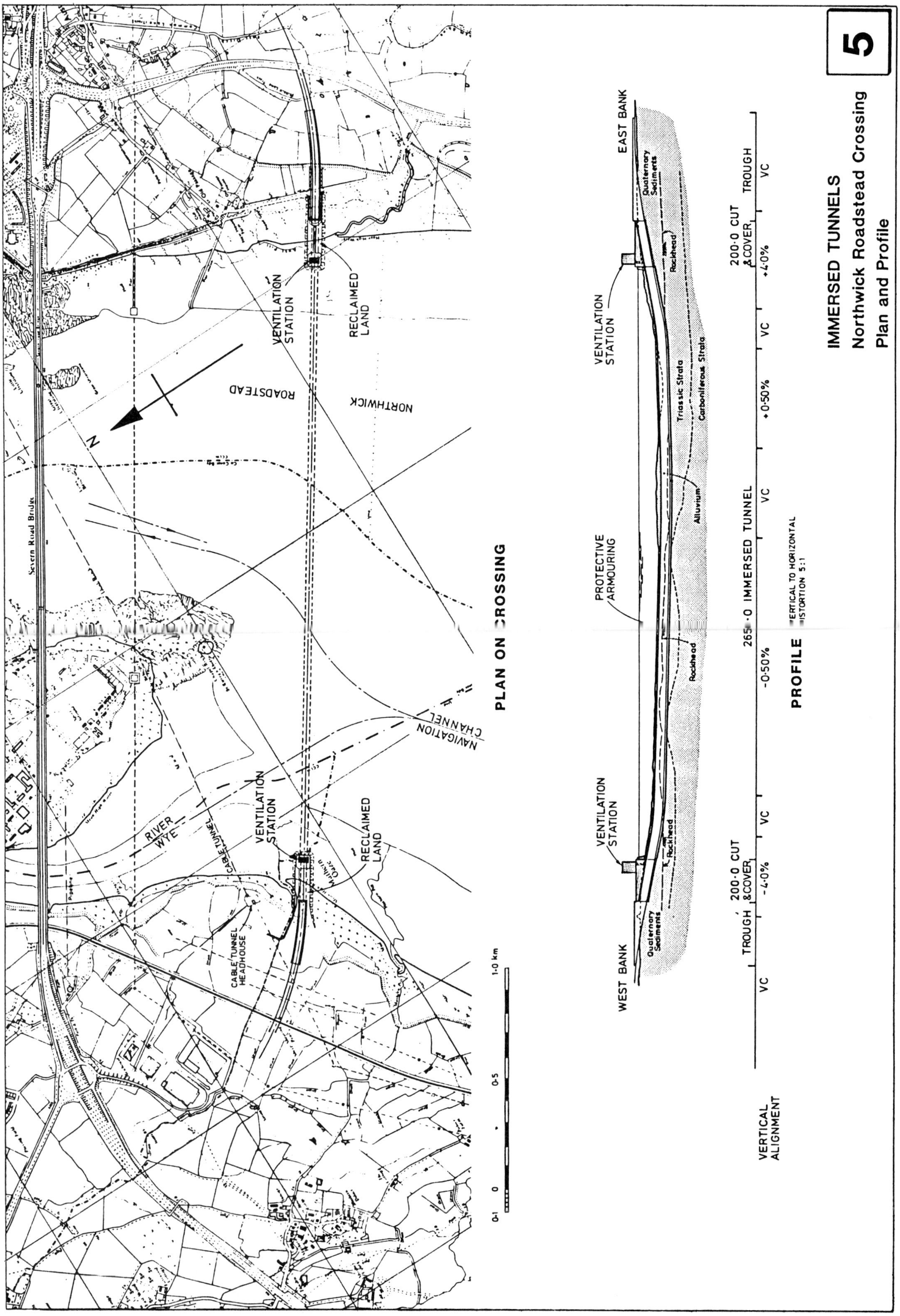

Northwick Roadstead Immersed Tunnel Crossing
Plan and Profile

5

- It would be difficult to provide emergency cross-adits between the two traffic ducts if phased construction were employed.

Services and Operation

- The 3.1 kilometres length of tunnel would impose high demands on operating and maintenance requirements.

- Emergency services could be faced with problems of access in single tube tunnels, particularly those carrying uni-directional traffic.

4.4 Highway Links and Interchanges

The characteristics of the links and interchanges, which are indicated in Figs. 2, 6, 7 and 8, are presented below in terms of ground conditions, geometric standards, construction and phasing.

The engineering aspects of the highway links are similar at each crossing, although the location of the connection points of the links to each crossing type may differ.

The ground conditions are generally good except on the low-lying coastal levels on each bank.

4.4.1 Newhouse to Aust and Northwick Roadstead Crossings

a) Links

- Generally alignments would be short in length, averaging approximately 2 kilometres on the west bank and 3 kilometres on the east bank, except that the links to Interchange 1 would be only approximately 500 metres in length.

- The links to Interchanges 2, 3 and 12 would pass mainly over low-lying ground.

b) Interchanges

Ground Conditions

- Interchanges 2 and 3 would be sited on low-lying ground.

- Interchanges 1, 11 and 12 would be sited on firm, higher ground.

Geometric Standards

- Interchanges 3 and 12 would be relatively unconstrained while Interchanges 1, 2 and 11 would have lower than desirable minimum standards.

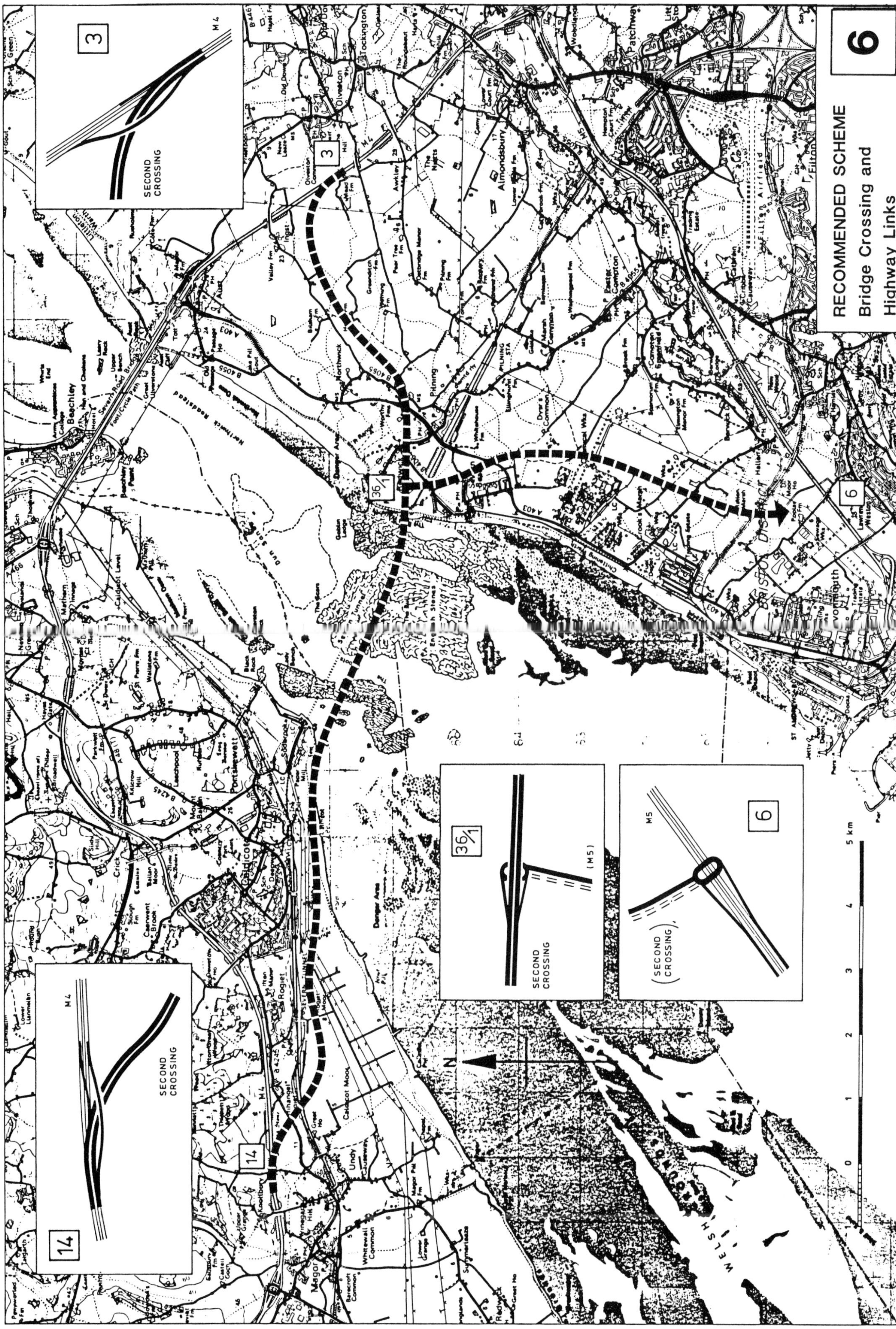

Recommended Scheme
Bridge Crossing and Highway Links

6

- The geometric standards of Interchange 11 would be reduced further if the driven tunnel portal position had to be relocated nearer to the M4 as a result of a site investigation.

Construction

- Interchanges 2, 3 and 12 would be sited on open ground and their construction would cause only slight disruption to existing M4 traffic.

- Interchange 11 would necessitate the demolition and reconstruction of existing motorway bridges with consequential lengthy periods of contraflow working.

- Interchange 1 would involve major changes to the layout of the existing Aust Interchange prior to construction of new carriageways. Access and working space would be very restricted and there would be severe disruption due to temporary rerouteing of all existing traffic movements.

Phasing

- Free flow interchanges would only be suitable for one-way single carriageway first phase construction.

4.4.2 English Stones Crossings

a) Links

- The links to Interchange 13 would be approximately 4 kilometres in length, 3 kilometres of which would be running across low-lying ground.

- The links to Interchange 14 would each be approximately 2 kilometres longer than those to Interchange 13. The links to Interchanges 3 and 6 would each be approximately 6 kilometres in length. The entire length of all links, except for one kilometre adjacent to the M4 at Interchange 14, would be located on the coastal levels.

b) Interchanges

Ground Conditions

- Interchanges 3 and 6 would be located on low-lying ground.

- Interchanges 13 and 14 would be located on firmer, higher ground.

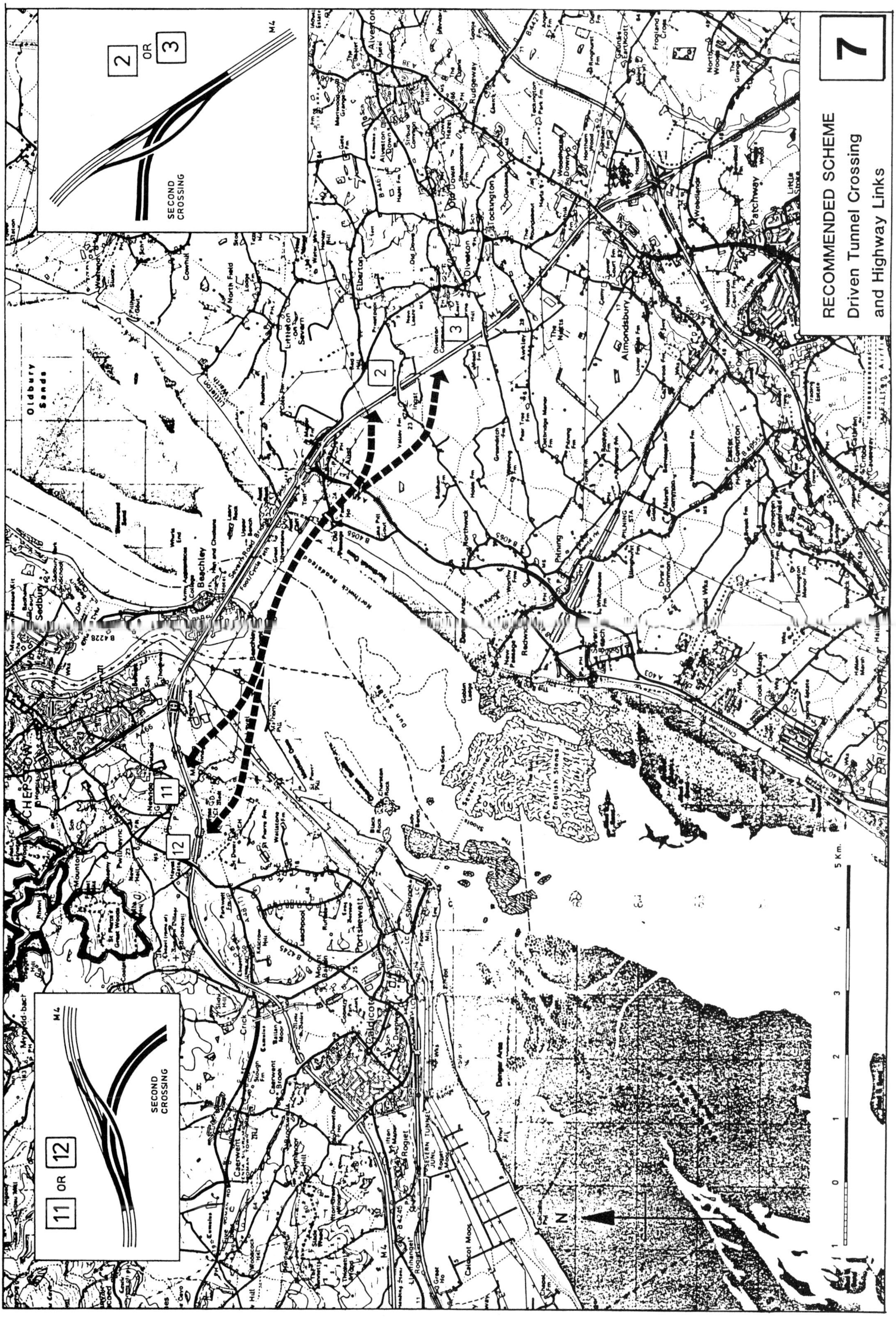

Recommended Scheme
Driven Tunnel Crossing and Highway Links

7

Geometric Standards

- Interchanges 3 and 14 would occupy relatively unconstrained sites.

- Interchange 13 would require a reduction in standard for free flow layouts.

Construction

- Interchanges 3 and 14 would be located on open ground and their construction would cause minimum disruption to M4 traffic.

- Interchange 6 would be located on open ground but its construction and the demolition of Lawrence Weston Road overbridge would involve considerable disruption of M5 traffic.

- Construction of Interchange 13, as a free flow layout, could introduce significant contraflow working on the M4.

- Interchange 13 for a single two-way carriageway would require the demoltion of Dewstow Road overbridge and hence, possible short term closure of the M4.

- Access for construction of Interchanges 13 and 14 would probably be via B4245, resulting in haulage through Magor, Undy, Rogiet and Caldicot.

Phasing

- The westbound carriageway of a dual two-lane motorway with free flow interchanges could be constructed as an initial phase.

- No element of a dual two-lane motorway within a free flow interchange could be developed from an existing single carriageway scheme. In the case of Interchanges 13 and 14, total demolition of the existing grade separated roundabout type junction and construction of a free flow interchange would be required.

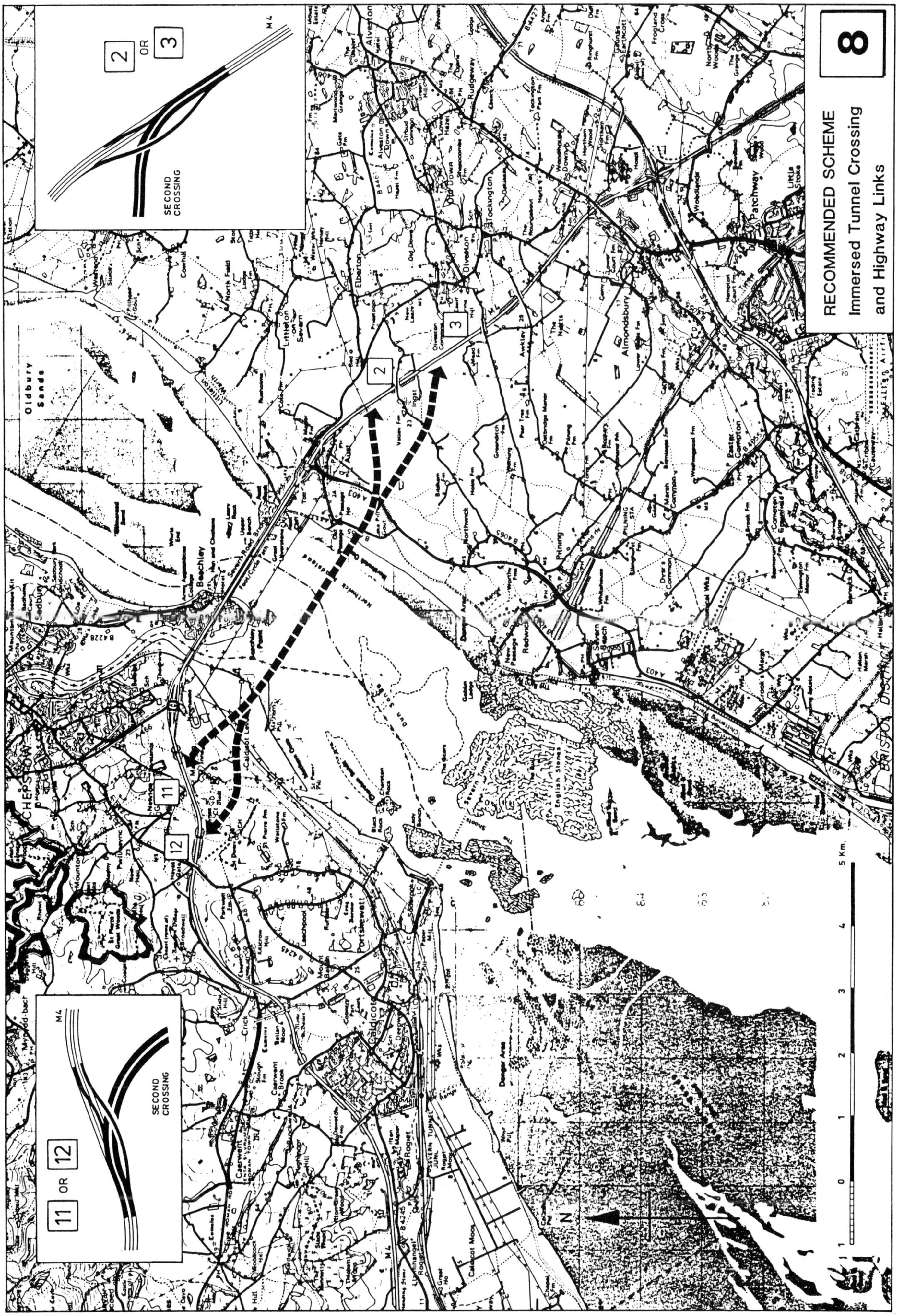

Recommended Scheme
Immersed Tunnel Crossing and Highway Links

8

5.0 PLANNING AND ENVIRONMENT

5.1 Bridge Schemes

The Newhouse to Aust bridge option adjacent to the existing Severn Bridge would result in little land take, with consequent minimal agricultural and ecological effects. This option would not conflict with existing planning policies. It would require the acquisition of approximately thirty Ministry of Defence homes associated with the Army Apprentices College on Beachley Point. Other houses at Beachley would suffer from significant short term construction noise. There would be some additional visual impact on occupiers at Beachley, although many of the houses affected are already overshadowed by the existing M4 viaduct. There would be some disturbance to an established salmon catching area near Aust Cliff and to the nearby geological Site of Special Scientific Interest on the cliff face. On the Avon bank, the highway links for a crossing with single or dual two-lane carriageway to motorway standards would result in slightly increased environmental impact on part of Aust village, but this would be a small increment on the impact from the existing M4. The one-way single carriageway with three lanes to motorway standard would have a negligible effect on Aust village.

An English Stones bridge crossing would intrude upon popular open estuarial views in the areas of Sudbrook Point, south of Portskewett, and the Binn Wall promenade, north of Severn Beach. However, the bridge would be a positive feature in the wider estuary context, although it would be relatively distant from the main vantage points. Ecological impact would be limited if viaducts rather than causeways were predominantly incorporated in the bridge design. The ecological impact would include disturbance to feeding birds along the shorelines, construction over existing mudflats and the loss of existing salt marsh adjacent to Sudbrook Point.

The highway links within Avon, which connect to Interchange 3 by passing to the north of Pilning, would create somewhat less noise and visual intrusion on the communities at the eastern end of the English Stones than would a route to the south of Pilning. All links from the English Stones bridge to Interchange 3 would involve substantial land take with consequent adverse agricultural, landscape with some local ecological impact and extensive conflict with Green Belt policies.

Those options incorporating highway links to both Interchanges 3 and 6 would require some 60 hectares of agricultural land and affect four communities in Avon. A junction of the routes to Interchanges 3 and 6 west of Redwick is preferred to other locations on environmental grounds.

Within Gwent the English Stones highway links to Interchange 14 would have, overall, somewhat less adverse planning and environmental impact than those to Interchange 13. Significant noise and visual impact on Rogiet and Caldicot would be avoided but more agricultural land would be required. Options to Interchange 13 would result in the loss of a significant part of the area of undeveloped land between Caldicot and Rogiet, which is preserved as a green wedge in current county and local planning policies. Ecologically, the highway link to Interchange 13 and the associated toll plaza would affect more extensive parts of the shoreline of the

Severn Estuary than links to Interchange 14. It is this shoreline area which accommodates substantial concentrations of birds, that the Nature Conservancy Council intends to incorporate within the proposed Gwent Levels Site of Special Scientific Interest.

5.2 Driven Tunnel Scheme

There should be no significant environmental impact associated with a driven tunnel at Northwick Roadstead.

On the Avon bank the highway links to Interchange 2 would require less agricultural land take than links to Interchange 3 and they would have somewhat less adverse landscape and ecological effect than Interchange 3 options, as a result of the shorter route lengths involved. The proximity to Aust of Interchange 2 routes would, however, be a disadvantage. All Avon bank highway links associated with the Northwick Roadstead crossings would conflict to some extent with Green Belt policies, but the conflict would be less serious with routes to Interchange 2. On the Gwent bank, routes to Interchange 11 would avoid the adverse impact of the Interchange 12 highway links on St. Pierre Park.

5.3 Immersed Tunnel Scheme

An immersed tunnel at Northwick Roadstead would have only minor environmental impact, although the approach roads south of Old Passage on the Avon bank would be visible from local vantage points.

The planning and environmental impact of the links would be similar to those described above in connection with the driven tunnel.

6.0 TRAFFIC OPERATIONS AND TRAFFIC MANAGEMENT

For the purposes of analysis a design year of 2010 was selected, with an assumed opening year of 1996 for a second crossing.

6.1 Dual Carriageway Crossings

A dual carriageway second crossing would result in approximately 70 per cent of the total cross-estuary traffic using the new crossing, signposted as the direct motorway route. Substantial reserve capacity would be available on the new crossing and relatively low flows would remain on the existing Severn Road Bridge and its immediate motorway approaches. A second crossing at the English Stones would therefore relieve about 19 kilometres of M4 of significant traffic flows. The provision of a new motorway standard crossing would be of especial benefit at times of accidents or other restrictions as it would provide significantly more flexibility to cope with abnormal traffic situations. The English Stones crossings would be slightly penalised in respect of flexibility by the greater response time to incidents inherent in the length of their approach links. Provision of a dual carriageway second crossing would also enable high-sided vehicles travelling in either direction to use a new wind-shielded bridge or tunnel. Thus, with an appropriate crossing control system and traffic management, a virtually uninterrupted motorway connection across the estuary could be maintained at all times. In general, both for normal conditions and for restricted traffic flow, a new dual carriageway crossing would provide a high level of service.

In tunnels, the dual carriageway standard would provide significantly better safety for the public and better access for emergency services in the event of a fire or major traffic incident, than schemes where only a single tube is available. However, because no hard-shoulder would be provided in tunnels a minor incident could cause significant hold up at times of heavy traffic.

If high traffic growth is sustained, improvement of M4 west of Almondsbury would be required by about 2010, in addition to the merge for the M5 South - M4 West movement at the Almondsbury interchange. These problems would not occur with schemes which have a link to M5 as this link reduces the flow on M4 West of Almondsbury. The connection to M5 would change traffic on the radial routes on the west and north sides of Bristol. In particular, there would be an increased use of A4, Portway, which may possibly overload certain junctions on this route. Conversely, however, there would be some relief on the M32 in the scale of its anticipated traffic overload as a result of the re-routeing of traffic in Bristol.

6.2 One-way Crossings

With a one-way two lane single carriageway second crossing, there would be reserve capacity on the motorway components of the two crossings. However, if high growth is sustained to the design year, the carriageway on the existing bridge, which would become the A466 link to Aust, would have a flow close to the upper limit design flow for a single carriageway with little spare capacity. A one-way three lane single carriageway which would provide satisfactory capacity in both directions would only be feasible for a bridge.

From the traffic management standpoint, new single direction crossing options would be adequate for normal operation but less flexible in their ability to handle the consequences of incidents and maintenance. A one-way tunnel or a wind-protected new bridge scheme would not provide wind protection to eastbound traffic, since this traffic would remain on the existing bridge. With the two-lane schemes, westbound traffic requiring access at Aust or Newhouse would also not be provided with wind protection. In the case of a single-direction tunnel at English Stones, the extremely long circuit imposed on the escort/patrol vehicles would be inefficient to operate.

Single direction tunnels would involve difficult access in the event of a fire or major incident and provide a significantly poorer level of safety than interconnected dual-tube tunnels. In addition, the problem of dealing with a long queue of vehicles in the event of temporary closure would be more significant on a single direction motorway than with a two-way crossing.

6.3 Two-way Single Carriageway Crossings

At the English Stones the two-way single carriageway crossing option linking M4 to M5 would have sufficient reserve capacity for normal traffic operations. In general this option would provide a reasonable balance between traffic demand and capacity on the new and existing crossings. However, with high traffic growth some overloading at peak August weekends and under normal operations in the latter part of the evaluation period, could be expected to occur. It is also apparent that M4-M5 options could result in significant traffic changes in the Bristol area and some of these effects would need further evaluation.

The single carriageway schemes at the Northwick Roadstead would leave rather more traffic on the existing bridge than the equivalent schemes at the English Stones. The overall system would consequently rely more heavily on traffic management to effect diversions between the two crossings. Some overloading on the existing bridge could recur by the design year during peak holiday periods, though the two crossing system overall would have adequate capacity. The single carriageway Northwick Roadstead crossing would not affect traffic volumes and routeings on the M4, M5 and in Bristol.

Although windshielding would substantially reduce the possibility of vehicle overturning, it would not reduce to the same extent other effects of crosswind speed on the carriageway. It has therefore to be expected that on account of the exposure inherent in an elevated bridge, a single carriageway two-way crossing would be prone to a greater number of road accidents than would normally be experienced on this type of road. Such accidents in periods of high winds would be more serious on a single carriageway than on a dual facility. In addition, the absence of the usual roadside verges on the crossing would exacerbate accident recovery work.

From the traffic management standpoint, single carriageway crossings would operate reasonably well and they could cater for some diversional routing for the majority of the time. However, the capacity provided would not be sufficient to accommodate an appreciable volume of diverted traffic and the English Stones schemes would result in longer travel routes for diverted M4 to M4 traffic.

Safety is an important consideration in a single-tube tunnel as access in the event of a fire or major incident is more difficult than with twin tubes. The single tube would provide a significantly poorer level of safety and in addition, the restricted cross-section would reduce its usefulness as a diversionary route for high traffic volumes.

7.0 SCHEME EVALUATION

7.1 Economic Evaluation

In the initial economic evaluation the costs and benefits of each scheme were compared. Separate analyses were carried out for the bridge schemes, driven tunnel schemes and immersed tunnel schemes to establish their economic worth and to derive a short-list of schemes for final evaluation.

Construction, maintenance and operating costs were estimated in 1983 prices and analysed according to the standard cost/benefit methodology of the Department of Transport, to derive for each scheme a cost deflated to 1979 prices discounted to 1979. These costs were considered in relation to the sum of the travel benefits of each scheme, also expressed in 1979 prices. The travel benefits were estimated considering both high and low growth scenarios according to the standard Departmental approach. Benefits considered included savings in time, vehicle operating costs and road accidents in normal traffic conditions with a second crossing together with extra savings as a result of avoidance of traffic delays that would otherwise arise for the following reasons:

- queueing in the existing toll plaza up to 2006
- maintenance of the structure and carriageways on the existing bridge
- traffic incidents on the existing bridge
- lane closures and traffic restrictions due to high winds.

The first two of these sources of extra benefits are estimated by accepted Departmental procedures whereas the last two are estimated by more experimental methods which are still subject to internal agreement.

The results of the economic evaluation clearly established for each type of crossing the limited number of schemes for overall assessment and these are listed in Table 7.1 together with the Net Present Value (NPV) attributed to each. At this stage the dual carriageway bridge schemes adjacent to the existing bridge were rejected as being uneconomic. Option numbers in Table 7.1 are not consecutive because a number of the original sequentially numbered options were discarded as the studies proceeded. Table 7.1 includes the latest estimates of scheme costs.

Two bridge schemes showed small positive NPV's under the high growth assumptions though most of the bridge schemes and all of the tunnel schemes had negative NPV's even under this scenario. Under the low growth scenario, all schemes had a pronounced negative value. There was however, some scope for improvement by further refinement of design proposals, through phasing of the second crossing or similar measures and these were considered in the final assessments.

Provision of hard shoulders and wind protection on bridges were additional design aspects that were subjected to detailed economic evaluation, which showed that in the case of hard shoulders the benefits on the bridge crossings were not of sufficient magnitude to justify the cost of a full width provision. However, on operational and safety grounds hard shoulders are desirable and it would be

TABLE 7.1: SCHEMES FOR OVERALL ASSESSMENT

Location	Option No. and carriageway standard	Growth Scenario	Benefits from travel savings and reductions in delay due to tolling and maintenance. £M	Additional Benefits from reduced delay due to incidents and high winds. £M	Expenditures on construction maintenance and operating £M	NPV £M
BRIDGE SCHEMES						
ADJACENT CROSSING M4-M4	28 1/2 D3M	High	21.65	8.07	37.42	-7.7
		Low	9.61	3.13		-24.68
ENGLISH STONES M4-M4	19 D2M	High	35.91	8.66	48.41	-3.84
		Low	20.86	3.46		-24.09
	19 1/2 D2M	High	26.81	4.39	35.68	-4.48
		Low	14.14	1.31		-20.23
ENGLISH STONES WITH BIFURCATED LINK M4-M4/M5	19A D2M/WS2	High	51.07	8.66	56.77	+2.96
		Low	34.87	3.46		-18.44
ENGLISH STONES M4-M5	13 WS2	High	37.97	7.79	41.23	+4.53
		Low	27.23	3.19		-10.81
DRIVEN TUNNEL SCHEMES						
NORTHWICK ROADSTEAD M4-M4	39 WS2	High	19.19	8.10	55.08	-27.79
		Low	9.04	3.29		-42.75
	29 D2M	High	22.55	8.66	93.50	-62.29
		Low	9.69	3.46		-80.35
	29 1/2 D2M	High	20.19	4.32	53.88	-29.36
		Low	9.44	1.31		-43.13
	29 1/2 D3M	High	20.50	6.12	54.30	-27.68
		Low	9.51	2.88		-41.91
IMMERSED TUNNEL SCHEMES						
NORTHWICK ROADSTEAD M4-M4	39 WS2	H	19.19	8.11	49.96	-22.66
		L	9.04	3.29		-37.63
	26 D2M	H	22.66	8.66	71.29	-39.97
		L	9.69	3.46		-58.14
	26 1/2 D2M	H	20.25	4.34	49.44	-24.85
		L	9.44	1.31		-38.69
	26 1/2 D3M	H	21.33	6.74	49.86	-21.79
		L	9.51	3.13		-37.22

worth considering the provision of narrow hard shoulders to achieve worthwhile cost savings without appreciable loss of benefit. The evaluation also showed that the provision of wind shielding could be justified on economic grounds for all two-way crossings. For one-way crossings the economic case for wind-shielding is marginal, but is still recommended.

7.2 Final Assessment

The short-listed schemes summarised above were the subject of confirmatory studies and further development in areas which improved traffic operations and economic return. The confirmatory studies included further wind tunnel testing of wind shielding devices and assessment of interference effects on the existing bridge of an adjacent second crossing bridge. The principal further developments included the following:

i) The link from the English Stones bridge crossing to the M5 which was considered in several alternative forms including the provision of a dual carriageway highway standard and a junction with the A403

ii) Phased construction of dual carriageway schemes

iii) Improvements in the one-way schemes to achieve a more balanced distribution of traffic flows and slightly lower cost.

7.2.1 Design of the Link to M5

The engineering studies indicated that several improvements and economies were possible for the M5 link road. These included the adoption of a lower profile for the link, introduction of an at-grade junction with A403 and upgrading of the link to dual carriageway standard. An analysis of the traffic effects and economic benefits of these changes was undertaken and the results are shown in Table 7.2.

The lower level profile and A403 junction improved the NPV of this scheme to approximately +£6M in the high growth and -£15M in the low growth scenario. Further improvement, in the form of a dualled link to M5 did not increase the benefits sufficiently to outweigh the additional cost. However, on route planning grounds it was considered that dualling of this link may be desirable. It would provide for possible increased local traffic growth in the event of acceleration of development in the Avonmouth/Severnside area as a result of the improved access to the motorway network.

7.2.2 Phasing of Dual Carriageway Schemes

Only the dual carriageway schemes lend themselves to phasing. Four possible construction sequencies were considered for phasing the provision of a dual carriageway English Stones bridge. In the case of the dual carriageway tunnels the only possible phasing would be the sequential construction of the two tunnels.

TABLE 7.2: ANALYSIS OF COSTS AND BENEFITS ASSOCIATED WITH CHANGES IN DESIGN OF THE M5 LINK ON AN ENGLISH STONES BRIDGE CROSSING, OPTION 19A

Option No. and carriageway standard	Growth Scenario	Benefits from travel savings and reductions in delay due to tolling and maintenance. £M	Additional Benefits from reduced delay due to incidents and high winds. £M	Expenditures on construction maintenance and operating £M	NPV £M
19A with low level single carriageway link to M5	High	51.07	8.66	56.02	+3.71
	Low	34.87	3.46		-17.69
As above but with A403 junction (19AJ)	High	51.86	8.66	54.38	+6.14
	Low	35.55	3.46		-15.37
19AJ but with a dual carriageway link to M5	High	52.00	8.66	55.96	+4.70
	Low	35.67	3.46		-16.83

English Stones Bridge

The evaluation showed that there was no worthwhile economic advantage to be gained from phasing the English Stones bridge schemes, principally because of the substantial bridge costs which must be carried in the first phase in any arrangement.

Driven Tunnels

The evaluation demonstrated that there are substantial economic advantages to be gained by phasing the driven tunnels, with the NPV of the scheme improving as the date for driving the second tunnel recedes. It was concluded from this that a driven tunnel scheme should be considered as a possible phased solution.

Immersed Tunnels

The advantages of phasing an immersed tunnel are rather less clear-cut than for a driven tunnel. This is principally because of the capital cost of the dry dock and other facilities required for the immersed tunnel construction method, which have to be carried in the first phase. The result is that the total cost of an immersed tunnel is significantly increased by phasing and the NPV of the overall tunnel provision deteriorates if the second phase is constructed less than 15 years after the initial provision. On balance it was concluded that the dual carriageway immersed tunnel should be regarded as an unphased scheme.

7.2.3 Evaluation of Bridge Schemes (See Figure 9)

The Newhouse to Aust bridge, adjacent to the existing structure, constructed with three-lane motorway standard carriageway, would be operated as a one-way motorway link westbound in conjunction with the existing bridge which would operate one-way eastbound. Together the two bridges would provide a motorway connection across the estuary.

In the final technical evaluation of the aerodynamic studies of the possible effects of an adjacent bridge, constructed between the CEGB cable crossing and the existing bridge, it was concluded that whilst it could be reasonably anticipated that the consequences for the existing bridge would not be of major proportions, it would be necessary to have contingency plans for strengthening its superstructure, to cover both the results of future investigations and allowancies for the degree of imprecision that would be associated with them. Such contingency plans could not be regarded as appropriate, however, as the existing bridge is already the subject of a strengthening programme. The difficulties and costs associated with contingency strengthening could not be contemplated unless the case for an adjacent crossing were to be totally compelling in comparison with other options.

Owing to the continued use of the existing bridge for eastbound traffic with this scheme it would not provide a completely wind protected crossing for high-sided vehicles and it would therefore fall short of providing the entirely secure crossing that South Wales economic development interests seek. This apart, the scheme would provide a satisfactory traffic link under most conditions and would have the minimum impact on local communities and on the environment. However, in the economic evaluation the scheme has a negative NPV even with the high growth scenario and is the least favourable of all the short-listed bridge schemes.

In view of the relatively low economic value of the scheme, its deficiency with respect to the security of the link and the difficulties attached to the additional contingency planning described above, Option 28 (the adjacent bridge) can not be recommended and it has been deleted from further consideration.

The English Stones bridge crossing was assessed with each of the possible alternative highway links and highway standards shown to be worthwhile in the economic evaluation.

The dual carriageway and one-way schemes for an English Stones crossing linking M4 to M4 were assessed and compared. The one-way second crossing scheme would leave more traffic on the existing bridge and would require the use of one carriageway of the existing bridge for traffic to and from Chepstow and A466. This would provide a worsening level of service after 2015. The restricted addition to capacity would also provide reduced flexibility for traffic management during maintenance works and major incidents. These deficiencies are reflected in the lower benefit estimates of the one-way scheme. The dual carriageway scheme would involve increased land take and noise impact on its route, but other environmental effects and the planning and economic development effects would be very similar for either of these schemes. In overall terms, the improvement in traffic operational conditions with the dual carriageway scheme, resulting in increased benefits, is considered to be worth the small increase in noise impact, the increased cost and the possibility of a lower NPV if the low growth scenario were to occur.

The dual carriageway scheme at the English Stones was assessed with and without the link to M5. The link to M5 would involve an additional 6.7 kilometres of new route by comparison with the scheme linking M4 to M4 only, with consequent increased farm severance and land take in the area between Redwick and Avonmouth. There would also be substantial additional noise and visual impact on the Avon bank, particularly at Severn Beach. On the Gwent bank and the estuary itself these two schemes would be identical, as would be their ecological impact. The link to M5 would have additional planning implications for the economic development balance between Bristol and Newport/south Gwent. The traffic effects of the M5 link would be to provide additional relief to M4, Almondsbury interchange and M5. The M5 link would

NEWHOUSE - AUST BRIDGE SCHEMES								
Option	Highway Standard	Crossing and Links			Existing Bridge Traffic	Total Construction Cost	NPV	
		Western Link	Crossing	Eastern Link			High Growth	Low Growth
28	½D3M	11N-A ←	A-B ←	B-1 ←	→	108·1	-7·7	-24·7

	Link 11N-A	Crossing A-B	Link B-1
Highway Standard	Cost		
½D3M	3·8	102·4	1·9

Link 14-E	
Highway Standard	Cost
D2M	21·2
½D2M	13·3
WS2	11·6

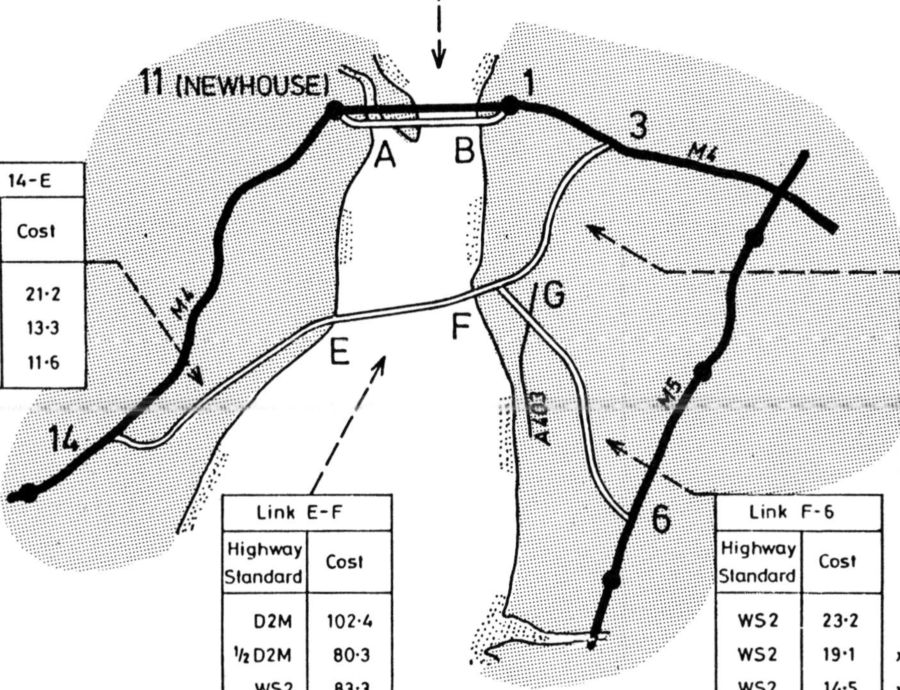

Link F-3	
Highway Standard	Cost
D2M	16·8
½D2M	11·5

Link E-F	
Highway Standard	Cost
D2M	102·4
½D2M	80·3
WS2	83·3

Link F-6		
Highway Standard	Cost	
WS2	23·2	
WS2	19·1	x Int at F
WS2	14·5	xx Int at F & G
D2AP	18·8	xx Int at F & G

ENGLISH STONES BRIDGE SCHEMES								
Option	Highway Standard	Crossings and Links			Existing Bridge Traffic	Total Construction Cost	NPV	
		Western Link	Crossing	Eastern Link			High Growth	Low Growth
13	WS2	14-E ⇄	E-F ⇄	F-6 ⇄	⇄	118·1	+4·5	-10·8
19	D2M	14-E ⇄	E-F ⇄	F-3 ⇄	⇄	140·4	-4·5	-24·7
19	½D2M	14-E ←	E-F ←	F-3 ←	⇄	105·1	-4·5	-20·2
19A	D2M	14-E ⇄	E-F ⇄	F-3 ⇄	⇄	159·5	+3·7	-17·7
	WS2			F-6_x ⇄				
19AJ	D2M	14-E ⇄	E-F ⇄	F-3 ⇄	⇄	154·9	+6·1	-15·4
	WS2			F-6_{xx} ⇄				
19AJD	D2M	14-E ⇄	E-F ⇄	F-3 ⇄	⇄	159·2	+4·7	-16·8
	D2AP			F-6_{xx} ⇄				

KEY
- Cost in £m at 1983 prices
- NPV in £m deflated and discounted to 1979 prices
- → indicates direction of traffic flow
- 1, 14 denote Interchanges
- E, F denote crossing reference points
- Int = Interchange

Short-listed Bridge Schemes

9

produce a 30 per cent improvement in travel benefits and consequent improvement in NPV. It was concluded from this assessment that the improvement in traffic operations and economic return would be worth the increased land take and environmental impact, which could be mitigated with appropriate amelioration works at the detailed design stage.

The scheme with the smallest NPV range was the single carriageway English Stones bridge linking M4 in Wales to M5 in Avon, with a positive NPV on high growth and a relatively small negative value on low growth. This was compared with the dual carriageway English Stones bridge scheme with connections to both M4 and M5 in Avon. On economic evaluation this is the 'next best' scheme.

The single carriageway scheme, however, has a number of disadvantages relative to the dual carriageway scheme. The single carriageway bridge would be prone to increased road accidents on account of the exposure inherent on an elevated bridge. The protection from wind shielding would significantly reduce, but not eliminate, crosswinds and both high sided and light vehicles may experience some buffetting from the wind, which on a single carriageway would increase the incidence of vehicle collision compared with a dual facility. Such collisions during high winds are likely to be more serious on a single carriageway crossing than on a dual facility. In addition, the absence of the usual roadside verges on the bridge over the 4.9 kilometres length of the crossing would make accident recovery more difficult. These safety disadvantages are not fully reflected in the standard COBA accident parameters. The single carriageway scheme would also provide only a limited facility for maintaining a reasonable level of service for crossing traffic during incidents and at times of holiday peak flow. It would have a similarly limited ability to accommodate future traffic growth and no scope for capacity enhancement unless built as the first phase of a dual carriageway. The scheme therefore would provide only restricted flexibility in operation. In planning terms the scheme would not achieve the important regional economic planning ojective for South Wales of a second crossing to reinforce the M4 corridor and it could even partially frustrate economic development in South Wales. The scheme would have serious strategic planning implications for the balance of development in Bristol and South Wales.

The dual carriageway scheme at English Stones with links to both M4 and M5 in Avon (Option 19AJ) has an NPV of +£6.14M on high growth and -£15.37 on low growth scenarios. This NPV is worse than the single carriageway scheme on low growth but it has none of the traffic operational and management disadvantages. It is also preferable on overall planning grounds, in that it would fully achieve the important economic planning ojective for South Wales of a second crossing reinforcing the M4 corridor. The link to M5 which provides an important component of the travel benefits, would in this scheme, as in the single carriageway scheme, change the accessibility relationship between South Wales and

Bristol, thereby introducing a new element into the planning considerations for Avon and Gwent. However, with the dual carriageway scheme, the impact of this link in planning terms would be much reduced in comparison with the corresponding impact of the single carriageway scheme, because of the improved M4 to M4 link with Option 19AJ. The dual carriageway scheme would have a greater environmental impact in Avon on account of the increased route length, agricultural land take and severance, together with increased impact on Redwick, on the Avon levels area and on the Green Belt north of Bristol.

The difference in NPV between the two schemes is small, with the dual carriageway scheme better on high growth by £1.6M but worse on low growth by £4.5M. The planning and traffic advantages achieved by the dual carriageway scheme more than outweigh the possibility of a reduced NPV and the increased environmental impact. The dual carriageway scheme, Option 19AJ, is therefore the preferred bridge scheme.

7.2.4 Evaluation of Driven Tunnel Schemes (See Figure 10)

The short-listed driven tunnel schemes were subjected to final detailed evaluation of the physical engineering, traffic, environmental, economic and cost considerations set out in the previous sections.

The final economic evaluation showed the 'best' driven tunnel scheme to be the one-way scheme (Option 29 or 30), comprising a single bore two-lane tunnel with the approaches a single carriageway of three-lane motorway standard. This was found to have the least negative NPV. By comparison the dual two-lane carriageway tunnel scheme would have an NPV of -£62.3M. However, the one-way tunnel would have substantial traffic operational disadvantages and significant potential safety disadvantages in comparison with a dual carriageway tunnel with cross passages. Phasing the construction of the driven tunnel has been shown to result in a significant improvement in NPV as the date of opening of the second bore recedes. Improvements in safety and operation could be achieved in a second phase.

The overall optimum driven tunnel scheme would therefore be a phased construction of the dual carriageway tunnel (Option 29 or 30), with the second bore opening some 10 to 15 years after the first.

7.2.5 Evaluation of Immersed Tunnel Schemes (See Figure 10)

The short-listed immersed tunnel schemes were subjected to final detailed evaluation of the engineering, traffic, environmental, economic and cost considerations set out in the previous sections.

The final economic evaluation showed the best immersed tunnel scheme to be the one-way scheme (Option 25 or 26). However, the one-way tunnel would have substantial traffic operational disadvantages and potential safety disadvantages in comparison with a dual carrriageway tunnel with cross passages. In the case of the immersed tunnel, because of high initial costs, phasing the construction has been shown to produce no advantage in NPV if the second tube is deferred by less than 15 years. However, a phased deferment of the second tube for longer than 15 years is not desirable from traffic operational considerations.

An additional important factor against phasing an immersed tunnel is the difficulty of achieving the cross passages between the two tunnels, that are so necessary to secure satisfactory conditions for tunnel operations and public safety.

Therefore, the overall optimum immersed tunnel scheme would be the dual carriageway scheme (Option 25 or 26) constructed in its entirety from the outset.

7.2.6 Financial Analysis

A financial analysis has been carried out on the recommended Second Severn Crossing Schemes based on the Department of Transport accounting practice for the existing Severn Bridge, as governed by the Severn Bridge Tolls Act 1965. It has been assumed that a new Tolls Act will be passed to coincide with the opening of a Second Severn Crossing and that thereafter both crossings would be operated as a single financial entity, with tolls at the same level on each crossing.

Alternative high and low inflation rates of 8 per cent and 3 per cent, respectively, were considered with real interest rates of 3 per cent assumed. High/low traffic forecasts consistent with those in the transport modelling/evaluation analyses have been considered.

The central analysis combines high traffic growth with low inflation and a pay back period of 40 years. Combinations of high/high and low/low would represent, respectively, the "most"/"least" favourable conditions in terms of the level of toll required.

Under the central assumptions the following tolls would be required for the revenue to meet capital charges, interest payments on the deficit, operating costs, maintenance costs and provision of a sinking fund to discharge future obligations.

	Toll Levels in 1984/85 Prices	
	Light vehicles	Heavy Vehicles
Required post-1996/97		
Bridge	£0.70	£1.40
Driven Tunnel	£1.15	£2.30
Immersed Tunnel	£0.95	£1.90

NORTHWICK ROADSTEAD DRIVEN TUNNEL SCHEME								
Option	Highway Standard Crossing / Link	Crossing and Links			Existing Bridge Traffic	Total Construction Cost	NPV	
		Western Link	Crossing	Eastern Link			High Growth	Low Growth
29	D2/D2M	11-C ⇄	C-D ⇄	D-2 ⇄	⇄	225·8	-62·3†	-80·4†
29	½D2/½D3M	11-C ←	C-D ←	D-2 ←	→	123·7	-27·7	-41·9
29	½D2/½D2M	11-C ←	C-D ←	D-2 ←	→	122·6	-29·4	-43·1
39	S2/WS2	11-C ⇄	C-D ⇄	D-2 ⇄	⇄	127·1	-27·8	-42·8

Link 11-C	
Highway Standard	Cost
D2M	6·1
½ D2M	4·2
½ D3M	4·1
WS2	2·3

Crossing C-D	
Highway Standard	Cost
D2	209·0
½ D2	111·1
S2	113·0

Link D-2	
Highway Standard	Cost
D2M	10·7
½ D2M	7·3
½ D3M	8·5
WS2	11·8

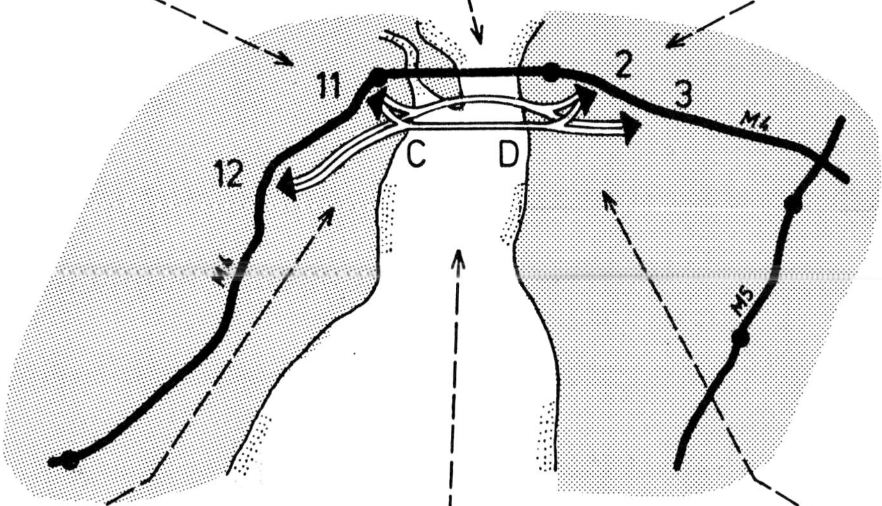

Link 11-C	
Highway Standard	Cost
D2M	10·3
½ D2M	6·7
½ D3M	6·7
WS2	3·7

Crossing C-D	
Highway Standard	Cost
D2	147·9
½ D2	102·9
S2	105·1

Link D-2	
Highway Standard	Cost
D2M	11·7
½ D2M	8·3
½ D3M	9·4
WS2	11·5

NORTHWICK ROADSTEAD IMMERSED TUNNEL SCHEME								
Option	Highway Standard Crossing / Link	Crossing and Links			Existing Bridge Traffic	Total Construction Cost	NPV	
		Western Link	Crossing	Eastern Link			High Growth	Low Growth
26	D2/D2M	11-C ⇄	C-D ⇄	D-2 ⇄	⇄	169·9	-40·0	-58·1
26	½D2/½D3M	11-C ←	C-D ←	D-2 ←	→	119·0	-21·8	-37·2
26	½D2/½D2M	11-C ←	C-D ←	D-2 ←	→	117·9	-24·9	-38·7
39	S2/WS2	11-C ⇄	C-D ⇄	D-2 ⇄	⇄	120·3	-22·7	-37·6

KEY
- Cost in £m at 1983 prices
- NPV in £m deflated and discounted to 1979 prices
- † NPV = -45·6 and -61·8 for high and low growth rate respectively, for 15 year phased construction
- → indicates direction of traffic flow
- 2, 11 denotes Interchanges
- C, D denotes crossing reference points
- Eastern Link connects to either Interchange 2 or 3
- Western Link connects to either Interchange 11 or 12

Short-listed Tunnel Schemes

10

8.0 RECOMMENDATIONS

8.1 Introduction

The analysis of the engineering, planning and environmental aspects, traffic operation and management and the financial appraisal of the complete schemes provides a basis for recommending a bridge, a driven tunnel and an immersed tunnel crossing.

There are, however, further considerations that are not readily quantified or assessed. Their importance may be considerable and therefore the main points are summarised below:

i) The provision of a second crossing will be important to maintain a reasonable level of road transport service for South Wales, without which there could be serious adverse economic repercussions. Over and above maintenance of the status quo, a second crossing is seen as having a small positive effect on regional development. The second crossing would therefore be supportive of regional economic policy. The NPV, ranging from +£6.1M at high growth to -£15.4M at low growth for an English Stones crossing scheme, has therefore to be viewed in the perspective of the Government's commitment to assisting peripheral and depressed regions, as indicated by the annual Government regional development grants and assistance to Wales amounting to an average of £82M per annum (in 1979 prices) over recent years.

ii) The estimate of benefit for avoiding high wind delays takes no account of economic knock-on effects, such as economic development lost due to a poor perception of the existing bridge, increased inventory cost of freight in transit, etc.

iii) The provision of a second crossing would contribute to the European Economic Community transport policy by both removing what could otherwise become a transport bottleneck and by improving the main transport link to two of the Community's peripheral regions - South Wales and Eire.

iv) The bridge has very rarely been closed to all traffic in the past. If for any reason that condition were to be experienced in the future for any extended period of time, the economic repercussions and costs would be substantial. Provision of a second crossing of dual carriageway standard would avoid such a possibility.

v) The economic value of the present crossing in 1996 has been conservatively estimated at £45M per annum (in 1979 prices discounted to 1979) in transport benefit alone. A small negative NPV such as that on the recommended bridge scheme therefore equates to about 4 months of the transport benefits of there being a Severn crossing.

vi) The possibility of a second crossing having a traffic generation effect has been considered and the potential benefits have been assessed at £1.5M to £2.5M, which would improve the economic return of the crossing.

The recommended schemes, described below, include the most effective and appropriate highway links to the motorway system on both banks. The planning and environmental issues are of greater significance for the highways than the crossings. Nevertheless it has been possible to propose routes which are satisfactory on these grounds assuming that there is a careful and sensitive approach to the final designs of the highways and related works.

The recommended schemes are shown on Figures 6, 7 and 8 and summarised in Figure 11.

8.2 Bridge

The crossing at the English Stones, consisting of 4 kilometres of approach viaducts founded on the English Stones and a cable stayed bridge over The Shoots, with a 456 metres main span, is recommended as the most appropriate bridge scheme and is shown in Figure 6. The relevant costs and net present values are summarised in Figure 11. The recommended highway standard for the bridge is that of dual two-lane motorway.

The feasibility of providing wind shielding has been established for this particular cable stayed bridge, as has the feasibility of an essentially maintenance-free deck with replaceable cables, combined with either a concrete or steel web and bottom flange system. Maintenance-free protection is feasible for the steel webs and bottom flange system using an "enclosure" system. Sufficient progress has been made in this study related to the proposed bridge crossing to have a confident view of the investigations, including wind tunnel testing that would be appropriate to the development of working systems for the wind shielding and maintenance concepts at the final design stage.

The highway links that are recommended are of dual two-lane carriageway motorway standard, connecting to the M4 in Gwent at Interchange 14, west of Caldicot, and to the M4 at Interchange 3 in Avon, east of Aust. Also recommended is an additional link to the M5, north of Avonmouth, connecting to the main crossing link west of Redwick and incorporating a subsidiary junction with the A403. According to traffic and cost-benefit assessments, the standard of this link could be a wide single two-way carriageway. A dual two-lane all purpose carriageway would, however, be appropriate for a link joining two motorways and would be adaptable to any increases in traffic flows resulting from future developments in Wales, Avonmouth and the West Country.

8.3 Driven Tunnel

The recommended driven tunnel crossing is sited some 600 metres south of the Severn Road Bridge on an alignment passing under Northwick Roadstead and the tip of Beachley Point. The tunnel would be 4.4 kilometres between portals and this scheme is illustrated on Figure 7. The relevant costs and net present values are summarised in Figure 11.

NORTHWICK ROADSTEAD DRIVEN TUNNEL SCHEME							
Option	Highway Standard	Cost of Crossing and Links			Total Construction Cost	NPV	
		Link 11-C	Crossing C-D	Link D-2		High Growth	Low Growth
29	D2M D2	6·1 —	— 209·0	10·7 —	225·8	-62·3*	-80·4*

NORTHWICK ROADSTEAD IMMERSED TUNNEL CROSSING							
Option	Highway Standard	Cost of Crossing and Links			Total Construction Cost	NPV	
		Link 11-C	Crossing C-D	Link D-2		High Growth	Low Growth
26	D2M D2	10·3 —	— 147·9	11·7 —	169·9	-40·0	-58·1

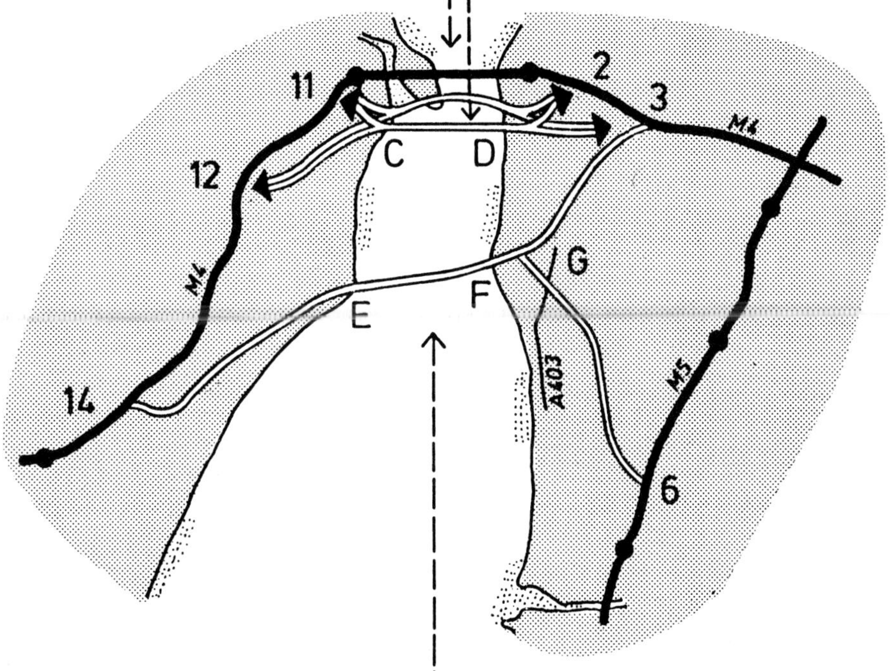

ENGLISH STONES BRIDGE SCHEME								
Option	Highway Standard	Cost of Crossing and Links				Total Construction Cost	NPV	
		Link 14-E	Crossing E-F	Link F-3	Link F-6		High Growth	Low Growth
19AJ	D2M WS2	21·2 —	102·4 —	16·8 —	— 14·5	154·9	+6·1	-15·4

KEY
- Cost in £m at 1983 prices
- NPV in £m deflated and discounted to 1979 prices
- *NPV = -45·6 and -61·8 for high and low growth rate respectively, for 15 year phased construction
- → indicates direction of traffic flow
- 2, 11 denote Interchanges
- C, D denote crossing reference points
- Eastern Link connects to either Interchange 2 or 3
- Western Link connects to either Interchange 11 or 12

The proposed alignment would enable advantage to be taken of Beachley Point for the location of shafts for both construction and ventilation. The feasibility of constructing 12 metre diameter bores, partly through the Triassic strata in the descending sections, but mainly through the much harder but more stable Lower Dolomite, has been established. A detailed site investigation would however, be required to determine the exact position and nature of two buried channels which are indicated by geological evidence.

The west bank section of the tunnel may require both cut and cover and soft ground tunnelling techniques before the rock tunnelling section is reached.

The ventilation and fire safety requirements are demanding for a long highway tunnel and the feasibility of satisfying these requirements by the provision of transverse ventilation with an additional ventilation station at Beachley has been established.

The highway standard of the tunnel would be a dual two-lane carriageway without hard shoulders. The corresponding bore diameter for one carriageway is approximately 12 metres, which is near the limit of feasibility in the Severn Estuary. Two bores are therefore required for the completed dual carriageway system.

The highway links that are recommended are of dual two-lane motorway standard. On the Gwent bank the connection to the M4 would be to either Interchange 11 or 12. On the Avon bank the connection to the M4 would be at either Interchange 2 or 3.

The construction of the two bores necessary for the dual two-lane carriageway tunnel would be largely independent and this would enable advantage to be taken by phasing the tunnel construction programme. Thus the first bore could be completed and carrying traffic, with the second bore added at a suitable later date.

There is, however, a balanced decision to be made between the safety, operational flexibility and wind shielding advantages of having a dual bore tunnel from the outset, and the economic and financial expenditure savings of phasing the opening of the second bore of the tunnel by some years. This decision would need further consideration before a final recommendation could be established and therefore both possibilities are put forward for consideration by the Department.

8.4 Immersed Tunnel

The recommended immersed tunnel crossing is located 1.2 kilometres downstream of the Severn Road Bridge and running approximately parallel to the bridge. The tunnel passes beneath Northwick Roadstead and is illustrated in Figure 8. The relevant costs and net present values are summarised in Figure 11. The recommended highway standard in the immersed tunnel is dual two-lane without hard shoulders.

A digital ground model of the geophysical survey data was used to establish that the trench would be excavated in sediments and rock which would be dredgeable, but it has been recognised that a small amount of hard rock might be encountered. The possible intrusion into the trench excavation of this hard rock has led to the recommendation that the minimum height rectangular tunnel cross-section should be employed on this crossing.

The feasibility of providing an effective ventilation system has been established. The minimum provision that has been considered appropriate for this crossing is the semi-transverse/transverse system.

The linking highways are recommended as being of dual two-lane motorway standard on both banks. The connection to the M4 on the Gwent bank would be at either Interchange 11 or 12. On the Avon bank the connection would be at either Interchange 2 or 3 on the M4.

8.5 Conclusions

The above recommendations for dual carriageway crossings and highway links for a bridge at the English Stones and for immersed and driven tunnels at Northwick Roadstead in the vicinity of the existing bridge, have been arrived at by taking a balanced view of the combined assessments of all aspects of the Study. The crossing locations themselves for the bridges and tunnels are respectively supported by both the cost-benefit analyses and the engineering studies.

There is some conflict, however, in the evidence and analyses relating to an opening date for a second crossing. The bridge scheme has positive cost benefit on the high growth scenario. High traffic growth has occurred in recent years and may continue. The tunnel schemes are significantly negative even on high growth. The bridge scheme is, however, also negative on the low growth evaluation.

The need for a second crossing at an early date must also be recognised as a response to the anticipated problem of traffic congestion on the present bridge in future years. The traffic studies have shown that if traffic growth continues at the NRTF high growth rate, congestion and delay at the existing bridge and toll plaza would occur on a significant number of occasions each year from the early 1990's onwards. With every passing year the duration of congestion and period of delay would lengthen. Drivers could be expected to take such avoiding action as is possible, but in the majority of cases they are likely to queue at the toll plaza rather than divert via Gloucester. Studies have shown that by 1996 delays of 15 minutes or more would be likely for several hundred hours per annum.

The result of this build up of congestion and delay would be an increasingly poor public perception of the service provided by the existing Severn Road Bridge and this would be very much to the detriment of the economy of South Wales. The economic disbenefits of persistent congestion at the bridge would be felt in many spheres of economic activity and would exceed the transport costs alone. In

Section 8.1 the additional economic and policy arguments supporting the need for a second crossing have been mentioned. Many of these arguments would equally support the case for an early opening date for the second crossing.

The high growth cost-benefits for an English Stones bridge crossing and the considerable weight of the above points leads to the recommendation of 1996 as the date by which it would be prudent to have a second crossing in operation. In fact an even earlier date would, if chosen now, keep open the option of that date should traffic growth and other issues show it to be necessary. It would also bring forward the date at which a Severn crossing protected from high winds would be available.

The Study is not required to choose between the bridge and tunnel options, but clearly the cost-benefit analysis favours the wind-shielded bridge scheme at the English Stones. The recommended additional link to the M5 would also provide further advantages to the national highway system.